# Mental Health Crisis in Higher Education

Peter J. O. Aloka
*University of the Witwatersrand, South Africa*

A volume in the Advances in Higher Education and Professional Development (AHEPD) Book Series

IGI Global
PUBLISHER of TIMELY KNOWLEDGE

Published in the United States of America by
IGI Global
Information Science Reference (an imprint of IGI Global)
701 E. Chocolate Avenue
Hershey PA, USA 17033
Tel: 717-533-8845
Fax: 717-533-8661
E-mail: cust@igi-global.com
Web site: http://www.igi-global.com



Library of Congress Cataloging-in-Publication Data

Names: Aloka, Peter, 1976- editor.
Title: Mental health crisis in higher education / edited by Peter Aloka.
Description: Hershey, PA : Information Science Reference, 2024. | Includes bibliographical references and index. | Summary: "This edited volume seeks to address the existing gap in the literature on student stress and mental health"-- Provided by publisher.
Identifiers: LCCN 2023055044 (print) | LCCN 2023055045 (ebook) | ISBN 9798369328330 (hardcover) | ISBN 9798369328347 (ebook)
Subjects: LCSH: College students--Mental health. | College students--Mental health services. | Education, Higher--Psychological aspects.
Classification: LCC RC451.4.S7 M424 2024 (print) | LCC RC451.4.S7 (ebook) | DDC 616.8900835--dc23/eng/20231227
LC record available at https://lccn.loc.gov/2023055044
LC ebook record available at https://lccn.loc.gov/2023055045

This book is published in the IGI Global book series Advances in Higher Education and Professional Development (AHEPD) (ISSN: 2327-6983; eISSN: 2327-6991)

British Cataloguing in Publication Data
A Cataloguing in Publication record for this book is available from the British Library.

# Advances in Higher Education and Professional Development (AHEPD) Book Series

Jared Keengwe
University of North Dakota, USA

ISSN:2327-6983
EISSN:2327-6991

Mission

As world economies continue to shift and change in response to global financial situations, job markets have begun to demand a more highly-skilled workforce. In many industries a college degree is the minimum requirement and further educational development is expected to advance. With these current trends in mind, the **Advances in Higher Education & Professional Development (AHEPD) Book Series** provides an outlet for researchers and academics to publish their research in these areas and to distribute these works to practitioners and other researchers.

**AHEPD** encompasses all research dealing with higher education pedagogy, development, and curriculum design, as well as all areas of professional development, regardless of focus.

Coverage

- Adult Education
- Assessment in Higher Education
- Career Training
- Coaching and Mentoring
- Continuing Professional Development
- Governance in Higher Education
- Higher Education Policy
- Pedagogy of Teaching Higher Education
- Vocational Education



The Advances in Higher Education and Professional Development (AHEPD) Book Series (ISSN 2327-6983) is published by IGI Global, 701 E. Chocolate Avenue, Hershey, PA 17033-1240, USA, www.igi-global.com. This series is composed of titles available for purchase individually; each title is edited to be contextually exclusive from any other title within the series. For pricing and ordering information please visit http://www.igi-global.com/book-series/advances-higher-education-professional-development/73681. Postmaster: Send all address changes to above address. 

## Titles in this Series

*For a list of additional titles in this series, please visit:*
*http://www.igi-global.com/book-series/advances-higher-education-professional-development/73681*

***Creating Diverse Experiences for Rural Appalachian Pre-Service Teachers***
Kimberly Dianne Cassidy (Shawnee State University, USA)
Information Science Reference • © 2024 • 300pp • H/C (ISBN: 9781668443699) • US $215.00

***Best Practices to Prepare Writers for Their Professional Paths***
Carissa A. Barker-Stucky (Carnegie Writers, Inc., USA) and Kemi Elufiede (Carnegie Writers, Inc., USA)
Information Science Reference • © 2024 • 300pp • H/C (ISBN: 9781668490242) • US $225.00

***Accessibility of Digital Higher Education in the Global South***
Pfano Mashau (University of KwaZulu-Natal, South Africa) and Tshililo Ruddy Farisani (University of KwaZulu-Natal, South Africa)
Information Science Reference • © 2024 • 371pp • H/C (ISBN: 9781668491799) • US $215.00

***Balance and Boundaries in Creating Meaningful Relationships in Online Higher Education***
Sarah H. Jarvie (Colorado Christian University, USA) and Cara Metz (The University of Arizona Global Campus, USA)
Information Science Reference • © 2024 • 340pp • H/C (ISBN: 9781668489086) • US $215.00

***Teaching Humanities With Cultural Responsiveness at HBCUs and HSIs***
DuEwa M. Frazier (Coppin State University, USA)
Information Science Reference • © 2024 • 270pp • H/C (ISBN: 9781668497821) • US $230.00

***Stabilizing and Empowering Women in Higher Education Realigning, Recentering, and Rebuilding***
Heidi L. Schnackenberg (SUNY Plattsburgh, USA) and Denise A. Simard (SUNY Plattsburgh, USA)
Information Science Reference • © 2023 • 303pp • H/C (ISBN: 9781668485972) • US $215.00

***Promoting Intercultural Agility and Leadership Development at Home and Abroad for First-Year Students***
Jon Stauff (South Dakota State University, USA) and Jill E. Blondin (Virginia Commonwealth University, USA)
Information Science Reference • © 2024 • 320pp • H/C (ISBN: 9781668488324) • US $215.00

***Practices and Perspectives of Teaching and Teacher Education in Africa***
Gideon Boadu (RMIT University, Melbourne, Australia) George Odhiambo (United Arab Emirates University, Al Ain, UAE) and Pegah Marandi (Excelsia College, Australia)
Information Science Reference • © 2023 • 284pp • H/C (ISBN: 9781668477229) • US $270.00

IGI Global
PUBLISHER of TIMELY KNOWLEDGE

701 East Chocolate Avenue, Hershey, PA 17033, USA
Tel: 717-533-8845 x100 • Fax: 717-533-8661
E-Mail: cust@igi-global.com • www.igi-global.com

# Table of Contents

# Detailed Table of Contents



There are increased mental health and well-being concerns among students at universities worldwide. By adopting a conceptual review of literature, this chapter analyzed well-being and mental health initiatives for students in universities. On the bases of the literature review in this chapter, it is concluded that there is need for supportive work environments, mental health in universal health coverage, creating opportunities for student engagement, mentorship at various academic departments building social networks, and finally, individual coping strategies are also useful in enhancing well-being and mental health of academic staff at universities. It is recommended that universities should develop holistic mentorship for students so that this can take care of all aspects of their lives.



This chapter presents the state of mental health of students in higher education institutions, help seeking behaviors, and available mental health support. Mental health problems have a profound impact on all aspects of the student's life at the individual, interpersonal, and even institutional level. The chapter also presents factors that have been associated with seeking help, including the social environment within the college/university. Colleges and universities offer a unique setting to address mental health problems among students, and therefore should develop programmes for mental health promotion and disease prevention for their students before they grow in severity and cause long-term problems.

Mental health problems can affect many areas of students' lives, reducing their quality of life, academic achievement, physical health, and satisfaction with the college experience; as well as negatively impacting relationships with friends and family members. These issues can also have long-term consequences for students, affecting their future employment, earning potential and overall health. Stress is a commonly used concept in today's world due to the rapid advancements in almost everything (technologies and human evolution), and the world is becoming increasingly stressful. Unfortunately, students who struggle with depression and anxiety are reluctant to seek help. Higher education institutions can use the content of this chapter to develop appropriate targeted coping mechanisms and strategies which can be used by student counsellors to alleviate stressors among students thereby assisting in the enhancement of holistical health and wellness, and the academic excellence of students worldwide.



This book chapter takes a proactive approach to address stress by introducing a preventive measure, a relatively new approach implemented on college students in Bangalore, India called the "wellbeing van." The chapter emphasizes the importance of not only managing and coping with stress, but also implementing strategies that promote overall well-being by tapping into the intrinsic factors of the student. The well-being van has shown promising results in reducing stress levels among students in academic institutions. Additionally, the chapter delves into the difficulties students face in maintaining social relationships, conforming to societal expectations, and finding their place. It provides valuable insights on how to foster healthy social dynamics and create supportive environments for students.



Students' mental well-being plays an important role in academic achievement in higher educational institutions. A good mental state enables us to fully enjoy and appreciate our environment and the people around us. We can resist stress better and tackle daily life challenges with a positive frame of mind. Good mental health also allows one to be productive and to use one's mental abilities to the full. However, being a student brings about a number of events that can lead to stress, such as living away from home, giving up a good job to be a student, and organising your finances, deadlines and exams, to name just a few. The content of this chapter can be used by divison of student support affairs in higher education institutions worldwide to develop targeted interventions and strategies for alleviating the risk factors of concern to the mental health of students in higher education institutions.

Implications for institutions, management, students, and parents are discussed. This chapter aims to comprehensively analyze stress and mental health challenges among higher education students, raising awareness and promoting strategies for a supportive environment, guided by the presented conceptual framework.



College is intended to prepare students to become successful members of society. However, the academic demands of college can trigger stress and mental health problems. College students are in a unique position where they have to juggle academics, a social life, and, often, part-time jobs. As a result, college students are a particularly vulnerable group when it comes to stress and mental health issues. One subset of students facing the struggles of college achievements are pre-med students. Pre-med students face numerous challenges that can negatively impact their mental health. The academic pressures, financial stress, lack of social support, and relationship challenges, among others, can increase the risk of depression, anxiety, and other mental health disorders. The team of contributing authors on this chapter will address mental health in the higher education environment. This chapter will present a program for educators, peer students, and staff to provide mental health assistance for the premedical student.



Standard-based tests are a common form of final assessment in secondary education worldwide, but they pose many challenges for students. They require not only academic competence, but also mental resilience, which is rarely instructed in school. This chapter argues for the inclusion of strong mental training during revision. for this, it will review the history and rationale of standard-based assessments, and how they relate to the political and social aspects of different countries. It will also examine the controversies and criticisms of this form of evaluation, and how it affects the students' emotions and

The emotional well-being of students at higher education institutions was examined in this chapter. The study used a conceptual review as its framework, and data from published results presented in this chapter showed that most students in higher education institutions faced emotional challenges as a result of their new environment, financial challenges, academic-related stress, anxiety, and depression. Furthermore, many students in higher education are still adjusting to their new experiences and finding their fit in order to achieve in their academic pursuits. It is recommended that higher education institutions adopt innovative techniques to increase students' emotional wellbeing, such as boosting student awareness, building and designing a culture of wellbeing, and providing digital mental services.



In the contemporary, fast-paced world, adolescents are confronted with unparalleled challenges and pressures to excel. The core objective of this chapter is to furnish readers, particularly mental health professionals and adults, with pragmatic methodologies to aid adolescents in navigating the challenges that beset their lives. In conclusion, this chapter serves as a valuable reservoir of knowledge for those who are concerned about the well-being of adolescents in today's fiercely competitive and demanding milieu. It furnishes a comprehensive comprehension of self-talk and its various manifestations, elucidating their profound influence on an individual's thoughts, emotions, and actions. Ultimately, the chapter advocates for a proactive approach to adolescent well-being, underscoring the primacy of prevention over remediation.



Mental health concerns among college students have become a growing issue in higher education institutions worldwide. The transition to college life often comes with various stressors, such as academic pressure, social adjustments, and financial challenges, which can negatively impact students' well-being. To address this issue, higher education institutions are increasingly focusing on promoting mental health and coping skills to foster student flourishing. This abstract explores the importance of implementing initiatives and programs that support mental health and coping skills on college campuses. Firstly, it is essential to understand the concept of flourishing, which encompasses positive emotions, engagement, meaning, positive relationships, and accomplishment. Promoting flourishing on campus involves creating an environment that not only addresses mental health issues but also nurtures students' overall well-being.

# Preface

It is with great pleasure that I present this edited reference book, *Mental Health Crisis in Higher Education*, a comprehensive exploration into the challenges, adjustments, and mental well-being of students navigating the complex landscape of higher education. As the editor of this compilation, I am honored to contribute to the discourse on an issue of paramount importance—students' mental health during their academic journey.

Higher education represents a critical juncture in an individual's life, marked by newfound independence, academic rigor, and the pursuit of personal and professional growth. The transition from secondary school to university can be both exhilarating and daunting, and the impact on students' stress and mental health cannot be overstated. Research indicates that a significant proportion of students face mental health challenges, often exacerbated by the stressors inherent in higher education institutions.

This edited volume seeks to address the existing gap in the literature on student stress and mental health. By bringing together scholars, experts, and practitioners, we aim to shed light on the multifaceted aspects of this crucial issue. The chapters in this book explore a wide range of topics, from barriers to coping with stress and adaptive coping mechanisms to gender differences in stress and mental health. We delve into the intricacies of mental health crises, the state of mental health awareness, and various dimensions of students' emotional well-being.

## ORGANIZATION OF THE BOOK

**Chapter 1:** This chapter conducts a conceptual review of literature to analyze well-being and mental health initiatives for students in universities globally. It emphasizes the need for supportive work environments, mental health in universal health coverage, opportunities for student engagement, mentorship, building social networks, and individual coping strategies. The conclusion advocates for holistic mentorship programs in universities to address all aspects of students' lives.

**Chapter 2:** Focusing on the state of mental health among students in higher education, this chapter explores help-seeking behaviors and available mental health support. It identifies the profound impact of mental health problems on various aspects of students' lives and recommends that colleges and universities develop programs for mental health promotion and disease prevention.

**Chapter 3:** This chapter examines how mental health problems affect different areas of students' lives and emphasizes the reluctance of students struggling with depression and anxiety to seek help. It delves into the consequences of these issues on academic achievement, physical health, and overall satisfaction with the college experience.

**Chapter 4:** Addressing stress proactively, this chapter introduces a preventive measure known as the "wellbeing van" implemented on college students in Bangalore, India. It explores the van's impact on reducing stress levels and provides insights into fostering healthy social dynamics and creating supportive environments for students.

**Chapter 5:** This chapter underscores the importance of students' mental well-being for academic achievement in higher education. It explores the challenges students face, such as living away from home and managing finances, and emphasizes the positive impact of good mental health on productivity and the use of mental abilities.

**Chapter 6:** Investigating factors affecting students' well-being, this chapter explores elements like sexual harassment, student unrest, family roles, and institutional environment. It aims to understand how these factors influence learners' well-being in higher education institutions, providing valuable insights for future directions.

**Chapter 7:** A qualitative study on emotional burden among student mothers, this chapter identifies coping strategies and measures to reduce emotional burden. It highlights the challenges faced by student mothers, including overwhelming responsibilities, and discusses implications and recommendations based on the findings.

**Chapter 8:** Conducting a conceptual review, this chapter addresses mental health disorders affecting students in higher education institutions. It recommends a proactive approach, suggesting that universities implement innovative programs to prevent poor mental health and provide targeted support for at-risk students.

**Chapter 9:** Focused on challenges faced by higher education students, this chapter explores stress's impact on various aspects of well-being and academic, physical, social, and psychological dimensions. It introduces a conceptual framework and discusses implications for institutions, management, students, and parents.

**Chapter 10:** This chapter addresses mental health issues among pre-med students in the higher education environment. It discusses the challenges they face, including academic pressures and relationship challenges, and presents a program for educators, peer students, and staff to provide mental health assistance.

**Chapter 11:** Arguing for the inclusion of strong mental training during revision for standard-based tests, this chapter reviews the history and rationale of such assessments. It suggests practical strategies for teachers, including mindfulness exercises, collaboration activities, feedback mechanisms, and the facilitation of healthy habits.

**Chapter 12:** This chapter explores the impact of stress during the COVID-19 pandemic on students of different genders. Using a textual narrative synthesis, it examines how students were affected and the strategies used to cope, providing a review from six different countries.

**Chapter 13:** Examining psychological well-being as a multidimensional concept, this chapter discusses essential elements and emphasizes the importance of proactive, resilience-focused mental health promotion efforts in higher education to assist students.

**Chapter 14:** Highlighting the importance of mental health awareness in higher education institutions, this chapter discusses the impact on students' well-being, academic progress, and overall campus environment. It advocates for campuses that prioritize student welfare, leading to improved performance and well-rounded individuals.

**Chapter 15:** Examining emotional well-being of students, this chapter uses a conceptual review framework. It discusses challenges students face in higher education and recommends innovative techniques to enhance emotional well-being, such as awareness campaigns and digital mental health services.

**Chapter 16:** Focused on adolescents, this chapter provides pragmatic methodologies to aid them in navigating challenges. It comprehensively explores self-talk and its influence on thoughts, emotions, and actions, advocating for a proactive approach to adolescent well-being.

**Chapter 17:** Addressing mental health concerns among college students, this chapter explores the importance of initiatives promoting mental health and coping skills on college campuses. It discusses the concept of flourishing and emphasizes creating environments nurturing overall student well-being.

**Chapter 18:** Providing an overview of support services for students' mental health in Namibian higher education institutions, this chapter examines counselling services, peer support programs, mental health awareness initiatives, and crisis intervention services. It analyzes institutional support mechanisms and provides recommendations for future practice.

**Chapter 19:** Emphasizing the importance of mental health in students' lives, this chapter discusses the psychological variables affecting students' mental well-being. It highlights the need for comprehensive services that address various challenges students face, ensuring their overall adjustment at school.

**Chapter 20:** Focusing on the transition from childhood to adulthood, this chapter discusses the importance of mental health in interpreting and interacting with the world. It explores the stress and fear accompanying matriculated students entering higher institutions and underscores the significance of psychological well-being in this transition.

Each chapter contributes unique insights and perspectives, offering a holistic understanding of the factors influencing students' mental health. Importantly, the findings presented herein have practical implications for higher education institutions, their management, students, and parents. It is our hope that this book will serve as a valuable resource for scholars, doctoral students, counselors, and the management of higher education institutions, providing guidance and fostering the development of effective mechanisms for student adjustment.

The collaborative effort of the authors in this volume reflects a commitment to advancing knowledge, promoting awareness, and contributing to the overall well-being of students in higher education. I extend my sincere gratitude to all the contributors for their insightful and thought-provoking chapters.

As we navigate the complex landscape of *Mental Health Crisis in Higher Education*, may this book serve as a catalyst for positive change and inspire further research and initiatives aimed at creating supportive environments for students in higher education.

Sincerely,

*Peter J.O. Aloka*
*University of the Witwatersrand*

# Chapter 1
# Well-Being and Mental Health Initiatives for Students in Universities

**Peter J. O. Aloka**
https://orcid.org/0000-0002-4298-9211
*University of the Witwatersrand, South Africa*

**Justine Momanyi Omare**
https://orcid.org/0000-0002-2909-9214
*Jaramogi Oginga Odinga University of Science and Technology, Kenya*

**Emmily Achieng Owuor**
*University of Nairobi, Kenya*

**Calvince Okongo**
*Rongo University, Kenya*

**Joshua Owino**
*Jaramogi Oginga Odinga University of Science and Technology, Kenya*

## ABSTRACT

*There are increased mental health and well-being concerns among students at universities worldwide. By adopting a conceptual review of literature, this chapter analyzed well-being and mental health initiatives for students in universities. On the bases of the literature review in this chapter, it is concluded that there is need for supportive work environments, mental health in universal health coverage, creating opportunities for student engagement, mentorship at various academic departments building social networks, and finally, individual coping strategies are also useful in enhancing well-being and mental health of academic staff at universities. It is recommended that universities should develop holistic mentorship for students so that this can take care of all aspects of their lives.*

DOI: 10.4018/979-8-3693-2833-0.ch001

## INTRODUCTON

The concept of wellbeing within the university teaching and learning environment has been undertaken in several studies. It is useful here to make the distinction between mental wellbeing and mental health. Stanton, et al., (2016) define wellbeing from their student participants that includes "social, physical and mental dimensions" that require "balance" in order to achieve a "sense of happiness and fulfilment" (p. 92). Well-being reflects a broader social, physical, and economic experiences. It is often indicative of how closely an individual can live their life in accordance with how they want to. Good well-being is associated with developing robust relationships, reaching individual potential, and being able to engage in activities of personal value and meaning (Nicholls, et al., 2022). The World Health Organization on the other hand uses the term well-being to define mental health as 'a state of well-being in which an individual realizes his or her own abilities, can cope with the normal stresses of life, can work productively and is able to make a contribution to his or her community' (WHO, 2018). Mental health encompasses a spectrum of experience, ranging from good mental health to mental illness. Good mental health is more than just the absence of mental illness, but rather the presence of particular skills, habits and capacities that enable an individual to effectively react to, or deal with the environment around them (Nicholls, et al., 2022). According to Karimzadeh, et al., (2017), mental health is used for describing 'the cognitive and emotional levels of well-being as well as lack of psychological disorder' (p. 4497). In fact, positive psychology defines mental health as one's ability to enjoy life, create balance between daily activities and attempt to achieve psychological well-being (p. 4498). Mental health in this research is conceptualized as the continuum of neurophysiological and cognitive state that is related to emotion, mood, thinking and behaviour. Mental wellbeing has been argued to have both positive and negative dimension (Franke, et al., 2017). Positive dimension of mental wellbeing is considered as a complete state of cognitive functioning whereby the individual can cope with adversity, whereas, the negative dimension refer to the psychological distress and psychiatric disorder (Schütte, et al., 2014).

## BACKGROUND

Students have major roles to perform at the universities including research, teaching, community service and administrative responsibility. Student members carry a significant responsibility of training and developing students to become future leaders of the country by obtaining tertiary education (Adewale & Abdulsalam, 2017). Their responsibility is not only teaching but they are also responsible for the academic achievement of their students. Student members are, therefore, expected to spend considerable amount of time writing proposals for research support and collaborating with other institutions for them to be able to get support for their research activities (Kyvik, 2013). The increasing quantity of students pursuing postgraduate studies has placed pressure on students to supervise large number of candidates at the same time. This has resulted into students suffering from burnout and stress (Adewale & Abdulsalam, 2017). Student members are expected to build their network and community with industry, government and civil society (Altback, 2013). They can do that by being part of societies and organizations formed in community to deal with those social issues. Student members also serve as social and cultural critics in society. The academic community also provide a valuable voice in analyzing the cultural, religious and other social issues in the society. These students' members still have to proceed with their daily academics responsibilities of teaching, conducting research, offering community service and being supervisors. They combine both their academic and administrative work and are still expected to give the best performance in all these responsibility (Adewale & Abdulsalam, 2017).

Students in higher education institutions (HEIs) are among the most hit by this trend as literature suggests that increasing workloads, poor work life balance, lack of management support and other factors results in workplace anxiety and stress which affect their mental wellbeing (Schlevis et al., 2016). Academics are encumbered with extensive tasks, including teaching and research, and the attainment of a balance is a challenge to the realization of healthy well-being. Regrettably, the structure and content of academic jobs has been reported as crucial factors plaguing their wellbeing. For instance, research reports that taking too much time on academic work could cause problems, including sleeping disorders, family conflict especially with one's spouse, loss of vigour and declining work motivation (Noor, 2011). Although an academic career was traditionally seen as one offering low-stress, security, safe employment and high social standing with opportunities to do satisfying, autonomous work, universities have increasingly been exposed to the consequences of a changing environment, the changing world of work, and the concomitant, increased levels of occupational stress. Evidence in the United Kingdom (Tytherleigh, et al., 2007). In addition, Ntshoe, et al., (2008) highlight the complexities of academic work, academics abandoning core teaching functions in order to give attention to miscellaneous tasks, and the distortion of roles, all of which may give rise to low staff morale. In Malaysia, the increase in the quantity of universities in this country has caused pressure for students to put more effort into their academic work (Ahsan, et al., 2010). This is due to the competitive pressure from other universities for each university to gain recognition as one of the best performing universities in the country. This has resulted into low satisfaction of students towards their work and has affected their physical and mental wellbeing (Ahsam & Abdullah et al., 2010). A study that was conducted in the UK to trace work related wellbeing of students' members has indicated that work demand experienced by students has increased overtime (Borritz et al., 2014). The resources that were traditionally designed to decrease stress level in the organisation such as role clarity and independence with ones' work have reduced overtime. Studies have demonstrated a poor mental state of students in the university (Borritz et al., 2014).

However, previous studies indicate that students at universities face poor mental and well-being issues at work. For example, Dinu et al., (2021) found that teaching workload increased during the pandemic, with 51% of respondents indicating that teaching took 41% – 80% of their time while 47.5% indicated no increase, suggesting that workload increase was not evenly distributed. Furthermore, they found that workload increased with seniority, thus increasing risk of burnout (Dinu et al., 2021). The rationale for this finding is that senior academics were more likely to be spending substantive amounts of time in meetings, developing plans to manage the impact of the pandemic. Similarly, De Gruyter indicated that the biggest shift was in the number of hours worked, which was largely driven by digital learning (Gewin, 2021). In South Africa, Banda and Malinga (2021) found that their teaching workload increased and that they were faced with substantial hurdles to implementing online learning, which included a lack of preparedness for online teaching, poor Internet connectivity, the instability of the electricity grid and the affordability of data. Other studies of students have identified teaching and research pressures, heavy administrative burden, lack of resources, managing e-mail, poor quality working relationships, unsatisfactory leadership and management, and lack of involvement in decision-making as particularly hazardous to well-being. Reflecting the increasing number of roles that academics are expected to fulfill, raole stressors such as overload and conflict have also been identified as particularly problematic with negative implications for well-being and job performance (Guthrie, et al., 2017). A combination of work-related (such as heavy workload, long hours, and university service), individual difference, and behavioral factors have been found to contribute to work-life conflict among students (Hogan, 2016). Moreover, another research by Gulliver, et al., (2019) argues that staff can become overloaded, often lacking relevant training and being confused about their role and what they can do, which creates some risks; assuming meetings are confidential when they cannot be so; and having difficulty in distinguishing between academic and pastoral/personal problems. Academics are well-placed but ill-equipped to effectively help due to stigma, lack of skills, weak mental health literacy, workload and/or their own mental health needs. A survey by Morrish (2019) highlighted the escalating crisis, that referrals to counseling and occupational health services had risen astronomically between 2009 and 2016, increases of 50% were common and in some universities had exceeded 300%.

According to Martineau, et al., (2017), a dedicated and accomplished group of individuals shaping young minds, conducting groundbreaking research, and advancing knowledge, faculty may face a hidden struggle with demanding workloads, intense expectations, teaching excellence, and administrative duties. The pressure to secure their career path and navigate a highly competitive academic landscape can indeed impact faculty members' mental well-being. As such, the mental health of academics is a pressing concern that demands attention, and this may exhibit repercussions on individuals and institutions. Morever, Corpuz, (2022) argues that employees experience emotional exhaustion and burnout. The demanding nature of academic work, coupled with the emotional investment required in teaching and student support, puts university employees at risk of emotional exhaustion and burnout. 4 Long working hours, insufficient support systems, and a lack of work-life balance contribute to this phenomenon. In another study, the national charity, Education Support, found that 77% of education staff were suffering from poor mental health and 72% from stress (Wray & Kinman, 2021). While the majority of literature focuses on schools, staff mental wellbeing is also a serious concern among those working in early years settings and in higher education. Pre-pandemic, 1 in 4 early years professionals were considering leaving the sector due to stress and mental health problems. While at the other end of the education trajectory, a survey by Morrish (2019) highlighted the escalating crisis: Data from 59 higher education institutions revealed that referrals to counseling and occupational health services had risen astronomically between 2009 and 2016, increases of 50% were common and in some universities had exceeded 300%. In addition, Kinman (2014) the overarching burden for higher education professionals is the perpetual pressure of "doing more with less"; a situation which is deemed unsustainable, yet inevitable, due to the marketisation of the sector. Furthermore, Oberle and Schonert-Reichl (2016) found an effect of teacher stress on the stress levels of their students which accounted for more than half of the variability in students' levels of the stress hormone, cortisol. Staff and student wellbeing are inextricably linked, and it therefore stands to reason that effective strategies for tackling student mental health, while also benefitting their academic progress, must consider and support the mental wellbeing of teaching staff. In a study from Brazil, Borges, et al., (2023) showed that the mental health of non-teaching technical and administrative staff was affected by contract and legal conditions, and common psychological alterations were identified. Furthermore, another study revealed that instability of working conditions, work overload, lack of employees, and absence of performance evaluation were among the frustrations those workers experienced in their daily routine. Kinman and Johnson (2019) indicated that university employees who reported higher levels of core self-evaluations and vigor had more positive perceptions of organizational change, were more satisfied with the changes implemented, and more actively involved in the change process. This process was documented where staff with more vigor perceived the changes more positively that, in turn, strengthened their self-evaluations over time. This highlights the importance of these individual differences as resources that can enhance the success of organizational change initiatives. Academic employees were found to be less satisfied with the organizational changes than support staff at both follow-up points and the link from vigor to satisfaction with change was also weaker for them. Moreover, Kinman (2019) reported that the level of over-commitment found among students was particularly high and this was a strong predictor of health status, confirming the risks of excessive striving at work over time. The negative effects of being overcommitted to work on mental health was compounded by a need for approval and esteem. To improve the well-being of academic employees, interventions are needed to restore the balance between efforts expended and rewards received from different domains and initiatives to reduce over-commitment to the job role are also required. This may be challenging in light of the effort needed for academics to meet institutional expectations for excellence across several domains.

Fontinha, et al., (2019) study in the United Kingdom revealed that academics had less favorable perceptions of their working conditions than support staff; they also reported lower levels of job control and organizational commitment and more work-related stress. The negative effects of job role were exacerbated by the longer hours that academics typically worked per week. Academics who had a better work-life balance tended to have more positive perceptions of their working conditions and be more committed to their organization. Interestingly, employees who worked up to 10 extra hours per week perceived a higher level of control, were typically more satisfied with their job and career, and reported better well-being than those who either worked no overtime, or who put in more hours. Johnson, et al., (2019) study reported that the stressors that were the strongest predictors of physical and psychological ill health were also examined, together with the main and moderating effects of resilience. Academics reported better physical health than nonstudents and were less troubled by their working conditions, relationships, pay, and benefits, but had a greater risk of work overload and work-life conflict. Although the stressors found to influence health status were similar for both groups, the overall findings highlight the need for different stress management initiatives to address the specific risk factors experienced by the two core staff groups. The study also provides insight into the role played by resilience; the authors argue that it may influence initial perceptions of work-related stressors as troublesome and enable individuals to cope with some stressors but not others. Job-related factors are likely to influence these processes.

However, Westerhof and Keyes' (2010) model argues that, mental illness and mental health are not opposites, but rather occur and overlap on separate continua. Levels of mental illness co-exist with levels of mental health, creating different states of subjective wellbeing. In this chapter, the concept of emotional wellbeing describes the presence or absence of emotional difficulties on the mental illness continuum. Mental health is the continuum between flourishing and languishing, that is, between functioning well and experiencing subjective feelings of incompleteness, emptiness, or stagnation. Mental health includes the following three core components: emotional health, psychological wellbeing and social wellbeing. The next section presents the synthesized literature review on well-being and mental health initiatives for students at universities.

## WELL-BEING AND MENTAL HEALTH INITIATIVES FOR STUDENTS AT UNIVERSITIES

From the ongoing discussion on well-being and mental health of students at universities, several initiatives have been proposed.

## Stepchange Support Interventions

This may involve establishing clear guidelines for workload distribution, providing training on stress management and resilience, and integrating mental health support services. For example, Wray and Kinman (2021) argues that some wellbeing initiatives were perceived by staff as tokenistic and ineffectual and, moreover, the perpetuation of a resilience narrative, which places the onus for mental wellbeing on the individual, was condemned. For staff, organizational level support was considered a priority, for example, having a manageable workload, increased autonomy, and feeling appreciated and respected. While counseling, coaching and mentoring services were valued by staff, provision was reported as often limited and access problematic. Thus, services are more likely to be culturally and contextually appropriate and inclusive of all members of the University community. Moreover, Arday (2022) advocates the need to diversify and modernize mental health approaches to accommodate the needs of expanding, multi-diverse University communities. A further recommendation from Stepchange urges for all support interventions to be monitored and evaluated on effectiveness and quality. Moreover, Corpuz, (2023) argues that, there is a significant need to implement effective policies and practices. Universities should develop and implement comprehensive policies and practices that address well-being in the workplace. Moreover, the study recommended that there is need for creating a culture of work appreciation and recognition, as well as offering opportunities for professional development and growth, are also important components of effective policies.

## Establish Supportive Work Environments

According to Corpuz, (2023), there is a need to establish supportive work environments. Therefore, on the basis of this, creating a supportive work environment involves fostering positive relationships, promoting open communication, and cultivating a culture of mutual respect and empathy. University administrators should encourage collaboration, provide opportunities for feedback and participation, and ensure that resources and support systems are readily available for employees. Second, school administrators must promote work-life balance. Recognizing the importance of work-life balance, universities can implement policies and practices that enable employees to effectively manage their professional and personal lives. This may include flexible working hours, remote work options, and access to wellness programs or resources. Encouraging boundaries, promoting time management skills, and destigmatizing self-care are also crucial in creating a healthy work-life balance. Moreover, Brewster, et al., (2022) recommended that instead, institutional policies, training and culture appear to (explicitly or implicitly) prioritise student wellbeing in a way which leads to staff wellbeing appearing to be in opposition to that of students. However, the findings also indicate that there is potential to move away from current conceptualizations of a positionality between the two. Identifying how structural and cultural challenges affect both staff and students has started to demonstrate how prioritizing an integrated approach to staff and student wellbeing may be beneficial for all. If a positive working culture and environment was associated with staff productivity, purpose, and wellbeing, it could enable greater pedagogical and pastoral support to enrich student learning and wellbeing.

## Mental Health in Universal Health Coverage

According to Fernandez, et al., (2016), the main themes of this framework revolve around integration of mental health in universal health coverage; ensuring promotion of mental health over the life course;

and implementation of these themes through leadership, advocacy, and data availability. In higher education, the evidence of the effectiveness of strategies to promote mental health remains inconclusive and mostly focused on students. Thus, suitable initiatives, services, and resources should ensure that work-environment stress is alleviated for all these parties. Although some initiatives are ubiquitous and can enhance the well-being of different universities and populations, it should be kept in mind that every campus is unique, and its particular experiences should be specifically considered to address its mental health needs. Moreover, Cottini and Lucifora (2013) argues that the influence of organizational culture on faculty well-being cannot be underestimated, as the psychological workplace environment is intricately connected to individual mental health. Therefore, workplaces can be sources of well-being, and a supportive workplace environment is associated with diminished levels of job dissatisfaction, burnout, and depression. Payne (2022) study established that staff training in mental health literacy (knowledge, skills, attributes, and understanding) was required. Specific training was recommended in pastoral care for personal tutors and for staff pedagogy on health professional programmes. Finally, teaching staff needed support when supporting students with poor mental health. Such training and support can be integrated into a preventative, university-wide, holistic policy for student mental health commensurate with the University Mental Health Charter.

## Faculty Ownership

According to Kennedy, (2022 faculty ownership can be fostered through inclusive and participatory processes in the mental health strategy, where faculty should be involved in the development and refinement of the guidelines, ensuring that their perspectives and experiences are heard and valued. In addition, creating opportunities for faculty engagement, such as establishing cross-disciplinary committees or task forces, possibly also with student and staff representation, can empower faculty to contribute actively and exhibit a sense of collective responsibility towards well-being. In addition, Desselle, et al., (2020) reiterate that institutional approaches to demonstrate support for faculty include providing resources for professional development in teaching, research, and service as well as appreciation, encouragement, and reassuring faculty of their value. Furthermore, fair distribution of tasks, transparency of tenure and promotion expectations, equitable appraisal and rewards, and timely, effective, inclusive communication and a leadership that embeds diversity and equity are all of the utmost importance. Moreover, Hughes and Spanner (2019) insist that universities should provide clear and fair policies which promote an open culture around mental health and wellbeing, encouraging staff to seek help if they need to.

## Staff Mentoring Services

According to Kibbe, et al., (2016), mentoring enhances productivity, efficiency, and motivation, and formal mentoring programs have an overall positive impact on junior faculty who are taken under the wings of mentors for guidance and motivation. Moreover, mentorship at various academic departments is key to career satisfaction and retention, as reported previously. Hence, universities should give more attention and consideration to mentorship and should acknowledge that faculty may be struggling due to a dearth of formal and/or informal support from their leadership. Aloka, (2022) study reiterate that barriers to work wellness among staff in higher education institutions include but are not limited to aspects such as personal barriers, environmental barriers, organizational barriers, and legal barriers. The study recommends that wellness programs should include the vision, mission, and values of the organization and that there should be enhanced transparency and staff consultation before implementation is done. Moreover, Dooris, (2009) also proposes a setting-based model recognizes that health is determined by an individual's environmental, economic, social, organizational, and cultural circumstances, and thus aims to improve the environment in which a person lives, studies or works. Setting-based approaches are therefore concerned with the structural and organizational factors that impact health as opposed to focusing on individual risk factors. Setting-based approaches include policies, social marketing, strategies to improve the built environment, and academic- and curriculum-based strategies.

## Individual Coping Strategies

From literature review, there exists numerous individual coping strategies that could be adopted by students in an effort to cope with poor well-being and mental health challenges. For example, Lashuel (2020) reported that balancing life with career means that faculty are able to set realistic expectations of their workload and are also able to advocate for a culture of declining additional responsibilities and opportunities in favor of making time for themselves, their family, and their research. Moreover, setting boundaries applies to working with students, delegating assignments, distributing the workload, cutting additional tasks, and using smart time-management approaches. This gives the opportunity to relax, unwind, and disengage from work in an era where work emails are accessible by smartphones, making everyone constantly available and reachable.

## Social Support

According to Petersen, et al., (2012), social support can mediate a decrease in feelings of depression and anxiety. Hence, building social networks and reducing loneliness along the academic path is vital and effective; it can improve work dynamics and help faculty to persist in a demanding environment through building collaborations and team work. Moreover, faculty must recognize that reaching out to others for mental health support is essential, whether it is colleagues in the workplace or professional counselors. Hall (2017) suggests that the issue of mental wellbeing amongst the employees cannot be tackled in isolation without recognizing the effect of the structure of an organization or the influence which revolves around management. Also, evidence has shown that students with mental health issues are not very comfortable disclosing or discussing this issue with the management and may suggest a broken tie with management, causing loss of integrity and trust. Hamilton (2019) study reported that insight was gained into the efforts expended by students and the powerful role played by job-specific demands in influencing their well-being, particularly in relation to student expectations and their learning capabilities. Academics generally considered more informal reward mechanisms relating to interactions with students and pedagogical activities to be particularly beneficial. These findings provide an explanation for the high level of over commitment students typically show to their work, as they strive to maintain informal, job-specific, and value-based sources of reward in the absence of more formalized institutional mechanisms.

## Holistic University Approach

According to Brewaster, et al., (2022), exemplifying the importance of a whole university approach to mental wellbeing, participants identified a predominantly reactive mental health culture in higher education focused on individual actions, services, and interventions, and dissociated from proactive, preventative, and strategic change across the whole university system. It was suggested that a focus on culture would help to de-individualize wellbeing, ensuring that the way in which community expectations shape what is possible within an organizational context. Moreover, Ryan, et al., (2023) study recommended that developing a whole-of-university approach to promoting student wellbeing is important for addressing the growing severity and prevalence of mental health difficulties across student populations. An essential part of this holistic approach is the development of institutional policies and strategy plans focused on providing wellbeing promoting social, physical, and digital environments, as well as strengthening community awareness and actions. In addition—and perhaps most important to the student experience—are policies and institutional strategies that foster development of engaging curricula and learning experiences. This might include a focus on curricula and learning experiences that create social connection, build self-efficacy, foster intrinsic motivation, and learning experiences that afford choice and flexibility.

## CONCLUSION AND RECOMMENDATION

On the bases of the literature review in this chapter, it is concluded that there is need for creating a culture of work appreciation and recognition, as well as offering opportunities for professional development and growth, are also important components of effective policies), establish Supportive Work Environments, thus, on the basis of this, creating a supportive work environment involves fostering positive relationships, promoting open communication, and cultivating a culture of mutual respect and empathy. In addition, Mental Health in Universal Health Coverage, Such training and support can be integrated into a preventative, university-wide, holistic policy for student mental health commensurate with the University Mental Health Charter. In addition, creating opportunities for faculty engagement, such as establishing cross-disciplinary committees or task forces, possibly also with student and staff representation, can empower faculty to contribute actively and exhibit a sense of collective responsibility towards well-being. Moreover, mentorship at various academic departments is key to career satisfaction and retention, as reported previously. Hence, universities should give more attention and consideration to mentorship and should acknowledge that faculty may be struggling due to a dearth of formal and/or informal support from their leadership. Hence, building social networks and reducing loneliness along the academic path is vital and effective; it can improve work dynamics and help faculty to persist in a demanding environment through building collaborations and team work. In addition, individual coping strategies are also useful in enhancing well-being and mental health of students at universities. Thus, from the chapter review of literature, it is recommended that Universities should develop holistic mentorship for students so that this can take care of all aspects of their lives. Moreover, wellness programs should include the vision, mission, and values of the organization and that there should be enhanced transparency and staff consultation before implementation is done.

## REFERENCES

Adewale, A. S., & Abdulsalam, I. (2017). Impact of higher education management and leadership. *Malaysian Online Journal of Educational Management*, *5*(2), 23–34. doi:10.22452/mojem.vol5no2.5

Aloka, P. J. O. (2022). Barriers to work wellness among students in higher education institutions. In C. Alexander & A. Tureen (Eds.), *Leadership Wellness and Mental Health Concerns in Higher Education* (pp. 22–42). IGI Global. doi:10.4018/978-1-7998-7693-9.ch002

Altbach, P. G. (2013). Advancing the national and global knowledge economy: The role of research universities in developing countries. *Studies in Higher Education*, *38*(3), 316–330. doi:10.1080/03075079.2013.773222

Arday, J. (2022). No one can see me cry: Understanding mental health issues for Black and minority ethnic staff in higher education. *Higher Education*, *83*(1), 79–102. doi:10.100710734-020-00636-w

Banda, B.C., & Malinga, W. (2021). Coronavirus (COVID-19) and women in higher education in a South African University: Academic and social implications. *African Journal of Gender, Society and Development*, *10*(1), 7–34. doi:10.31920/2634-3622/2021/v10n1a1

Borges, L. O., Motta, G. M. V., Garcia-Primo, G. M., Barros, S. C., & Heleno, C. T. (2023). Working Conditions and Mental Health in a Brazilian University. *International Journal of Environmental Research and Public Health*, *20*(2), 1536. doi:10.3390/ijerph20021536 PMID:36674290

Brewster, L., Jones, E., Priestley, M., Wilbraham, S. J., Spanner, L., & Hughes, G. (2022). 'Look after the staff and they would look after the students' cultures of wellbeing and mental health in the university setting. *Journal of Further and Higher Education*, *46*(4), 548–560. doi:10.1080/0309877X.2021.1986473

Corpuz, J. C. G. (2022). Protecting the minority: How do we protect the minority in times of crisis? *Journal of Primary Care & Community Health*, *13*, 21501319221108999. doi:10.1177/21501319221108999 PMID:35748429

Corpuz, J. C. G. (2023). Enhancing Well-Being in the University Workplace: The Context of Higher Educational Institution. *Journal of Primary Care & Community Health*, *14*, 21501319231181488. doi:10.1177/21501319231181488 PMID:37326366

Corpuz, J. C. G. (2023, April). Workplace mental health in schools. *Workplace Health & Safety*, *71*(4), 160–161. doi:10.1177/21650799221147171 PMID:36695164

Cottini, E., & Lucifora, C. (2013). Mental health and working conditions in Europe. *Industrial & Labor Relations Review*, *66*(4), 958–988. doi:10.1177/001979391306600409

Desselle, S. P., Darbishire, P. L., & Clubbs, B. H. (2020). Pharmacy Faculty Burnout: Cause for Concern that Requires Our Support and Use of Best Evidence. *Innovations in Pharmacy*, *11*(3), 1–10. doi:10.24926/iip.v11i3.3274 PMID:34007640

Dinu, L. M., Dommett, E. J., Baykoca, A., Mehta, K. J., Everett, S., Foster, J. L. H., & Byrom, N. C. (2021). A case study investigating mental wellbeing of university academics during the covid-19 pandemic. *Education Sciences*, *11*(11), 702–710. doi:10.3390/educsci11110702

Dooris, M. (2009). Holistic and sustainable health improvement: The contribution of the settingsbased approach to health promotion. *Perspectives in Public Health*, *129*(1), 29–36. doi:10.1177/1757913908098881 PMID:19338133

Fernandez, A., Howse, E., Rubio-Valera, M., Thorncraft, K., Noone, J., Luu, X., Veness, B., Leech, M., Llewellyn, G., & Salvador-Carulla, L. (2016). Setting-based interventions to promote mental health at the university: A systematic review. *International Journal of Public Health*, *61*(7), 797–807. doi:10.100700038-016-0846-4 PMID:27364779

Fontinha, R., Easton, S., & Van Laar, D. (2019). Overtime and Quality of Working Life in Academics and Nonacademics: The Role of Perceived Work-Life Balance. *International Journal of Stress Management, 26*(2), 173–183. doi:10.1037tr0000067

Franke, F., Huffmeier, J., Montano, D., & Reeske, A. (2017). Leadership, followers' mental health and job performance in organizations: A comprehensive meta-analysis from an occupational health perspective. *Journal of Organizational Behavior, 38*(3), 327–350. doi:10.1002/job.2124

Gewin, V. (2021). Pandemic burnout is rampant in academia. *Nature, 591*(7850), 491–493. doi:10.1038/d41586-021-00663-2 PMID:33723408

Gulliver, A., Farrer, L., Bennet, K., & Griffiths, K. M. (2019). University staff mental health literacy, stigma and their experience of students with mental health problems. *Journal of Further and Higher Education, 43*(3), 434–442. doi:10.1080/0309877X.2017.1367370

Guthrie, S., Lichten, C., van Belle, J., Ball, S., Knack, A., & Hofman, J. (2017). *Understanding mental health in the research environment.* Rand Corporation. Retrieved fromhttps., www.rand.org/pubs/research_reports/RR2022.html

Hall, R. (2017). *The rise ofacademic ill-health.* Wonkhe. https://wonkhe.com/blogs/therise-of-academic-ill-health/

Hamilton, J. E. (2019). Cash or Kudos: Addressing the Effort-Reward Imbalance for Academic Employees. *International Journal of Stress Management, 26*(2), 193–203. doi:10.1037tr0000107

Hogan, V., Hogan, M., & Hodgins, M. (2016). A study of workaholism in Irish academics. *Occupational Medicine, 66*(6), 460–465. doi:10.1093/occmed/kqw032 PMID:27170737

Hughes, G., & Spanner, L. (2019). *The University Mental Health Charter.* Student Minds. https://www.studentminds.org.uk/uploads/3/7/8/4/3784584/191208_umhc_artwork.pdf

Johnson, S. J., Willis, S. M., & Evans, J. (2019). An Examination of Stressors, Strain, and Resilience in Academic and Non-Academic U.K. University Job Roles. *International Journal of Stress Management, 26*(2), 162–172. doi:10.1037tr0000096

Karimzadeh, M., Rostami, M., Teymouri, R., Moazzen, Z., & Tahmasebi, S. (2017). The association between parental mental health and behavioral disorders in pre-school children. *Electronic Physician, 9*(6), 4497–4502. doi:10.19082/4497 PMID:28848622

Kennedy, D. R., Clapp, P., DeLuca, J. L., Filtz, T. M., Kroon, L., Lamberts, J. T., Oliphant, C. M., Prescott, W. A., & Ray, S. D. (2022). Enhancing Pharmacy Faculty Well-Being and Productivity While Reducing Burnout. *American Journal of Pharmaceutical Education, 86*(5), 8764. doi:10.5688/ajpe8764 PMID:34507961

Kibbe, M. R., Pellegrini, C. A., Townsend, C. M. Jr, Helenowski, I. B., & Patti, M. G. (2016). Characterization of Mentorship Programs in Departments of Surgery in the United States. *JAMA Surgery, 151*(10), 900–906. doi:10.1001/jamasurg.2016.1670 PMID:27383863

Kinman, G. (2014). Doing more with less? Work and wellbeing in academics. *Somatechnics, 4*(2), 219–235. doi:10.3366oma.2014.0129

Kinman, G. (2019). Effort-reward imbalance in academic employees: Examining different reward systems. *International Journal of Stress Management*, *26*(2), 184–192. doi:10.1037tr0000128

Kinman, G., & Johnson, S. (2019). Special section on well-being in academic employees. *International Journal of Stress Management*, *26*(2), 159–161. doi:10.1037tr0000131

Kyvik, S. (2013). The academic researcher role: Enhancing expectations and improved performance. *Higher Education*, *65*(4), 525–538. doi:10.100710734-012-9561-0

Lashuel, H. A. (2020). What about faculty? *eLife*, *9*, e54551. doi:10.7554/eLife.54551 PMID:31912781

Martineau, M., Beauchamp, G., & Marcotte, D. (2017). Efficacy of mental health prevention and promotion strategies in higher education. *Sante Mentale au Quebec*, *42*, 165–182. doi:10.7202/1040249ar PMID:28792567

Morrish, L. (2019). *Pressure Vessels: The Epidemic of poor mental health among higher education staff.* Higher Education Policy Institute. https://www.hepi.ac.uk/wp-content/uploads/2019/05/HEPI-Pressure-Vessels-Occasional-Paper-20.pdf

Nicholls, H., Nicholls, M., Tekin, S., Lamb, D., & Billings, J. (2022). The impact of working in academia on researchers' mental health and well-being: A systematic review and qualitative meta-synthesis. *PLoS One*, *17*(5), e0268890. doi:10.1371/journal.pone.0268890 PMID:35613147

Noor, K. M. (2011). Work-life balance and intention to leave among academics in Malaysian public higher education institutions. *International Journal of Business and Social Science*, *2*(11), 1–12.

Ntshoe, I., Higgs, P., Higgs, L. G., & Wolhuter, C. C. (2008). The changing academic profession in higher education and new managerialism and corporatism in South Africa. *South African Journal of Higher Education*, *22*(2), 391–403. doi:10.4314ajhe.v22i2.25793

Oberle, E., & Schonert-Reichl, K. A. (2016). Stress contagion in the classroom? The link between classroom teacher burnout and morning cortisol in elementary school students. *Social Science & Medicine*, *159*, 30–37. doi:10.1016/j.socscimed.2016.04.031 PMID:27156042

Payne, H. (2022). Teaching Staff and Student Perceptions of Staff Support for Student Mental Health: A University Case Study. *Education Sciences*, *12*(4), 237–249. doi:10.3390/educsci12040237

Petersen, A. M., Riccaboni, M., Stanley, H. E., & Pammolli, F. (2012). Persistence and uncertainty in the academic career. *Proceedings of the National Academy of Sciences of the United States of America*, *109*(14), 5213–5218. doi:10.1073/pnas.1121429109 PMID:22431620

Ryan, T., Marangell, S., & Baik, C. (2023). Examining Mental Health and Wellbeing Policies in Australian Universities. In K. Coleman, D. Uzhegova, B. Blaher, & S. Arkoudis (Eds.), *The Educational Turn. Rethinking Higher Education*. Springer. doi:10.1007/978-981-19-8951-3_12

Schelvis, R. M. C., Wiezer, N. M., Blatter, B. M., van Genabeek, J. A., Oude Hengel, K. M., Bohlmeijer, E. T., & van der Beek, A. J. (2016). Evaluating the implementation process of a participatory organizational level occupational health intervention in schools. *BMC Public Health*, *16*(1), 1212. doi:10.118612889-016-3869-0 PMID:27905904

Schütte, S., Chastang, J. F., Parent-Thirion, A., Vermeylen, G., & Niedhammer, I. (2014). Social inequalities in psychological well-being: A European comparison. *Community Mental Health Journal, 50*(8), 987–990. doi:10.100710597-014-9725-8 PMID:24664367

Stanton, A., Zandvliet, D., Dhaliwal, R., & Black, T. (2016). Understanding students" experiences of wellbeing in learning environments. *Higher Education Studies, 6*(3), 90–99. doi:10.5539/hes.v6n3p90

Tytherleigh, M. Y., Webb, C., Cooper, C. L., & Ricketts, C. (2007). Occupational stress in UK higher education institutions: A comparative study of all staff categories. *Higher Education Research & Development, 24*(1), 41–61. doi:10.1080/0729436052000318569

Westerhof, G. J., & Keyes, C. L. M. (2010). Mental illness and mental health: The two continua model across the lifespan. *Journal of Adult Development, 17*(2), 110–119. doi:10.100710804-009-9082-y PMID:20502508

World Health Organization. (2018). *Mental health atlas 2017.* WHO Regional Office for the Eastern Mediterranean.

Wray, S., & Kinman, G. (2021). *Supporting Staff Wellbeing in Higher Education.* Education Support. https://www.educationsupport.org.uk/media/x4jdvxpl/es-supporting-staff-wellbeing-in-he-report.pdf

# Chapter 2
# State of Mental Health of Students in Universities

**Damaris Auma Ochanda**
https://orcid.org/0000-0002-0363-8662
*Masinde Muliro University of Science and Technology, Kenya*

## ABSTRACT

*This chapter presents the state of mental health of students in higher education institutions, help seeking behaviors, and available mental health support. Mental health problems have a profound impact on all aspects of the student's life at the individual, interpersonal, and even institutional level. The chapter also presents factors that have been associated with seeking help, including the social environment within the college/university. Colleges and universities offer a unique setting to address mental health problems among students, and therefore should develop programmes for mental health promotion and disease prevention for their students before they grow in severity and cause long-term problems.*

## INTRODUCTION

Globally, mental health problems are increasingly becoming common and are associated with impaired level of functioning accompanied with reduced quality of life (Kessler, et al., 2011). Mental health is paramount for student's adjustment and coping during their academic journey. Mental health problems may on the other hand have a serious impact on a student's life, affecting capacity to organize highly demanding study hours, socialize, and perform academically (Pacheco, et al., 2017). Many students have been shown to experience the first onset of mental health problems or an exacerbation of these symptoms during their college life. This is related to coping with academic pressure, having to deal with the stressful tasks of separation and individuation from family while some students may have to attend to numerous work and family responsibilities (Pedrelli et al., 2015). Students in higher education are also passing through critical developmental period in their lives where they transit from late adolescents to early adulthood therefore the need to understand the state of their mental health. Further, Lipson et al., (2022) affirms that colleges and universities have many unique opportunities for identifying risks and

DOI: 10.4018/979-8-3693-2833-0.ch002

delivering prevention and intervention to students in need making higher education an ideal setting to address mental health during a psychosocially significant period of life.

## BACKGROUND

The World Health Organization (WHO) (2022) defines mental health as a state of mental well-being that enables people to cope with the stresses of life, realize their abilities, learn well, work well, and contribute to their community. Mental health is an integral component of health and well-being that underpins our individual and collective abilities to make decisions, build relationships and shape the world we live in. Further, it is a basic human right and is crucial to personal, community and socio-economic development. Patel et al. (2018) affirms that mental health exists on a complex continuum with experiences ranging from an optimal state of well-being to debilitating states of great suffering and emotional pain and is therefore not defined by the presence or absence of a mental disorder. Mental health is more than the absence of mental disorders and is experienced differently from one person to the next at varying degrees of difficulty and distress (WHO, 2022). Mental health means that one is able to connect, function, cope and thrive in whichever situation or surrounding environment and it is as important as one's physical health (WHO, 2022). In our context, mental health therefore enables the student to connect with those in their environment, function academically, cope with the ever changing circumstances and thrive holistically as a student.

Despite its importance, it is only of recent that mental health was included in the world's global agenda. The Millennium Development Goals (MDGs) omitted mental health, this saw global leaders championing for its inclusion in Sustainable Development Goal (SDG) 3 which targets by 2030 to reduce by one third premature mortality from non-communicable diseases and promote mental health and well-being (Votruba et al., 2016). A study on Global Burden of Disease done in 2013 found that mental and substance use disorders had increased over the preceding 3 years to account for 11% of Daily-Adjusted Life Years (DALYs) compared with 7.8% in 2010, and these disorders alone accounted for 21.2% of Years Lived with Disability (YLDs) worldwide. This makes mental illness a major challenge and a key developmental issue for both low, middle and high-income countries (Votruba et al., 2016). The World Mental Health Report by WHO (2022) indicates that mental disorders are the leading cause of years lived with disability, accounting for one in every six YLDs globally. Mental health also enables one to develop relationships, perform activities of daily living and adjust to situations, any impairment and lack of access to appropriate support may result to mental health conditions. The mental health conditions lead to disturbance in thoughts and feelings, changes in behaviours, compromise physical health and disruption of relationships, school drop outs or interference with livelihoods. Studies done in the United States of America (USA), Canada, Australia, Turkey and other countries have shown an increase in issues affecting mental health of students in higher education (Okoro et al., 2022). Mental health of students is a key area of focus for all stakeholders particularly towards identifying risks and appropriate preventive strategies.

## FACTORS ASSOCIATED WITH MENTAL HEALTH OF STUDENTS IN HIGHER EDUCATION INSTITUTIONS

An increase in issues affecting mental health of students in higher education institutions has been documented and linked to different factors including transitioning at a young age to higher education institutions, increase in expectations, responsibility, moving away from family (Tett et al., 2017), and increasing financial pressures on students associated with declines in public funding to sustain the students while studying (Hassel & Ridout, 2018). This is affirmed by Eleftheriades et al. (2020) who reported that financial strain increases need insecurity related to food and housing and is higher among student-parents.

Education and expectations of academic performance have also been associated with significant sources of stress to students. A survey conducted by Organization for Economic Co-operation and Development (OECD) involving 72 countries and consisting of 540,000 student respondents revealed that 66% of the students reported feeling stressed about poor grades and 59% reported that they often worry that taking a test will be difficult. The OECD further found that 55% of students feel very anxious about taking a test, even when they are well prepared, further 37% of the students reported feeling very tense when studying (Organization for Economic Co-operation and Development, 2017). Academic experience and expectations leads to stress and anxiety among the students contributing to interference with mental health during their studies. Bernal-Morales et al. (2015) further notes that depression and anxiety can adversely affect academic progress and achievement.

Sexual victimization as a factor has been positively associated with mental health problems of university students including suicidal ideation, depressive feelings, psychological distress, and risk taking behaviours. For university students of all genders and degree levels, Rape, Abuse & Incest National Network (RAINN) in Eleftheriades et al. (2020) cites a sexual assault frequency of 11.2% with 23.1% sexual assault frequency among female undergraduates while male students noted to be much more likely to be sexually assaulted than their non-student counterparts.

According to Eleftheriades et al. (2020) bullying is another factor that negatively impacts mental health and in higher education bullying can be perpetrated by peers or by those in authority such as supervisors, professors and mentors. Supervisor-student bullying can take different forms including academic exploitation whereby a supervisor takes credit for a student's work or making inappropriate, discriminatory, or derogatory comments. Students can often feel as if they have no means of recourse due to the hierarchical nature of higher education which makes it difficult for them to report these negative experiences due to fear of the consequences, or because they believe their experience is normal. A study by Harrison et al. (2022) to investigate students' perceptions and experiences of bullying in UK higher education revealed that bullying is either perpetrated by individuals or by groups of students. In a one-to-one situation bullying may be intentional, goal-directed and linked to personal gain and at group level it may involve active exclusion and isolation of individuals by the groups which includes ignoring the student, neglecting to give them important information and restricting their involvement in non-academic activities. The bullying as a stressor predisposes the student to mental health problems.

## PREVALENCE OF MENTAL HEALTH PROBLEMS AMONG STUDENTS

Globally, mental health problems among students has been on the rise. As affirmed by Eleftheriades et al. (2020), there is growing evidence suggesting that the prevalence and or severity of university mental health issues has been increasing over the past half-century. A review of prevalence rates for psychological distress in university students globally reported rates of around one in ten in Nigeria and China, approximately one in five in Denmark, Norway and Japan, more than one in four in France and Turkey, and more than a third in Poland and Bulgaria (Sharp & Theiler, 2018). According to Sanci et al. (2022) young adults entering university have been reported to experience mental health problems and severe psychological distress at rates even higher than age-matched peers in the general population. Research suggests that common mental illnesses, including anxiety and depression, are higher in university cohorts when compared to same-aged peers in the general community, suggesting there are other additional factors that may put students at risk. These may include academic pressures and greater external expectations on performance, financial pressures of living, being from a rural or regional location, being part of a racial minority and being gender diverse (Gulliver et al., 2023). Similarly, study by Lipson et al. (2019) showed that suicidal ideations steadily increased over the past decade, from 5.8% in 2007 to 10.8% in 2016–2017 among students in US universities.

Studies on prevalence on mental health problems indicate that half of adult psychiatric illnesses, including major depression, anxiety disorders, and substance abuse, start by age of 14 years with 75% presenting by age of 25 years (Basta et al., 2022; Oswalt, et al., 2020). Mental Health conditions among college students has several effects including negatively affecting quality of life, decrease physical health, and wellbeing, and impeding academic success. For example, depression and anxiety are associated with decreased Grade Point Average (GPA), acute infectious illness, increased alcohol consumption, smoking, increased self-injurious behaviors, withdrawal from college, suicidal ideation, and suicide (Oswalt, et al., 2020).

Studies conducted before and during the COVID-19 pandemic have consistently found a high prevalence of anxiety and mood disorders among university or college students (Wang, 2020). University years are a peak period for the onset of these disorders related to stressors driven by academic demands, shift in social roles and instability of educational and occupational opportunities which increase vulnerability of the students to mental health problems (Auerbach, et al., 2018). Epidemiological studies suggest that 12–50% of college students meet criteria for one or more common mental disorders (Hunt & Eisenberg, 2010). Further, Bruffaerts et al., (2018) in their study reported that one in every third freshmen had a mental health problem in the past one year which was associated with reduced academic performance.

Bantjes et al. (2019) in their study in South Africa to determine the life time and 12-month prevalence of common medical disorders among university students, showed that 38.5% of the respondents reported at least one lifetime disorder, the most common of which was major depressive disorder. The 12-month prevalence of any common mental disorder was 31.5%, with generalized anxiety disorder being the most common. These results were higher than the 30% and 17% respectively found among a nationally representative sample of the country's general population. Kitzrow (2009) notes that of recent, students are joining college more overwhelmed compared to those of earlier years and thus increasing demand for strengthening of mental health support programmes. In their survey of university students seeking services in the counselling centers Gallagher et al. (2000) reported that, university and college counseling centers have reported a shift in the needs of students seeking counseling services from more benign developmental and informational needs, to more severe psychological problems with approximately 16% of counseling center clients having severe psychological problems. On the other hand, 84% of counseling centers indicated that the number of students with severe psychological problems was on the rise and therefore a concern. Ninety-four percent of directors of the counselling centers also noted an increase in the number of students coming for counseling who were already taking psychiatric medications. They estimated that 17% of counseling center clients take psychiatric medication, in contrast to 9% in 1994. These findings show that students in institutions of higher learning suffer a range of mental health problems which requires the institutions to identify appropriate preventive strategies and support systems that the students can easily access services from. Kitzrow (2009) confirms a high incidence and serious nature of mental health problems among college students with student affairs administrators reporting that they were spending more time dealing with troubled students and had seen marked increases in serious mental health problems among students including eating Disorders, Drug Abuse, Alcohol Abuse, Classroom Disruption, Gambling and Suicide Attempts. Evidence therefore shows that mental health problems among students in higher education institutions is on the increase which calls more attention to be paid in supporting the psychological wellbeing of the young adults as they transition into and through their tertiary education.

## EFFECTS OF MENTAL HEALTH PROBLEMS ON STUDENTS

Mental health enhances the ability of a student to adjust, cope and take control of their life while in college. Mental health problems have a profound impact on all aspects of the student's life both at the individual, interpersonal and even institutional level. At the *individual level*, mental health problems can affect all aspects of the student's life including physical, emotional, cognitive, and interpersonal functioning. Mental health problems may also have a negative impact on academic performance and ability to continue and complete studies. Further, depression and elevated levels of psychological distress among university students negatively impacts their academic performance and course completion (Sharp & Theiler, 2018), interferes with interpersonal relationships and is linked to suicide risks and workplace performance issues (Sanci et al., 2022). At individual level, students with higher levels of psychological distress are characterized by higher test anxiety, lower academic self-efficacy, and less effective time management and use of study resources. They are also less likely to persist when faced with distraction or difficulty and less likely seek for academic assistance (Kitzrow, 2009). Bantjes et al. (2019) affirms that mental illness has a profound and deleterious effect on social adjustment to university life, impeding academic attainment and leads to adverse health outcomes including death by suicide.

At the *interpersonal level*, students with mental health problems may affect many other people on campus including roommates, class-mates, faculty and staff, in terms of disruptive, disturbing or even dangerous behavior with the potential to physically harm themselves or someone else. Brooker et al. (2017) affirms that psychological distress negatively affects the individual student's emotion or behavior which can sometimes manifest in disturbing, disruptive or aggressive behavior towards student peers and university staff. Similarly, the needs of troubled students can be demanding and require extra attention and time from administrators, faculty, and staff. Students' mental health problems also impact *institutions* in terms of legal challenges related to risk management issues and mental health services provided by the institution. Several institutions have found themselves battling lawsuits alleging inadequate or negligent treatment of mental health problems (Kitzrow, 2009). Mental health affects all the aspects of the student's life and there is therefore a growing concern of the need for effective prevention, early detection, and treatment approaches for common mental disorders among students in higher education institutions.

## STUDENTS' LIFE AND MENTAL HEALTH

Joining higher education exposes the student to several stressors which may affect their mental health. For these young people transition starts before entering university, and includes navigating changes between academic years, and then graduating and entering the world of work or postgraduate study. Throughout their college life, students must make sense of who they are and how they fit into academic life (Tett et al., 2017). Students face adjustment challenges when they join the higher education system. Some students are able to adjust relatively well to their new environment, whilst for others, the adjustment involves a great amount of emotional maladjustment and personal stress which predisposes them to mental health problems. Higher education institutions provide a transition period for young people and coincides with a critical developmental phase of individuation and separation from family. The young person also develops new social connections, achieves increased autonomy and responsibility. Through this transition, students face new challenges, such as making important independent decisions about their lives and studies, adjusting to the academic demands of the new learning environment, and interacting with a diverse range of new people. In addition, many students must, often for the first time, leave their family homes and distance themselves from their support networks (Hernández-Torrano et al., 2020).

According to Duffy et al (2019) during the transition period, the brain undergoes accelerated development and is at heightened sensitivity to risk exposures including psychosocial stressors, recreational drugs, alcohol binging, and sleep disruption which are commonly encountered by university students. Moreover, more than 75% of mental disorders emerge by early adulthood and are associated with a substantial delay in treatment (Duffy et al., 2019; Votruba et al., 2016). Undiagnosed, untreated or inadequately treated mental illness is associated with progression to more complex disorders, college dropout, addiction, and self-harm. Studies further describe university as a period of 'heightened distress' (Bewick et al., 2010). The transition to university coincides with a high-risk period for maladaptive coping, onset of mental disorders and academic failure. Similarly, this period also represents an important window of opportunity for prevention and timely intervention. Thus, universities need to take a leading role in recognizing the importance of developing of an integrated system of mental health care for student (Duffy et al., 2019). Understanding the state of mental health of students in higher education institutions will facilitate the development of systems to prevent and address their mental health issues.

According to Gall et al. (2000) some students struggle to adjust to university life and this exposes them to 'acute stressors', due to the initial intense strain on wellbeing at the start of university. In their study among university students in USA, Conley et al. (2020) measured the students' psychological wellbeing at three time points during their first year. Findings showed that the participants had high psychological distress and reduced psychological wellbeing at the midpoint of their first year compared to the week before starting university. Further, there was little improvement by the end of the academic year. The transition into university life exposes students to stressors particularly in their first year as they attempt to adjust. Conley et al. (2020) notes that university presents significant challenges for students making it difficult for students to recover their initial coping level. Transitioning to institutions of higher education for these young students forces them to leave their families, friends and comfort zones and has been described as an experience of 'loss.' The students feel a loss of their former identities, social networks and even place. At the same time, they face challenges related to developing a new identity (Sanne et al., 2020). For successful coping, the student must adjust to academic demands as well as develop autonomy and confidence in learning through developing a 'learner identity' (Briggs et al., 2012). Adjustment during transition also calls on the student's ability to acquire a sense of belonging (Thomas, 2012). Students therefore are exposed to different stressors that may affect their mental health during the initial periods of their university lives as they struggle to adjust and fit into this new environment and new academic demands. The stressors and expectations for these students change from time to time as the student adjusts into university life and with changing demands from the academic programme from one year to another. Further the students experience less academic support with increasing academic pressure due to assessments counting towards their final degree as they progress with their studies. Cage et al. (2021) noted that Students experience different strains and fluctuating stress levels throughout their studies. This is supported by studies which have shown that mental health of students in universities fluctuate from one year to another with students in the USA on a four-year degree programme having poorest psychological functioning in the first 2 years of study, with improvements in the final 2 years (Conley et al., 2020), while in England for students on a three-year programme, university life triggered anxiety, with fluctuating psychological wellbeing, and higher rates of depression reported in the final year of study (Bewick et al., 2010). These study findings show that students in universities experience different mental health related issues from joining the institution and throughout their academic journey. This calls upon university administration to deliberately develop mental health care programmes that aim at preventing mental illness and promoting well-being of the students.

## HELP SEEKING FOR MENTAL HEALTH AMONG STUDENTS IN HIGHER EDUCATION INSTITUTIONS

Students seeking services from the counseling centers have consistently presented with severe concerns including suicidal tendencies, substance abuse, history of psychiatric treatment or hospitalization, depression and anxiety. In the state of mental health disturbance, the students require to seek for help because lack of diagnosis, support and treatment result to deterioration of the student's mental and health status (Duffy et al., 2019). Baik et al. (2019) notes that the high prevalence of mental health problems among university students is a critical issue for both universities and their wider communities due to the negative impact on every aspect of students' physical, cognitive, emotional and interpersonal functioning. In particular, prolonged psychological distress impacts the student's capacity to learn and impairs their academic participation by impairing information processing, attention, memory, decision-making, motivation, and impulse control. Help seeking is therefore important to enable the affected student access prompt mental care and support. Further, seeking timely mental health support is critical to the students' wellbeing.

Seeking for prompt support is linked to mental health literacy. According to Kutcher et al. (2016), mental health literacy refers to the ability to use mental health information to recognize, manage and prevent mental health disorders and make informed decisions about help-seeking and professional support. Rickwood et al. (2005) notes that *Help-seeking* is "a behavior of actively seeking help from other people," which includes discussing one's problem with another person to obtain support or guidance. The sources can be formal (e.g., people who have accredited professional background in the relevant field) or informal (e.g. parents and other family members). University students may have limited mental health literacy skills, therefore leading to poor help seeking attitudes, and a lack of both the intention to seek help and actual help seeking behaviour. Mental health literacy also encompasses help seeking knowledge, or an understanding of what formal sources (psychologists, psychiatrists, counsellors, general practitioners, etc.) are available, the processes surrounding help seeking and knowing when to seek help. Therefore, poor help seeking knowledge reduces help seeking behaviour, presumably because individuals are unable to recognise symptoms of mental illness and are unaware of available treatments. Action for help seeking behaviour requires a person to have both high help seeking knowledge and intentions to disclose. Intentions to disclose by university students are strongly influenced by internal beliefs about stigma, fear of potential repercussions socially or academically and feelings of social isolation and lack of belonging (Gulliver et al., 2023).

The universities and communities require information on the state of students' help seeking behavior from existing institutional mental health structures and support systems for development of appropriate preventive and mental health promotion strategies. A study conducted by Sanci et al. (2022) in Australia reported that despite the different health services that are available to students, whether on campus, in the general community, or online, almost one quarter of students indicated that there were times in the previous 12 months when they needed mental or emotional support but could not get it. On the contrary other studies report that most students with mental health problems do not seek and receive help, and that their help-seeking patterns vary with types of mental health issues (Bourdon et al., 2020). Further, Ning et al. (2022) notes that, in the context of higher education, students often try to conceal or solve their mental health challenges by themselves. Professional help is in most instances the last resort that university students tap into when they are in psychological crisis. However, research shows that students' higher levels of depressive symptoms reduce their likelihood of seeking help from parents and friends, as their levels of withdrawal and indifference toward help-seeking tend to increase together with their depression, which makes it increasingly difficult for students to articulate their feelings and reach out for help.

A study on mental distress, help Seeking, and use of health services among university students at Norwegian universities and colleges revealed that 40% of the participants gave physical health problems and 15% reported mental health problems as the main reason for their visit to the general practitioner (GP), 10.4% had been to a psychologist/ psychotherapist, three out of four of these at least as frequently as once a month. All help-seeking patterns, particularly use of health clinic/nurse and mental health services, were more common in female than male students. Further, students living in campus housing were more likely to use mental health services at their campus than students living off campus. This study also showed that students with the highest symptom burden sought help from psychologists/ therapists and GP three to five times more often than those with a lower symptom burden. Also students who experience the highest symptom burden and are most dependent on these services are less satisfied than healthier and less frequent users, this could be due to long waiting lists, unmet needs in therapy, and often the mental condition itself; depressed people, for example, often experience low energy and motivation, are generally pessimistic about their treatment and future outcomes (Sæther et al., 2021).

Similarly, other studies reveal poor help seeking behavior among students compared to the general population. A study conducted in Ethiopia among students who are at risk for common mental disorders (CMDs) showed that, 78.4% of the students had sought some form of help either from formal or informal sources while the remaining 21.6% had not sought any form of help. This is because one of the core symptoms of CMDs is hopelessness, which might further hinder the help-seeking intention of the students with CMDs. Of those who had a history of previous help seeking 92%, reported that the consultations were helpful. Further the study also revealed that informal sources (parents, partners, religious leaders, and friends) were the most frequently accessed sources of help by students than the formal sources (Kukoyi et al., 2022; Ning, et al., 2022; Gebreegziabher et al., 2019). Students' help seeking is also associated with the information they have on mental health and having a positive attitude towards utilization of mental health services while the lack of qualified mental health personnel restricts them from seeking care (Kukoyi et al., 2022). Poor help seeking among students who need mental health treatment or psychological support has also been reported in universities in China. Although the Chinese central government has emphasized university students' mental health education and built infrastructure to provide student counseling services inside higher education institutions, most university students do not access on-campus mental health support (Ning et al., 2022).

## FACTORS INFLUENCING HELP SEEKING FOR MENTAL HEALTH AMONG STUDENTS

Prompt help seeking for mental health problems is linked to good outcomes. Several factors have been associated with help seeking among students. In their study Velasco et al. (2020), reported that among these factors, mental health literacy and prior mental health care were most cited facilitators for help-seeking for mental health problems. Specifically, timely access to mental health was facilitated by having a previous positive experience with mental health services or help-seeking, being familiar with the sources of help, and good symptom and problem recognition. Higher engagement with the community and having a trusting and committed relationship with relevant adults such as parents, school teachers and counsellors also facilitated seeking help among adolescents. Another factor that facilitates help seeking for mental health among students is the social environment within the university/college. In their study, Dong et al. (2022) reported that one component of the college experience that encouraged help-seeking was the social support provided by other students and by campuses, often through greater visibility of resources or greater communication about mental health in general with the participants reporting more open conversation about mental health in college compared to high school. In the same study, participants reported that being in college provided distance from their home life in ways that could make it easier to seek help. For example, some talked about their relationships with their families as stressors to their mental health due to high familial expectations for academic success. Gulliver et al. (2023) notes that connectedness with university, belonging and group identity have a significant impact on attitudes towards help seeking and subsequent help seeking behaviours. These shared identities and feelings of belonging have been shown to improve a range of psychological and behavioural outcomes, such as elevated self-esteem, social competence, resilience and reduced loneliness thus enhancing students' help seeking behavior.

On the other hand, several barriers have been associated with help seeking among universities students who need mental health services. Ning et al. (2022) in their study among university students in China reported that a lack of trust in counselors, stigma towards mental illness, low mental health literacy, and inaccessibility to mental health services were four major barriers that impeded students from timely help seeking from professional mental health services. Similarly, in their study Kukoyi et al. (2022) reported stigma and cost as the most identified barriers that hinder mental health service utilization by students. According to Velasco et al. (2020), stigma is the primary obstacle to help-seeking for mental problems while the second most mentioned barrier was associated to family beliefs toward mental health services and treatment. Further, problems related to mental health literacy lead to poor recognition of mental health conditions of self and others and lack of awareness of available sources of help. Other barriers to help seeking include problems regarding service and personnel availability and other structural factors (such as cost, transportation and waiting times). Lastly, higher levels of psychological distress, suicidal ideation and depressive symptoms are linked to lower help-seeking behaviours. Dong et al. (2022) notes that college students in general report barriers to mental health treatment including skepticism about the effectiveness of treatment, a perceived lack of urgency, unfamiliarity with service options, confusion about health insurance, and concerns about parents discovering that the student is seeking treatment. Administrators in higher education institutions should be cognizant to the factors that promote help seeking and the barriers and develop strategies that enhance students' access to mental health services when needed.

## STATE OF MENTAL HEALTH SUPPORT FOR STUDENTS IN HIGHER EDUCATION INSTITUTIONS

Studies have shown that an increasing number of students in higher education institutions do experience mental health problems and have poor help seeking behaviors. This calls on the institutions to make deliberate efforts in providing mental health interventions and support for the students. Sæther et al. (2021) notes that colleges and universities offer a unique setting to address mental health problems among students and intervene before they grow in severity and cause long-term problems. Understanding the state of support for students creates an opportunity for universities to understand where to begin when developing structures and systems to improve mental health of the students. The mental health programmes can be integrated (offered by the student welfare organization on campus) or divided (both on campus and in community or specialized health care), and referral to specialized health care outside campus. In their study, Sæther et al. (2021) found that between-campus differences in use of health care services was related to available services and not necessarily demand. This means that accessibility to care for a student seeking help for a mental problem depends on service availability and the student may also miss the care when required. Further, group based and not individualized mental health initiatives have become increasingly implemented and popular among students. Groups do offer social and psychological support and opportunity for students to interact and share experiences. Group therapy is not only useful in students with psychiatric disorder or psychopathology, but helps improve general factors like autonomy, socialization, self-esteem, and improved interpersonal skills.

Globally, delays in accessing professional support among students with mental health problems are common. The ratio of counsellors to students on campus is still low in universities thus contributing to delays in students' access to mental health services. This has also been reported in universities in China where despite guidelines issued by Ministry of Education of on-campus counselors to student ratio that should not be lower than 1:4000, and that each higher institution should have at least two on-campus counselor, even with hired part-time counselors to meet these requirements, the ratio is still low. For example, Tsinghua University, China's very top university, has 38,000 students, but only 11 full-time and 21 part-time counselors, which leads to 4027 counseling times per counselor each year. Once students sign up for a counseling service on campus, though it is for free, the waiting time could range from a week to months, depending on the urgency of the case and the turnover of the counselors (Ning et al. 2022).

Improving mental health and well-being of students in institutions of higher education requires strategies that enhance mental health literacy and reduce stigma based on the collective values of contribution, compassion and acceptance rather than the normative expectations that further impose stress, shame and fear among students (Ning et al., 2022). Kukoyi et al. (2022) recommends that mental health services should be made affordable and at a subsidized rate because poverty and the lack of a social safety net for mental health service consumers have been found to increase the burden of mental disorders and lead to poor mental health outcomes. Therefore, higher education institutions should adopt strategies that reduce costs and thus increase access .to mental health services by the students.

## FUTURE RESEARCH DIRECTION

Understanding the magnitude of mental health problems and state of mental health of university students is important for all stakeholders in higher education institutions including parents and the students.

Consulted studies have shown that there is increasing prevalence of mental health problems among college/university students due to several factors including the students joining universities at a young age (a period when important developmental processes are taking place), high academic expectations and adjustments that the students go through as they transition into college life. Colleges and universities offer a unique setting to address mental health problems among students and studies have shown that help seeking which is linked to mental health literacy among the students plays a major role in connecting the student to mental health services. Stigma on the other hand has been cited as the main barrier to help seeking among students with mental health problems. Evidence shows that delays in accessing professional support among students with mental health problems are common within higher education institutions and this could contribute to poor mental health outcomes. The current study recommends that higher education institutions should deliberately adopt strategies to promote mental health, help seeking among students and prevent mental health problems. The strategies should also endeavor to improve access of students to mental health interventions to enhance prompt help seeking, diagnosis and care. Further research should explore challenges faced by higher education institutions in provision of mental health support and services for their students.

## CONCLUSION

Mental health and wellbeing of students is a topic that should concern stakeholders in institutions of higher education. Studies have shown an increase in the prevalence of mental health problems among students in colleges/universities which is associated with key developmental period in their life and increasing familial and academic demands that they face. The extent of the impact of mental health problems among students is at individual, interpersonal and institutional level. Help seeking is key to linking the students to mental health services and support and is affected by different factors most important is mental health literacy. Stigma is the most cited barrier to help seeking among students. Further delay and lack of services when needed impede students from accessing care. The administrators in higher education institutions should therefore recognise the increasing prevalence of mental health problems among the student population and purpose to deliberately put in structures to promote mental health and enhance access of students to mental health services when needed.

## REFERENCES

Auerbach, R. P., Mortier, P., Bruffaerts, R., Alonso, J., Benjet, C., Cuijpers, P., Demyttenaere, K., Ebert, D. D., Green, J. G., Hasking, P., Murray, E., Nock, M. K., Pinder-Amaker, S., Sampson, N. A., Stein, D. J., Vilagut, G., Zaslavsky, A. M., & Kessler, R. C. (2018). WHO World Mental Health Surveys International College Student Project: Prevalence and distribution of mental disorders. *Journal of Abnormal Psychology, 127*(7), 623–638. doi:10.1037/abn0000362 PMID:30211576

Baik, C., Larcombe, W., & Brooker, A. (2019). How universities can enhance student mental wellbeing: The student perspective. *Higher Education Research & Development, 38*(4), 674–687. doi:10.1080/07294360.2019.1576596

Basta, M., Micheli, K., Koutra, K., Fountoulaki, M., Dafermos, V., Drakaki, M., & Vgontzas, A. N. (2022). Depression and anxiety symptoms in adolescents and young adults in Greece: Prevalence and associated factors. *Journal of Affective Disorders Reports, 8*, 100334. Advance online publication. doi:10.1016/j.jadr.2022.100334

Bernal-Morales, B., Rodríguez-Landa, J. F., & Pulido-Criollo, F. (2015). *Impact of anxiety and depression symptoms on scholar performance in high school and university students, a fresh look at anxiety disorders*. London, UK: IntechOpen. doi:10.5772/60711

Bewick, B., Koutsopoulou, G., Miles, J., Slaa, E., & Barkham, M. (2010). Changes in Undergraduate Students' Psychological Well-being as They Progress through University. *Studies in Higher Education, 35*(6), 633–645. doi:10.1080/03075070903216643

Bourdon, J. L., Moore, A. A., Long, E. C., Kendler, K. S., & Dick, D. M. (2020). The relationship between on-campus service utilization and common mental health concerns in undergraduate college students. *Psychological Services, 17*(1), 118–126. doi:10.1037er0000296 PMID:30299149

Briggs, A. R. J., Clark, J., & Hall, I. (2012). Building Bridges: Understanding Student Transition to University. *Quality in Higher Education, 18*(1), 3–21. doi:10.1080/13538322.2011.614468

Bruffaerts, R., Mortier, P., Kiekens, G., Auerbach, R. P., Cuijpers, P., Demyttenaere, K., Green, J. G., Nock, M. K., & Kessler, R. C. (2018). Mental health problems in college freshmen: Prevalence and academic functioning. *Journal of Affective Disorders, 225*(1), 97–103. doi:10.1016/j.jad.2017.07.044 PMID:28802728

Cage, E., Jones, E., Ryan, G., Hughes, G., & Spanner, L. (2021). Student mental health and transitions into, through and out of university: Student and staff perspectives. *Journal of Further and Higher Education, 45*(8), 1076–1089. doi:10.1080/0309877X.2021.1875203

Conley, C. S., Shapiro, J. B., Huguenel, B. M., & Kirsch, A. C. (2020). Navigating the College Years: Developmental Trajectories and Gender Differences in Psychological Functioning, Cognitive-Affective Strategies, and Social Well-Being. *Emerging Adulthood, 8*(2), 103–117. doi:10.1177/2167696818791603

Dong, H., Dai, J., Lipson, S. K., & Curry, L. (2022). Help-seeking for mental health services in Asian American college students: Anexploratory qualitative study. *Journal of American College Health, 70*(8), 2303–2310. doi:10.1080/07448481.2020.1851234 PMID:33289588

Duffy, A., Saunders, K. E. A., Malhi, G. S., Patten, S., Cipriani, A., McNevin, S. H., MacDonald, E., & Geddes, J. (2019). Mental health care for university students: A way forward? The Lancet. *The Lancet. Psychiatry, 6*(11), 885–887. doi:10.1016/S2215-0366(19)30275-5 PMID:31324561

Eleftheriades, R., Fiala, C., & Pasic, M. D. (2020). The challenges and mental health issues of academic trainees. *F1000 Research, 9*, 104. https://www.ncbi.nlm.nih.gov/pmc/articles/PMC7199285/pdf/f1000research-9-23184.pdf. doi:10.12688/f1000research.21066.1 PMID:32419927

Gall, T. L., Evans, D. R., & Bellerose, S. (2000). Transition to First-Year University: Patterns of Change in Adjustment across Life Domains and Time. *Journal of Social and Clinical Psychology, 19*(4), 544–567. doi:10.1521/jscp.2000.19.4.544

Gallagher, R., Gill, A., & Sysko, H. (2000). *National survey of counseling center directors*. International Association of Counseling Services.

Gebreegziabher, Y., Girma, E., & Tesfaye, M. (2019). Help-seeking behavior of Jimma university students with common mental disorders: A crosssectional study. *PLoS One*, *14*(2), e0212657. doi:10.1371/journal.pone.0212657 PMID:30794639

Gulliver, A., Wysoke, T., Calear, A. L., & Farrer, L. M. (2023). Factors Associated with Engagement in University Life, and Help Seeking Attitudes and Behaviour in First Year Undergraduate Students. *International Journal of Environmental Research and Public Health*, *20*(1), 120. doi:10.3390/ijerph20010120 PMID:36612442

Harrison, E. D., Hulme, J. A., & Fox, C. L. (2022). A Thematic Analysis of Students' Perceptions and Experiences of Bullying in UK Higher Education. *Europe's Journal of Psychology*, *18*(1), 1841–0413. ejop.psychopen.eu. doi:10.5964/ejop.3669 PMID:35330856

Hassel, S., & Ridout, N. (2018). An Investigation of First-Year Students' and Lecturers' Expectations of University Education. *Frontiers in Psychology*. doi:10.3389/fpsyg.2017.02218

Hernández-Torrano, D., Ibrayeva, L., Sparks, J., Lim, N., Clementi, A., Almukhambetova, A., Nurtayev, Y., & Muratkyzy, A. (2020). Mental Health and Well-Being of University Students: A Bibliometric Mapping of the Literature. *Frontiers in Psychology*, *11*, 1226. doi:10.3389/fpsyg.2020.01226 PMID:32581976

Hunt, J., & Eisenberg, D. (2010). Mental Health Problems and Help-Seeking Behavior Among College Students. *The Journal of Adolescent Health*, *46*(1), 3–10. doi:10.1016/j.jadohealth.2009.08.008 PMID:20123251

Kessler, R. C., Aguilar-Gaxiola, S., Alonso, J., Chatterji, S., Ormel, J., Üstün, T. B., & Wang, P. S. (2011). *The global burden of mental disorders: An update from the WHO World Mental Health (WMH)*. Surveys.

Kitzrow, M. A. (2009). The Mental Health Needs of Today's College Students: Challenges and Recommendations. *NASPA Journal*, *46*(4), 646–660. doi:10.2202/1949-6605.5037

Kukoyi, O., Orok, E., Oluwafemi, F., Oluwadare, T., Oni, O., Bamitale, T., Jaiyesimi, B., Ojo, T., & Eze, H. (2022). *Factors affecting the utilization of mental health services among undergraduate students in a Nigerian University. Heliyon*. Cell Press. doi:10.1016/j.heliyon.2022.e11476

Kutcher, S., Wei, Y., & Coniglio, C. (2016). Mental health literacy: Past, present and future. *Canadian Journal of Psychiatry*, *61*(3), 154–158. doi:10.1177/0706743715616609 PMID:27254090

Lipson, S. K., Lattie, E. G., & Eisenberg, D. (2019). Increased Rates of Mental Health Service Utilization by U.S. College Students: 10-Year Population-Level Trends (2007–2017). *Psychiatric Services (Washington, D.C.)*, *70*(1), 60–63. doi:10.1176/appi.ps.201800332 PMID:30394183

Lipson, S. K., Zhou, S., Abelson, S., Heinze, J., Jirsa, M., Morigney, J., Patterson, A., Singhd, M., & Eisenberg, D. (2022, June 01). Trends in College Student Mental Health and Help-Seeking by Race/Ethnicity: Findings from the national Healthy Minds Study, 2013–2021. *Journal of Affective Disorders*, *306*, 138–147. doi:10.1016/j.jad.2022.03.038 PMID:35307411

Ning, X., Wong, J. P. H., Huang, S., Fu, Y., Gong, X., Zhang, L., Hilario, C., Fung, K. P. L., Yu, M., Poon, M. K. L., Cheng, S., Gao, J., & Jia, C.-X. (2022). Chinese University Students' Perspectives on Help-Seeking and Mental Health Counseling. *International Journal of Environmental Research and Public Health, 19*(14), 8259. doi:10.3390/ijerph19148259 PMID:35886103

Organization for Economic Co-operation and Development. (2017). PISA 2015 Results (Volume III). Paris, France.

Oswalt, S. B., Lederer, A., Chestnut-Steich, K., Day, C., Halbritter, A., & Ortiz, D. (2020). Trends in college students' mental health diagnoses and utilization of services, 2009–2015. *Journal of American College Health, 68*(1), 41–51. doi:10.1080/07448481.2018.1515748 PMID:30355071

Pacheco, J. P., Giacomin, H. T., Tam, W. W., Ribeiro, T. B., Arab, C., & Bezerra, I. M. (2017). Mental health problems among medical students in Brazil: a systematic review and meta-analysis. *Brazillian Journal of Psychiatry.* https://www.scielo.br/j/rbp/a/FsKx7VwgRVSvwS638BqhbmK/#

Patel, V., Saxena, S., Lund, C., Thornicroft, G., Baingana, F., & Bolton, P. (2018). The Lancet Commission on Global Mental Health and Sustainable Development. *Lancet, 392*(10157), 1598. Doi: 31612-x. doi:10.1016/S0140-6736(18)

Pedrelli, P., Nyer, M., Yeung, A., Zulauf, C., & Wilens, T. (2015). College Students: Mental Health Problems and Treatment Considerations. *Academic Psychiatry, 39*(5), 503–511. doi:10.100740596-014-0205-9 PMID:25142250

Rickwood, D., Deane, F. P., Wilson, C. J., & Ciarrochi, J. (2005). Young people's help-seeking for mental health problems. *Australian e-Journal for the Advancement of Mental Health, 4*(3), 218–251. doi:10.5172/jamh.4.3.218

Sæther, M. H., Sivertsen, B., & Bjerkeset, O. (2021). Mental Distress, Help Seeking, and Use of Health Services Among University Students. The SHoT-Study 2018, Norway. *Frontiers in Psychiatry, 12*, 727237. doi:10.3389/fpsyt.2021.727237 PMID:34744820

Sanci, L., Williams, I., Russell, M., Chondros, P., Duncan, A., Tarzia, L., Peter, D., Lim, M. S. Y., Tomyn, A., & Minas, H. (2022). Towards a health promoting university: Descriptive findings on health, wellbeing and academic performance amongst university students in Australia. *BMC Public Health, 22*(1), 2430. doi:10.118612889-022-14690-9 PMID:36575509

Sharp, J., & Theiler, S. (2018). A Review of Psychological Distress Among University Students: Pervasiveness, Implications and Potential Points of Intervention. *International Journal for the Advancement of Counseling, 40*(3), 193–212. doi:10.100710447-018-9321-7

Tett, L., Cree, V. E., & Christie, H. (2017). From Further to Higher Education: Transition as an on-Going Process. *Higher Education, 73*(3), 389–406. doi:10.100710734-016-0101-1

Thomas, L. (2012). Building Student Engagement and Belonging in Higher Education at a Time of Change. *Paul Hamlyn Foundation, 100*, 1–99.

van Herpen, S. G. A., Meeuwisse, M., Hofman, W. H. A., & Severiens, S. E. (2020). A head start in higher education: The effect of a transition intervention on interaction, sense of belonging, and academic performance. *Studies in Higher Education, 45*(4), 862–877. doi:10.1080/03075079.2019.1572088

Velasco, A. A., Cruz, I. S. S., Billings, J., Jimenez, M., & Rowe, S. (2020). What are the barriers, facilitators and interventions targeting help-seeking behaviours for common mental health problems in adolescents? A systematic review. *BMC Psychiatry*, *20*(1), 293. doi:10.118612888-020-02659-0 PMID:32527236

Votruba, N., & Thornicroft, G. (2016). Sustainable development goals and mental health: Learnings from the contribution of the FundaMentalSDG global initiative. *Global Mental Health (Cambridge, England)*, *3*, e26. doi:10.1017/gmh.2016.20 PMID:28596894

Wang, X., Hegde, S., Son, C., Keller, B., Smith, A., & Sasangohar, F. (2020). Investigating mental health of US college students during the COVID-19 pandemic: Cross-sectional survey study. *Journal of Medical Internet Research*, *22*(9), e22817. doi:10.2196/22817 PMID:32897868

WHO. (2022). *World mental health report: transforming mental health for all*. Geneva: World Health Organization.

# Chapter 3
# Maladaptive Coping Mechanisms

**Daniel Opotamutale Opotamutale**
https://orcid.org/0000-0002-8913-056X
*University of Namibia, Namibia*

**Fillemon Shekutamba Albanus**
https://orcid.org/0000-0003-1516-2523
*University of Namibia, Namibia*

## ABSTRACT

*Mental health problems can affect many areas of students' lives, reducing their quality of life, academic achievement, physical health, and satisfaction with the college experience; as well as negatively impacting relationships with friends and family members. These issues can also have long-term consequences for students, affecting their future employment, earning potential and overall health. Stress is a commonly used concept in today's world due to the rapid advancements in almost everything (technologies and human evolution), and the world is becoming increasingly stressful. Unfortunately, students who struggle with depression and anxiety are reluctant to seek help. Higher education institutions can use the content of this chapter to develop appropriate targeted coping mechanisms and strategies which can be used by student counsellors to alleviate stressors among students thereby assisting in the enhancement of holistical health and wellness, and the academic excellence of students worldwide.*

## INTRODUCTION

Stress is a major mental health problem affecting university and college students globally. A minimal degree of stress and strains may not be a point of concern (Chang, 2017). However, if the student feels extreme stress before and during an examination, it is a point of concern for mental health. It is reported that, annually, 20% of students in the 18–24 age group commit suicide owing to examination-related stress, as well as less time to socialise and be involved in active relaxation activities which has a nega-

DOI: 10.4018/979-8-3693-2833-0.ch003

tive effect of examination outcomes Go, (2016). Therefore, stress presents a serious threat to students' academic achievement.

Kwaah and Essilfe (2017) reported that coping mechanism are one of the necessary measures for preventing the harmful effects of prolonged stress. Moreover, coping mechanism is multidimensional and involve various strategies some of which are more functional than others (Kwaah & Essilfe, 2017). Students with poor coping mechanisms and personality types such as type A personality may be at risk of suffering additional stress, leading to negative patterns of behaviour, the development of psychosomatic symptoms and decreased academic performance (Akinci et al., 2018).

Preventing stress encompasses strategies that the student can undertake to reduce stress and its impact. Such strategies include aspects such as eating a well-balanced diet, avoiding the consumption of alcohol and related drug abuse, and enough sleep – at least eight hours a night is recommended (Bondarchuk et al., 2023). Furthermore, Bondarchuk et al., (2023) reported that exercising is one of the best strategies a student needs to consider when dealing stress as this will help to ease the body muscles, which becomes tense when one is stressed, by increasing blood circulation and thereby increasing the student's thinking capacity. Additionally, active study skills can help to ease stress by developing the confidence in the student to control their work leading to success. Finally, student counsellors can help students cope with stress by supporting them to make better study choices as well as to make changes that help decrease them stress levels (, (Bondarchuk et al., 2023).

Stress is a physical or emotional reaction to stressors that emanate either from external or internal the student (American Psychological Association, 2020). Such reactions influence almost every systemic aspect of the human body, affecting individuals' emotions and attitudes (American Psychological Association, 2020). On the other hand, stressors could take the form of human beings, locations or situations which may actually precipitate stress in somebody, but with specific emphasis on negative academic stress. However, a certain amount of stress or tension is recognised as assisting an individual to function on a higher level in certain situations, even though in the event that the tension accumulates they may be powerless to deal with the extreme emotions of stress that arise (Gustems-Carnicer et al., 2019).

Academic stress occurs when educational associated stipulations transcend the accommodative materials accessible to the person involved (Scott et al., 2019). The availability, existence and seriousness of the academic stressors, including the inability to handle or deal with extreme academic achievements and ultimatums, could affect the level of the stress reaction or feedback encountered (Levin, 2021).

Scientists have reported various causes of stress within higher education institutions which entail personal, environmental and adaptive or coping components (Alkhawaldeh et al., 2023). Personal characteristics are important here; for example, students with greater amounts of neuroticism, a human trait distinguished by anxiousness and pessimism, have been shown to experience greater amounts of stress (Rettew et al. (2021). Moreover, students who are introspective and tend to isolate themselves from the communal situations may be more vulnerable to stress than students who are extroverts and enjoy communicating and social interaction (Gao et al., 2020). Students who have access to college or university resources like proper educational support networks or services could be more equipped to cope with stress thus increasing academic accomplishments (Amanvermez et al., 2020).

Al Battashi et al. (2021) reported that some of the factors that significantly precipitate and are connected with greater stress levels are the usage of smart phones and sleeping habits. The amount of stress within university and college student populations has been considered and properly recorded, showing consistency with regard to the aetiology and impact of the levels of stress and tension being encountered (Levin, 2021). In spite of this, all over the authorities, acquiring better grade scores, heavy workloads, excessive homework tasks, anxiety over deadlines, money problems or shortage and eventually receiving individual degrees all lead to emotions of stress (Ashipala & Shilunga, 2023; Levin, 2021). Shatimwene et al. (2020) found that the two-week block system was too short and could not provide students with sufficient time for learning and practising the needed tasks; thus, the students often failed to differentiate between the theoretical and practical teaching. Students are often expected to attend the practical teaching while occupied with theoretical teaching, which leads to the developmental of stress among nursing students in particular (Shatimwene et al, 2020).

Consequently, students are at higher risk of substandard academic performance, as well as significant educational stress, which exacerbates stress patterns and maladaptive coping mechanisms and diminishes student wellness (Scott et al., 2019). Hence, it is essential to identify, acknowledge and manage the adverse side effects that stress imposes on academic achievement, as well as personal and societal wellness, in order to prolong the professional and private lives of the students (Gustems-Carnicer et. al., 2019).

## BACKGROUND

Good Therapy (2018) reported that maladaptive coping mechanisms are fruitless and unsuccessful or ineffective and have unplanned negative outcomes (Good Therapy, 2018). Furthermore, coping mechanisms prevent students from remaining emotionally, physically and psychologically stable in distressing situations (Sutton, 2020). Nevertheless, existing literature describes coping mechanisms as adaptive or maladaptive, whereby avoiding coping is also categorised as a maladaptive coping style (Niu et al 2022). Therefore, students utilise avoidance coping mechanisms in an attempt to avoid facing the problem by its very nature, including the psychological harm correlated to the difficulty or problem, and stress or stressors. As a result, avoidance coping mechanism retains the students in state of negation against the negative existing problem, stress or stressors being experienced (Goldman & Bell, 2022; Niu et al 2022). For this reason, maladaptive coping mechanisms do not avoid the aetiologies of stressors, but rather offer only a short-term solution to stress; even though they seem to work temporarily, the continuous use of such mechanisms negatively affects students' psychological wellness (Sutton, 2020).

On the other hand, adaptive coping mechanisms are usually considered to be healthy and efficient strategies for controlling frustrating situations (Good Therapy, 2018). Therefore, the adaptive coping mechanisms which set out to be a healthy state of stress resolution entail a social support network, tranquillity, problem resolution, as well as physical exercise (Good Therapy, 2018). A support network that offers social and psychological support is beneficial in relieving individuals' stress feelings; in addition, the utilisation of a social support network is believed to enhance people's ability to manage when experiencing stress (Santiago et al., 2022). Equally, psychological support acts as a shielding mechanism, because it counteracts the negative influence of stress (Cleveland Clinic, 2020). According to Butler et al., (2020), problem-focused resolution aims at eliminating and diminishing the aetiologies of the stressors, subsequently decreasing the amount of stress being experienced by particular individuals. Hence, maladaptive coping mechanisms are inefficient and have the likely detrimental chronic or prolonged implications, while adaptive coping mechanisms are efficient and enable prolonged wellness among individuals generally and students in particular (Levin, 2021).

Coping strategies are more than a significant trigger of stress in a university student's life. Coping strategies are described as the mechanisms which people utilise in managing stress and negative feelings or thoughts (Crego et al., 2016). Students who make use of avoidance coping methods, like alcohol and drug misuse are more likely to encounter stress than students that utilise good coping styles, like searching for communal support networks and participating in physical exercises (Compas et al., 2019; Makarowski et al., 2020). Therefore, this indicates that the course of actions students takes to deal with distress could have a huge influence on their own stress intensification and overall wellness. Compas et al., (2019) labelled coping models of stress and resilience that people could utilise during periods of stress as coping models (Karugahe & Lambert, 2021). These include, firstly, searching for social support, secondly, attempting to find resolutions to the issue, and thirdly, attempting to prevent problem (Karugahe & Lambert, 2021). Equally important, Ashipala et al. (2023) reported that academics (students) should also be motivated to sustain a record of all the things such as academic overload that trigger them to feel stressed, anxious or worried, and to learn to say 'no' to activities that they are not able to deal with.

The theory or notion of coping was derived in psychology between the years 1940 and 1950 (Lazarus & Folkman, 2020). Lazarus and Folkman (2020) described coping as the continual evolving mindfulness and attitudinal attempts in controlling particular external or internal stress factors which are considered to be burdensome. Coping is defined as the knowledgeable or effective process that operates as the steady evaluation and re-evaluation of a person's surrounding or circumstances (Goldman & Bell, 2022). Lazarus and Folkman (2020) discussed the actual factors that affect students' coping capabilities, which are identified as coping assets, and are often referred to as defensive factors. Defensive factors comprise social skills, problem-solving abilities, good faith, wellness and vitality, (Goldman & Bell, 2022; Lazarus & Folkman, 2020). The risk factors entail the impact of cultural and traditional standards and norms of feelings, attitudes and environmental limitations, for example assets and the intensity of the stress (Goldman & Bell, 2022; Lazarus & Folkman, 2020).

The approaches students use to respond to stress or stressors are often referred to as coping mechanisms or techniques (Lazarus & Folkman, 2020). Coping mechanisms were traditionally explained by relating ideas and attitudes associated with coping in similar individuals directed towards coping with the stress (Wright, 2020). Literature categorises coping mechanisms as follows: emotion-based coping mechanisms and problem-based coping mechanisms (Lazarus & Folkman, 2020). Emotion-based coping mechanisms normally do not include mitigating spiritual distress or re-examining an experience which led to spiritual or psychological stress (Lazarus & Folkman, 2020). Students might take part in emotion-based coping mechanisms like attempting to view the best in a negative situation (Goldman & Bell, 2022). In addition, the objective of emotion-based coping mechanism is to assist students in remaining confident and buoyant prior to or when experiencing negative stressors or stress (Goldman & Bell, 2022).

In contrast, problem-based coping mechanisms are the preferred mechanisms, as an alternative to psychological circumvention. In addition, problem-based coping mechanisms are regarded as ideal coping strategies in terms of which students may engage in certain exercises to address the problem, negative habits, stress or stressors (Goldman & Bell, 2022). Problem-based coping mechanisms are often utilised when students perceive themselves to be mentally unwell (American Psychological Association, 2020); Goldman & Bell, 2022). Coping is multifaceted and includes several different mechanisms or strategies with some being more efficient than others (Kwaah & Essilfie, 2017). Thus, students often tend to have poor coping mechanisms and differences in disposition which may lead to additional stress in particular students, causing a negative stereotyped attitude, a decline in academic achievement, and psychoneurotic signs and symptoms (Akoro, 2018).

## UNDERSTANDING MALADAPTIVE COPING MECHANISMS

Examples of maladaptive coping strategies include avoidance behaviours like drinking, emotional numbing, gambling, and social withdrawal. Emotional masking, negative judgments, overcompensation, and relying on the same approach over and over to similar situations are also forms of maladaptive coping. According to Goldman and Bell (2022), students in colleges and universities are most likely to participate in maladaptive coping mechanisms. Consequently, students who are lonely or leading a single lifestyle often tend to utilise avoidance mechanisms as well a social support mechanism remarkably smaller than students living with family members (Alkhawaldeh et al., 2023). Additionally, the incidence of heavy drinking and drinking habits at universities and colleges have been a significant concern recently (Levin, 2021). Heavy drinking is described as the excessive intake of alcohol (more than five drinks) by both men and women in no more than two (2) hours for sedentary people, which could trigger a blood alcohol level of 0.08 (National Institute on Alcohol Abuse and Alcoholism, 2020). Despite the detrimental health impacts which often result from heavy drinking, higher education students still persist in participating in excessive drug and alcohol use (Levin, 2021). Alcohol and drugs are taken by approximately 50% of university and college students, and roughly 80% of those particular students drink alcohol (Galbicsek, 2020).

Moreover, Norman and Ford (2018) found that increased awareness of educational stress leads to students seemingly becoming involved in heavy drinking and drug abuse as a stress coping technique or mechanism. Heavy drinking on the part of higher education students in dealing with distress is a major worry. Consuming drugs and alcohol offer only a temporary relief from stress emotions; however, most students utilise drugs and alcohols as a coping technique (Chen & Feeley, 2016). Nevertheless, higher academic students appear to be relieving their distress through heavy drinking, and are literally putting themselves their health and wellbeing at risk (Levin, 2021). Additionally, the National Institute on Alcohol Abuse and Alcoholism (2020) revealed that educational issues are linked to heavy drinking, with approximately one quarter of higher education students missing lectures, performing negatively in assessments, tasks and assignment, collapsing in lectures and getting substandard marks, thus leading to enhanced degrees of stress which students were attempting to circumvent in the first place.

Physical fitness is a wider notion which entails recreation and physical exercise as part of day surviving, professionals, spare time for travelling in order to relax (Stults-Kolehmainen et al. 2022). Hence, the US Department of Health and Human Services (2018) recommends approximately 150 to 300 minutes of average intensity, or 75 to 150 minutes of high intensity cardio-respiratory exercises per week. However, this advice was only successfully achieved by 45.6% of university or college students (American College Health Association, 2019). Notwithstanding, evidence suggests that physical exercise has a favourable effect on stress, thus being an effective coping technique for stress. There thus appears to be a significant correlation between stress and physical exercise, increasing psychological wellness and stress coping ability (Stults-Kolehmainen & Sinha, 2022).

Despite the good wellness results involved in physical fitness, there is still an inverted relationship between physical exercise and stress (Stults-Kolehmainen et al. 2022). Consequently, greater amounts of stress are interrelated with minimal involvement in physical exercise and vice versa (Levin, 2021). Oswalt and Riddock (2017) indicate that mentees who described themselves as depressed stated that they did not train repeatedly and viewed themselves as only slightly healthy. In addition, the negative impact stress has on physical fitness could offer awareness and the reason for less than 50% of mentees exercising as suggested (Levin, 2021).

Moreover, sleep plays a very significant part in daily operations and task execution (Levin, 2021). Despite the fact that students need approximately eight hours of bed rest every night, university and college students reported average bed rest of only seven hours every night (Kloss et al., 2016). Therefore, given students' sleeping patterns, higher education institutions face numerous noticeable insomnias among college students which put them at risk factor of insomnia as well almost worldwide (Atteraya., 2020). Similarly, stress and sleep issues are crucial aspects impeding the academic accomplishments of tutees (American College Health Association, 2019). As a result, this precipitates the development of stress emotions, which is a huge driver to inadequate sleep routines among students (Sakhelashvili et al., 2023). Bologna (2019) reported that lack of sleep and distress or stress are directly linked, therefore the emotions often lead to students encountering sleeping difficulties; in turn, insomnia increases the degree of nervousness and distressed emotions.

Nonetheless, Wulandari, (2021) reported a relationship between educational inspiration, grade point average and insomnia. Insomnia could be caused by different kinds of academic stress or stressors, such as lesson plans, educational prerequisites, due dates, lack of finances, and examinations (Wulandari, 2021). Accordingly, students sometimes perceive themselves as unready and constantly stressed out or panicking and all of a sudden start to apply the all-nighter to replace the wasted time (Levin, 2021). The all-nighter is described as a night during which an individual study a particular subject instead of sleeping resting, for example the all-nighter (Merriam-Webster, 2020, All-nighter section). Hence, studying excessive quantities of data within a short duration could negatively influence the academic achievements of such students, causing immediate memory to fade prior to examinations (Earnest, 2016). Additionally, focusing and problem analysis, including logical thinking or reasoning abilities, are often damaged by insomnia, and students may encounter problems with concentration and the comprehension of the given academic work (Earnest, 2016). Wherefore, staying awake all night long, with the intention of studying and finishing the rest of the work, could significantly increase the magnitude of distress that students in higher education institutions might encounter (Levin, 2021).

Henceforth, higher education institution students' involvement in the abuse of prescription drugs, particularly in times of greater academic overload or distress in meeting academic requirements is an increasing concern in universities and colleges worldwide (Norman & Ford, 2019). Juergens (2020) concluded that even though the prescription stimulants are aimed at overcoming the impact of short attention span or hyper activeness, certain stimulants like Adderall, Concerta, Vyvanse, Dexedrine and Ritalin are misused by students to increase their attention span and focus.

Norman and Ford (2019) have shown that college and university students who have a lower grade point average (GPA) have an enhanced likeliness to participate in prescription drugs abuse, and roughly 10 to 35% of students abused prescription drugs in order to perform better academically. Furthermore, students at graduate colleges and universities are conceivably more at risk of misusing prescription drugs than fellow students who intend to form part of the postgraduate workforce (Norman & Ford, 2019). Moreover, exacting graduate academic demands might affect students' engagement in prescription drug abuse and therefore the stress to accomplish academic success rises in the half-semester and the last exam weeks increasing stress levels (Norman & Ford, 2019) and eventually increasing the probability of students partaking in prescription drug abuse (Norman & Ford, 2019).

Academic honesty is the utilisation, creation, and transmission of data in a moral, truthful and accountable fashion (Brown et al., 2019, p. 4). Academic honesty is endorsed as a leading proposition in higher educational institutions (universities and colleges); however, academic fraud is common undermining the foundations of almost all the higher educational institutions (Levin, 2021). Muhammad Asyraf Haziq Rossliet al. (2021) showed that the incidence of academic cheating or fraud in higher education institutions has been an issue of great concern.

## Stages of Stress or Stressors Coping Process

According to Wickrama et al., (2016), in situations where coping efforts are unsuccessful, the consequences are personalised emotions of anxiety, and simultaneous physical signs and symptoms of stress. These physiological signs and symptoms happen as a result of the stimulation of neurotransmitters (Wickrama et al., 2016). Wickrama et al. (2016), expressed the physiological feedback to stress in the conception known as the General Adaptation Syndrome (GAS), which entails the three subsequent stages described below:

### Stage 1: The Alarm Response Stage

In this stage, the human body reacts to stressors with the defence reactions activated by the hormones from the adrenal cortex (Wickrama et al. 2016). For instance, if one encounters danger the body's biological response entails an endurance state. This stage is therefore distinguished by a fight or flight reaction, a physical process which alerts the human body as to when and how to respond when encountering a dangerous situation (Wickrama et al. 2016). As a result, this results in a firm and persistent biological stress reaction. And, when the stressors are not eradicated, then automatically the human body progresses into the succeeding second stage.

### Stage 2: The Resistance/Rebelliousness Stage

In this stage, the individual's body resists the stressors till the stressors disappear (Wickrama et al. 2016). When the first threat appears, the parasympathetic nervous system decreases the stress reaction. The adrenal cortex also causes blood pressure to fall and the heart rate to regulate (Wickrama et al. 2016). Despite the body being in the recovery stage, it stays aware until the stressor is no longer a problem. However, when it is long-term stressors such as stressful work or a toxic relationship, then the body automatically stays in a greater attentive state and the hormones of stress rise. Consequently, when the stressors do not fade, the human body attempts to make changes to handle the stressors, leading to insomnia, inattentiveness and moodiness, which then drives an individual's body to the following third stage.

### Stage 3: The Exhaustion/Weariness Stage

In this stage, the influences of unceasing stressors which lead to a person's body capability to be unsuccessful in completing the stress cycles resulting in repetitive stress reactions (Wickrama et al. 2016). Eventually, the lack of support and therapeutic treatment or intervention leads to long-term or chronic stress and could cause chronic wellness problems such as nervousness, tiredness, distress, abdominal pain, mental exhaustion and sudden death (Wickrama et al. 2016).

## A BIOPSYCHOSOCIAL HEALTH MODEL

In this book chapter a Biopsychosocial Health Model will be used to show the interface between the biological, psychological and social factors that are involved in mental illness. The biopsychosocial health model methodically describes the complex cooperation of the three prime parts; namely, the biological, psychological and social factors involved in the evolution of mental illness. This theory is important in backing up the review of the related literature, and in the discussion of the following: The three stages of stress or the stress-coping process, the three major realms of psychological functioning that are affected by stress, and effective coping mechanisms for stressors among students in higher education institutions. Last but not least, the personal or self-management strategies that promote psychological adjustment with be discussed, and the chapter will conclude by making recommendations based on the discussion. The Biopsychosocial Health Model (Fig. 1) comprises the various biological, psychological and social factors that contribute to mental health/illness among students in higher education institutions.

*Figure 1. The Biopsychosocial Health Model of the factors associated with mental health*
*(Murray et al. 2022)*

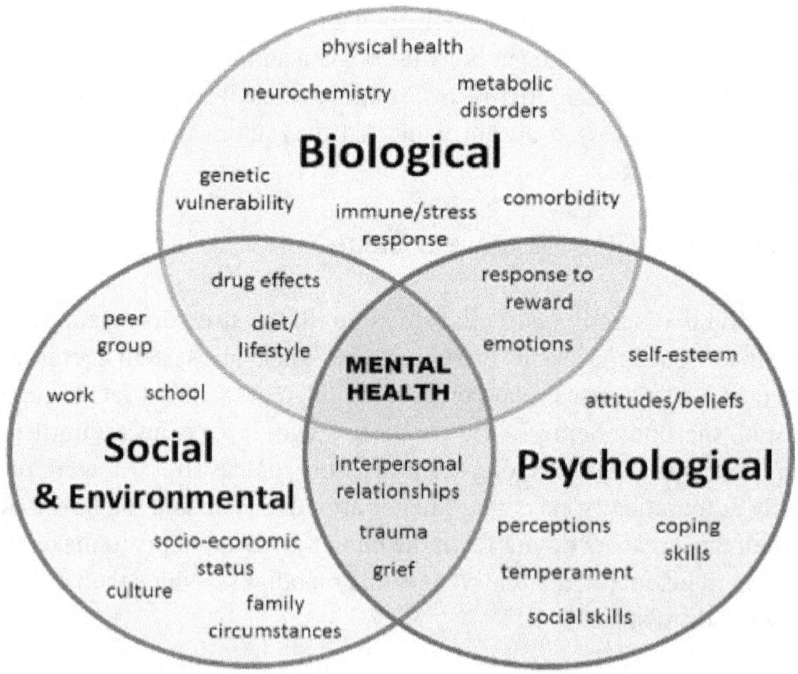


### Types of Coping Mechanisms

#### Adaptive Coping Mechanisms

Adaptive coping mechanisms are positive, supportive, and life-enhancing stress management tools. These actions bring joy and comfort to your life while reducing stressful emotions, leaving you feeling more balanced and at ease.

Those with adaptive coping mechanisms tend to have positive outlooks, and dealing with challenges head-on builds self-confidence and self-esteem. Instead of avoiding their problems, they acknowledge the presenting issues and move forward with a solution in mind. These individuals can experience stress-related growth, meaning their stressors help improve emotional regulation and mitigate negative self-talk.1

Adaptive coping mechanisms examples include:

- Practicing yoga
- Seeking support
- Using relaxation techniques
- Problem-solving
- Using humor
- Physical activities
- Being creative

## Maladaptive Coping Mechanisms

Maladaptive coping mechanisms are harmful and can worsen stress and difficult emotions. These techniques are counterproductive because, while they may appear helpful, individuals often experience more problems than benefits.

Individuals with histories of anxiety, depression, and other mental health concerns may lean toward these coping styles because their symptoms can cloud thinking, feeling, and decision-making. They may lack emotional self-regulation skills central to healthy coping and understanding how to manage problems in life.2

Examples of maladaptive coping mechanisms include:

- Substance use
- Gambling
- Impulsivity
- Self-harm
- Emotional numbing
- Withdrawing from others
- Rationalizing bad behavior
- Escaping or distracting from the problem
- Overindulging (i.e., overeating, overspending, etc.)

## Emotion-Based Coping

Emotion-based coping strategies reduce reactive emotions to a stressor rather than the stressor itself. These skills help individuals manage their feelings and responses before tackling the problem. Emotion-based coping offers space to process their emotions, often through techniques like talk therapy, narrative therapy, or art therapy.

Examples of emotion-focused coping strategies include:

- **Journaling:** Writing thoughts, feelings, and emotions down can help people address stress without judgment. They can pour their emotions onto a blank page and unload their fear, anxiety, or depression. Journaling allows individuals to record their reactions, reflect, and find opportunities for emotional growth.
- **Yoga:** Yoga allows individuals to express emotions through their bodies and find balance. Processing emotions becomes easier when individuals focus on maintaining emotional equilibrium.
- **Meditation:** Meditation involves focusing attention and achieving a state of deep relaxation, often through techniques like guided imagery or mantra repetition.
- **Deep breathing:** Breathwork is a simple yet effective coping mechanism that involves taking slow, deep breaths to activate a relaxation response, reduce stress, and promote a sense of calm.
- **Mindfulness:** Mindfulness means cultivating self-awareness and being fully present in the moment without judgment. These skills can help individuals reduce stress and improve overall well-being.

## Problem-Based Coping

Problem-based coping strategies involve directly facing, addressing, and reducing an issue. Individuals can feel empowered by these tools because they take a problem and apply solutions. They gain a sense of control, productivity, and self-confidence.

Examples of problem-focused coping mechanisms include:

- **Researching the topic:** Researching and gathering data can be educational and empowering. Doing so gives structure and a timeline to follow when tackling a problem.
- **Creating a to-do list:** Creating a to-do list can place additional foundation blocks an individual needs to resolve their problem. Items on the to-do list are generally clear, leaving little room for gray areas and distraction.
- **Asking for support:** Seeking support from trusted individuals, friends, family, or professionals offers opportunities to share your struggles and gain guidance, comfort, or advice during challenging times.
- **Changing the situation:** Actively modifying your circumstances is another problem-focused approach to relieving stress or adversity. Doing so may involve planning to leave, setting boundaries, or implementing strategies to address the root cause.
- **Prioritizing:** Prioritizing means organizing tasks or responsibilities according to importance. This approach helps you effectively manage your time and resources, reducing overwhelm and promoting a sense of control.

## Social Coping

Social coping involves seeking assistance and support from others to manage stress and adversity. This coping mechanism can take various forms, like talking to a trusted friend or family member, participating in a support group, or seeking professional help.

Social coping can provide emotional and instrumental guidance, a sense of belonging, and opportunities for learning and growth. Individuals can also broaden their perspectives and gain new insights into their experiences, leading to improved resilience and overall well-being.

### Avoidance Coping

Avoidance coping is a behavioral mechanism aimed at avoiding or suppressing sources of stress rather than addressing them. Avoidance coping can take many forms, including denial, substance abuse, procrastination, or distraction.

Avoidance coping can provide temporary relief but exacerbate stress, leading to adverse physical and mental health outcomes. Individuals relying on avoidance coping may find themselves experiencing chronic anxiety, guilt, or low self-esteem.

## Effective Coping Mechanisms for Stressors experienced by Students in Higher Education Institutions

- Thoughts: Negative feelings, beliefs or contemplation could be persistent and deafening, so teach yourself how to disrupt the stressors, and never attempt to shut them off; however, never allow the stressors to take control of you.
- Do one job at a time; For instance, when walking or spending time with close relatives or friends you could switch off your cell phone in order to fully interact with the loved ones.
- Establish your own objectives; objectives do not have to be forceful. However, call your relatives instead of waiting for the mobile phone to ring. Ensure that for any objectives that you plan, accomplishing them will enhance self-esteem and a feeling of fulfilment.
- Maintain a journal; revealing yourself regarding the encountering of difficult days could assist one to have clues as to how to relieve pressure and even increase the body's defence against illness.
- Always share a smile; often times, life becomes humourless, therefore when you sense anything which makes you laugh or smile, share it with your relatives, friends and loved ones.
- Sacrifice; sacrificing is known as a win-to-win exercise, as assisting other people makes one feel loved and pleased with themselves.
- Look after your health; have a well balance diet, watch films, talk to your relatives or friends that it has been a while without speaking to one another since childhood, settle down on park or beach benches and inhale the scents of the beautiful flowers including the refreshing ocean view.

## Personal or Self-Management Strategies That Promote Psychological Adjustments

- Exercise: consistent physical exercise improves emotional wellness and could minimise unhappiness and anxiety.
- Practising daily lives; shutting your eyes, imagining yourself in another place and taking slow deep breaths could be extremely helpful in preventing emotional suppression.
- Having a hobby; choosing and enjoying a hobby leads to a well-balanced lifestyle permitting one to enjoy doing what one loves, consequently, eliminating the excessive tension of daily stressors and retaining the activeness of the mind.

- Think properly about your own psychological wellness and evaluate your psychological well-being consistently.
- Think about the particular needs or stressors or distress that you are experiencing and how the stressors are influencing you.
- Allow yourself to take a break from your doubts and worries.
- Sacrifice part of each day for the well-being of brain health, as well as to become energised and confidence.

## Future Steps for Overcoming Stress or Stressors Experienced for Students in Higher Education Institutions

### Step 1: Do not Get Too Concerned About Things That You Do Not Have Power Over

It is important to know your own personal boundaries, learn to welcome life as it is, and attempt searching for good techniques regarding every stressor or issue you encounter.

### Step 2: Talk About Your Stressors or Concerns

Plainly stating or sharing what your stressors or issues are, could aid one in overcoming them all by finding appropriate solutions; however, storing up the stressors might actually worsen the situation. As an individual, you need to talk about your emotions to your friends and family members, or they could be communicated to the responsible counsellors of the academic organisation who habitually deal with common stress issues among students.

### Step 3: Search for More Information Regarding Your Stressors or Issues

There might be prescribed sources available to address the particular stress issue. Significantly there are websites where one is able to read about or watch videos on solutions to stressors or problems.

### Step 3: Set or Establish Priorities

When you feel depressed or stressed out due to excessive responsibilities at hand, then normalise these by preparing a scheduled to-do list, and properly organize it with considerations of the significance and need.

### Step 4: Arrange Items Based on Outlook

Examine your surroundings and evaluate how other people are managing. Often there is somebody going through worse stressors than yours, and most people cope well, so why do you think you will not be able to do so?

### Step 5: Attempt to Ignore Your Stressors

Certain stressors or worries naturally fade with time, as memories of situations fade. Hence, the stressors that would have happened yesterday might fade by tomorrow morning. Also spend time doing the things you love, ensure you have enough sleep and observe how you wake up feeling the next morning. Moreover, write down all your stressors in a diary. This will reassure you that you are dealing with them after finishing examinations and other tasks.

## FUTURE RESEARCH DIRECTIONS

Most studies on this subject matter have focused on the causes, signs and symptoms of stress and their impact. There is a limited- research evidence on the adoption of effective techniques for mitigating stress or stressors within higher education institutions. Therefore, there is still a significant need to explore efficient techniques to properly alleviate and prevent stressors or high stress levels among students in higher education institutions worldwide.

## SOLUTIONS AND RECOMMENDATIONS

Students battling with stress require the full support of their relatives, friends, and co-students including ordinary people to allow them to cope effectively. Moreover, students need to clearly comprehend the reality regarding the physical health and the route of stress or stressors in order to search for appropriate effective strategies. Students battling with stress or stressors should be encouraged to open up and speak out about their stress or stressors. Data regarding stress or stressors needs to be available for access by students battling with stress or stressors globally in colleges and universities. Such data should be in line with students' comprehensive capacity in order to enhance their knowledge of the stress or stressors. Students are also advised to disengage from all the things that are triggering frustration, concern or anxiety, and to learn to ignore the things that they have no control over. In most instances, college and university student counsellors or committees responsible for helping students who suffer from stress seem not to be actively involved in searching for students who may be presenting with the obvious signs/symptoms of stress, thereby leaving students in lonely and basically becoming more indecisive about opening up about the problems they are encountering. Hence, student counsellors or committees at higher education institutions should regularly and actively search for students who may be experiencing stress, rather than waiting for such students to open up to them themselves about their personal difficulties/stressors.

## CONCLUSION

Mental health problems can affect many areas of students' lives, reducing their quality of life, academic achievement, physical health, and satisfaction with the college experience, and negatively impacting relationships with friends and family members. These issues can also have long-term consequences for students, affecting their future employment, earning potential and overall health. Stressors encountered by students are mainly due to academic-related overload, educational migration (going to higher education institutions such as universities or colleges), financial burden, lack of holistic support from friends, families and lack of regular active institutional support of students across global colleges and universities. Thus, student counsellors or committees in the higher educational institutions should constantly and actively aid their academics to best mitigate or cope stress or stressors. Higher education institutions can use the content of this chapter to develop appropriate targeted coping mechanisms and strategies which can be used by student counsellors to alleviate stressors among students thereby assisting in the enhancement of holistical health and wellness, and the academic excellence of students worldwide.

## REFERENCES

Akinci, Z., Yurcu, G., & Ekin, Y. (2018). Relationships between student personality traits, mobbing, and depression within the context of sustainable tourism education: The case of a faculty of tourism. [Al]. *Sustainability (Basel)*, *10*(10), 3418. doi:10.3390u10103418

Alkhawaldeh, A., Al Omari, O., Al Aldawi, S., Al Hashmi, I., Ann Ballad, C., Ibrahim, A., Al Sabei, S., Alsaraireh, A., Al Qadire, M., & ALBashtawy, M. (2023). Stress Factors, Stress Levels, and Coping Mechanisms among University Students. *TheScientificWorldJournal*, *2023*, 2023. doi:10.1155/2023/2026971 PMID:37426577

Amanvermez, Y., Rahmadiana, M., Karyotaki, E., de Wit, L., Ebert, D. D., Kessler, R. C., & Cuijpers, P. (2020). Stress management interventions for college students: A systematic review and meta-analysis. *Clinical Psychology: Science and Practice*. https://psycnet.apa.org/doi/10.1111/cpsp.12342

American College Health Association. (2019). Academic impacts. *American College Health Association*. https://www.acha.org/documents/ncha/NCHAII_SPRING_2019_US_REFERENCE_GROUP_EXECUTIVE_SUMMARY.pdf

American Psychological Association. (2020a). *Coping strategy*. American Psychological Association. https://dictionary.apa.org/coping-strategy

American Psychological Association. (2020b). *Stress*. American Psychological Association. https://dictionary.apa.org/stress

Ashipala, D. O., Albanus, F. S., & Nghole, T. M. (2023). Overview and management of burnout among academics. In A. ul Haque (Ed.), Handbook of research on dissecting and dismantling occupational stress in modern organizations (pp. 200-215). IGI Global. doi:10.4018/978-1-6684-6543-1.ch015

Ashipala, D. O., & Shilunga, A. P. (2023). Overview and management of anxiety. In S. G. Taukeni (Ed.), *Acceleration of the biopsychosocial model in public health* (pp. 194–210). IGI Global.

AtterayaM. S. (2020). Acculturation stressors and academic adjustment among Nepalese students in South Korean higher education institutions. doi:10.1101/2020.12.07.414441

Battashi, N., Al Omari, O., Sawalha, M., Al Maktoumi, S., Alsuleitini, A., & Al Qadire, M. (2021). The relationship between smartphone use, insomnia, stress, and anxiety among university students: A cross-sectional study. *Clinical Nursing Research*, *30*(6), 734–740. doi:10.1177/1054773820983161 PMID:33375850

Bhargava, D., & Trivedi, H. (2018). A study of causes of stress and stress management among youth. *IRA-International Journal of Management & Social Sciences, 11*(03), 108–117. doi:10.21013/jmss.v11.n3.p1

Biggs, A., Brough, P., & Drummond, S. (2017). Lazarus and Folkman's psychological stress and coping theory. In C. Cooper & J. C. Quick (Eds.), *The handbook of stress and health: A guide to research and practice* (pp. 349–364). Wiley. doi:10.1002/9781118993811.ch21

Bologna, C. (2019). The scary ways an all-nighter messes with your body and brain. *HuffPost.* https://www.huffpost.com/entry/what-happens-when-you-pull-an-allnighter_l_5dd5b559e4b010f3f1d21d30

Bondarchuk, O., Balakhtar, V., Pinchuk, N., Pustovalov, I., & Pavlenok, K. (2023). Adaptation of coping strategies to reduce the impact of stress and Lonelines on the psychological well-being of adults. *Journal of Law and Sustainable Development, 11*(10), e1852. doi:10.55908dgs.v11i10.1852

Brown, T., Bourke-Taylor, H., Isbel, S., Gustafsson, L., McKinstry, C., Logan, A., & Etherington, J. (2019). Establishing similarities and differences among the self-reported academic integrity of Australian occupational therapy undergraduate and graduate-entry Master's students. *The Open Journal of Occupational Therapy, 7*(3), 1–16. doi:10.15453/2168-6408.1558

Butler, F. C., & Martin, J. A. (2020). Research in Occupational Stress and Well Being: Vol. 123-146. Struggling to survive: Non-family member employees, the family, and stress in family firm startups. Emerald. doi:10.1108/S1479-355520200000018006

Chang, K. H., Lu, F. J., Chyi, T., Hsu, Y. W., Chan, S. W., & Wang, E. T. (2017). Examining the stress-burnout relationship: The mediating role of negative thoughts. *PeerJ, 5*, e4181. doi:10.7717/peerj.4181 PMID:29302397

Cleveland Clinic. (2020, September 10). *Stressors: Coping Skills and Strategies.* Cleveland Clinic. https://my.clevelandclinic.org/health/articles/6392-stress-coping-with-lifes-stressors

Compas, B. E., Vreeland, A., & Henry, L. (2019). Coping models of stress and resilience. The Oxford Handbook of Stress and Mental Health, 584-600. Oxford Press. doi:10.1093/oxfordhb/9780190681777.013.27

Crego, A., Carrillo-Diaz, M., Armfield, J. M., & Romero, M. (2016). Stress and academic performance in dental students: The role of coping strategies and examination-related self-efficacy. *Journal of Dental Education, 80*(2), 165–172. doi:10.1002/j.0022-0337.2016.80.2.tb06072.x PMID:26834134

Earnest, D. (2016). Studying: Is it bad for your health to pull an all-nighter? *Texas A&M.* https://www.sciencedaily.com/releases/2016/09/160919162837.htm epidemic.html

Galbicsek, C. (2020). College alcoholism. *Alcohol Rehab Guide.* https://www.alcoholrehabguide.org/resources/collegealcoholabuse/#:~:text=Roughly%20 80%20percent%20of%20college, alcohol%20 in%20too%20little%20time.

Gao, W., Ping, S., & Liu, X. (2020). Gender differences in depression, anxiety, and stress among college students: A longitudinal study from China. *Journal of Affective Disorders, 263*, 292–300. doi:10.1016/j.jad.2019.11.121 PMID:31818792

Go, M. (2016). The effects of entrance examination stress on suicide ideation among college entrance examinees - Moderating effect of social support. *Health & Welfare, 18*, 55. doi:10.23948/kshw.2016.12.18.55

Goldman, J. A., & Bell, S. C. B. (2022). Student and faculty coping and impacts on academic success in response to COVID-19. *Journal of Interdisciplinary Studies in Education, 11*(1), 74–91.

Good Therapy. (2018, September 26). Coping Mechanisms. *Good Therapy.* https://www.goodtherapy.org/blog/psychpedia/coping-mechanisms

Gustems-Carnicer, J., Calderón, C., & Calderón-Garrido, D. (2019). Stress, coping strategies and academic achievement in teacher education students. *European Journal of Teacher Education, 42*(3), 375–390. doi:10.1080/02619768.2019.1576629

Juergens, J. (2020). *Prescription study aid abuse.* Addiction Center. https://www.addictioncenter.com/college/prescription-study-aid-abuse/

Karugahe, W., & Lambert, J. (2021). Gender, role in domestic violence as victim or perpetrator and coping strategies in Uganda: Implications for gender-inclusive counsellors. *Asia Pacific Journal of Counselling and Psychotherapy, 12*(1), 58–72. doi:10.1080/21507686.2021.1876113

Kloss, J. D., Nash, C. O., Walsh, C. M., Culnan, E., Horsey, S., & Sexton-Radek, K. (2016). A "Sleep 101" program for college students improves sleep hygiene knowledge and reduces maladaptive beliefs about sleep. *Behavioral Medicine (Washington, D.C.), 42*(1), 48–56. doi:10.1080/08964289.2014.969186 PMID:25268924

Kwaah, C. Y., & Essilfie, G. (2017). Stress and coping strategies among distance education students at the University of Cape Coast, Ghana. *Turkish Online Journal of Distance Education, 18*(3), 120–134. doi:10.17718/tojde.328942

Levin, D. J. (2021). *Academic stressors, perceived stress, and coping strategies among undergraduate students* [Senior Honours Projects, James Madison University]. https://commons.lib.jmu.edu/honors202029/128

Madsen, T. (2020). Between frustration and education: Transitioning students' stress and coping through the lens of semiotic cultural psychology. *Theory & Psychology, 31*(1), 61–83. doi:10.1177/0959354320944496

Makarowski, R., Piotrowski, A., Predoiu, R., Görner, K., Predoiu, A., Mitrache, G., & Nikkhah-Farkhani, Z. (2020). Stress and coping during the COVID-19 pandemic among martial arts athletes: A cross-cultural study. *Archives of Budo, 16*, 161–171.

Merriam-Webster. (2020). All-nighter. *Merriam-Webster.* https://www.merriamwebster.com/dictionary/all-nighter

Muhammad Asyraf Haziq Rossli, K. M. (2021). Determinants of academic fraud in higher education institutions: A fraud triangle perspective. *Psychology (Savannah, Ga.), 58*(2), 3879–3892. doi:10.17762/pae.v58i2.2653

Murray, J., & DeBerard, S. (2022). *Biopsychosocial model and health.* Biopsychosocial Model and Health., doi:10.4324/9780367198459-REPRW63-1

National Institute on Alcohol Abuse and Alcoholism (NIH). (2020). College Drinking. *National Institute on Alcohol Abuse and Alcoholism.* https://www.niaaa.nih.gov/publications/brochures-and-fact-sheets/college-drinking

Niu, X., & Snyder, H. R. (2022). The role of maladaptive emotion regulation in the bidirectional relation between sleep and depression in college students during the COVID-19 pandemic. *Anxiety, Stress, and Coping*, *36*(1), 83–96. doi:10.1080/10615806.2022.2073441 PMID:35536737

Norman, L., & Ford, J. (2018). Undergraduate prescription stimulant misuse: The impact of academic strain. *Substance Use & Misuse*, *53*(9), 1482–1491. doi:10.1080/10826084.2017.1413393 PMID:29313737

Norman, L. B., & Ford, J. A. (2019). Undergraduate prescription stimulant misuse and academic strain: The role of college major and graduate school plans. *Journal of Drug Issues*, *49*(4), 756–771. doi:10.1177/0022042619870504

Norman, L. B., & Ford, J. A. (2019). Undergraduate prescription stimulant misuse and academic strain: The role of college major and graduate school plans. *Journal of Drug Issues*, *49*(4), 756–771. doi:10.1177/0022042619870504

Rettew, D. C., McGinnis, E. W., Copeland, W., Nardone, H. Y., Bai, Y., Rettew, J., Devadenam, V., & Hudziak, J. J. (2021). Personality trait predictors of adjustment during the COVID pandemic among college students. *PLoS One*, *16*(3), e0248895. doi:10.1371/journal.pone.0248895 PMID:33730075

Rosario, M. G. L. D. (2023). Stress and coping strategies and academic performance of teacher education students. *Journal for Educators, Teachers and Trainers, 14*(3). https://jett.labosfor.com/

Sakhelashvili, I., & Spruyt, K. (2023). The interaction between stress and sleep disorders among foreign medical students in Georgia. *Sleep Medicine*, *110*, 225–230. doi:10.1016/j.sleep.2023.08.021 PMID:37647713

SantiagoP. H.SoaresG. H.SmithersL. G.RobertsR.JamiesonL. (2022). Psychological network of stress, coping and social support in an Aboriginal population. https://doi.org/ doi:10.31234/osf.io/cz59w

Scott, B., Modna, Y., Khashchuk, D., & Duke, J. (2019). The Interrelationship between perceived stress level, sleep quality, and academic performance among students of a Caribbean Medical School. *Anatomy Physiology & Biochemistry International Journal*, *6*(1), 555676.

Shatimwene, G. P., Ashipala, D. O., & Kamenye, E. (2020). Experiences of student nurses on the use of the two-week block system at the satellite campus of a higher education institution in Namibia. *International Journal of Higher Education*, *9*(3), 222–231. doi:10.5430/ijhe.v9n3p222

Stults-Kolehmainen, M., Gilson, T., SantaBarbara, N., McKee, P., Sinha, R., Bartholomew, J., Boullosa, D., Budnick, C., Bueno, F. A., Haughton, A., Barker, J., & Ash, G. (2022). Qualitative and quantitative evidence of motivation states for physical activity, exercise and being sedentary from university student focus groups. *SportRxiv*. doi:10.51224/SRXIV.189

Sutton, A. (2020). Living the good life: A meta-analysis of authenticity, well-being and engagement. *Personality and Individual Differences*, *153*, 109645. doi:10.1016/j.paid.2019.109645

*Tremendously, adv*. (2023). Oxford English Dictionary. doi:10.1093/OED/4986167386

US Department of Health and Human Services. (2018). *President's council on sports, fitness & nutrition*. US DoHHS.

Wickrama, T., Wickrama, K., Banford, A., & Lambert, J. (2016). PTSD symptoms among tsunami exposed mothers in Sri Lanka: The role of disaster exposure, culturally specific coping strategies, and recovery efforts. *Anxiety, Stress, and Coping*, *30*(4), 415–427. doi:10.1080/10615806.2016.1271121 PMID:27960534

Wright, R. R. (2020). Directed coping: A key to coping effectively? *Stress and Health*, *37*(3), 466–475. doi:10.1002mi.3009 PMID:33220167

WulandariP. H. (2021). Nothing good happens after midnight: The relationship between circadian disruption due to insomnia and lack of sleep to increased risk of cardiovascular diseases. doi:10.22541/au.161360164.47679831/v1

## ADDITIONAL READING

McLean, L., Gaul, D., & Penco, R. (2022). Perceived social support and stress: A study of 1st year students in Ireland. *International Journal of Mental Health and Addiction*, 1–21. 10.1007%2Fs11469-021-00710-z PMID:35103049

Rettew, D. C., McGinnis, E. W., Copeland, W., Nardone, H. Y., Bai, Y., Rettew, J., Devadenam, V., & Hudziak, J. J. (2021). Personality trait predictors of adjustment during the COVID pandemic among college students. *PLoS One*, *16*(3), e0248895. doi:10.1371/journal.pone.0248895 PMID:33730075

## KEY TERMS AND DEFINITIONS

**Coping Mechanisms:** Are habitually described as the methods or manners in which an individual customary reacts to stress, through the interrelations of ideas or emotions, and attitudes linked to coping similar individuals over time and in-between various situations (Biggs et al., 2017).

**Maladaptive Coping Mechanisms:** Refers to inefficient coping methods or techniques which can be unsuccessful or can sustain inadvertent negative outcomes (Good Therapy, 2018). For instance, in this book chapter, maladaptive coping mechanisms entail attitudes to alcohol, the usage of unprescribed medications or stimulants, lack of physical exercise and academic theft.

**Stress:** Is referred to as the physical or emotional reaction to internal or external stressors that entail innovations influencing almost each systematic aspect of the human body, affecting individuals' emotions and attitudes (American Psychological Association, 2020).

**Stressors:** This referred to environment stimulus that tremendously causes stress (Oxford English Dictionary, 2023).

# Chapter 4
# The Wellbeing Van:
## A Strength-Based Model for Student Engagement and Promoting Student Wellbeing

**Rithu Paul**
https://orcid.org/0000-0002-6193-8356
*Jyoti Nivas Pre-University College, India*

**Aneesh Kumar**
https://orcid.org/0000-0003-1081-7201
*Christ University, India*

**Sruthi Suresh**
https://orcid.org/0000-0002-2505-9872
*Christ University, India*

## ABSTRACT

*This book chapter takes a proactive approach to address stress by introducing a preventive measure, a relatively new approach implemented on college students in Bangalore, India called the "wellbeing van." The chapter emphasizes the importance of not only managing and coping with stress, but also implementing strategies that promote overall well-being by tapping into the intrinsic factors of the student. The well-being van has shown promising results in reducing stress levels among students in academic institutions. Additionally, the chapter delves into the difficulties students face in maintaining social relationships, conforming to societal expectations, and finding their place. It provides valuable insights on how to foster healthy social dynamics and create supportive environments for students.*

DOI: 10.4018/979-8-3693-2833-0.ch004

## INTRODUCTION

Intrinsic factors play a crucial role in shaping student wellbeing, particularly in relation to stress. Factors such as coping strategies, self-efficacy, mindset, emotional intelligence, self-care practices, and perceived control significantly influence how students experience and manage stress. Effective coping strategies, a strong sense of self-efficacy, and a growth mindset contribute to students' ability to navigate stressors and maintain a positive outlook. Emotional intelligence empowers students to recognize and regulate their emotions, fostering resilience and adaptive responses to stress. Engaging in self-care practices provides students with the tools to nurture their physical and mental wellbeing, mitigating the negative impact of stress. Lastly, a sense of control over their academic tasks and responsibilities empowers students to approach stress with confidence and actively seek solutions. Recognizing and nurturing these intrinsic factors is vital for promoting student wellbeing and equipping them with the skills to effectively manage stress.

This book chapter takes a proactive approach to addressing stress by introducing a preventive measure, a relatively new approach implemented on college students in Bangalore, India called the "Wellbeing van." Drawing inspiration from the PERMA model developed by Martin Seligman, the chapter emphasizes the importance of not only managing and coping with stress but also implementing strategies that promote overall wellbeing by tapping into the intrinsic factors of the student. The wellbeing van has shown promising results in reducing stress levels among students in academic institutions. Additionally, the chapter delves into the difficulty's students face in maintaining social relationships, conforming to societal expectations, and finding their place. It provides valuable insights on how to foster healthy social dynamics and create supportive environments for students.

The positive schooling approach aims to integrate student wellbeing, virtues, and academic achievement in the learning process. With the growing importance of holistic learning experiences for students, it becomes essential for researchers and educators to explore the positive schooling approach. The current chapter identifies the key concepts that foster wellbeing and flourishing among students that paves way for students to enhance their intrinsic factors. A deeper understanding of these concepts and their relevance is obtained by examining the existing theories and literature in the field of positive schooling. The ecological systems theory by Bronfenbrenner (1977) highlights the importance of various stakeholders in this holistic learning process. The chapter provides insights into a strength-based model focusing on using character strengths as a tool to promote wellbeing and flourishing among students. The model delineates the process that enables students to shift from the state of languishing to flourishing. The model named Wellbeing Van discusses the role of students in actively promoting wellbeing and flourishing within their peer groups. The model used strategies like social media, small group discussion and campus-wide activities to help students learn, live, and embed wellbeing. The Wellbeing Van is set in the strength-based model and enables readers to explore the feasibility of such programs before implementing them in their institutions. Practical solutions for educational institutions are suggested based on this model.

Student engagement and well-being in schools and colleges have been a topic of concern for educators and adults working with young people (Boulton et al., 2019; Zepke, 2014). Effectively engaging students in academic and socioemotional learning ensure better learning outcomes and learners for a meaningful life (Wang and Hofkens, 2020; Weissberg and Cascarino, 2013). Engagement experiences within a learning environment including classroom experiences, teacher-student interaction, school climate, and peer interaction help young people to grow and flourish (Zepke and Leach, 2010). Engaging young people is not an easy task. It requires a sound understanding of the developmental needs and generational demands of adolescents and young adults. We need strong culturally competent and evidence-based models to work with young people.

The COVID-19 pandemic and associated restrictions which lead to widespread social isolation have impacted health and mental health worldwide (Brooks et al., 2020). While these restrictions have been challenging for people of all ages, they may be particularly difficult for adolescents, who at this developmental stage rely heavily on their peer connections for emotional support and social development (Ellis and Zarbatany 2017). Quarantine and social distance measures impede peer or social interaction. These measures may have a serious impact on adolescent mental health (Rapee et al., 2019). However, there is a need to examine the long-term psychological impact of the COVID-19 pandemic among adolescents through longitudinal studies as most current information is limited to retrospective and self-report measures (e.g., Hawke et al., 2020). The recovery and restoration from the pandemic need to place well-being at the forefront. Educators, academic leaders, and parents are concerned about learning losses, disengagement, and rising mental health issues among students in the post-pandemic context.

In the current chapter, we explore ways to engage youth by optimally channelizing their untapped enthusiasm and potential, which often goes unnoticed by the adults in the environment. Our ideas and values attached to traditional teaching and learning methods have contributed to our misconceptions of student engagement and learning. For instance, educators often plan class activities, content, and assessment without even understanding the learning needs. The learners who are average or below in class performance may rarely get attention from the teacher. Sometimes the focus point while working with these students would be to look at the deficits that they have rather than their strengths or potential. These learners thereby may develop poor self-concept, negative coping strategies, be disengaged, and fail to try the opportunities available. Learning is an equally or sometimes more social-emotional domain than just the cognitive aspect. Hence engagement in the learning environment begets well-being and academic outcomes.

Creating a space for engagement and connection in the classroom helps the student be part of the learning process and reduce their stress. Engaged students contribute to class discussions, which help develop self-confidence and motivation, which in turn enhances their well-being and buffers mental health risks. Creating opportunities for learners to engage in meaningful activities, helping them make positive connections with peers and adults in their environment, and fostering their strengths help them to be happier and flourish in their lives. In this chapter, we will review some existing models in practice for improving the well-being of the youth through engagement. Providing a deeper insight into adolescent behaviour and coping mechanisms. This is explored through the lens of Bronfenbrenner's ecological system theory. Some practical strategies to employ and promote flourishing among this age group are outlined at the end of the chapter. We will further discuss the proposed model of flourishing in detail in explaining sociocultural influences on the learning of the student.

Before we see how the proposed model of The Wellbeing Van is put into practice, let us lay the foundation of how it all began. In the next section, we explore the various models of youth engagement and character strengths to gain insight into resources that are required to understand flourishing.

## ENGAGING YOUTH

The group that falls under the label of late adolescents, teens, young adults, youth, or emerging adults are of target focus in the chapter. The literature considers adolescence as a time of crisis, confusion, and the most vulnerable period in an individual's development (Steinberg, & Silk, 2002). With the changes happening around them, young people face immense challenges in their lives. The current youth in our high schools, colleges, and university classrooms belong to a generation called generation Z or post-millennials different from the adults working with them. These students are born into the era of technology and change. While they are technologically advanced, entrepreneurial, and adaptive to change, they are vulnerable to many challenges like mental health risks, social engagement, and career choices (Beck, & Wright, 2019; Schwieger, & Ladwig, 2018). Communicating, teaching, and working with the current generation of youth requires more informed and planned activities. Focusing on their strengths and creating more meaningful engagement has been found to be more effective (Seemiller & Clayton, 2019).

Waters et al. (2009), observed that adolescents and young adulthood as a time of exploration and making a meaningful or informed commitment. Young people develop a better sense of self, and the crisis at this stage facilitates exploration. They invest their energy in being more independent and responsible (Arnett, 2007). If guided and mentored, youth can be agents or drivers of change. Providing such opportunities for growth enhances their well-being (Bouvet, Cosmini, Palaktsoglou, & Vanzo, 2017). Effective engagement would help them develop themselves and contribute back to the community by being effective citizens and good human beings (Cicognani et al., 2008). Hence, the role of adults in the environment would be able to provide opportunities to develop meaningful connections to develop a better sense of self (Whitlock, 2007).

## MODELS OF EFFECTIVE YOUTH ENGAGEMENT

### The Six Cs of the Positive Youth Development Framework

Positive youth development (PYD) provides a framework for professionals and adults working with young people. Researchers put forth different PYD models and their corresponding constructs, including Benson's 40 developmental assets, Catalano's 15 PYD factors, the socioemotional learning approach (CASEL, www.casel.org; see also Weissberg, Durlak, Domitrovich, & Gullotta, 2015), and the "being" approach (Shek et al., 2019). Lerner's 5Cs and 6Cs model is the most widely researched models (Heck & Subramaniam, 2009). These models proposed key attributes namely competence, confidence, connection, character, caring, and contribution that can be nurtured among adolescents.

Each of the six attributes outlined by the model focuses on an essential aspect of adolescent development. Competence refers to the adolescent's abilities in different domains, including academic, social, cognitive, and vocational. Confidence addresses the adolescent's overall self-worth and self-efficacy. Connection focuses on the adolescent's ability to develop and maintain positive relationships with their family members, peers, and the larger society. Character refers to the adolescent's awareness of and adherence to morals, values, cultural, and societal norms. Caring or compassion highlights the adolescent's ability to be sympathetic and empathetic towards others. This model states that if these 5Cs have been nurtured, adolescents are most likely to exhibit the sixth C of contribution, contributing to society through their personal development and actions (Mercier et al., 2019; Shek et al., 2019). However, most interventions and programs based on this model included only a few of these attributes instead of the complete model. Further, studies examining the sixth C, contribution, were conducted more often than any other attributes (Shek et al., 2019).

## Character Strengths

### The Values in Action (VIA) Model

As the importance of PYD grew, the need to focus and build "good character" became important. Competent and confident youth without character may not know where and when to use their abilities. Character is multidimensional and comprises positive traits. Hence, researchers Peterson and Seligman proposed the Values in Action (VIA) (2004) based on their intensive study of character strengths. Character strength is defined as "a behavioural and motivational disposition leading to excellence and flourishing"

In the VIA model, the 24 strengths are categorized under six virtues, namely Transcendence, Wisdom, Humanity, Courage, Temperance, and Justice. Transcendence relates to how individuals connect with the world around them in a meaningful way and include the strengths of appreciation of beauty and excellence, gratitude, hope, spirituality, and humour. The virtue of wisdom has strengths pertinent to seeking and gaining knowledge, such as creativity, curiosity, judgment, perspective, and love of learning. Humanity refers to those strengths that contribute to interpersonal relationships, including social intelligence, kindness, and love. Courage includes the strengths of zest, honesty, bravery, and perseverance. The virtue of temperance relates to strengths that help regulate an individual's habits, such as self-regulation, humility, forgiveness, and prudence. Finally, justice includes the strengths of fairness, teamwork, and leadership. Although all the strengths are present in every individual, the signature strengths and weaker strengths vary from person to person, and they guide individual behaviour.

*The Clifton Strengths* (Clifton, Anderson, & Schreiner, 2002), formerly known as the Strengths Quest Program, is based on the core idea of identifying and honing one's talents into strengths. The program starts off with an initial assessment using the Clifton Strengths Finder which helps students identify the five themes that are most applicable to them out of the 34 talent themes. Students then undertake in-depth training in their identified talents and work towards building them into their strengths. In the next two stages of the program, students work on the identified strengths, start owning them, and gradually observe how they are integrated into their daily life (Clifton et al., 2002).

It is well-established that character strengths help students to thrive (Park, 2004). However, if we observe models of PYD and VIA character strengths focus on the thriving of young individuals where they look at strengths rather than deficits (Gradišek). Both models focus on helping youth build and strengthen their resources to flourish in life and eventually contribute to society (Park, 2004). Both models see youth as agents of change, as resources waiting to be developed (Bowers et al., 2010; Roth & Brooks-Gunn, 2003). We have understood the theories that help enhance student engagement thereby reducing stress and promoting flourishing in them.

According to the theory of character strengths, everyone has unique strengths, which accommodate individual differences and allow for diversity within a classroom. Additionally, research shows that strengths promote psychological and subjective well-being, flourishing, and child development. They also act as protective factors against the aftermath of a negative event and help individuals stay resilient. Thus, using character strengths as a vehicle for flourishing is ideal, especially in the school environment.

## ROLE OF LEARNING ENVIRONMENT

If we think of great school and college memories, we will remember laughing along with our peers and teachers; the joyful experiences in the classroom. Everyday experiences shape our values, perspectives, and largely our identity. Schools and education settings play a vital role in a student's life by providing a safe and positive environment that builds strengths. Promoting student engagement is crucial for their behavioural, social, and academic development (Griffiths et al., 2012). Meaningful and carefully planned activities to engage students can create positive school culture that helps students develop healthy coping mechanisms. Student engagement activities should not just be limited to academics and getting higher scores. Focusing on the behavioural, social, and emotional engagement of students enhances holistic development (Appleton, Christenson, & Furlong, 2008). These components of students' engagement boost academic growth, create a strong sense of connection and belongingness with school, and promote well-being (Griffiths et al., 2012; Ramshe, Ghazanfari, & Ghonsooly, 2019; Wang & Eccles, 2012). Students who feel disconnected from their peers and school are at a high risk of involving in substance use, violence, and delinquent behaviours (Copeland et al., 2018).

Traditional school-based interventions largely aim to address a deficit or fix a concern among students or in the school environment. Positive schooling interventions call for the need to move away from the deficit approach of fixing problems and emphasize the need to focus on holistic development and positive school culture (Williams & Kumar, 2018). Designing an intervention or model should be evidence-based and culturally informed. An intervention or model may fail if it does not consider specific cultural aspects. Meticulous planning and execution increase the likelihood of success of the intervention.

### Positive Education Model

What is it we want out of our life? All of us would answer that question with two things–happiness and being a good person. Seligman and Csikszentmihalyi (2000) captured this in their definition of a Good Life which comprises of positive subjective feelings, positive individual traits, and positive institutions that enable the other two. Positive Education or Positive Schooling is an initiative to create a positive institution.

So, what does positive education do? Positive Education aims at two goals, namely promoting flourishing and positive mental health. The positive schooling model, which was developed in the early 2000s, encourages schools to focus on promoting learning through individual students' strengths and personal motivations. With the main purpose of enhancing well-being and creating a safe environment for them, this approach incorporates concepts of engendered learning, customized learning goals, learning as a cooperative process, positive change, and student well-being (Kumar & Mohideen, 2021; Singh, 2018). Research shows the benefits of promoting a positive school culture that helps students in school adjustment, performance, and social functioning (Shoshani & Slone, 2013).

Various theorists have analytically investigated positive schooling, giving us a wider perspective on the concept. For example, (Diener et al., 2010) compared the concept of positive schooling to the different levels in a house. They stated that the house is built on a foundation of care, trust, and respect for diversity promoting a secure and supportive environment for children to explore and flourish. On the next two floors of the house are plans, motivations, and goals that dynamically contribute to how and why a child engages in the learning process. At the third level, children develop a spirit of enquiry centered around the hope that develops because of having a safe and engaging learning environment.

Going through these different levels in their schooling, students develop a sense of commitment and responsibility to contribute effectively to society in their own unique ways.

So, how do we make positive education work? Creating a positive culture within the school needs to be an intentional and planned activity (Thomas, Jose, & Kumar, 2018). Character strengths are the key tools through which we can promote positive education. Geelong Grammar School (GGS) Project is a great example of an effort to integrate positive psychology into a school-wide system (Seligman et al., 2009). GGS Model for Positive Education as an applied framework of positive education (Norrish et al., 2013). The GGS model is derived from the Penn Resiliency Program and Positive Psychology Programme. The GGS provides a strong framework for positive schooling and its benefits.

The Geelong Grammar School Model (Institute of Positive Education, n.d.) for Positive Education outlined earlier focuses on using character strengths as a means for a student to 'flourish'. The model identifies flourishing as the desired outcome that can be achieved by nurturing one's and others' well-being through character strengths. It highlights the importance of recognizing everyone's 24 VIA character strengths and using them to foster well-being. Further, as well-being appears to be a non-measurable concept, six measurable domains of well-being are included in this model, i.e. positive relationships, emotions, health, engagement, accomplishment, and purpose. Finally, the implementation of this model is based on four critical ongoing processes, i.e. learn it, live it, teach it, and embed it. Research evidence shows that positive schooling contributes to student well-being and development, middle school adjustment, school performance, social functioning (Shoshani & Slone, 2013), and school discipline (Day-Vines & Terriquez, 2008).

## The Wellbeing Van: Proposed Model of Flourishing

Thus, we began developing a model on student engagement and flourishing called "The Well-being Van", as part of the Student Mental Health and Positive Schooling research project.

*Figure 1. Diagrammatical representation of the proposed model of flourishing through character strengths*

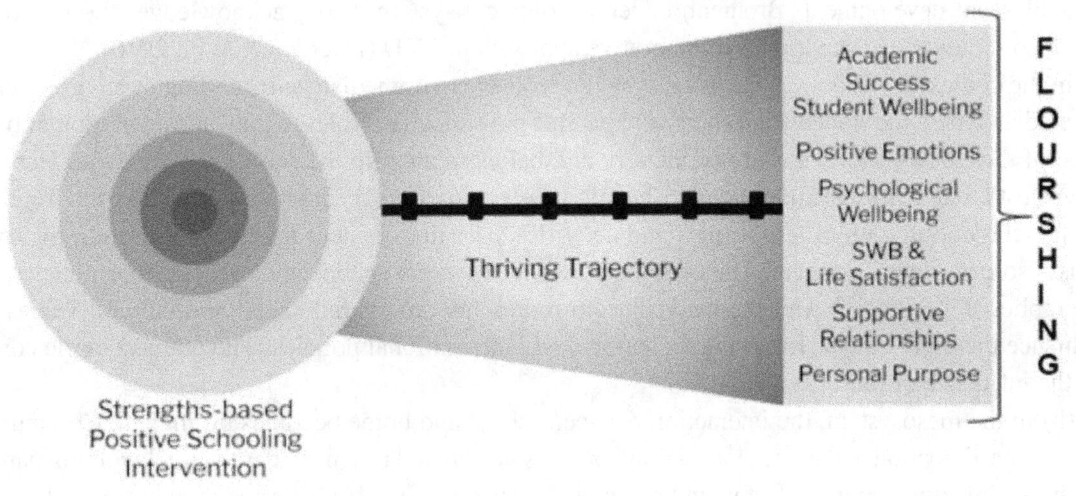

Before we go into HOW strengths are utilized to flourish, let us first set the stage for a positive school. We propose that we view the learning environment of the student–i.e., school, from a socio-ecological-developmental lens. This is mainly because, as we know, behavior and development do not occur in isolation but involve the interplay and influence of a host of different individual, social, and ecological factors. The proposed model draws inspiration from Bronfenbrenner's ecological system theory which placed the individual and his or her relationships with social environments in concentric circles (Bronfenbrenner, 1976).

## Understanding a Positive Learning Ecosystem Using Bronfenbrenner's Theory

The ecological system theory highlights that development does not occur in isolation but is a dynamic process involving multiple environmental systems (Bronfenbrenner, 1976). This model suggests we can understand an individual's environment by looking at it as five concentrically placed circles. With the individual at the center, each circle represents one environmental system that influences development. The five circles are the microsystem, which represents immediate and direct influences, such as family and friends; the mesosystem, which represents the interaction of two or more microsystems, such as school and home, the exosystem, which represents the larger social system that has an indirect influence on the child but the child does not have any influence on the system, such as the media, educational policy, or legal system, the macrosystem, which represents the broader culture in which the child and people around him or her lives, such as the ethnic proportion and socioeconomic status of the country or society that the child lives, and the chronosystem, which represents the changes that happen to the child or the aforementioned systems (Analisah & Indartono, 2019; Bronfenbrenner, 1976).

When developing programs to promote positive adolescent development, it is essential to note that adolescents do not live in isolation but in a dynamic set of environments that comprise a range of factors in the home, school, neighbourhood, and the larger community environment. Bower and Griffin (2011) highlight the importance of parental involvement in the increase of students' social competence and performance. Moreover, Epstein (1995) discusses the importance of the school-parent-teacher relationship which would help foster a sense of community of holistic learning among students. When there is a collaborative effort amongst these environments, it significantly influences the impact of a program on adolescent development. Bronfenbrenner's ecological system theory acknowledges the role of the larger community and supports a collaborative approach to PYD (Duerden & Witt, 2010).

In the context of school (a) the microsystem involves the immediate surrounding or environment of the student where the students, teachers, and parents have specified roles to play during particular times. Each of these roles shows a sense of identity and belongingness in the school environment. Here, the innermost circle represents the student. The microsystem involves the immediate learning environment, i.e. the classroom, with different roles and activities. The mesosystem involves interacting microsystems – so peer interaction, etc. The exosystem would represent school-wide practices or policies, like assemblies, for instance. And the macrosystem represents the overall social and cultural values that influence the inner circles, for example, national and international policies. The outmost circle considers the influence of time.

(b) In the mesosystem, the interaction between school and home becomes prominent. Communication and participation in the decision-making process play a vital role in student's life. Involving parents, teachers, and administrative staff in understanding the needs of the students and their concerns becomes relevant. Interactions among peers and teachers increase a sense of connectedness with the school that helps the student develop a positive relationship with the school. Involving students in the decision-making process by the school authorities further helps the student to be actively involved and engaged throughout their schooling. Moreover, integrating student-centered approaches further increases collaboration among peers, teachers, and school authorities.

(c) The exosystem however involves the role of other external factors that play a role in the child's development. They are not directly linked to the school, however, have a huge influence on the child. For example, a parent's work environment indirectly affects the child when discussions of workplace conflicts and disagreements take place. Moreover, a family's social network also seems to have an influence on the child's development. Another example is the physical school environment which includes, the size of the classroom, paint colours used on the walls, and so on has an influence on the student's connection with the school.

(d) The macrosystem, regulating how the other three systems -the microsystem, the mesosystem, and the exosystem operate, create a societal blueprint of a culture that needs to develop or that develops in a child. The child or student learns about the lifestyle, knowledge of different things, opportunities, and so on. Here, the school cultures take form, ensuring to create a caring, positive school climate for students.

(e) The chronosystem entails the characteristics of change over time in the individual. In terms of how the child or student utilizes these interactions and engages in the development of society.

Bronfenbrenner's ecological model assumes that creating a sense of connection and belongingness helps satisfy the student's need for autonomy and competence. Hence creating a positive culture within the school through creating routines, practices, and policies would establish an ecosystem and climate for flourishing (Paul & Kumar, 2021).

Now that we have understood the school and its various interconnected spheres of influence let us look at a positive education intervention structure. Based on Seligman's pioneer positive schooling program at Geelong Grammar School in Australia, Norrish (2013) came up with an applied framework of positive education. The framework identifies six different well-being domains – positive emotions, relationships, purpose, engagement, accomplishment, and health. A positive schooling intervention that targets all these domains ostensibly leads to flourishing. As we mentioned earlier, these six domains are all underpinned by character strengths, so character strengths are used to impart and cultivate flourishing in the students. The framework uses three ways to do this. While Norrish's framework does not use the ecological systems theory, in our model, we are mapping the three methods onto Bronfenbrenner's levels to make it more explicit and targeted during intervention designing. Teach it – where strengths are taught to students and teachers –acting on the individual and microsystem levels. Live it – where teachers are encouraged to become role models for students to emulate – micro and mesosystem levels. And Embed it – school-wide practices – exosystem level.

We have an integrated and targeted positive schooling intervention that addresses the individual, interpersonal, and school-wide well-being domains. While each domain can be targeted at all ecosystem levels, we have tabulated a limited number of them here, drawing from previous research. This is the intervention, the input for positive education. What is the outcome? Flourishing. The concepts of hedonic, eudemonic, and thriving contribute to a multidimensional and holistic definition of well-being. Simply put, it is feeling good and doing good. Common outcome measures of flourishing include grades, positive-negative emotions, life satisfaction, and psychological well-being, to name a few.

While there are few differences between thriving and flourishing, scholars largely agree that they are very similar constructs. So, we propose, that the thriving trajectory is the process that over time, leads from the character strengths to flourishing. Now the thriving trajectory is characterized by six indicators.

And these six indicators almost perfectly map onto the six virtues that character strengths have been grouped into. This is the initial mapping that we have done, on a theoretical basis.

So, coming back to the model, let us follow one of the domains. Let us take the domain of positive accomplishment, which uses the character strength of perseverance falling under the virtue of courage, - goal setting, growth-based training, grit, etc. So, our model proposes that these activities, the character virtue of courage are developed, helping the student develop capacities in intentional self-regulation, thus resulting in the various flourishing outcomes.

What does this model mean? It captures the process of change more explicitly. This would help us understand why specific interventions work and might also aid in extending the positive effects of positive schooling programs. Secondly, it provides a blueprint for future interventions that take a strength-based whole school approach.

*Model in practice.* As discussed throughout this chapter, adolescence is a sensitive phase that holds immense opportunities to grow and reach potential. Different theories outlined above highlight various factors contributing to this development, including the individual's strengths, a positive school environment, and the larger society. A common thread that entwines all these aspects is adolescents' activities, be it in school, at home, or in the community. Most adolescents and young adults have some amount of free time in their daily lives. Some may be engaged in extracurricular activities such as sports or art classes, whereas others may attend extra classes such as private tuition. Similarly, some adolescents or young adults may spend their free time outdoors hanging out with friends or visiting places. However, others may be at home with their family, siblings, or digital friends. How adolescents and young adults spend their leisure time is significant to their growth and development. Just as this is a time of immense growth, it is also a period that is prone to risk-taking and engaging in unhealthy behaviors and coping mechanisms. Research has shown that providing adolescents and young adults opportunities to participate in structured activities organized by adults with set rules and goals can be beneficial (Duerden & Witt, 2010; Larson, 2000).

There are certain key features to be kept in mind to run a successful program to promote positive development among adolescents. The list of eight key features suggested by Eccles and Gootman (2003) are (a) physical and psychological safety, (b) appropriate structure, (c) supportive relationships, (d) opportunities to belong, (e) positive social norms, (f) support for efficacy and mattering, (g) opportunities for skill-building, and (h) integration of family, school, and community efforts (Duerden & Witt, 2010). Schools and educational institutions around the globe strive to provide such structured and engaging activities for adolescents in various forms.

## The Well-Being Van

The Well-being van was an initiative of the Student Mental Health and Positive schooling project, major research conducted by a team at the authors' Department. The idea of the Well-being Van was propagated from the positive schooling study group. The goal of the Well-being Van was to promote positive psychology practices among college students. The Well-being Van launched its social media page with a vision to reach out to the common youth to promote student well-being. Providing interactive activities and food for thought about each character strength discussed.

The Well-being Van works differently from other study groups where the focus is research and academia. It looks at the application of positive psychology in everyday life. The principle is "having fun with learning." The study group incorporated different names based on cartoon characters for different groups. For example, the general meeting of the group was called '*minions*'. The minions were a way of huddles together, playing games, and discussing the course of the Well-being Van and how we could take it forward. Then presenting the agenda in creative and interactive ways. The icebreakers usually included games that focused on creative thinking, teamwork, relationship building, and so on. Furthermore, each team performed different tasks pertaining to research, social media, and community development.

The Well-being Van was divided into three wings with different functions for each. (a) the Research wing updates the team with the current trends in the field of positive psychology and character strengths. They also paid attention to various interventions to be used in schools and colleges, (b) the social media wing handled the Instagram page keeping it relevant to pique the interest of the youth, involving fun puzzles, and questions. The social media handle was an attempt to keep the youth outside the campus well-informed and aware of the use of positive psychology and character strengths in life and how it promotes well-being and happiness. The social media wing was further worked on website development. The purpose of the website is to reach out to both the youth as well the academic front to keep them informed and updated about positive schooling and character strengths. And how they play a role in enhancing the well-being of children and youth. Thus, helping them lead a life full of potential, meaning, and purpose, (c) the community wing focused on spreading awareness on positive schooling methods and use of character strengths for the youth in the college. There would be exhibitions conducted, which created a platform for the youth to explore character strengths in the things they like to do, for example, identifying strengths of their favourite character in a book, or movie, in art forms that they practice. There were weekly discussions held on topics that could help enhance happiness, well-being, and general outlook towards life. Topics of discussion included, healthy ways of coping, self-care, hope, storytelling method, and more.

Moreover, discussions were portrayed in a fun, innovative, and interactive manner by applying the principles of positive psychology in these sessions. Some ways we used to incorporate fun into our interactions were agents' names given to each of us and we created commandments to be followed which included statements like "*You shall promise to HAVE FUN*", "*you shall never stop learning*", "*you shall be a pillar of support to your fellow agents*" and so on. There were regular check-ins done and agents were given space to reflect on their journey in the Well-being Van.

The Well-being Van has successfully been running for three years now. The youth has been helping each other develop and grow as they progress in their life. The Well-being Van is a place to explore and interact with the youth who are creating small waves of change with a vision to make the current generation lead a happy and satisfying life. Below there are a few reflections from some of the youth who were part of the well-being van.

## Reflections From the Students

*Working for The Well-being Van has taught us a lot of things - teamwork, consistency, the lack of it and how to get back, etc. The Well-being Van is not just another Instagram page, it's a curation of so many ideas, so many hours of discussion, so many ups and downs. Not only did we learn more about positive psychology, but also how to run an Instagram page. Some of us got comfortable with showing our faces in the videos while others got comfortable in penning down their thoughts in the form of poems or doodles. Basically, we learned that growth lies outside our comfort zone and we are happy to have tried it! (V.P., female, personal communication, 2018)*

*Being an agent of The Well-being Van not only provided you to learn about positive psychology and positive schooling, and it also helped you grow as a person. It helped push your limits and adorn different caps while taking on different roles. It gave us a lot of confidence and provided a space for not only professional but also personal growth. Joining the well-being van was one of the best decisions that I have made, and it helped me come out of my shell and discover a side of me that I did not know existed before. It also made us understand the effort that goes into making just one post or reel and made us appreciate the content on Instagram better (M.R., female, personal communication, 2019)*

*Working with the well-being van as an agent was a really good experience. This helped in learning so many things which I would have never tried before. It helped me to feel good about myself when I found hidden talent in me. It also made me explore positive psychology and extend the limits of knowledge. So, by creating the content for Instagram I got an opportunity to give back little from my side to society. This was a wonderful journey where each step was moving towards success in one way with ups and downs with the support of all fellow agents. Most of the time, the content which was put on was relatable to us in one way or another and helped us to build a concrete understanding of theoretical concepts with the application. (N.S., female, personal communication, 2021)*

## Strengths of a Strength-Based Model

The Well-being Van model strives to encourage the holistic development of the adolescent and young adults. These existing models use adolescent and young adult involvement in physical, service-oriented, and community-based activities to help them become productive and contribute to society. Simultaneously, involvement in these activities can be said to improve adolescent well-being, and interpersonal relationships, and help them create their identity. This would create a sense of meaning and belonging among the students helping them with effective management of their stress. Student reflections and research evidence has shown the impact these models have had on adolescents and young adults. Most of them report a better understanding of self, improvement in interpersonal skills, and ability to think critically, reflect and comprehend a wider range of concepts. Students involved in The Well-being Van also reported experiencing positive emotions and obtaining insight into subject-matter content because of their involvement in the activities. These are similar to the outcomes discussed in the proposed model. Let us explore some of the outcomes of the Well-being Van.

### Youth as Drivers of Change

Here, youth members become the agents of change, creating a positive culture by utilizing their strengths of character in their everyday life. Each member contributes to society by living and embedding character strengths in their everyday life. They inspire other members, friends, and family to bring about a change in their outlook towards life. The Well-being van is self-sufficient as the students work towards the mission and vision of the group. The well-being van followed a tier system of having members from each year that helps in the sustenance of the group throughout.

### Social Media as a Tool of Engagement

The current world works on a tap of a screen, all information is available to you. And most of us spend our time online, interacting with friends, family, and others. We use social media to keep ourselves updated about others and increase our awareness about various new topics. Youth comparatively spend a large amount of time on social media apps (Beyens et al., 2020; Gunita & John, 2018; Riehm et al., 2019). Using this as a tool, 'The Well-being Van' utilizes the strengths of such a medium to interact, build awareness and create a dialogue on positive schooling methods and character strengths among adolescents and emerging adults. A recent study by Liu et al. (2020) indicates flourishing in adolescents with the active use of social media. Highlighting the use of such tools helps in reaching out to adolescents and youth in promoting positive mental health in this current generation. Moreover, it creates a space for discussion and engagement about such topics invigorating young minds.

### Use of Reflective Practice

Every activity conducted was followed by a note of reflection. This gave the agents to think and reflect on their progress in the well-being van as well as in their academic life. The process of reflection was carried out through writing, which helped the students express their thoughts and feelings about the minions and activities, the discussions after the minions provided insight into and helped in the better working of 'the well-being van'. This practice of reflection became an effective tool in understanding about self and others.

### The Role of Mentors/Adults

Although the well-being van is run by the students, help of a facilitator is much required. Here, the role of the mentor is to facilitate the learning process to develop a growth mindset and grit in students. Here, the facilitator takes a back seat and enjoys the process of growth and change. They provide support to the students when required encouraging the strength of love for learning.

## Outcomes of Focusing on Well-Being and Flourishing

The 'Well-being Van' is the application of the proposed model of thriving looking at youth as change agents that learn and grow in the process, helping them flourish in different aspects of life. For instance, the students who were part of the Well-being Van felt a sense of positive accomplishment, where they utilized their character strength of perseverance with practices like goal setting, encouraging growth-based training, enhancing grit and so on. The aim of these activities was to develop the character of the virtue of courage that helps the student develop capacities in intentional self-regulation which could result in various flourishing outcomes. Similarly, many such character strengths were aimed to be developed among these youth members. The proposed model captures the process of change vividly through its application as you can see in the well-being van. This helps us understand why specific interventions work, extending the effects of positive schooling programs. The application of these models provides us with a blueprint for future interventions that take a school-wide strength-based approach.

Throughout the entire journey, efforts were put into practice to make the youth in the well-being van experience and build more positive emotions, be engaged in the van by tapping on their strength of curiosity, commitment, and determination. Utilizing their top strengths to the fullest potential as well as improving on their other strengths of character. Through this, they reported having developed a sense of positive accomplishment and purpose which helped them change their perspectives by developing a growth mindset. Also, finding a sense of meaning and purpose by being part of the well-being van has been said to have improved their subjective well-being (Park, Park, & Peterson, 2010). The Wellbeing Van became a source of support that further helped in building positive relationships leading to meaningful interaction.

Applying such school-wide practices accommodates individual differences and allows for diversity within a classroom. Additionally, research shows that strengths promote psychological and subjective well-being (Azañedo et al., 2021; Gillham et al., 2011), flourishing (Jafari, 2020), and child development. They also act as protective factors against the aftermath of a negative event and help individuals stay resilient ((Martínez-Martí & Ruch, 2016). Thus, using character strengths as a vehicle for flourishing is ideal, especially in the school environment.

## IMPLICATIONS FOR RESEARCH AND PRACTICE

Although character strengths and flourishing are widely researched, it is still a relatively new topic of exploration. Various researchers experiment with different theoretical frameworks and interventions even though there are some immediate outcomes, the impact of these programs from a longitudinal perspective is comparatively moving at a slow rate i.e, the interventions that are aimed for three or four months do show some improvement in students, however, the progress is slow. Flourishing is universal concept, however, the path to achieve this is not the same in every culture. Therefore, it calls for a tailored made programs and interventions. Tailor-made refers to culturally informed practices that are relevant and looks at youth development from an alternative perspective that could enhance academic, affective, behavioural, and cognitive engagement in classrooms.

Even though the programs are customised some factors can still be uniform such as building a community and strengthening the values, emphasising on the use of positive language and strengths in the meetings, through which we can develop a sense of belonginess among the youth. Ultimately helping them flourish in all endeavours of their life.

Furthermore, youth being involved in such activities and programs helps in creating a sense of service to build a community of care and belongingness, thereby contributing to the society at large. Schools and institutions would be empowered with such youth builds, self-confidence, courage, and leadership qualities in them.

## CONCLUSION

In perspective, a school environment that promotes love, care, and belongingness paves a path for increasing student engagement. This helps students develop a positive attitude towards their school environment thereby promoting their well-being. The chapter highlights the role of character strengths in building youth engagement. Although this chapter addresses youth engagement, the reader can apply some of the concepts discussed in everyday life, taking the idea of positive schooling beyond this chapter and into their daily routine.

## THINKING QUESTIONS

Do you think there will be cultural differences in implementing The Wellbeing Van in different institutions?

Do you think improving wellbeing of youth will help them develop better coping mechanisms towards stress?

## REFERENCES


Akram, M., & Rana, S. (2013). Positive schooling and subjective well-being of Pakistani children (A qualitative study). *Pakistan Journal of Social and Clinical Psychology, 11*(1), 42–51.

Analisah, C. D., & Indartono, S. (2019). Ecological theory: preventing student bullying to promote culture of peace. *Joint Proceedings of the International Conference on Social Science and Character Education (IcoSSCE 2018) and International Conference on Social Studies, Moral, and Character Education (ICSMC 2018)*. Atlantis Press. 10.2991/icossce-icsmc-18.2019.44

Appleton, J. J., Christenson, S. L., & Furlong, M. J. (2008). Student engagement with school: Critical conceptual and methodological issues of the construct. *Psychology in the Schools, 45*(5), 369–386. doi:10.1002/pits.20303

Arnett, J. J. (2007). Emerging adulthood: What is it, and what is it good for? *Child Development Perspectives, 1*(2), 68–73. doi:10.1111/j.1750-8606.2007.00016.x

Azañedo, C. M., Artola, T., Sastre, S., & Alvarado, J. M. (2021). Character strengths predict subjective well-being, psychological well-being, and psychopathological symptoms, over and above functional social support. *Frontiers in Psychology, 12*, 661278. Advance online publication. doi:10.3389/fpsyg.2021.661278 PMID:34621205

Beck, L., & Wright, A. (2019). iGen: What you should know about post-millennial students. *College and University, 94*(1), 21–26.

Beyens, I., Pouwels, J. L., van Driel, I. I., Keijsers, L., & Valkenburg, P. M. (2020). The effect of social media on well-being differs from adolescent to adolescent. *Scientific Reports, 10*(1), 10763. doi:10.103841598-020-67727-7 PMID:32612108

Boulton, C. A., Hughes, E., Kent, C., Smith, J. R., & Williams, H. T. (2019). Student engagement and wellbeing over time at a higher education institution. *PLoS One, 14*(11), e0225770. doi:10.1371/journal.pone.0225770 PMID:31774878

Bouvet, E., Cosmini, D., Palaktsoglou, M., & Vanzo, L. (2017). 'Doing good' in Italian through student community engagement: The benefits of language placements. *Australian Review of Applied Linguistics, 40*(2), 159–175. doi:10.1075/aral.40.2.05bou

Bowers, E. P., Li, Y., Kiely, M. K., Brittian, A., Lerner, J. V., & Lerner, R. M. (2010). The five Cs model of positive youth development: A longitudinal analysis of confirmatory factor structure and measurement invariance. *Journal of Youth and Adolescence, 39*(7), 720–735. doi:10.100710964-010-9530-9 PMID:20397040

Bronfenbrenner, U. (1976). The experimental ecology of education. *Educational Researcher, 5*(9), 5–15. doi:10.2307/1174755

Catalano, R. F., Berglund, M. L., Ryan, J. A., Lonczak, H. S., & Hawkins, J. D. (2004). Positive youth development in the United States: Research findings on evaluations of positive youth development programs. *The Annals of the American Academy of Political and Social Science, 591*(1), 98–124. doi:10.1177/0002716203260102

Central Board of Secondary Education. (2018). *Mainstreaming health and physical education.* CBSE. http://cbseacademic.nic.in/web_material/Circulars/2018/Health%20and%20Physical%20Education%20(HPE)%20IX-XII.pdf

Central Board of Secondary Education. (n.d.). *About CBSE.* CBSE. https://www.cbse.gov.in/newsite/aboutCbse.html

Cicognani, E., Pirini, C., Keyes, C., Joshanloo, M., Rostami, R., & Nosratabadi, M. (2008). Social participation, sense of community and social well-being: A study on American, Italian, and Iranian university students. *Social Indicators Research, 89*(1), 97–112. doi:10.100711205-007-9222-3

Clifton, D. O., Anderson, E., & Schreiner, L. A. (2002). *StrengthsQuest.* The Gallup Organization.

Copeland, M., Fisher, J. C., Moody, J., & Feinberg, M. E. (2018). Different kinds of lonely: Dimensions of isolation and substance use in adolescence. *Journal of Youth and Adolescence, 47*(8), 1755–1770. doi:10.100710964-018-0860-3 PMID:29774451

Day-Vines, N., & Terriquez, V. (2008). A strengths-based approach to promoting prosocial behavior among African American and Latino students. *Professional School Counseling, 12*(2), 170–175. doi:10.5330/PSC.n.2010-12.170

Diener, E., Wirtz, D., Tov, W., Kim-Prieto, C., Choi, D. W., Oishi, S., & Biswas-Diener, R. (2010). New well-being measures: Short scales to assess flourishing and positive and negative feelings. *Social Indicators Research, 97*(2), 143–156. doi:10.100711205-009-9493-y

Duerden, M. D., & Witt, P. A. (2010). An ecological systems theory perspective on youth programming. *Journal of Park and Recreation Administration, 28*(2), 108–120.

Epstein, J. L. (1995). School/family/community partnerships. *Phi Delta Kappan, 76*(9), 701.

Gillham, J., Adams-Deutsch, Z., Werner, J., Reivich, K., Coulter-Heindl, V., Linkins, M., Winder, B., Peterson, C., Park, N., Abenavoli, R., Contero, A., & Seligman, M. E. P. (2011). Character strengths predict subjective well-being during adolescence. *The Journal of Positive Psychology, 6*(1), 31–44. doi:10.1080/17439760.2010.536773

Gradišek, P. (2021). Character strengths of first-year student teachers and the 5 Cs of the Positive Youth Development framework: A mixed-methods study. In Kozina, A & Wiium, Z (Eds). Positive youth development in contexts (pp. 127). Pedagoški inštitut/Educational Research Institute. doi:10.32320/978-961-270-341-7.127-150

Griffiths, A. J., Lilles, E., Furlong, M. J., & Sidhwa, J. (2012). The relations of adolescent student engagement with troubling and high-risk behaviors. In S. Christenson, A. L. Reschly, & C. Wylie (Eds.), *Handbook of research on student engagement* (Vol. 840). Springer. doi:10.1007/978-1-4614-2018-7_27

Guinta, M. R., & John, R. M. (2018). Social media and adolescent health. *Pediatric Nursing, 44*(4), 196–201.

Hall, G. S. (1904). Adolescence in literature, biography, and history. In G. S. Hall (Ed.), *Adolescence: Its psychology and its relations to physiology, anthropology, sociology, sex, crime, religion and education* (Vol. 1, pp. 513–589). D Appleton & Company. doi:10.1037/10616-008

Han, H. (2018). The VIA inventory of strengths, positive youth development, and moral education. *The Journal of Positive Psychology, 14*(1), 32–40. doi:10.1080/17439760.2018.1528378

Hayden, M., Hemmens, A., Mcintosh, S., Sandoval-Hernandez, A., & Thompson, J. (2017). *The impact of creativity, activity, and service (CAS) on students and communities: Non-technical report for the International Baccalaureate Organization.* University of Bath. https://www.ibo.org/globalassets/publications/ib-research/dp/cas-finalreport-2017-en.pdf

Heck, K. E., & Subramaniam, A. (2009). Youth development frameworks [Monograph]. *4-H Center for Youth Development Monograph: University of California.* https://youthrex.com/wp-content/uploads/2019/02/1224.pdf

Jafari, F. (2020). The mediating role of self-compassion in relation between character strengths and flourishing in college students. *International Journal of Happiness and Development, 6*(1), 76–93. doi:10.1504/IJHD.2020.108755

Kierstead, J. (1980). *Montessori and Dewey: A comparison of their theory and practice* (ED198506). ERIC. https://eric.ed.gov/?id=ED198506

Kumar, P. A., & Mohideen, F. (2021). Strengths-Based Positive Schooling Interventions: A Scoping Review. *Contemporary School Psychology, 25*(1), 86–98. doi:10.100740688-019-00260-1

Larson, R. W. (2000). Toward a psychology of positive youth development. *The American Psychologist, 55*(1), 170–183. doi:10.1037/0003-066X.55.1.170 PMID:11392861

Martínez-Martí, M. L., & Ruch, W. (2016). Character strengths predict resilience over and above positive affect, self-efficacy, optimism, social support, self-esteem, and life satisfaction. *The Journal of Positive Psychology, 12*(2), 110–119. doi:10.1080/17439760.2016.1163403

Mercier, J., Powell, C., Langdon-Pole, G., Finau, D., Hicks, K., Bourchier, L., & Hampton, J. (2019). The five Cs of positive youth development in an Aotearoa/New Zealand program context. *Journal of Youth Development, 14*(4), 36–58. doi:10.5195/jyd.2019.774

Norrish, J. M., Williams, P., O'Connor, M., & Robinson, J. (2013). An applied framework for positive education. *International Journal of Wellbeing, 3*(2), 147–161.

Park, N. (2004). Character strengths and positive youth development. *The Annals of the American Academy of Political and Social Science, 591*(1), 40–54. doi:10.1177/0002716203260079

Park, N., Park, M., & Peterson, C. (2010). When is the search for meaning related to life satisfaction? *Applied Psychology. Health and Well-Being, 2*(1), 1–13. doi:10.1111/j.1758-0854.2009.01024.x PMID:23457083

Paul, R., & Kumar, A. (2021). Creating a positive school culture through new educational practices. In C. B. Gaines & K. M. Hutson (Eds.), *Promoting Positive Learning Experiences in Middle School Education* (pp. 149–166). IGI Global. doi:10.4018/978-1-7998-7057-9.ch008

Perron, N. C. (2017). Bronfenbrenner's ecological systems theory. *College student Development. Applying Theory to Practice on the Diverse Campus, 197*(23), 1–10.

Peterson, C., & Seligman, M. E. (2004). *Character strengths and virtues: A handbook and classification*. Oxford University Press.

Ramshe, M. H., Ghazanfari, M., & Ghonsooly, B. (2019). The Role of Personal Best Goals in EFL Learners' Behavioural, Cognitive, and Emotional Engagement. *International Journal of Instruction, 12*(1), 1627–1638. doi:10.29333/iji.2019.121103a

Riehm, K. E., Feder, K. A., Tormohlen, K. N., Crum, R. M., Young, A. S., Green, K. M., Pacek, L. R., La Flair, L. N., & Mojtabai, R. (2019). Associations between time spent using social media and internalizing and externalizing problems among US youth. *JAMA Psychiatry, 76*(12), 1266. doi:10.1001/jamapsychiatry.2019.2325 PMID:31509167

Roth, J. L., & Brooks-Gunn, J. (2003). What exactly is a youth development program? Answers from research and practice. *Applied Developmental Science, 7*(2), 94–111. doi:10.1207/S1532480XADS0702_6

Schwieger, D., & Ladwig, C. (2018). Reaching and retaining the next generation: Adapting to the expectations of Gen Z in the classroom. *Information Systems Education Journal, 16*(3), 45–54.

Seemiller, C., & Clayton, J. (2019). Developing the strengths of generation Z college students. *Journal of College and Character, 20*(3), 268–275. doi:10.1080/2194587X.2019.1631187

Seligman, M. E., Ernst, R. M., Gillham, J., Reivicha, K., & Linkinsd, M. (2009). Positive education: Positive psychology and classroom interventions. *Oxford Review of Education, 35*(3), 293–311. doi:10.1080/03054980902934563

Seligman, M. E. P., & Csikszentmihalyi, M. (2000). Positive psychology: An introduction. *The American Psychologist, 55*(1), 5–14. doi:10.1037/0003-066X.55.1.5 PMID:11392865

Shek, D. T., Dou, D., Zhu, X., & Chai, W. (2019). Positive youth development: Current perspectives. *Adolescent Health, Medicine and Therapeutics, 10*, 131–141. doi:10.2147/AHMT.S179946 PMID:31572041

Shoshani, A., & Slone, M. (2013). Middle school transition from the strengths perspective: Young adolescents' character strengths, subjective well-being, and school adjustment. *Journal of Happiness Studies, 14*(4), 1163–1181. doi:10.100710902-012-9374-y

Singh, S. (2018). Positive schooling and resilience. *Indian Journal of Positive Psychology, 9*(2), 311–316.

Snyder, C. R., & Lopez, S. J. (2007). *Positive psychology: The scientific and practical explorations of human strengths*. Sage Publications, Inc.

Steinberg, L., & Silk, J. S. (2002). *Parenting adolescents* (Vol. 1). Handbook of parenting.

Thomas, S., Jose, K. A., & Kumar, A. (2018). *Child Friendly Schools: Challenges and Issues in Creating a Positive and Protective School Environment. Positive Schooling and Child Development, 233*. Springer.

VIA Institute on Character. (n.d.). *The 24 Character Strengths*. VIA. https://www.viacharacter.org/character-strengths

Wang, M. T., & Eccles, J. S. (2012). Adolescent behavioral, emotional, and cognitive engagement trajectories in school and their differential relations to educational success. *Journal of Research on Adolescence, 22*(1), 31–39. doi:10.1111/j.1532-7795.2011.00753.x PMID:22822296

Waters, S. K., Cross, D. S., & Runions, K. (2009). Social and ecological structures supporting adolescent connectedness to school: A theoretical model. *The Journal of School Health, 79*(11), 516–524. doi:10.1111/j.1746-1561.2009.00443.x PMID:19840228

Weissberg, R. P., Durlak, J. A., Domitrovich, C. E., & Gullotta, T. P. (2015). Social and emotional learning: Past, present, and future. In J. A. Durlak, C. E. Domitrovich, R. P. Weissberg, & T. P. Gullotta (Eds.), *Handbook of social and emotional learning: Research and practice* (pp. 3–19).

Whitlock, J. (2007). The role of adults, public space, and power in adolescent community connectedness. *Journal of Community Psychology, 35*(4), 499–518. doi:10.1002/jcop.20161

Williams, J., & Kumar, A. (2018). *From Deficit to a Strength Model. Character Strength Development: Perspectives from Positive Psychology, 353*. Sage Publication.

Zepke, N. (2014). Student engagement research in higher education: Questioning an academic orthodoxy. *Teaching in Higher Education, 19*(6), 697–708. doi:10.1080/13562517.2014.901956

Zepke, N., & Leach, L. (2010). Improving student engagement: Ten proposals for action. *Active Learning in Higher Education, 11*(3), 167–177. doi:10.1177/1469787410379680

# Chapter 5
# Risk Factors of Mental Health of Students in Higher Education Institutions

**Daniel Opotamutale Opotamutale**
https://orcid.org/0000-0002-8913-056X
*University of Namibia, Namibia*

**Fillemon Shekutamba Albanus**
https://orcid.org/0000-0003-1516-2523
*University of Namibia, Namibia*

## ABSTRACT

*Students' mental well-being plays an important role in academic achievement in higher educational institutions. A good mental state enables us to fully enjoy and appreciate our environment and the people around us. We can resist stress better and tackle daily life challenges with a positive frame of mind. Good mental health also allows one to be productive and to use one's mental abilities to the full. However, being a student brings about a number of events that can lead to stress, such as living away from home, giving up a good job to be a student, and organising your finances, deadlines and exams, to name just a few. The content of this chapter can be used by divison of student support affairs in higher education institutions worldwide to develop targeted interventions and strategies for alleviating the risk factors of concern to the mental health of students in higher education institutions.*

## INTRODUCTION

Good mental health allows students to be productive academically and use their mental abilities to the full while appreciating their environment and the people around them. Mental health-related problems have become a significant point of concern, gaining attention and interest from the healthcare and higher education institutions and organisations (Limone & Toto, 2022). Existing evidence has shown that the prevalence of mental health problems, including self-harm and suicides within higher education

DOI: 10.4018/979-8-3693-2833-0.ch005

institutions (universities and college students), is rapidly increasing (Campbell et al., 2022). Moreover, institutions have implemented protocols for ensuring that mental issues among the public are dealt with legitimately to achieve high standards of mental health among students (Limone & Toto, 2022). The majority of the current population who fall victim to mental illnesses in the academic environment comprise college and university students (Larson et al., 2022). Although most colleges and universities have campus services available, majority of students who might get to benefit from mental health services do not sustain the care; almost half of students who presents positive for depression, for example, do not receive treatment (Lattie et al., 2022).

An extensive international survey of about 14,000 students across 19 universities in eight countries found that 35% of students met the diagnostic category for at least one general mental health condition (Auerbach et al., 2016). Hence, the rise in depression levels among university students is reported to be 12.9% higher than among the general public (Lim et al., 2018). The symptoms of mental ill-health predominantly emerge in adolescence and young adulthood (Auerbach et al., 2018; Bhatia et al., 2020). There is a rise in need for appropriate professional interventions to support students' mental health across all global higher education institutions. However, there is limited research on mental health focusing on the risk factors that predispose students to mental health illness in higher education institutions. Therefore, the purpose of this book chapter is to provide an overview of the risk factors for students' mental health in higher education institutions with specific emphasis on effective strategies that may be devised to mitigate these factors.

## BACKGROUND

There is an urgent need to contextualise the concept of mental health, as it remains one of the fundamental standards in human evolution. Despite this, the concept mental health means to the entire aspects of human evolution is an exclusive notion prime to it (Wren-Lewis & Alexandrova, 2021). Mental health is a multidimensional concept that refers to both physical and psychological health because both the body and the mind contribute to illness and health (Acutt & Hattingh, 2016). Therefore, a narrow definition of mental health is that mental health refers to an absence of cognitive illness (Wren-Lewis & Alexandrova, 2021). In addition, an important mental health definition refers to the state of extensive good health in social and individual daily living situations (Wren-Lewis & Alexandrova, 2021). Additionally, mental health can be described as an individual's state of well-being. Such an individual has insight into their own abilities and limitations and can cope with daily stress in life, can work productively and has the ability to contribute fruitfully to the well-being of fellow workers, family and community (Acutt & Hattingh, 2016).

Younger students studying in higher educational institutions are largely at risk of developing mental illness, which may reoccur throughout their entire lifespan (O'Keeffe et al., 2023). Therefore, the stress that students encounter due to the academic pressure of their studies can place them at risk of developing a mental illness (O'Keeffe et., 2023). Hence, various risk factors have been recognised as predisposing them to mental illness. Financial problems or distress is one of the major triggers of mental illness among students (Kandasamy et al., 2020). Moreover, financial problems are triggered by a shortage of capital or money which involves individual, family, and other kinds of financial issues, as cited in Kandasamy et al. (2020). Financial problems are linked to pedagogical and financial freedom, and risk handling, as students in higher education institutions are helpless when it comes to accessing various options to obtain adequate financial help which would support their expenses (Daud et al. 2018). As a result, dealing with loans themselves and all these types of financial issues can lead to the development of depression or stress and anxiety in students (Kandasamy et al., 2020; Ashipala & Shilunga, 2023).

The general health condition of a particular student is another factor which may trigger mental illness among students in higher educational institutions; adolescents and teenagers are impacted by chronic health conditions that can result to mental health problems (Delamater et al., 2017). Persistent illness like diabetes mellitus (DM) and cancer result in mental disorders, as students are reluctant to admit the reality of their illness, leading to mental depletion, often resulting in suicidal ideations among students (Delamater et al., 2017; Kandasamy et al., 2020). According to Kindred, & Bates, (2023) students had higher levels of anxiety and appeared to be less happy than the general public during the period of the coronavirus 19 outbreak. Social relationships are another factor that students in their first semester at higher institutions encounter as they navigate transformation action; most are able to navigate this process while others struggle to cope (McKinnon-Crowley et al., 2021). Additionally, greater competition in achieving educational successes may cause mental strain or depression in students in achieving their main missions and visions (McKinnon-Crowley et al., 2021). Furthermore, age may translate into some form of obstacle for particular students in higher education institutions that are reluctant to admit younger students (Birhanu Ayalew, 2022).

There are various factors that put students/people more at risk of developing mental health problems in higher education institutions. These factors are classified into categories, namely: educational risk factors, societal risk factors, cognitive risk factors, lifestyle risk factors and biological risk factors (Allott et al. 2020).

## Educational Risk Factors

In the educational sectors, several factors such as the duration of study, poor performances or results, job arrangements and higher education projects could be determining factors for the mental wellness of students (Limone & Toto, 2022). Moreover, the complexity of module content may exacerbate the prevailing risk factors of work overload, greater anxiety and distress (mental illness), when compared to other causes such as nursing and medicine which include intensive clinical practice (Fares et al., 2016). Similarly, Kiziela et al. (2018) argued that newly enrolled students majoring in medicine and nursing frequently lack the necessary resilience to deal with the workload and syllabus before registering at colleges, resulting in mental breakdown. According to Dalton et al. (2022), medicine and nursing students are at risk of developing distress in their educational journey.

Ruzhenkova, (2020) reported that students studying in exotic regions where foreign language are used show a greater propensity for anxiety and depression as first-year students. In contrast, students in their final year encounter a greater degree of mental illness (Ruzhenkova, 2020). At the same time, students in higher education institutions experience some form of mental illness because of the difficulty in coping with a college way of life, due to previous family experiences, loneliness, and social distance (Ruzhenkova, 2020). Also, Ishii et al. (2018) argued that poor grades or substandard academic performance could be associated with harmful effects to the students' mental health. Hence, a negative relationship among students and lecturers or tutors leads to a decline in students' mental health (Ishii et al., 2018).

## Societal Risk Factors

Undergraduate students in higher education institutions are at greater risk of developing severe depression, leading to anxiety, poor self-esteem and mental illness owing to individual separation, lack of social interaction and lack of friendship (Loades et al., 2020). Limone and Toto (2022) pointed out that several societal drawbacks like inappropriate housing and poverty are risks for mental problems among students. Additionally, poverty is accompanied by substandard academic performance, concentration-related problems, anxiety, schizophrenia, distress, criminality, and other correspondent mental health illness among students (Loades et al., 2020). Moreover, students from low-income households increases the opportunities or the risk of suffering from mental health issues due to the instilled inside strain and willingness to eradicate from poverty (Loades et al., 2020). Skilbred-Fjeld et al. (2020) and Jochman et al. (2019) stated that persecution and social injustice within higher institutions inflicts mental trauma, distress and anxiety, depression and declining self-confidence which could lead to self-harm or suicidal ideation among students.

## Cognitive Factors

Young adulthood trauma, violence, and negligence negatively affect students' perceptions and minds including the way they interrelate with fellow population in the academic environment (Limone & Toto, 2021).

Students, particularly females who have experienced a trauma event like abuse or mistreatment, could experience post-traumatic stress disorders (PTSDs), depression or distress and eventually poor intellectual and social development resulting in mental illness (Limone et al., 2021). Hassanzadeh et al. (2017) revealed that frustrating activities lead to the major emotional problems like anxiety, depression and distress or emotional strain. Therefore, severe and chronic educational distress like extreme fear of academic failure causes a deficiency of mental health in students, leading to low educational participation by students (Hassanzadeh et al., 2017). Stressful life circumstances encountered by undergraduate students may result in psychological displeasure and complications, which may trigger different psychological health illnesses like increased blood pressure and asthma (Limone & Toto, 2022).

## Lifestyle Risk Factors

Many undergraduates in higher education change their attitudes and behaviours to excessive alcohol consumption, cigarette smoking, unhealthy dietary intake, lack of exercise and drug abuse all of which pose serious threats to mental health (Pedersen et al., 2020). Equally fascinating, Cai et al. (2017) indicated that due to institutional or communal linkages, most students, particularly male students smoke, failing to realise that institutional smoking is closely linked to mental illness. Mofatteh (2021) indicated that some of the risk factors which lead to students suffering from poor mental wellness include staying far from home, educational and monetary problems, and lack of an emotional support network from friends and family members. In addition, lack of money has a serious impact on students' mental wellness (Mofatteh, 2021).

Alcohol and drugs abuse by students alter their intellectual defences towards academic strain or distress in the institutional environment (Mofatteh, 2021). Excessive alcohol intake is linked to poor mental attitudes or behaviour like missing lessons or classes, negligence, self-abuse, physical abuse, the satisfaction of offensive copulation actions, shyness and remorse as a result of consternation and depression (Rosenthal et al., 2018). Also, misuse or excessive consumption of alcohol and drugs, for instance marijuana, is linked to monomania or delusions which negatively affect students' well-being and cause devastating mental illnesses in students (Dammeyer, 2018).

Furthermore, in higher education institutions students develop poor sleeping patterns which may lead to mental disorders and illness (Rosenthal et al., 2018). Many students do not get adequate rest, triggering sleep deficits, with the risk of depression, distress and decreased mood (Rosenthal et al., 2018). Limone and Toto (2022) alleged that lack of engagement in physical activities is another precipitating risk factor that leads to mental health disturbances among students in higher education institutions.

### Biological Risk Factors

An individual's cognitive wellness is related to family history, such as the incidence of bipolar mood disorder, schizophrenia, psychosis, anxiety and distress (Grant & Chamberlain, 2020).

Students growing up in abusive surroundings background or being harassed by parents are at increased risk of developing distress or depression which then develops into mental illness at a later stage (Grant & Chamberlain, 2020). Nevertheless, Kenney and Müller (2017) state if the students' parents had poor eating habits, were exposed to various natural pollutants, had long-term stress, poor pre-infancy ingestion, thus family genetic traits are correlated and leading them to mental health disorders. Campbell et al. (2022) indicated that the student group at most risk of experiencing suicidal ideation are day students, lesbian, gay, bisexual and trans-sexual students, and foreign students.

Furthermore, higher risk of suicidal thoughts among this group of students could be triggered by the accessibility of services provided to these cohorts, which are inadequate compared to those given to the overall student population. Equally important, the largest rates of mental illness and suicide were experienced by students between the ages of 20 and 24, and graduates were particularly susceptible (Campbell., et al 2022). Students with long-term illnesses for instance diabetic mellitus and cancer that precipitate students to injustice, stigma, depression, distress and decreased self-assurance leading to intellectual disabilities and bullying or humiliating students mentally unstable (Dammeyer, 2018).

## HEALTH BELIEF MODEL

In this chapter, a Health Belief Model will be used to explain the various contributory risk factors for mental health among students in higher education institutions. The Health Belief Model (HBM) refers to the psycho-sociological health attitudes or behaviour modification model initiated to explicate and predict health-allied behaviours, specifically with regard to the uptake of health systems (Panahi, 2018).

Furthermore, the theory of a Health Belief Model entails an interface between behaviours and attitudes and their effect on health. The Health Belief Model synthesises health decisions into steps and provides a catalogue of variables which affect health activity; it does not offer a model of how accurately these works. The likelihood of taking recommended action is based on the following elements: perceived severity of disease, perceived susceptibility to disease, perceived benefits of action, perceived barriers to action as well as cues to action. This theory of Panahi, (2018) is important in backing up the results, discussion, and conclusion of the study to make recommendations on the findings.

*Figure 1. The theory of a health belief model on the risk factors of mental health*
*Source: (Panahi, 2018)*

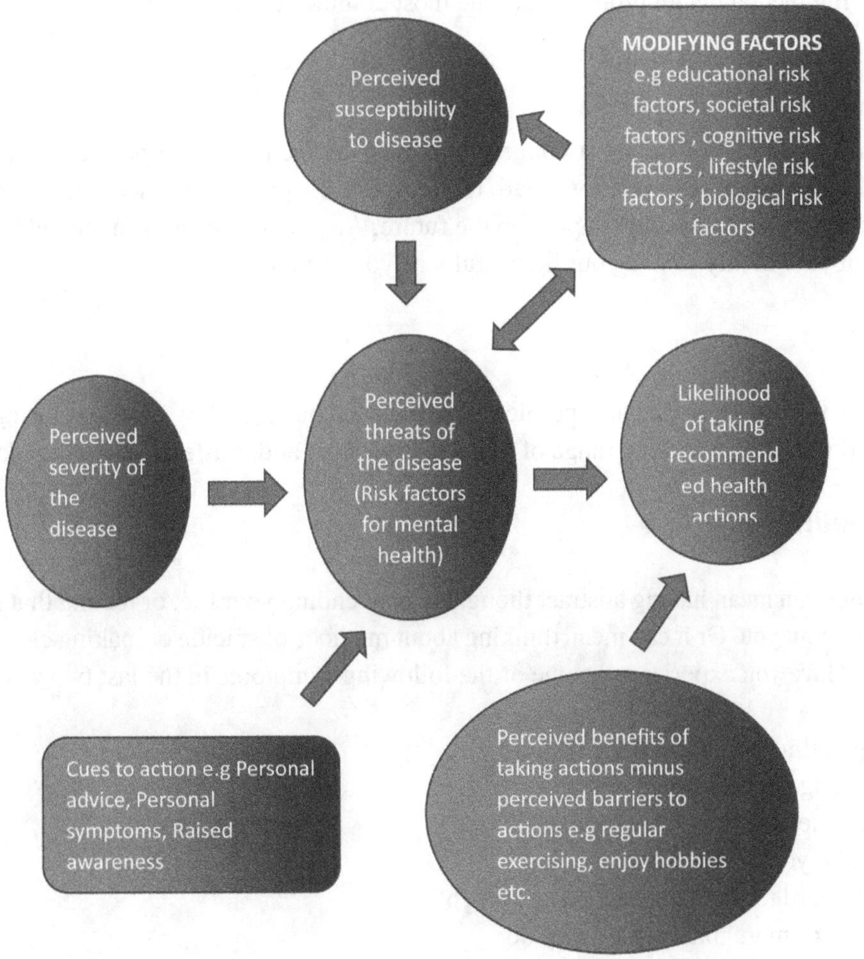


## THE LINKS BETWEEN VARIOUS CONTRIBUTORY RISK FACTORS AND THE MENTAL HEALTH OF STUDENTS IN HIGHER EDUCATION INSTITUTIONS: INFLUENCE ON PSYCHOLOGICAL ADJUSTMENT AND ITS IMPACT ON ACADEMIC ACHIEVEMENT

Societal risk factors such as poverty are proportionally linked to educational risk factors like substandard academic performance, poor intellectual and concentration-related problems, anxiety, and other related mental health illness among students.

Moreover, cognitive risk factors like frustrating activities result in anxiety, depression, distress or emotional strain, and are directly related to lifestyle risk factors such as alcohol and drug abuse by students as intellectual defence.

Mental health problems can affect many areas of students' lives, reducing their quality of life, academic achievement, physical health, and satisfaction with the college experience, and negatively impacting on relationships with friends and family members. These issues may also have long-term consequences for students, affecting their future employment, earning potential, and overall health.

The following mental health problems are the most common among students.

## Anxiety

Anxiety disorders are one of the most commonly diagnosed mental health problems among students. Anxiety is what we feel when we are worried, tense or afraid – particularly about things that are about to happen, or which we think could happen in the future. Anxiety can become a mental health problem if it impacts on your ability to live your life as fully as you want to.

## Depression

Depression is a type of mental health problem that involves having a low mood or losing interest and enjoyment in things. It can cause a range of other changes too, and if affects your everyday living.

## Suicidal Feelings

Suicidal feelings can mean having abstract thoughts about ending your life, or feeling that people would be better off without you. Or it can mean thinking about methods of suicide or making clear plans to take your own life. Have you experienced some of the following symptoms in the last two weeks?

- Ongoing feelings of sadness
- Being on edge or snapping at people
- Low self-esteem
- Feeling like you're not "good enough"
- Finding it hard to sleep or sleeping too much
- Eating less or more than you usually do
- Low energy
- Difficulty remembering things
- Feeling like you don't want to do anything.
- Having suicidal thoughts
- Feeling physically ill without knowing why
- Isolating or avoiding friends
- Changes in weight

Unfortunately, students who struggle with depression and anxiety are reluctant to seek help. This increases the risk of harmful outcomes, such as dropping out of college, poor academic performance, suicide and substance abuse.

Several signs that may indicate that an individual may be a candidate for risk factors for mental health include one or more of the following:

- Doing poorly in school
- Teasing others

- Showing excessive amounts of anger
- Being excessively jealous
- Appearing conceited
- Hesitating to try new things.

Here are some situations or risk factors that could trigger a mental health breakdown for college students:

- Relationship breakup
- Sexual assault
- Peer relationship difficulties
- Sexual identity adjustment difficulties
- Drug or alcohol use
- Family history of depression
- Stressful life events
- Comparison of own academic, athletic or social performance with that of peers
- Fears of disappointing parents because of grades or career path choice

### What Are the Warning Signs of Suicide?

- Ignoring class work or skipping classes
- Withdrawing from friends and wanting to be left alone
- Giving away possessions
- Talking about suicide
- Doing risky or self-destructive things, such as using drugs or driving recklessly
- Increasing use of alcohol or drugs
- Saying goodbye to people as if they won't be seeing them again.

N.B. This is not an exhaustive list. Be alert to behaviour and personality changes that can provide clues to a student's state of well-being.

## EXAM ANXIETY

Most people naturally feel anxious before an exam. Some anxiety before and during an exam enhances your performance. Sometimes, too much adrenaline is released, and you may begin to feel distress. Then anxiety can get in the way of performing well.

Exam anxiety is the experience of feeling an intense moment of fear or panic before and/or during an exam or assessment. Exam anxiety is a psychological condition that causes extreme distress and anxiety during exam times. Most people experience a certain degree of anxiety and stress before or during the exam, but this negatively affects learning and performance in insurmountable situations. Excessive anxiety and fear make concentration difficult, and the person makes a lot of effort to remember the subject they are working on.

There are two types of anxiety:

- **Low anxiety:** Students who experience low anxiety may feel a little nervous about an upcoming exam but are still able to focus their attention on their studies or the questions asked during the assessment. Usually, low anxiety students are not struck with intrusive thoughts or feel debilitated by the exam.
- **High anxiety:** Students who experience high anxiety show an immediate anxiety reaction when exposed to the feared test situation. They attempt to avoid the situation by not showing up to the exam or may endure it but with extreme fear. High anxiety can tip some into a sense of panic: "I just really can't do this!"

## How to Deal With Exam Anxiety?

- In order to manage anxiety, one needs to find a suitable motivation.
- It is necessary to direct existing anxiety in a positive direction without turning anxiety into fear of the future.
- A person needs to spend time in his spare time focusing on what they love.
- The person should take up a hobby that will diffuse anxiety.

Exam anxiety causes various levels of physical, cognitive, behavioural and emotional symptoms. Potential physical symptoms could include:

- Heart palpitations
- Sweating
- Tremors
- Symptoms such as dry mouth and nausea

Potential cognitive symptoms could include:

- Persistently comparing yourself to others
- Blanking out (feeling as if you can't remember any important information)
- Negative thoughts about yourself
- Flashbacks or persisting thoughts about past performances
- Dread of the consequences of failure
- Pressured thoughts related to "needing to study more" or "study harder"

Potential emotional symptoms may include:

- Irritation or anger towards oneself (or the test administrator)
- Excessive fear
- Shame
- Disappointment in oneself
- Sadness

## What Causes Exam Anxiety?

Like with most anxiety conditions, there doesn't appear to be a single cause of test anxiety. Instead, it's more likely that this anxiety emerges from a combination of factors. There are several causes of exam anxiety:

- **Fear of failure:** Many people measure their confidence and self-worth based on their performance. As a result, these individuals may internalise any perceived instances of failure as them being a failure.
- **Lack of preparedness or awareness:** In some cases, you may feel unprepared for a test. You may not have studied well enough, or you may not have studied the right material.
- **Struggling with testing in the past:** A history of issues with testing and performance may trigger negative thoughts about yourself and your ability to succeed. These thought patterns can spiral into anxiety, reinforcing a vicious cycle of nervousness before future tests.
- **External pressure:** If a parent, coach or teacher has overly high expectations for your behaviour, you may feel even more responsible for impressing them. This pressure may exacerbate anxiety.
- **Unrealistic fears:** Having unfounded worries, such as believing loved ones won't think you're smart or that your entire career will be doomed if you fail an exam, can exacerbate test anxiety.
- **Other anxiety symptoms or an anxiety disorder:** Anxiety can compound itself, meaning that if you struggle with anxiety in one area of your life, it can undoubtedly bleed into other areas.

## Ways to Overcome Test Anxiety

Although exam anxiety can feel frustrating, practising different relaxation and cognitive strategies can help you feel less nervous. Commit to trying new ways to cope with exam anxiety. Practising them often will help them become more second nature in your routine. But if you are dealing with test anxiety, consider trying these tips:

1. Study efficiently and in ways that work best for you.

Everyone studies differently, but rather than focus on how your peers' study, try to focus on doing more of what works for you. Try to prioritise active, rather than passive, engagement.

2. Start studying early and in the same place.

Waiting until the last minute to study will only increase your test-related stress. The best way to manage test anxiety is by making sure you are well prepared. Start by setting a realistic time frame for learning the required material, then find a place that's conducive to learning.

3. Get to the examination room early.

Arriving at the examination room early enough can reduce your anxiety. This can give you space to unwind, practise some relaxation exercises, locate the testing room, and find a seat where you will be able to focus.

4. Challenge perfectionistic thoughts.

The goal is not about achieving perfection and having that goal will only lead to burnout and frustration. It is okay to make mistakes. Remind yourself that perfectionism is not everything before, during and after the test.

5. Do not sacrifice sleep.

Many people spend the night before a test cramming in information. But poor sleep can wreak havoc on your physical and emotional well-being. Furthermore, good sleep can help solidify memory and concentration, both of which are essential for a key performance.

6. Read the instructions carefully.

Read the instructions thoroughly and if you have any questions ask for clarification before you get started. You are also more likely to catch careless mistakes when you take your time reading and fully comprehending the content and what is being asked in each section.

7. Keep track of time during the exam.

Monitor the time regularly but avoid constantly checking it as this can distract you and further increase your test anxiety. Moreover, if you are uncertain about a tough question, do not dwell on it. Keep in mind that you can get several answers wrong and still do well.

## SELF HELP TIPS

"Self-care is how you take your power back."

Self-care is important to maintaining a healthy relationship with yourself. It means doing things to take care of our minds, bodies and souls by engaging in activities that promote well-being and reduce stress. Doing so enhances our ability to live fully, vibrantly and effectively. The practice of self-care also reminds both you and others that your needs are valid and a priority

## THE EFFECTS OF POOR MENTAL HEALTH OF STUDENTS IN HIGHER EDUCATION INSTITUTIONS

The consequent risk effects of poor mental health problems among students varies, and might be as follows:

- Substandard or low academic participation as a result of dysfunctional responses triggered by temporary or chronic stressors and psychological problems.
- Abandoning or dropping out from school (college or university) due to alcohol or substance abuse and dependence.

- Risk of suicidal ideations and self-harm/ harm to others due to mood disorders and inflated manic and depressive feelings and destructive behaviours.
- Schizophrenia and other psychotic disorders related to the advancement of students' poor mental health and serious distortions in all spheres of the students' functioning (mind, speech, perceptions and emotions, leading to delusions and hallucinations).
- Dissociative and somatoform disorders related to disturbances in a student's sense of identification, memory and consciousness, including inexplicable physical signs and symptoms.
- Personality and impulse control disorders due to deviant behaviours like aggression, suspicion, disinterest, dependence, avoidance, obsessive gambling and manipulation.
- Eating disorders, obesity and sleep disorders related to excessive behaviours.
- Cognitive disorders related to psychoses and impairments that result from organic brain damage as a result of genetics, injuries or processes of aging.
- Violence and abuse due to aggression and sexual abuse on the part of other people.
- Gender-identity disorders and sexual disorders related to dysfunctional gender identification and sexual functioning.

## Mental Health and Wellbeing Tips and Strategies to Continue Looking After Ourselves and Each Other During These Difficult Times

1. Maintain a daily routine: try to get up at a consistent time and follow a daily plan.
2. Acknowledge your feelings. If you are overwhelmed, please contact the Directorate of Student Affairs.
3. It helps to make a list of things that you can do, that you are in control of: Studying, doing chores, exercising, doing things that you may have been putting off due to a lack of time.
4. Journaling your feelings; doing poetry; reading; undertaking creative exercises (drawing, colouring, artwork), listening to music, taking up a new hobby, are all useful activities to engage in.
5. Do something that you enjoy doing, or which makes you feel good, every day.
6. Loneliness and feelings of depression may be very real for you. Apart from the suggestions above, try to reach out to loved ones and supportive people through technology, where possible.
7. As much as possible, show compassion and kindness to one other times of fear, isolation (both physical and social) and uncertainty are when it is most important that we strengthen our sense of community by connecting with and supporting each other.
8. Connection – think of creative ways to stay connected with others, including social media, email and phone.
9. Stay connected with your values. Don't let fear or anxiety drive your interactions with others. We are all in this together!

## Is My Response Warranted?

Check to see if the situation warrants the response you're having. Examine the facts. While our emotions are always valid, they are not always justified. Look to see if your emotional response matches the circumstances.

## Am I Being Effective?

Examine whether what you're doing is helping or hurting the situation. If it's making things worse, do the opposite of whatever it is you feel like doing. Commit to it. If you want to stay home and isolate, force yourself to go out where there are people. If you're angry and want to yell, try avoiding the person who your anger is directed towards.

Take note: You are unique, spend time with yourself to assess what works for you

## AIM TO THRIVE

- **Establish healthy habits that work for you:** Schedule stress reduction physical activity and healthy eating like you schedule classes and homework.
- **Build resilience and coping skills:** Practise deep breathing, mindfulness, gratitude and changing negative thoughts into positive ones.
- **Find local mental health support:** Explore your student resources and locate counselling services (Directorate of Student Affairs), or other care providers *(see list).*
- **Grow and maintain support systems:** Get involved in campus life, meet new people and connect with positive people in your life.
- **Seek help!:** Don't wait until the problem escalates for you to seek help. Get professional help immediately if your symptoms or emotions are affecting concentration or functioning.

## STRATEGIES FOR MITIGATING RISK FACTORS FOR STUDENTS' MENTAL HEALTH IN HIGHER EDUCATION INSTITUTIONS

- **Act, belong and commit:** Act involves striving to keep yourself physically, socially and psychologically fit or as energetic as possible. Therefore, physical activities and exercise reduce anxiety, strain and frustration. Exercising also increases self-esteem. In addition, activities avail one of other individuals in non-clinical or greater geographical settings. Belong entails properly linking with the public or the society, meeting new friends, and talking to neighbours. Commit includes the ability to handle threats or challenges, and getting involved in societal issues and voluntarism.
- **Setting realistic attitudes:** Be pragmatic and cheerful; accept problems, difficulties and hardships and move on with life.
- **Self-esteem and confidence:** Instead of focusing on what you lack, you should target standards that make you a better individual, a respected colleague and a loveable family member and friend.
- **Maintaining emotional support:** Sustaining close bonds with family members, friends and the community to establish firm supportive connections for assistance, as well as assisting others.

Strategies for assisting students and higher education institutions with emotional or behavioural issues to enable students to deal with the mental health issues that may occur from educational, societal, lifestyle, cognitive and biological risk factors.

- **Day-dreaming and practising relaxation techniques:** Closing your eyes and meditating to move yourself into a dream situation, and practising slow, deep breathing techniques.

## SOLUTIONS AND RECOMMENDATIONS

To address the risk factors for students' mental health in higher education institutions and promote mental well-being among students the following is suggested:

1. Incorporating mental health education.

This strategy will aim to increase understanding of mental health issues, lessen the stigma associated with them, and give students the knowledge and abilities to better manage their own mental health and support others. It also gives students access to useful tools and techniques for stress management and resilience building. This can include time management techniques, relaxation exercises and mindfulness techniques. Additionally, students should be aware of the crisis hotlines, support groups and counselling services that are locally available and are accessible both on and off campus.

2. Mental health screening and assessment.

Mental health issues must be addressed effectively, whether in educational institutions or other settings. Mental health screening will help to identify students who may be at risk of various mental health conditions, such as depression, anxiety, or substance use disorders, at an early stage. Early identification allows for timely intervention and the prevention of more severe issues. By identifying students with emerging mental health issues, institutions can intervene before crises occur, reducing the risk of academic disruptions, dropout or serious health consequences.

3. Interactive learning.

Encourage real-life case studies and interactive role play to allow students to apply their knowledge and skills in practical scenarios. Also, invite mental health professionals, individuals with lived experience, or advocacy organisations to give guest lectures and share their insights and stories. This will help students develop self-awareness regarding their own mental health and well-being. Encourage self-reflection and self-assessment.

## FUTURE RESEARCH DIRECTIONS

Future research in the field of mental health among students in higher education institutions is essential for a better understanding, and addressing and preventing mental health challenges. Hence, a longitudinal study is encouraged in order to conduct a long-term study to track students' mental health from admission to graduation and beyond. This research can help identify trends, risk factors and protective factors that influence mental health problems over a period of time. Furthermore, future researchers are encouraged to investigate how cultural, racial and gender identities intersect with mental health experiences among students. Research should explore how different cultural backgrounds and identities impact stressors, coping mechanisms and help-seeking behaviours.

## CONCLUSION

There are factors which predisposes college students to stresses in society, particularly among undergraduates where mental wellbeing is often impaired and prevents individuals from making great social connections. Undergraduates often encounter mental disorder, which is concerning and prompts the examination of reasons behind this trend. Such reasons include the way students socialise with others, their thoughts and emotions, their body, their day-by-day propensities, and how well they do in school. Whether or not one does well at university is determined by distinctive feelings. When undergraduates feel disturbed or uncertain owing to things not going as they wished, it can make them feel on edge or down for a period of time, and they might later develop a chronic mental health condition. Moving to a new setting, like at a university, may require students to adjust to a distinctive way of living, which can in turn influence the way they live their everyday lives. Often, undergraduates engage in substance abuse which can be unsafe for them. An individual's family history of assets, long-term illnesses, and brain injury moreover lead increase risk of developing mental illness. So, society should act quickly to address the issues that can cause mental wellbeing issues for undergraduates, thus contributing to building a society which in the future will have great mental well-being. The content of this chapter can be used by the directorate of student support affairs in higher education institutions worldwide to develop targeted interventions and strategies for alleviating the risk factors of concern to the mental health of students in higher education institutions.

## REFERENCES

Acutt, J., & Hattingh, S. B. (2016). *Occupational health: Management and practice for health practitioners* (5th ed.). Juta.

Allott, K., & Lin, A. (2020). Cognitive risk factors for psychosis. *Risk Factors for Psychosis*, 269-287. doi:10.1016/B978-0-12-813201-2.00014-4

Ashipala, D. O., & Shilunga, A. P. (2023). Overview and Management of Anxiety. In *Acceleration of the Biopsychosocial Model in Public Health* (pp. 194–210). IGI Global.

Auerbach, R. P., Alonso, J., Axinn, W. G., Cuijpers, P., Ebert, D. D., Green, J. G., Hwang, I., Kessler, R. C., Liu, H., Mortier, P., Nock, M. K., Pinder-Amaker, S., Sampson, N. A., Aguilar-Gaxiola, S., Al-Hamzawi, A., Andrade, L. H., Benjet, C., Caldas-de-Almeida, J. M., Demyttenaere, K, & Bruffaerts, R. (2016). Mental disorders among college students in the World Health Organization world mental health surveys. *Psychological Medicine*, *46*(14), 2955–2970. doi:10.1017/S0033291716001665 PMID:27484622

Auerbach, R. P., Mortier, P., Bruffaerts, R., Alonso, J., Benjet, C., Cuijpers, P., Demyttenaere, K., Ebert, D. D., Green, J. G., Hasking, P., Murray, E., Nock, M. K., Pinder-Amaker, S., Sampson, N. A., Stein, D. J., Vilagut, G., Zaslavsky, A. M., & Kessler, R. C. (2018). WHO world mental health surveys international college student project: Prevalence and distribution of mental disorders. *Journal of Abnormal Psychology*, *127*(7), 623–638. doi:10.1037/abn0000362 PMID:30211576

BhatiaD.RoerigM.MaraniH.KingM.Morales-VazquezM.AllinS. (2020). *Rapid*.

Birhanu Ayalew, M. (2022). *Socialization experiences among undergraduate students in higher learning institutions (HLI)*. Higher Education - New Approaches to Accreditation, Digitalization, and Globalization in the Age of Covid. doi:10.5772/intechopen.99007

Cai, D., Zhu, M., Lin, M., Zhang, X. C., & Margraf, J. (2017). The bidirectional relationship between positive mental health and social rhythm in college students: A three-year longitudinal study. *Frontiers in Psychology*, *8*, 1119. doi:10.3389/fpsyg.2017.01119 PMID:28713318

Campbell, F., Blank, L., Cantrell, A., Baxter, S., Blackmore, C., Dixon, J., & Goyder, E. (2022). Factors that influence mental health of university and college students in the UK: A systematic review. *BMC Public Health*, *22*(1), 1–22. doi:10.118612889-022-13943-x PMID:36123714

Chernomas, W. M., & Shapiro, C. (2013). Stress, depression, and anxiety among undergraduate nursing students. *International Journal of Nursing Education Scholarship*, *10*(1), 255–266. doi:10.1515/ijnes-2012-0032 PMID:24200536

Dalton, J. (2022). A review of moral distress in nursing students: Causes and educational methods to address it. *Proceedings of the 2022 AERA Annual Meeting*. Aera. 10.3102/1892355

Dammeyer, J. (2018). *Mental health and psychosocial well-being in deaf and hard-of-Hearing students*. Oxford Scholarship Online. doi:10.1093/oso/9780190880545.003.0021

Daud, N., Norwani, N. M., & Yusof, R. (2018). Students financial problems in higher education institutions. *International Journal of Academic Research in Business & Social Sciences*, *8*(10). doi:10.6007/IJARBSS/v8-i10/5312

Delamater, A. M., Guzman, A., & Aparicio, K. (2017). Mental health issues in children and adolescents with chronic illness. *International Journal of Human Rights in Healthcare*, *10*(3), 163–173. doi:10.1108/IJHRH-05-2017-0020

Fares, J., Al Tabosh, H., Saadeddin, Z., El Mouhayyar, C., & Aridi, H. (2016). Stress, burnout and coping strategies in preclinical medical students. *North American Journal of Medical Sciences*, *8*(2), 75. doi:10.4103/1947-2714.177299 PMID:27042604

Grant, J. E., & Chamberlain, S. R. (2020). Family history of substance use disorders: Significance for mental health in young adults who gamble. *Journal of Behavioral Addictions*, *9*(2), 289–297. doi:10.1556/2006.2020.00017 PMID:32516117

Hassanzadeh, A., Heidari, Z., Feizi, A., Hassanzadeh Keshteli, A., Roohafza, H., Afshar, H., & Adibi, P. (2017). Association of stressful life events with psychological problems: A large-scale community-based study using grouped outcomes latent factor regression with latent predictors. *Computational and Mathematical Methods in Medicine*, *3457103*, 1–12. doi:10.1155/2017/3457103 PMID:29312459

Ishii, T., Tachikawa, H., Shiratori, Y., Hori, T., Aiba, M., Kuga, K., & Arai, T. (2018). What kinds of factors affect the academic outcomes of university students with mental disorders? A retrospective study based on medical records. *Asian Journal of Psychiatry*, *32*, 67–72. doi:10.1016/j.ajp.2017.11.017 PMID:29216609

Jochman, J. C., Cheadle, J. E., Goosby, B. J., Tomaso, C., Kozikowski, C., & Nelson, T. (2019). Mental health outcomes of discrimination among college students on a predominately White campus: A prospective study. *Socius: Sociological Research for a Dynamic World, 5*, 1–16. doi:10.1177/2378023119842728 PMID:31819906

Kandasamy, N., Indraah, K., Tukiman, N. A., Khalil Kusairi, F. W. K., Amir Sjarif, S. I., & Shahrul Nizar, M. S. S. (2020). Factors that influence mental illness among students in public universities. *Journal of Business and Economic Analysis, 3*(1), 77–90. doi:10.1142/j_10.36924sbe.2020.3106

Kenney, M., & Müller, R. (2017). Of rats and women: Narratives of motherhood in environmental epigenetics. *Biosocieties, 12*(1), 23–46. doi:10.105741292-016-0002-7

Kindred, R., & Bates, G. W. (2023). The Influence of the COVID-19 Pandemic on Social Anxiety: A Systematic Review. *International Journal of Environmental Research and Public Health, 20*(3), 2362. doi:10.3390/ijerph20032362 PMID:36767728

Kiziela, A., Viliūnienė, R., Friborg, O., & Navickas, A. (2018). Distress and resilience associated with workload of medical students. *Journal of Mental Health (Abingdon, England), 28*(3), 319–323. doi:10.1080/09638237.2018.1521922 PMID:30449227

Kumar, N. (2022). Mental health and well-being. Mental. *Applied Psychology. Health and Well-Being*, 1–23. doi:10.4324/9781003350651-1

Larson, L. R., Mullenbach, L. E., Browning, M. H., Rigolon, A., Thomsen, J., Metcalf, E. C., Reigner, N. P., Sharaievska, I., McAnirlin, O., D'Antonio, A., Cloutier, S., Helbich, M., & Labib, S. M. (2022). Greenspace and park use associated with less emotional distress among college students in the United States during the COVID-19 pandemic. *Environmental Research, 204*, 112367. doi:10.1016/j.envres.2021.112367 PMID:34774510

Lattie, E. G., Cohen, K. A., Hersch, E., Williams, K. D., Kruzan, K. P., MacIver, C., Hermes, J., Maddi, K., Kwasny, M., & Mohr, D. C. (2022). Uptake and effectiveness of a self-guided mobile app platform for college student mental health. *Internet Interventions : the Application of Information Technology in Mental and Behavioural Health, 27*, 100493. doi:10.1016/j.invent.2021.100493 PMID:35036331

Lim, A. Y., Lee, S. H., Jeon, Y., Yoo, R., & Jung, H. Y. (2018). Job-seeking stress, mental health problems, and the role of perceived social support in university graduates in Korea. *Journal of Korean Medical Science, 33*(19), e149. doi:10.3346/jkms.2018.33.e149 PMID:29736162

Limone, P., & Toto, G. A. (2021). Psychological and emotional effects of digital technology on children in Covid-19 pandemic. *Brain Sciences, 11*(9), 1126. doi:10.3390/brainsci11091126 PMID:34573148

Limone, P., & Toto, G. A. (2022). Factors that predispose undergraduates to mental issues: A cumulative literature review for future research perspectives. *Frontiers in Public Health, 10*, 10. doi:10.3389/fpubh.2022.831349 PMID:35252101

Limone, P., Zeffferino, R., Toto, G. A., & Tomei, G. (2021). Work stress, mental health and validation of professional stress scale (PSS) in an Italian-speaking teachers' sample. *Healthcare (Basel), 9*(11), 1434. doi:10.3390/healthcare9111434 PMID:34828481

Loades, M. E., Chatburn, E., Higson-Sweeney, N., Reynolds, S., Shafran, R., Brigden, A., Linney, C., McManus, M. N., Borwick, C., & Crawley, E. (2020). Rapid systematic review: The impact of social isolation and loneliness on the mental health of children and adolescents in the context of COVID-19. *Journal of the American Academy of Child and Adolescent Psychiatry, 59*(11), 1218–1239. doi:10.1016/j.jaac.2020.05.009 PMID:32504808

McKinnon-Crowley, S. (2021). College belonging: How first-year and first-generation college students navigate campus life by Lisa M. Nunn. *Review of Higher Education, 45*(2), 270–273. doi:10.1353/rhe.2021.0024

Mofatteh, M. (2021). Risk factors associated with stress, anxiety, and depression among university undergraduate students. *AIMS Public Health, 8*(1), 36–65. doi:10.3934/publichealth.2021004 PMID:33575406

O'Keeffe, P., Haralambous, B., Egan, R., Heales, E., Baskarathas, S., Thompson, S., & Jerono, C. (2023). Reimagining social work placements in the COVID-19 pandemic. *British Journal of Social Work, 53*(1), 448–470. doi:10.1093/bjsw/bcac124

Panahi, R. (2018). The factors associated to high risk behaviors in Sanandaj city students based on health belief model. *Journal of Health Education and Health Promotion*, 393-402. doi:10.30699/acadpub.ijhehp.6.4.393

Pedersen, A. L., Lindekilde, C. R., Andersen, K., Hjorth, P., & Gildberg, F. A. (2020). Health behaviours of forensic mental health service users, in relation to smoking, alcohol consumption, dietary behaviours and physical activity—A mixed methods systematic review. *Journal of Psychiatric and Mental Health Nursing, 28*(3), 444–461. doi:10.1111/jpm.12688 PMID:32916759

Rosenthal, S. R., Clark, M. A., Marshall, B. D., Buka, S. L., Carey, K. B., Shepardson, R. L., & Carey, M. P. (2018). Alcohol consequences, not quantity, predict major depression onset among first-year female college students. *Addictive Behaviors, 85*, 70–76. doi:10.1016/j.addbeh.2018.05.021 PMID:29860191

Ruzhenkova, V. V. (2020). Prevalence and dynamics of depression and anxiety in local and foreign medical students for a 6- year training period. *International Journal of Early Childhood Special Education, 12*(1), 606–611. doi:10.9756/INT-JECSE/V12I1.201044

Skilbred-Fjeld, S., Reme, S. E., & Mossige, S. (2020). Cyberbullying involvement and mental health problems among late adolescents. *Cyberpsychology (Brno), 14*(1), 1–16. doi:10.5817/CP2020-1-5

Teague, R. G. (2023). Infusing KM in global higher education: How effective KM program supports critical tacit knowledge retention within a US higher education institution. In L. J. Jones-Esan, V. Nadda, & K. S. Albright (Eds.), *Knowledge management and research innovation in global higher education institutions* (pp. 236–250). IGI Global.

Wren-Lewis, S., & Alexandrova, A. (2021, December). Mental health without well-being. *Journal of Medicine and Philosophy: A Forum for Bioethics and Philosophy of Medicine, 46*(6), 684–703.

## KEY TERM DEFINITIONS

**Achievement:** The act of successfully completing a task, reaching a goal, or attaining a specific result, often through effort, skill or determination (*Higher Education*, 2023).

**Higher Education Institutions:** A higher education institution encompasses various types of education delivered in postsecondary institutions of learning and usually awarding, at the end of a course of study, a named degree, diploma, or certificate of higher studies. Higher education institutions include universities and colleges and various professional schools that prepare students for law, theology, medicine, business, music, and art. Higher education institutions also include teacher-training schools, junior colleges, and institutes of technology (Teague, 2023).

**Mental Health:** Mental health is a state of complete well-being that enables the fulfilment of one's full potential in occupational, social and relational functioning (Kumar, 2022).

**Risk Factors:** Refers to attributes, characteristics or exposures that increase an individual's likelihood of academic failure or failure to complete high school.

**Student:** One who is enrolled or attends classes at a school, college or university.

# Chapter 6
# External Factors Affecting the Well-Being of Students in Higher Education Institutions

**Pamela Awuor Onyango**
*University of Nairobi, Kenya*

## ABSTRACT

*Studies have revealed that several factors affect the well-being of students in higher education institutions. The current chapter investigates some of the factors which include sexual harassment, student unrest, role of the family, and institutional environment. The main purpose of this chapter is to explore how the factors affect the well being of learners in higher education institutions. The chapter presents introduction of the study, its background, as well as the external factors affecting well being of students in higher education institutions together with future direction and the conclusion of the study.*

## INTRODUCTION

Advancing learner well being has become an important Educational agenda globally as a result of its broad benefits (Joing et al., 2020). Consequently, studies show that several learners in Higher Education encounter well being issues like depression and anxiety, psychological and emotional distress and heightened burnout (Baik et al., 2019). Universities are widely acknowledged as institutions where health and well-being can be nurtured to boost academic output, career transitions and enduring desirable health behaviours (Sanci et al. 2022). These Institutions are conscious of the need to assist and advance the health and well-being of learners to enhance opportunities for educational success and readiness to progress to the workforce (Duffy et al., 2019). The current study therefore intends to investigate the external factors affecting well-being of students in Higher Education Institutions by giving the background of the study in the next section.

DOI: 10.4018/979-8-3693-2833-0.ch006

## BACKGROUND

There is need to acknowledge the physical, societal, emotive and intellectual condition of learners in institutions, since this contributes to their well-being (Anderson & Graham, 2016). Scientists have endeavoured to portray the intricacy of the humanistic and philosophical nature of well being (Hascher & Waber, 2021). Well being is regarded as a condition of having constructive feelings and acquiring the ability realize one's full potential (Simons & Baldwins, 2021). In a study done by Anderson and Graham (2016), well-being was used to refer to mental, physical and social dimensions that need to be balanced, and that learners conceive their well-being as being loved, respected, happy, safe and healthy. Some scholars indicate that there is no common definition of well-being because the context and connotation depends on each individual, community and culture (Agrawal & Sharma, 2021). There are others who believe that there is a common consensus regarding the significance of student well-being despite the fact that a comprehensible definition of 'well- being' has not yet been realized (Douwes, 2023). Universities across the globe are facing a predicament of well-being (Riva et al., 2020). On the whole, school life remains paramount because through it, the learners interact and produce a cultural fusion that originates from the family, territorial, national and institutional influences (Wang et al., 2018). Therefore, there is need to scrutinize external factors which affect well being of students in Higher Education Institutions. The next section gives a general overview regarding external factors affecting well-being of students in Higher Education Institutions.

## EXTERNAL FACTORS AFFECTING WELL-BEING OF STUDENTS IN HIGHER EDUCATION INSTITUTIONS

Although University Education is important and lucrative, learners face several challenges and obstacles as they pursue their education (Luescher et al., 2017). Since learners require a positive learning experience (Durisic & Bunijevac, 2017), universities need to support their well-being in order to realize their fundamental aim of offering high quality academic experiences and successful graduation outcomes (Baik et al., 2019). Higher education plays a very important role in enabling the youth to engage in social reconstruction and economic development (Bijaraniya, 2022). Therefore, learners' well-being becomes a critical factor, as well as connection to a myriad of desirable outcomes related to academia and health (Amholt et al., 2020). The well-being of learners has consistently been associated with satisfaction or experiences within Higher Education (Wornast, 2018). Children visualize well-being as favourable experiences in their life (Vujcic et al., 2019). The next section explores four external factors which affect the well being of student in Higher Education Institutions, namely sexual harassment, student unrest, role of the family and institutional environment.

## SEXUAL HARASSMENT

Sexual harassment refers to a collection of behaviours and practices which are sexual in nature like sexual jokes, undesirable sexual advances or utterances, showing pictures or posters representing women, sexual assault or physical contact (Vuckovic et al., 2017). The act is also perceived as behavior in the form of undesirable comments or physical approach in the public space (Suprihatin & Azis, 2020). Sexual harassment is also regarded as any unwanted sexual advance, unsolicited request for sexual favour, physical or verbal conduct or gesture which is sexual in nature or any other conduct of sexual description that might logically be perceived or expected to give rise to offense, intimidation or humiliation of the person (WHO, 2016). Nevertheless, Gyawal (2021) contends that there are several acts which are considered as sexual harassment, and that it is not easy to come across a single most meaning. According to Galdi and Guizzo (2021), sexual harassment is sometimes performed non-verbally through winking, verbally by calling pet names or physically in the form of touch. Orfan et al., (2022) contend that sexual harassment can also be executed online and offline. Other forms of sexual harassment include verbal expression of sexual suggestion where male learners make undesirable sexual jokes to the female learners who are indeed disinterested. These may also involve sending WhatsApp messages, asking for sex, physical undesired touches, physical attempts of rape and sending of verbal sexual images (Ayo, 2019). Findings by Klein et al., (2022) demonstrate that sexual misconduct tends to focus on acquaintance rape without paying attention to less highly noticeable forms of harm. Sexual harassment is a contemporary silent issue in the academic setting (Saiman, 2018) which may be a product of power gap between men and women in social circumstances (Weinberg & Nielsen, 2017).

Sexual violence amongst university and college students is a common problem which needs serious attention by administrators, academics and policy makers (Perez- Trujillo, 2019). The vice has gained the attention of researchers globally due to the increase in incidences of sexual violations that are reported in Educational Institutions (Naom, 2020). The structures of the university consist of a combination of formal relations (like professional rank, institutional hierarchy, and student teacher correspondence) and informal power relations like career success which are possible areas of investigating sexual harassment among employee and students who share a similar context (Agardh et. al., 2022). According to Bezabeh (2016), sexual harassment in learning institutions is an inappropriate part of learning encounter which is not new. It pervades institutions of Higher Education worldwide where it affects individuals, groups and organizations (Bondestan & Lundqvisk, 2020). Not to mention, sexual harassment has been recognized as a common public health problem which is masked in most organizations (Oni et al., 2019). Study findings by Srikanth (2018) reveal that sexual harassment is the demonstration of harmful relationship which is considered as a breach of dignity, right to equality and right to social security pledged to human beings in every social organization and also a contravention of peaceful existence and right to life warranted by the law. Coupled with discrimination, sexual harassment is deemed to be closely linked to several chronic stressors that need to be incorporated alongside cumulative adversity so that the marginalized groups are fully represented (Jirek et al., 2018). Surprisingly, sexual harassment has been underreported because it is not viewed as a breach of human rights in the Institutions of Higher learning (Bondestan & Lundqvisk, 2020).

Research indicates that sexual harassment may as well take place anywhere including university and workplace and mostly involves anyone who has the opportunity to carry out the evildoing (Putrah, 2023). The context of the college places students at risk of lowered parental monitoring, escalated use of alcohol, heightened sexual vulnerability to peer norms about sexual violence (Mellins et al., 2017). It is evident that sexual harassment causes numerous effects to the learner and the integrity of the university (Ayo, 2019). Students who have experienced sexual harassment are much more likely to feel endangered by sexual misconduct and to exhibit negative views of its responses as compared to none harassed ones (Klein et al., 2022). Nine out of ten countries in the world have laws against sexual harassment but six out of ten do not have sufficient laws regarding it in schools and higher education (Tavares & Wodon, 2018). Originally, sexual harassment was perceived as women's encounter with unpopular workplace sexual attention (Wood et al, 2018). Other study findings indicate that both men and women are targets of sexual harassment although evidence shows that such harassment is predominantly aimed at women (Quick & Mcfadyen, 2017). All in all, study findings still indicate that women encounter sexual harassment quite often, as compared to men (Rosenthal et al., 2016). Studies by Wood et al. (2021) indicate that most sexual harassers tend to be men. Several students who are sexually harassed rarely achieve academic satisfaction (Rosenthal et al., 2016). This may be because sexual harassment negatively affects class attendance as those who encounter it take a relatively longer time before resuming classes and also find it difficult to concentrate in class (Ayo, 2019). Further, institutional circumstances cause victimization of female learners who are poor academically and hence easily lend themselves to immoral acts in exchange of success in academic performance, just like learners who have weak moral values that engage in sexual manipulation by institutional teachers (Mshenga, 2022).

Gender based violence and sexual harassment in Higher Education are perceived as symptoms of institutional failure (Drazoa, 2018). Recently, a systematic review scrutinized sexual harassment in Higher Education and the results indicated that exposed learners were likely to face post-traumatic stress disorder, impaired career opportunities, anxiety and increased alcohol use as part of the consequences (Bondestam & Lundqvist, 2020). In a study conducted by Gyawali (2021), it was found that sexual harassment of learners by teachers, relatives, neighbours, friends and peers leads to insomnia, humiliation, tension, frustration, irritation and fear. Supplementary observation by Bezabeh (2016) indicates that sexual harassment agitates the learners' physical and psychological well-being as well as academic achievement. Other effects of sexual harassment include trauma, stress, anxiety, frustration and irritation of the victims (Utkina & Efimova, 2022). Sexual harassment is linked to undesirable well being indicators like suicidality, substance use and depression, and stakeholders need to recognize its possible consequences for the learner well being (Crowley et al., 2021). Researchers contend that sexual harassment is a heightening epidemic in schools in most countries and view it therefore as a dangerous factor for long lasting complications like low self-esteem (Ondicho et al., 2018). It is important to recognize that the relationship between sexual violence and depression is well understood although the temporal features of the connection have not been well demonstrated (Tsai et al., 2016). This section concludes by exploring some recommendations which may be useful in addressing sexual harassment. Firstly, the interrogation of the cardinal processes of sexual harassment which involve characteristics and incentives of the perpetrators, forms one step towards addressing sexual harassment (Voth Schrag, 2017). Other suggestions have been put forward for the need to constitute consistent definitions of the diverse types of sexual violence and sexual harassment to ease the understanding of widespread presence and differences in commonness and the composition of preventive measures (Fedina, Holmes, and Backes, 2018). Lastly, provision of help and support in the form of rehabilitation and follow up for individuals who encounter sexual harassment is paramount (Bondestam and Lundqvist, 2020). The next section explores how student unrest affects well being of students in higher education istitutions.

## STUDENT UNREST

Students form the foundation of the growth and future of a country, and are expected to lead a disciplined life since the future of a country depends on them (Das, 2017). They constitute a meaningful societal class because they have a very significant role to play and each nation considers them as the hope of tomorrow (Choudhary, 2018). Universities worldwide have been experiencing growth in student unrest

(Thamtanajit, 2022) despite the fact that calmness is key to the prosperity of any entity (Nyamberega, 2018). According to Etaneki and Okolie (2020), university learners protest is a global occurrence which is bothersome to parents, the government and the learners too. The problem of indiscipline and unrest amongst students has grown alarmingly, reflecting emerging disorder in the society and manifesting itself in the form of agitations and antisocial behaviour (Das, 2017). Student unrest is considered as deliberate, disruptive, destructive and contradictory behavior of learners in universities, who destroy property due to demand on particular issues from institutional authority (Anho et al., 2023). According to Oyoo (2017), university unrest is common across the globe, although it is pronounced more in the developing countries. Falki (2021) also believes that the greatest problem facing Higher Education is student unrest. If there is anything predictable among Higher Institution learners, it is the fact that they are bound to riot in any academic session, leading to constant closure of institutions, which negatively affects curriculum coverage (Davies et al., 2016). Universities worldwide have gone through crises beyond social and organizational unrests (Omodan & Dube, 2019). The most pronounced among them being the one masterminded by students and their leaders, who often view the university management as an authority that must be challenged in order to listen to them (Bunni, 2020). Students in all categories of learning institutions such as universities, professional colleges, degree colleges and higher secondary schools seem to be involved in violent activities which interrupt the educational environment (Das, 2017). The unrests are downgrading and unpleasant yet as they plan the episode, the students forget that education as a process, involves a number of investment levels (Segametsi, 2017). Student discipline and unrest has unquestionably acquired alarming proportions and turned out to be a serious matter for parents, educationists, administrators and the entire society (Choudhary, 2018). Research findings indicate that universities worldwide have experienced crises, in addition to social and organizational dissatisfaction among university authorities, staff unions and student unions (Omodan & Dube, 2019). The violent protests are a universal occurrence which leads to anxiety, destruction of property and injury to people (Langley, 2018). Instant implications are usually on the learners themselves who always report that they feel stressed and anxious in the midst of unrest, in addition to symptoms of stress disorder (Ni et al., 2020).

According to Odebode (2018), the reasons for student protests are quite many, and numerous studies attribute the causes to a wide range of internal and external factors which could be predominantly related to the institutional system or based on pressing and trending matters in the society and universal community. Twenge et al. (2021) suggest that learner protests demonstrate the deep seated dissatisfaction they feel about the state of Higher Education as they increasingly speak about issues which matter to them, which is an admirable commitment to justice, but may affect the students' psychological behavior. Choudhary (2018) thinks that student unrest is caused by the poor and deteriorating conditions of the university and low administrative and academic standards which generate perennial acts of indiscipline among the learners.

Most of the protests in institutions of higher learning are linked to university management methods with diverse charges that the university officials are predominantly autocratic in their association with their subordinates (Omodan, 2016). The constant dissatisfaction of students which results from disagreements between students and institutional authority has caused deaths, destruction of property and lengthened academic sessions (Akparep, 2019). Students engage in turbulence, strikes, boycott of classes, arson, violence and destruction of property. Additionally, they use unjustified means to acquire examinations and tests, abuse the teachers, break or burn institutional property, intimidate invigilators and also insult staff in the name of demanding for rights and freedom, which is either legitimate or illegitimate (Falki,

2021). Additional findings by Das (2017) indicate that student indiscipline and unrest also takes the form of sexual assault, rioting, stealing, lying drug abuse, and many more.

The most instant implication of unrest is usually on the learners, as some experience stress disorder symptoms (Rink & Lipinska, 2020). The long lived effects of unrest can be disastrous, as they can cause reduced enrolment, dropout and lowered recognition and trust by the society, which may destroy the reputation of the university, leading to difficulty in attracting faculty and top students (Klemenčič & Park, 2018). It is also important to note that student unrest negatively affects academic achievement because it causes vandalization of property; learners interrupt peace, interfere with infrastructural development, engage in illegal activities within the tertiary institutions that interfere with academic accomplishments (Chikendu, 2022). Study findings by Sanjay (2019) established that student unrest affects the whole society because the learners develop anxiety and frustration and the parents and guardians are not quite aware when exactly their children will complete the degree course due to interruption. Potgieter et al. (2019) also believe the psychological connotation of student unrest is not only confined to the students but to all stakeholders as well as the identity of such institutions. Other outcomes of student unrest include death, destruction of property and fluctuation of the university calendar (Onivehu, 2021). Furthermore, failure in student protest negotiations has destabilized campus life and interfered with teaching and learning (Langley, 2018). Student dissatisfaction and frustration has also degraded student teacher relationship (Das, 2017).

Research findings in a study conducted by Chiluba (2019) established that the consequences of student protest were violence, dismantling of property, interference with academic activities, undertaking the examinations without completion of the course outline, punishment and suspension of learners and their leaders. Chikendu (2022) established that student dissatisfaction leads to the establishment of criminal gangs, low academic performance, breaking of laws and regulation and engagement in cultism. Davies et al. (2016) attest that upon graduation, some employers consider the graduates as half-baked and unemployable people who need to be subjected to a sequence of teaching and training in order to measure up to the required standards as a result of several factors like student unrest. Finally, Alorani and Alradaydeh (2018) recommend the need to take care of learners' psychological needs holistically and effectively. The university authorities and management also need to engage consensus building, collaborative management style, teamwork and organizational relationship in the management process to alleviate social unrest, which leads to the realization of peace and calmness(Omodan, 2023). According to Birya (2020), collegial relationships among university stakeholders may lead to improved cooperation and communication, which can be used to resolve disputes before they escalate into crises. The next section deals with the role of the family in the well being of students in higher education institutions.

## ROLE OF THE FAMILY

The word 'family' generally includes children, parents, siblings, extended members of the family (Jabbari &Rouster, 2023). According to Kustiani and Fauziyah (2019) the family is a composition of father, mother and children only. On the contrary, Khatoom and Sharma (2021) believe that the family is made up of either parents and their children only or parents, children and relatives who live together. Some scholars argue that the family is made up of relatives and beloved ones who elicit positive relationships (Zhigunova, 2017). Even so, the family is the primary social establishment in the society whose function is to produce upcoming generation, to provide love and affection to the children and to facilitate the socialization process (Upali, 2017). It is also considered as a small society that reflects how the composition of the developing family life will influence the organization of future community life (Astuti et al., 2017). Although the well being of children is marjorly the responsibility of the family, the conventional role it undertakes has changed extraordinarily as a result of various interconnected factors (Upali, 2017).

Family connections are persistent and significant for well being across lifetime (Thomas et al., 2017). Therefore, learners need a very stable family environment, for it positively influences their quality of life (Chavez et al., 2018). The students' psychological well-being is strengthened by increased social support (Abaid et al., 2020) and the parents and family members play an important role in determining the character and nature of children (Maunah, 2019). Furthermore, the family relationship is important conditioning factors for adolescent well-being (McMahon et al., 2020). The family continues supporting the lives of young people as they transit to adulthood because they still depend on their parents (Lindell et al., 2018). Adolescents who are brought up in extremely unstable family contexts achieve poor developmental outcomes (Thomas et al., 2017).

To a greater extent, the family is regarded as the initial and one of the most prominent institutions in shaping the life of an individual (Sowani & Lavalekar, 2020). Other than that, the family has been entrusted with the responsibility of ensuring that learners achieve a status of well-being (Upali, 2017). It also influences the composition of human values and its social values are linked to the socialization and development of value based familiarization of young people (Lazurenko, et al., 2021). Supportive and secure family interconnections provide advice, care and love while conversely, stressful family associations are weighed down with erroneous demands and repeated critical feedback (Gunn & Eberhardt, 2019). The association of children with other people, their emotional response to social situations and performance of actions proposed by adults is mostly influenced by the family (Busyigina et al., 2019).

The involvement of the family in educational matters plays a very important role in the development of children, and parents need to create a conducive atmosphere which fosters the development of their potential and self-confidence (Wulandary, 2017). Empirical studies indicate that parental support accounts for a vital ingredient that strengthens learners' physical well-being, psychological well-being and self-worth (Thomas et al., 2017). Other studies have also highlighted the importance of family environment in strengthening the psychological well-being of its members (Sowani & Lavalekar, 2020). Literally, involvement of parents is used to refer to the motivated participation of parents in several activities that are geared towards promoting development and learning of their children (Ma et al., 2016). This is because early adulthood is a significant short-lived period of life during which the youth mould their independent identity as their connections with other family members become intricate (Sowani & Lavalekar, 2020). Parental involvement can be investigated in keeping with the realms of their association with their children either at home or at school (Hornby & Blackwell, 2018). Parents who are enthusiastically involved in the education of their children positively influence their levels of motivation, behavior and achievement (Taseer, 2023).

Emotional support gained from the family is beneficial in educational outcomes because it strengthens psychological well-being and helps much in learners' engagement (Roksa & Kinsley, 2019). Other study findings also indicate that family support is the most essential social support across all ages and plays a significant role in determining the mental health of college students (Newhart, 2019). Moreover, Gans and Johnson (2016) strongly support the impact of family functioning on the adjustment of college students. Newhart (2019) believes that particular family relationships like attachment affect the adjustment of students to college. Arshad and Shahzadi (2016) believe that the family has immense accountability in socializing children to become groomed, productive and educated societal members. Attitudes of family members and friends can impact on a learner's motivation, persistence and success in college in addition to influencing the student's learning, especially if their beliefs are incompatible with the practices in the college environment (Green et al., 2017). Over and above that, a highly adjusted family function which is grounded on close relationship between parents and their children contributes to a fairly positive, balanced development and an increased level of well-being (King et al., 2018).

According to Kayla et al. (2018), the influence of the family affects the entire family, especially children, adolescents once they leave home. Gasper et al. (2021) posit that families which have resilient skills and social support contribute to better child well- being. Equivalently, adolescence well-being thrives on parent–child relationship which is based on communication, trust and absence of alienation (Monaco, 2019). A family environment that promotes development and quality of life of adolescents needs to inculcate good communication (Bireda, 2017). Parents too play an important role in influencing the well-being of children (Fallesen & Gähler, 2020) since they provide social support in the form of facilitation, inspiration and also involve themselves in activities with their children (Kalya et al. 2018). Finally, research indicates that parents are the key players in the lives of children and their main objective is to institute an active care giver role in them (Rafferty et al., 2020). The current study recommends the need to attempt to achieve a good family well being with negligible conflict, open communication and close emotional connectedness, as this produces individuals who are mentally and physically healthy (Gunn & Eberhardt, 2019). There is also need to ensure that the learner receives positive family support, since this turns out to be a predictor of learning effectiveness that provides motivation and engagement, especially during pandemics (Yang et al., 2022). Parents should be warm and supportive because this mitigates the influences of family financial constrains on mental health challenges in early and middle childhood, with top levels of supportive- parent child association, which is a very significant prediction of child development (Kirby et al, 2020). The next section explores the role of institutional environment in the well being of students in higher education institutions .

## INSTITUTIONAL ENVIRONMENT

According to Barden and Caleb (2019), a learner's overall experience in Higher Education is strongly influenced by the learning experiences and teaching environment. Various researchers believe that Universities are environments that support and amplify the well being of learners (Riva et al., 2020). Furthermore, research indicates that there are two dimensions of the institutional environment; the first emphasizes factors which promote the teaching and learning process like the organization of the school climate and teacher quality while the second one concerns interpersonal relationships like coexistence between tutors and learner, and the learners and their peers (Wang, & Degol, 2016). Other research findings also indicate that the institutional environment consists of common constituents which are related to either safety or physical comfort, dedication and support networks between teachers and the learners (Shukla et al., 2019). The interactions which arise from school life can be visualized as school climate, which points out how individuals perceive the emotional, social, physical environment of an institution, coupled with association among diverse members of the community, like the policies, norms and activities that guide institutions including constructs like safety, academic expectations, inclusion and social support (Wang et al. 2018). Further, Rudasill et al. (2018) perceive the school climate as the cognitive and affective perceptions with reference to social interactions relationships, safety, beliefs and values. Muhammad (2020) believes that the learning environment is anything related to education concerning the institution like classmates, relationship with tutors and the culture of the program. Research findings by Kurniawati and Hafina (2020) indicate that studies about climate in institutional contexts analyze the classroom set up, which can be viewed as the kind of environment designed by teachers and learners in addition to the psychosocial features of classroom life. According to Adan et al. (2022), institutional environment refers to a combination of formal laws, institutional norms, teaching methodology, rules and regulations, customs, values and behavior. Some reseaarchers believe that there is neither a single meaning ascribed to school climate construct nor a general definition although others have opted for a theoretical and abstract definition (Grazia & Molinari, 2021). Others also argue that although the significance of school climate is acknowledged, there are neither common consent regarding the variables which constitute it nor how to measure them (Grazia and Molinari, 2021).

Since learners spend most of their life in the institutions, the quality of the environment is quite important (Bakır-Ayğar &. Kaya, 2017). The learning environment is dictated by the institutional climate, which is considered as the nature of relationship among individuals in an institution (Kalkan & Dagli, 2021). It is crucial to establish the influence of the teaching and learning conditions and experiences as well as the association between learners and staff on learner well being (Riva et al., 2020). Learner- instructor associations are considered as significant and essential expressive mutual associations that can be blossomed to nurture purposeful and enduring communication (Wang & Guan, 2020). As a result, teacher learner rapport is reasonably significant for the success of the learner because it creates a feeling of attachment and safety in addition to feelings of encouragement and respect from educators, which makes the learners eager to attain emotional, educational, behavioural and intellectual objective (Rafsanjani et al., 2019). Clearness, affirmation, proximity, affection, hilarity, friendship to learners and compliment are examples of behaviors that teachers may use to communicate positively to learners (Frisby, 2019). It is agreeable that favourable teacher- learner interpersonal associations strongly facilitate widespread worthwhile student teacher related end results which include well-being, hope, success, motivation, achievement, learning, engagement, among many others (Havik & Westergård, 2020) because teaching is a profession which is relational (McIntyre et al., 2020). The association between learners and tutors is significant because both are tasked with the responsibility of realizing a successful instructional and leaning exercise (Delos & Torio, 2021). A healthy school environment can emphatically impact on the learners' resilience, well-being and moral identity (Rieki et al., 2017).

Improving the institutional climate can be a game plan to improve the learner self-efficacy and other features of learner well-being (Wong, et al., 2021). The learning environment can also influence a learner's psychological well-being (Muhammad, 2020). There exists a positive relationship between learning environment and academic achievement, and learners who acquire positive perception of their learning environment realize improved academic achievement (Jaffery & Kishwar, 2019). Likewise, Bakır-Ayğar and Kaya (2017) affirm that learners' perception of the institutional climate is positively related to their school belonging. Kalkan and Dağlı (2021) posit that students who have a sense of belonging to the school develop heathy relationships with their companions and teachers. Garcia (2020) also postulates that institutions with positive institutional climate have limited behavioural problems, heightened academic achievement and school commitment. Similar study findings also demonstrate that a healthy school climate reduces learner misconduct and classroom misbehavior (Martinez et al., 2020), institutional violations (Magier et al. 2020) and negative attitude (Charlton et al., 2021). According to Reaves et al. (2018), a good institutional climate prevents undesirable consequences like problem behaviours. A humble, comprehensives, caring and safe learning context inspires learners' well-being (Schonert-Reichl &Kimberly 2017). Good peer relationship and communication can be improved in the institutional environment by fostering quality cooperation, which is important in realizing goals that are shared by cooperative group members (Blair& Perry, 2019). Another recommendation from Zhao et al. (2017) indicates that if social support is utilized, it may foster the realization of peer relationships, since this makes individuals develop a sense of trust in others, which ultimately impacts on their interpersonal relationships that heightens the development of prosocial behaviours.

## FUTURE RESEARCH DIRECTION

There is need for intensified research regarding all the possible factors that affect the well being of students in Higher Education Institution as well as how to address ensuing challenges. Causes of sexual harassment like limited financial dependence, especially for women, need to be handled with the importance they deserve. Stakeholders in education should work around all the matters that appertain to the welfare of learners and address their concerns before matters get out of hand. The association between family members needs to be fruitful because it plays a very significant role in the learner well being. Families need to accommodate the needs of the learners through out. Finally, the study recommends that Institutions of Higher learning should ensure that all mechanisms that enable smooth learner adjustment in the Institution are put in place.

## CONCLUSION

The current chapter may not exhaust the external factors which affect the well being of students in Higher Education since they are are quite numerous. Firstly, sexual harassment has been singled out as a serious public health menace which is covert in Institutions (Oni et al., 2019). Secondly, student unrest is a problem which poses diverse implications on institutional management (Anho et al., 2023). Thirdly, there are many family processes that impact on the whole family, the most affected being the children (Kayala et al., 2018). In conclusion therefore, the current study recommends the need for thorough investigation of external factors which affect learners in Institutions of Higher learning and implementation of remedies towards the challenges faced by the students.

## REFERENCES

Acosta, J., Chinman, P., Ebener, P., Malone, A., Phillips, A., & Wilks, A. (2019). Understanding the relationship between perceived school climate and bullying: A mediator analysis. *Journal of School Violence*, *18*(2), 200–215. doi:10.1080/15388220.2018.1453820 PMID:30778279

Adan, M., Ansari, A., & Yasmeen, B. (2022). The effects of institutional environment on academic performance at higher level of learning: A case of Punjab University Lahore. *Bulletin of Business and Economics*, *11*(1), 104–112.

Agardh, A., Priebe, G., Emmelin, M., & Palmiere, J. (2020). Sexual harassment among employees and students at a large Swedish university: Who are exposed, to what, by whom and where – a cross-sectional prevalence study. *BMC Public Health*, *22*(1), 1–14. PMID:31898494

Agrawal, S., & Sharma, N. (2021). *Barriers and role of higher educational institutes in students' mental well-being: A critical analysis*. Atlantis Press International.

Akparep, J. (2019). An examination of the causes of students-management conflicts in university for development studies from 1999 to 2009 January. *Open Journal of Leadership*, *8*(2), 75–94. doi:10.4236/ojl.2019.82005

Alorani, O., & Alradaydeh, M. (2018). Spiritual well-being, perceived social support, and life satisfaction among university students. *International Journal of Adolescence and Youth*, *23*(3), 291–298. doi:10.1080/02673843.2017.1352522

Amholt, T., Dammeyer, J., Carter, R., & Niclasen, J. (2020). *Child indicators research*. Springer.

Anderson, D. L., & Graham, A. P. (2016). Improving student wellbeing: Having a say at school. *school effectiveness and school improvement, 27*(3), 348-366.

Anho, J., Kporhobo, J., & Aweto, J. (2023). Students unrest in Nigerian universities: Types, causes and administrative strategies to the challenges. *World Journal of Advanced Research and Reviews*, *18*(03), 376–385. doi:10.30574/wjarr.2023.18.3.1072

Arshad, M., Shahzadi, E., & Mahmood, A. (2016). Parents Involvement at University Level Education: Students Perception in Under Developing Country. *European Scientific Journal*, *12*(22), 294–304. doi:10.19044/esj.2016.v12n22p294

Astuti, B., Sugiyatno, S., & Aminah, S. (2017). The development of early childhood sex education materials for early childhood education (ECE) teachers. [Jurnal Pendidikan dan Pemberdayaan Masyarakat]. *JPPM*, *4*(2), 113–120. doi:10.21831/jppm.v4i2.14869

Awodiji, O. (2023). Students' unrest in higher education: A perspective from The 4IR in book: A compendium of response to student unrest in African Universities. (pp.185-318): Axiom Academic Publishers (PTY) Ltd.

Ayo, V. (2019). *Effects of sexual harassment on the academic performance of female students at Makerere University*. [Unpublished Bachelor's Degree Dissertation, Makerere University, Uganda].

Baik, C., Larcombe, W., & Brooker, A. (2019). How universities can enhance student mental wellbeing: The student perspective. *Higher Education Research & Development*, *38*(7), 1–14. doi:10.1080/07294360.2019.1576596

Bakır-Ayğar, B., & Kaya, A. (2017). Ortaokul öğrencilerinin okul aidiyet duygusu ile okul temelli yalnızlıkarasındaki ilişkide okul ikliminin aracılık rolü. *E-Uluslararası Eğitim Araştırmaları Dergisi*, *8*(1), 14–27.

Banyard, V., Demers, J., Cohn, E., Edwards, K. M., Moynihan, M. M., Walsh, W. A., & Ward, S. K. (2020). Academic correlates of unwanted sexual contact, intercourse, stalking, and intimate partner violence: An understudied but Important Consequence for College Students. *Journal of Interpersonal Violence*, *35*(21-22), 4375–4392. doi:10.1177/0886260517715022 PMID:29294800

Barden, N., & Caleb, R. (2019). *Student mental health and wellbeing in higher education: A Practical Guide*.Sage eds.

Bezabeh, T. S. (2016). *Exploring institutional policies and female students' coping strategies on sexual harassment: A case study of Adi Haki Campus*. [Unpublished Master's thesis, Mekelle University, Ethiopia].

Bijaraniya, B. (2022). Student's unrest In Higher Education: Nature, cause and effect. *International Journal of Advanced Research in Commerce, Management &. Social Science*, *5*(3), 176–180.

Bireda, A. D., & Pillay, J. (2018). Perceived parent–child communication and well-being among Ethiopian Adolescents. *International Journal of Adolescence and Youth*, *23*(1), 109–117. doi:10.1080/02673843.2017.1299016

Birya, G. D. (2020). *The role of communication in crisis management in institutions of higher learning in Kenya: A case of Daystar University student unrest.* [Doctoral dissertation, Daystar University, Kenya].

Blair, B. L., & Perry, N. B. (2019). Parental sensitivity and friendship development: The mediating role of cooperation. *Social Development*, *28*(1), 106–119. doi:10.1111ode.12332

Bondestam, F., & Lundqvist, M. (2020). Sexual harassment in higher education – A systematic review. *Eur J High Educ*, *10*(4), 397–419. doi:10.1080/21568235.2020.1729833

Buni, I. (2020). Managing students' unrest in Universities: Unmasking the threat and success implication through Ubuntu. *Multicultural Education*, *6*(2), 27–38.

Busygina, A., Rudenko, I., Arkhipova, I., Firsova, T., & Murtazina, D. & Shichiyakh. (2019). Study of the features of family education in the process of social adaptation of a child. *Revista de Ciencias Sociales y Humanidades*, *4*(13), 346–352.

Carrico, B. A. (2016). *The effects of students' perceptions of campus safety and security on student enrollment.* [Unpublished PhD dissertation Marshall University, USA].

Charlton, T., Moulton, C., Sabey, V., & West, R. (2021). A systematic review of the efects of schoolwide intervention programs on student and teacher perceptions of school climate. *Journal of Positive Behavior Interventions*, *23*(3), 185–200. doi:10.1177/1098300720940168

Chávez-Flores, Y. V., Hidalgo-Rasmussen, C. A., & Navarro, S. M. (n.d.). Intrafamily relationships and health-related quality of life in Mexican adolescents who harm themselves without suicidal intent. *Salud y Sociedad*, *9*(2), 130–144.

Chemutai, B., Onkware, K., & Iteyo, C. (2020). Nature of student unrest in secondary schools in Kericho County Kenya. *International Journal of Social Sciences and Humanities Invention*, *7*(11), 6293–6307. doi:10.18535/ijsshi/v7i011.04

Chikendu, E. (2022). Student's unrest and academic achievements in Tertiary Institutions In Nigeria. *International Journal of Research Publication and Reviews*, *3*(5), 2452–2457.

Chiluba, B. C. (2019). Strategies for social engagement: The University of Zambia student unrests. *International Journal of Research and Innovation in Social Science*, *3*(7), 267–271.

Choudhary, K. (2018). Student unrest:Causes and cure. *International Journal of Advance Research in Science and Engineering*, *7*(4), 755–762.

Connolly, J., Josephson, W., Schnoll, J., Simkins-Strong, E., Pepler, D., MacPherson, A., Weiser, J., Moran, M., & Jiang, D. (2015). Evaluation of a youth-led program for preventing bullying, sexual harassment, and dating aggression in Middle Schools. *The Journal of Early Adolescence*, *35*(3), 403–434. doi:10.1177/0272431614535090

Corradi, A. (2021). Safety in numbers: Security on campus and the importance of the corporatization of Universities. *Security Journal*, *35*(11), 1–21.

Crowley, B. Z., Cornell, D., & Konold, T. (2021). School climate moderates the association between sexual harassment and student well-being. *School Mental Health*, *13*(4), 695–706. doi:10.100712310-021-09449-3

Dahlum, S., & Wig, T. (2021). Chaos on campus: Universities and Mass Political Protest. *Comparative Political Studies*, *54*(1), 3–32. doi:10.1177/0010414020919902

Das, D. (2017). Student indiscipline and student unrest in relation to their socioeconomic background political influence and academic achievement. *International Journal of Humanities and Social Science*, *6*(2), 92–98.

Davies, K., Ekwere, G., & Uyanga, U. (2016). Factors influencing students unrest in institutions of higher learning and its implications on the academic performance of students in University of Uyo, Akwa Ibom State, Nigeria. *Research in Pedagogy*, *6*(1), 26–42. doi:10.17810/2015.21

Delos Reyes, R. D. G., & Torio, V. A. G. (2021). The relationship of expert teacher–learner rapport and learner autonomy in the CVIF-dynamic learning program. *The Asia-Pacific Education Researcher*, *30*(5), 471–481. doi:10.100740299-020-00532-y

Douwes, R., Metselaar, J., Hendrika, G., Pijnenborg, M., & Boonstra, N. (2023). Well-being of students in higher education: The importance of a student perspective. *Cogent Education*, *10*(1), 1–17. doi:10.1080/2331186X.2023.2190697

Drazoa, C. (2018). Sexual harassment at African Higher Education Institutions. *Industry and Higher Education*, *94*(4), 4–5. doi:10.6017/ihe.2018.0.10553

Dufy, A., Saunders, K. E., Malhi, G. S., Patten, S., Cipriani, A., & McNevin, S. H. (2019). Mental health care for university students: A way forward? *The Lancet. Psychiatry*, *6*(11), 885–887. doi:10.1016/S2215-0366(19)30275-5 PMID:31324561

Durisic, M. & Bunijevac, M. (2017). Parental involvement as a important factor for successful Education. *c e p s Journal, 7*(3), 137-153.

Ekpoh, U., Edet, O., & Ukpong, N. (2020). Security challenges in Universities: Implications for safe school environment. *Journal of Educational and Social Research*, *10*(6), 112–124. doi:10.36941/jesr-2020-0113

Etaneki, A. F., & Okolie, U. C. (2020). students ' unrest : An evaluation of influencing factors and control in tertiary educational institutions in Delta State, Nigeria. *Journal Plus Education*, *25*(1), 192–210.

Falki, S. (2021). Student unrest- Its causes and remedies. *International Journal of Indian Psychology*, *9*(2), 442–469.

Fallesen, P., & Gähler, M. (2020). Family type and parents' time with children: Longitudinal evidence for Denmark. *Acta Sociologica, 63*(4), 361–380. doi:10.1177/0001699319868522

Fedina, L., Holmes, J. L., & Backes, B. L. (2018). Campus sexual assault: A systematic review of prevalence research from 2000 to 2015. *Trauma, Violence & Abuse, 19*(1), 76–93. doi:10.1177/1524838016631129 PMID:26906086

Fogelgarn, R., & Burns, E. A. (2020). What constrains passionate teaching? A heuristic exploration. *Issues in Educational Research, 30*(2), 493–511.

Frisby, B. N. (2019). The influence of emotional contagion on student perceptions of instructor rapport, emotional support, emotion work, valence, and cognitive learning. *Communication Studies, 70*(4), 492–506. doi:10.1080/10510974.2019.1622584

Galdi, S., & Guizzo, F. (2021). Media-induced sexual harassment: The routes from sexually objectifying media to sexual harassment. *Sex Roles, 84*(11), 645–669. doi:10.100711199-020-01196-0

Gans, S. E., & Johnson, V. K. (2016). Cortisol response to family interaction as a predictor for adjustment. *Journal of Family Psychology, 30*(7), 812–821. doi:10.1037/fam0000238 PMID:27559928

Garcia, S. L. (2020). *Attending anyway: A qualitative case study of the intersections of family stress, school climate, and school attendance choices within a Northeast Urban High School.* [Unpublished doctoral dissertation, Concordia University, USA].

García, V. T., Fernández, B. G., & Ruiz-Gallardo, J. R. (2018). Home-based family Involvement and academic achievement: A case study in Primary Education. *Educational Studies, 44*(3), 361–375. doi: 10.1080/03055698.2017.1373636

García-Hernández, R. J., Hernández-Sánchez, J. E., & García-Martínez, V. (2020). Sexual harassment in a Higher Education Institution. *Multidisciplinary Journal of Gender Studies, 9*(3), 210–233. doi:10.17583/generos.2020.5609

Gargiulo, I., Garcia, X., Benages-Albert, M., Martinez, J., Pfeffer, K., & Vall-Casas, P. (2020). *Women's safety perception assessment in an urban stream corridor: Developing a safety map based on qualitative GIS. Landscape and urban planning*. Springer.

Gaspar, T., Gomez-Baya, D., Trindade, J, & Botelho Guedes, F., Cerqueira, A., & Margarida G. de Matos. (2021). Relationship between family functioning, parents' psychosocial factors, and children's well-being. *Journal of Family Issues, 0*(0), 1–18.

Glariana, E., & Solar, B. (2015). Status of schools safety and security among elementary schools in the fifthy class municipality. *Asia Pacific Journal of Multidisciplinary Research, 3*(5), 10–18.

Grazia, V., & Molinari, L. (2021). School climate multidimensionality and measurement: A systematic literature review. *Research Papers in Education, 36*(5), 561–587. doi:10.1080/02671522.2019.1697735

Green, R. A., Conlon, E. G., & Morrissey, S. A. (2017). Task values and self-efficacy beliefs of undergraduate psychology students. *Australian Journal of Psychology, 69*(2), 112–120. doi:10.1111/ajpy.12125

Guan, S.-S. A., & Fuligni, A. J. (2015). Changes in parent, sibling, and peer support during the transition to young adulthood. *Journal of Research on Adolescence, 26*(2), 286–299. doi:10.1111/jora.12191

Gunn, H. E., & Eberhardt, K. R. (2019). Family dynamics in sleep health and hypertension. *Current Hypertension Reports, 21*(5), 39. doi:10.100711906-019-0944-9 PMID:30982174

Gyawali, K. (2021). Sexual harassment and its effects on mental health of the teenage school girls in lalitpur and Rupandehi District. *Journal of Balkumari College, 10*(1), 39–47. doi:10.3126/jbkc.v10i1.42092

Hascher, T., & Waber, J. (2021). Teacher well being: A systematic review of the research literature from the Year 2000-2019. *Educational Research Review, 34*(8), 10041. doi:10.1016/j.edurev.2021.100411

Havik, T., & Westergård, E. (2020). Do teachers matter? Students' perceptions of classroom interactions and student engagement. *Scandinavian Journal of Educational Research, 64*(4), 488–507. doi:10.1080/00313831.2019.1577754

Hernández, C., Jiménez, M., & Guadarrama, E. (2015). La percepción del hostigamiento y acoso sexual en mujeres estudiantes en dos instituciones de educación superior. *Revista de la Educación Superior, 44*(176), 63–82. doi:10.1016/j.resu.2015.12.004

Hirsch, J., & Khan, S. (2020). *Sexual citizens: A landmark study of sex, power and assault on Campus.* W.W. Norton and Company Independent Publishers.

Hornby, G., & Blackwell, I. (2018). Barriers to parental involvement in Education: An Update. *Educational Review, 70*(1), 109–119. doi:10.1080/00131911.2018.1388612

Hughes, G., Panjwani, M., Tulcidas, P., & Byrom, N. (2018). *Student mental health: The role and experience of academics.* Student Minds.

Huppert, F. A. (2017). *Challenges in defining and measuring well-being and their implications for policy. In future directions in well-being.* Springer.

Jabbari, B., & Rouster, A. S. (2023). *Family dynamics.* StatPearls Publishing.

Jackson, C., & Sundaram, V. (2020). *Lad culture in Higher Education: Sexism, sexual harassment and violence.* Routledge. doi:10.4324/9780203702901

Jaffery, A., & Kishwar, M. (2019). Student's perception of educational environment and their academic performance; Are they related? *Pakistan Armed Forces Medical Journal, 69*(6), 1267–1271.

Jirek, S. L., & Saunders, D. G. (2018). Cumulative adversity as a correlate of posttraumatic growth: The effects of multiple traumas, discrimination, and sexual harassment. *Journal of Aggression, Maltreatment & Trauma, 27*(6), 612–630. doi:10.1080/10926771.2017.1420720

Joing, I., Vors, O., & Potdevin, F. (2020). The subjective well-being of students in diferent parts of the school premises in French middle schools. *Child Indicators Research, 13*(4), 1469–1487. doi:10.100712187-019-09714-7

Kalkan, F., & Dağlı, E. (2021). The relationships between school climate school belonging and school burnout in secondary school students. *International Journal of Contemporary Educational Research, 8*(4), 59–79. doi:10.33200/ijcer.878682

Kayla, N., Kayla, S., Amy, M., & Samuel, A. (2018). College students' pereption of family influence impacting their health and lifestyle. *TEACH Journal of Christian Educ*, *12*(2), 10.

Khatoon, A., & Sharma, M. (2021). Relationship between family environment and academic achievement. *Elementary Education Online*, *20*(1), 3202–3207.

King, V., Boyd, L. M., & Pragg, B. (2018). Parent–adolescent closeness, family belonging, and adolescent well-being across family structures. *Journal of Family Issues*, *39*(7), 2007–2036. doi:10.1177/0192513X17739048 PMID:29805189

Kirby, N., Wright, B., & Allgar, V. (2020). Child mental health and resilience in the context of socioeconomic disadvantage: Results from the Born in Bradford cohort study. *European Child & Adolescent Psychiatry*, *29*(4), 467–477. doi:10.100700787-019-01348-y PMID:31243580

Klein, L. B., Stoner, M. C. D., Bhushan, N. L., Mulholland, G. E., Fisher, B. S., Kupper, L. L., Alam, I. Z., & Martin, S. L. (2022). Sexual harassment of students at institutions of Higher Education: Variations in students' experiences, knowledge, and perceptions across institutions. *Feminist Criminology*, *17*(3), 322–342. doi:10.1177/15570851211062572

Klemenčič, M., & Park, B. (2018). *Student politics: Between representation and activism. (Handbook on Politics and Higher Education)*. Edward Edgar.

Kurniawati, K. D., & Hafina, A. (2020). *The analysis of classroom climate in the perspective of peace psychology*. Atlantis Press. doi:10.2991/assehr.k.200130.093

Kustiani, A., & Fauziyah, P. Y. (2019). Analysis of factors affecting parental participation towards early childhood education program. *Journal of Nonformal Education*, *5*(1), 47–56. doi:10.15294/jne.v5i1.18333

Langley, E. (2018). *Study on triggers that lead to student protests and violent behaviours at the University of Kwazulu-Natal*. [Unpublished Master of Commerce Dissertation, University of Kwa Zulu Natal, South Africa].

Latcheva, R. (2017). Sexual harassment in the European Union: A Pervasive But Still Hidden Form of Gender-Based Violence. *Journal of Interpersonal Violence*, *32*(12), 1821–1852. doi:10.1177/0886260517698948 PMID:30156991

Lazurenko, N., Korolyova, K., Voloshina, I Svischeva (2021). The role of family in the students' educational achievement. *Revista on line de Política e Gestão Educacional, 2*(7), 3986-3997.

Lee, M. F. & Syaid, S. (2017). Factors contributing towards Malaysian Technical University (MTU) students' mental health. *Pertanika J. Soc. Sci. & Hum. 25*(S), 93 – 100.

Li, X., Zhang, C., & Li, W. (2015). Does the visibility of greenery increase perceived safety in urban areas? Evidence from the place pulse 1.0 Dataset. *ISPRS International Journal of Geo-Information*, *4*(3), 1166–1183. doi:10.3390/ijgi4031166

Lindell, A. K., & Nicole, C. (2018). Continuity and change in the family system across the transition from adolescence to emerging adulthood. *Marriage & Family Review*, *53*(4), 388–416. doi:10.1080/01494929.2016.1184212

Lipson, S. K., & Eisenberg, D. (2018). Mental health and academic attitudes and expectations in university populations: Results from the healthy minds study. *Journal of Mental Health (Abingdon, England)*, *27*(3), 205–213. doi:10.1080/09638237.2017.1417567 PMID:29265935

Luescher, T., Loader, L., & Mugume, T. (2017). Feesmustfall: An internet-age student movement in South Africa and the case of The University of The Free State. *Politikon: South African Journal of Political Studies*, *44*(2), 231–245. doi:10.1080/02589346.2016.1238644

Ma, X., Shen, J., Krenn, H. Y., Hu, S., & Yuan, J. (2016). A meta-analysis of the relationship between learning outcomes and parental involvement during early childhood education and early elementary education. *Educational Psychology Review*, *28*(4), 771–801. doi:10.100710648-015-9351-1

Maier, S. L., & DePrince, B. T. (2020). College students' fear of crime and perception of safety: The influence of personal and University prevention measures. *Journal of Criminal Justice Education*, *31*(1), 63–81. doi:10.1080/10511253.2019.1656757

Mangus, L., Somers, C., Yoon, J., Partridge, T., & Pernice, F. (2021). Examination of college student achievement within an ecological framework. *Journal of Adult and Continuing Education*, *27*(2), 231–247. doi:10.1177/1477971420963434

Maringe, F., & Chiramba, O. (2022). Disruptions in higher education: Mitigating issues of access and success in the COVID-19 pandemic. *South African Journal of Higher Education*, *36*(4), 6–20. doi:10.20853/36-4-5382

Mart'ınez-Fern'andez, M. J., Díaz-Aguado, M. J., Chacón, J. C., & Martín-Babarro, J. (2021). Student misbehaviour and school climate: A multilevel study. *Psicologia Educativa*, *27*(1), 1–11. doi:10.5093/psed2020a10

Maunah, B. (2019). The contribution of family and community education in realizing the goals of school education. *American Journal of Education and Learning*, *4*(2), 292–301. doi:10.20448/804.4.2.292.301

McIntyre, N. A., Mulder, K. T., & Mainhard, M. T. (2020). Looking to relate: Teacher gaze and culture in student-rated teacher interpersonal behaviour. *Social Psychology of Education*, *23*(2), 411–431. doi:10.100711218-019-09541-2

McMahon, G., Creaven, A., & Gallgher, S. (2020). Stressful life events and adolescent well being: The role of parents and peer relationships. *Stress and Health*, *36*(3), 299–310. doi:10.1002mi.2923 PMID:31920010

Mellins, C. A., Walsh, K., Sarvet, A. L., Wall, M., Gilbert, L., Santelli, J. S., Thompson, M., Wilson, P. A., Khan, S., Benson, S., Bah, K., Kaufman, K. A., Reardon, L., & Hirsch, J. S. (2017). Sexual assault incidents among college undergraduates: Prevalence and factors associated with risk. *PLoS One*, *12*(11), 1–23. doi:10.1371/journal.pone.0186471 PMID:29117226

Mohd, N. M. N., Nahar, H. S., Alrazi, B., & Taha, R. (2019). Stress among accounting students: A preliminary study of Malaysian Universities. *Journal of Business and Social Development*, *7*(1), 9–19.

Mónaco, E., Schoeps, K., & Montoya-Castilla, I. (2019). Attachment styles and well-being in adolescents: How does emotional development affect this relationship? *International Journal of Environmental Research and Public Health, 16*(14), 2554. doi:10.3390/ijerph16142554 PMID:31319570

Mshenga, R. (2022). Effect of sexual harassment affect students. *International Journal of Novel Research in Healthcare and Nursing*, *9*(3), 160–165.

Mubita, K. (2021). Understanding school safety and security: Conceptualization and definition. *Journal of Lexicography and Terminology*, *5*(1), 76–86.

Muhammad, B. M.(2020). The effect of learning environment towardspsychological wellbeing and academic achievement of University Students. *Palarch's Journal of Archaeology of Egypt/Egyptology 17*(2), 1-11.

Muthonde, C. K. (2022). Sexual harassment and related policy in Higher Institutions of Learning in Kenya. In L. A. Wakiaga (Ed.), *Women's contribution to Higher Education and social transformation. Implications for policy and praxis from Kenya* (pp. 51–67). Springer International Publishing. doi:10.1007/978-3-030-95622-6_4

Naom, O. (2020). *Influence of sexual harassment on High School Students' self-esteem in selected Secondary Schools in Nyamira and Kiambu Counties, Kenya.* [Unpublished PhD Thesis, Kenyatta University, Kenya].

Newhart, S. (2019). *The influence of family functioning on social competence, social support, and mental health among college students.* [Unpublished Doctor of Education Dissertation, The College of William and Mary, Virginia].

Ni, Y., Yao, X., Leung, K., Yau, C., Leung, C., Lun, P., & Leung, G. (2020). Depression and post-traumatic stress during major social unrest in Hong Kong: A 10-year prospective cohort study. *Lancet, 395*(10220), 273–284. doi:10.1016/S0140-6736(19)33160-5 PMID:31928765

Nurrokhmanti, H., Claramita, M., & Utomo, P. S. (2016). Among students' internal factors, should motivation be used as one of recruitments for admission of medical students in Indonesia? *Indosesian Journal of Medical Education*, *5*(2), 59–66.

Nyamberega (2018). Factors influencing student unrest in Kenya's Secondary Schools:A survey of selected Counties. *The International Journal of Humanities & Social Studies*, *6*(4), 346-356.

Odebode, A. (2019). Factors responsible for students' unrest in Nigerian tertiary institutions: Implications for counselling practices. *Mimbar Pendidikan: Jurnal Indonesia untuk Kajian Pendidikan, 4*(2), 93–102.

Oladipo, S. A., Awoyinfa, J. O., & Adefarakan, O. S. (2018). Institutional critical factors in University Personnel Security. [IJIBS]. *International Journal of Innovative Business Strategies*, *4*(2), 219–227. doi:10.20533/ijibs.2046.3626.2018.0031

Omodan, B. (2023). Addressing the underside of student unrest in South African universities using collegial leadership as approach. *Transformation in Higher Education*, *8*(0), 27. doi:10.4102/the.v8i0.273

Omodan, B. I. (2016). *Influence of trade unionism on management of Tertiary Institutions in Ekiti State.* [M.Ed. Thesis, Ekiti State University, Ado Ekiti, Nigeria].

Omodan, B. I., & Dube, B. (2019). Bridging the dichotomous gaps between trade unions and management of Tertiary Institutions in Nigeria. *Journal of Social Studies Education Research, 10*(1), 285–300.

Ondicho, N. K., Njuguna, F. W., & Kombo, K. (2019). Prevalence of students' sexual harassment in Secondary Schools in Nyamira and Kiambu Counties, Kenya. *Journal of Education, 7*(3), 1–21.

Oni, H., Tshitangano, T., & Akinsola, H. (2019). Sexual harassment and victimization of students: A case study of a higher Education Institution In South Africa. *African Health Sciences, 19*(1), 1478–1485. doi:10.4314/ahs.v19i1.21 PMID:31148975

Onivehu, A. (2021). Causes, consequences and control of student protests. *Sociální Pedagogika. Social Education, 9*(1), 8–21.

Orfan, S., Ibrahim, F., & Noori, A. (2022). Sexual harassment of higher education female students in Afghanistan: A case study. *Issues in Educational Research, 32*(2), 659–680.

Owusu, G. A., Akoto, J. S., & Abnory, M. M. (2016). Is our safety and security guaranteed on University of Cape Coast Campus? Undergraduates Students' Perceptions. *International Journal of Higher Education, 5*(4), 75–85.

Oyoo, E. (2017). *Indicators of Mental Status of University Students at the onset of Unrest: A Case of Kisii University, Kenya.* [Unpublished Phd Thesis, Rongo University, Kenya].

Perez-Trujillo, M., Jaramillo-Sierra, A., & Quintane, E. (2019). Connectedness as a protective factor of sexual victimisation among University Students. *Victims & Offenders, 14*(7), 895–919. doi:10.1080/15564886.2019.1655121

Potgieter, M., Pilcher, L. A., Tekane, R. R., Louw, I., & Fletcher, L. (2019). Lessons learnt from teaching and learning during disruptions. In: Schultz, M., Schmid, S., Lawrie, G. (eds) Research and practice in Chemistry Education. Springer, Singapore. doi:10.1007/978-981-13-6998-8_6

Puckett, K. (2022). Safety and Security On Campus: *Student perceptions and influence on enrollment.* [Unpublished MA Thesis, Electronic Theses and Dissertations. East Tennessee State University, USA].

Putrah, A. (2023). Students' reception towards sexual harassment case of Gen-Z At a Private Universityin Depok. *IJAMESC, 1*(2), 35–44.

Quick, J. C., & McFadyen, M. A. (2017). Sexual harassment: Have we made any progress? *Journal of Occupational Health Psychology, 22*(3), 286–298. doi:10.1037/ocp0000054 PMID:27732009

Rafferty, K. A., Beck, G., & McGuire, M. (2020). When facing hopeful and hopeless experiences: Using snyder's hope theory to understand parents' caregiving experiences for their medically complex child. *Journal of Pediatric Health Care, 34*(6), 542–549. doi:10.1016/j.pedhc.2020.06.003 PMID:32771340

Rafsanjani, M. A., Pamungkas, H. P., & Rahmawati, E. D. (2019). Does teacher-student relationship mediate the relation between student misbehavior and teacher psychological well-being? *Journal of Accounting And Business Education, 4*(1), 34–44. doi:10.26675/jabe.v4i1.8411

Ranganathan, M., Wamoyi, J., Pearson, I., & Stockl, H. (2020). Measurement and Prevalence of Sexual Harassment In Low- And Middle-Income Countries: A Systematic Review and Meta-Analysis. *BMJ Open, 11*(6), 1–15. PMID:34168030

Reaves, S., McMahon, S. D., Duffy, S. N., & Ruiz, L. (2018). The Test of Time: A Meta-Analytic Review of The Relation Between School Climate And Problem Behavior. *Aggression and Violent Behavior, 39*, 100–108. doi:10.1016/j.avb.2018.01.006

Rehman, A. U., Bhuttah, T. M., & You, X. (2020). Linking burnout to psychological well-being: The mediating role of social support and learning motivation. *Psychology Research and Behavior Management, 13*, 545–554. doi:10.2147/PRBM.S250961 PMID:32753983

Riekie, H., Aldridge, J. M., & Afari, E. (2017). The Role of the School Climate in High School Students' Mental Health and Identity Formation: A South Australian study. *British Educational Research Journal, 43*(1), 95–123. doi:10.1002/berj.3254

Rink, J., & Lipinska, G. (2020). Evidence of Distinct Profiles Of ICD-11 Post-Traumatic Stress Disorder (PTSD) And Complex PTSD In A South African Sample. *European Journal of Psychotraumatology, 11*(1), 1818965. doi:10.1080/20008198.2020.1818965 PMID:33282146

Riva, E., Freeman, R., Schrock, L., Jelicic, V., Ozer, C.-T., & Caleb, R. (2020). Student Wellbeing in the Teaching and Learning Environment: A Study Exploring Student and Staff Perspectives. *Higher Education Studies, 10*(4), 103–115. doi:10.5539/hes.v10n4p103

Roksa, J., & Kinsley, P. (2019). The Role of Family Support in Facilitating Academic Success of Low-Income. *Research in Higher Education, 60*(4), 415–437. doi:10.100711162-018-9517-z

Rosenthal, M., Smidt, A., & Freyd, J. (2016). Still Second Class: Sexual Harassment of Graduate Students. *Psychology of Women Quarterly, 40*(3), 364–377. doi:10.1177/0361684316644838 PMID:27821904

Rudasill, K. M., Snyder, K. E., Levinson, H., & Adelson, J. L. (2018). Systems View of School Climate: A Theoretical Framework for Research. *Educational Psychology Review, 30*(1), 35–60. doi:10.100710648-017-9401-y

(2022). RUDN. *Journal of Political Science, 24*(1), 166–174.

Sanjay, K. (2019). Causes and Consequences of Unrest Among Phd Scholars: A Study On Regular Phd Students in Himachal Pradesh. *The Journal of Progressive Education, 12*(2), 119–127.

Savolainen, T. (2023). A Safe Learning Environment from The Perspective of Laurea University of Applied Sciences Safety, Security and Risk Management Students and Staff. *Heliyon, 9*(3), 1–14. doi:10.1016/j.heliyon.2023.e12836 PMID:36895344

Schonert-Reichl, K. A. (2017). Social and Emotional Learning and Teachers. *The Future of Children, 27*(1), 137–155. doi:10.1353/foc.2017.0007

Schuck, A. M. (2016). Evaluating the Impact of Crime and Discipline on Student Success in Postsecondary Education. *Research in Higher Education, 58*(1), 77–97. doi:10.100711162-016-9419-x

Segametsi, B. (2017). Students' Unrest in Tertiary Institutions of Botswana: Implications on Teaching and Learning. [Unpublished Masters in Higher Education, Botho University, Botswana].

Shariati, A., & Guerette, R. T. (2019). Resident students' perception of safety in on- campus residential facilities: Does crime prevention through environmental design (CPTED) make a difference? *Journal of School Violence*, *18*(4), 570–584. doi:10.1080/15388220.2019.1617721

Shukla, K. D., Waasdorp, T. E., Lindstrom Johnson, S., Orozco Solis, M. G., Nguyen, A. J., Rodríguez, C. C., & Bradshaw, C. P. (2019). Does School Climate Mean the Same Thing in The United States as in Mexico? A Focus On Measurement Invariance. *Journal of Psychoeducational Assessment*, *37*(1), 55–68. doi:10.1177/0734282917731459

Simons, G., & Baldwin, D. S. (2021). A Critical Review Of The Definition Of 'Wellbeing' for Doctors and Their Patients In A Post Covid-19 Era. *The International Journal of Social Psychiatry*, *67*(8), 984–991. doi:10.1177/00207640211032259 PMID:34240644

Sowani, D., & Lavalekar, A. (2020). Exploring Psychological Well-Being of College Students In Maharashtra in Relation to Their Family Environment. *Indian Journal of Positive Psychology*, *11*(3), 197–202.

Srikanth, A. (2018). Incidents of Sexual Harassment at Educational Institutions in India: Preventive Measures and Grievance Handling. *Asian Review of Social Sciences*, *7*(3), 108–113. doi:10.51983/arss-2018.7.3.1458

Stanton, A., Zandvliet, D., Dhaliwal, R., & Black, T. (2016). Understanding Students" Experiences of Wellbeing In Learning Environments. *Higher Education Studies*, *6*(3), 90–99. doi:10.5539/hes.v6n3p90

Suprihatin & Azis, A. (2020). Pelecehan Seksual pada Jurnalis Perempuan di Indonesia. *Jurnal Studi Gender*, *13*(2), 413–434.

Svane, D., Evans, N. S., & Carter, M.-A. (2019). Wicked Wellbeing: Examining The Disconnect Between The Rhetoric and Reality of Wellbeing Interventions In Schools. *Australian Journal of Education*, *63*(2), 209–231. doi:10.1177/0004944119843144

Taseer, N. A., Khan, S. A., Yasir, W., Kishwer, R., & Iqbal, K. (2023). Impact of Family Involvement on Academic Achievement at Higher Secondary Level. *Journal of Social Sciences Review*, *3*(2), 1–10. doi:10.54183/jssr.v3i2.231

Thamtanajit, K. (2022). Prolonged Protests And Student Achievement: Evidence From Political Unrest In Thailand. *Eastern Economic Journal*, *48*(2), 226–250. doi:10.105741302-022-00216-z

Thomas, P. A., Liu, H., & Umberson, D. (2017). Family Relationships and Well-Being. *Innovation in Aging*, *1*(3), 1–11. doi:10.1093/geroni/igx025 PMID:29795792

Tsai, A., & William, R. (2016). Prospective Study of The Mental Health Consequences of Sexual Violence Among Women Living With HIV In Rural Uganda. *Journal of Interpersonal Violence*, *31*(8), 1531–1553. doi:10.1177/0886260514567966 PMID:25586914

Twenge, J. M., Cooper, C., & Thomas, E. (2021). Anxiety And Depressive Symptoms In US Census Bureau Assessments of Adults: Trends From 2019 To Fall 2020 across Demographic Groups. *Journal of Anxiety Disorders*, *83*, 102455. doi:10.1016/j.janxdis.2021.102455 PMID:34332230

Upali, P. (2017). Impact of Family on Children's Wellbeing. *Journal of Sociology and Social Work, 5*(1), 149–158.

Utkina,V & Efimova, A. (2022). *Career Barriers In Ghana: Evidence From Female Civil Servants.*

Van Rijswijk, L., & Haans, A. (2018). Illuminating For Safety: Investigating The Role Of Lighting Appraisals on The Perception Of Safety In The Urban Environment. *Environment and Behavior, 50*(8), 889–912. doi:10.1177/0013916517718888 PMID:30245528

Voth Schrag, R. J. (2017). Campus based sexual assault and dating violence: A review of study contexts and participants. *Affilia, 32*(1), 67–80. doi:10.1177/0886109916644644

Vuckovic, M., Altvater, A., Helgesson, S., & Kloss, K. (2017). Sexual harassment and gender-based violence in Tanzania's public service. *International Journal of Workplace Health Management, 10*(2), 116–133. doi:10.1108/IJWHM-02-2015-0011

Vujcic, M. T., Brajsa-Zganec, A., & Franc, R. (2019). Children And Young Peoples' Views On Well-Being: A Qualitative Study. *Child Indicators Research, 12*(3), 791–819. doi:10.100712187-018-9559-y

Wang, C., Boyanton, D., Ross, A. S. M., Liu, J. L., Sullivan, K., & Anh Do, K. (2018). School Climate, Victimization, and Mental Health Outcomes Among Elementary School Students In China. *School Psychology International, 39*(6), 587–605. doi:10.1177/0143034318805517

Wang, M. T., & Degol, J. L. (2016). School climate: A review of the construct, measurement, and impact on student outcomes. *Educational Psychology Review, 28*(2), 315–352. doi:10.100710648-015-9319-1

Wang, Y., & Guan, H. (2020). Exploring Demotivation Factors Of Chinese Learners Of English As a Foreign Language Based on Positive Psychology. *Revista Argentina de Clínica Psicológica, 29*(1), 851.

Weinberg, J., & Nielsen, L. (2017). What is sexual harassment? An empirical study of perceptions of ordinary people and judges. *Saint Louis University Public Law Review, 36*(1), 39–58.

Wen, C. I. (2019). Factors affecting students' subjective well-being: The relationship between religion, cultural intelligence, personality traits and subjective well-being (SWB) (December 30, 2019). *J. Mgt. Mkt. Review, 4*(4), 234–241. doi:10.35609/jmmr.2019.4.4(2)

Wong, D., & Kulwant, K. (2021). The longitudinal relationship of school climate with adolescent social and emotional health. *BMC Public Health, 21*(1), 207–215. doi:10.118612889-021-10245-6 PMID:33485308

Wood, L., Hoefer, S., Kammer-Kerwick, M., Parra-Cardona, J. R., & Busch-Armendariz, N. (2021). Sexual harassment at institutions of higher education: Prevalence, risk, and extent. *Journal of Interpersonal Violence, 36*(9-10), 4520–4544. doi:10.1177/0886260518791228 PMID:30071790

World Health Organization. (2016). Working for health and growth: investing in the health workforce. Report of the High- Level Commission on Health Employment and Economic Growth, Geneva, Switzerland. WHO.

Wornast, T. (2018). *Exploring student well-being in Higher Education.* [Unpublished PhD Thesis, Canteburry Christ University, UK].

Yang, Y., Liu, K., Li, M., & Li, S. (2022). Students' affective engagement, parental involvement, and teacher support in emergency remote teaching during the COVID-19 pandemic: Evidence from a cross-sectional survey in China. *Journal of Research on Technology in Education, 54*(sup1), S148-S164.

Zhao, K. L., Yang, M. Y., Miao, L. T., Liu, S., & Zhang, L. (2017). The effect of attachment on college students' internet altruistic behavior: Mediating model of trust and empathy. *Chinese J. Ergon, 23*, 23–28.

Zhigunova, M. (2017). Matrimonial installations of modern students (On the Example of the City of Barnaul). *Herald of Omsk University. Series. Historical Studies (Melbourne, Vic.), 3*(15), 183–188.

# Chapter 7
# Emotional Burden Among Student Mothers:
## Emotional Burden, Coping Strategies, Ways of Helping Student Mothers Combine Multiple Roles

**Monica Anne Achieng Oyoo**
https://orcid.org/0009-0005-6276-1846
*Maseno University, Kenya*

## ABSTRACT

*This study aimed to find out the emotional burden among student mothers, coping strategies, and measures that can be taken to reduce the emotional burden. This is qualitative study adopted a feminist and interpretive paradigm approach. Purposive and snowball sampling techniques were used to select 13 student mothers of ages between 14-26 years. A structured interview was used to collect data for the study. The findings showed that student mothers suffered emotional burden due to the overwhelming responsibilities and lack of understanding. The data also revealed that the student mothers coped with the emotional burden through acceptance, avoidance, sharing with friends and spiritual leaders, and planning. The implications and recommendations are discussed.*

## INTRODUCTION

The current trend of economy requires that every individual be independent as the times that women depended on men are long gone. It is therefore not plausible for any female, married or not to end their education due to motherhood. Research has it that domestic violence is prevalent in households where a wife has to depend on a man for livelihood. Findings of a study by Dahal, Joshi & Swahnberg (2022) suggest that the subjugation of women occurs due to practices based on gender differences and can lead to interpersonal and socio-cultural violence. Similarly, World Health Organization (WHO), (2009) established that sex trafficking, as an example of the outcome of inequality and violence, occurs due to the disadvantageous

DOI: 10.4018/979-8-3693-2833-0.ch007

position of women compounded by poverty and illiteracy. The differences between sexes were exhibited in the attainment of education and professional jobs, ownership of assets and feminization of poverty.

It therefore becomes necessary for the woman to obtain a higher education to attain the necessary qualification and certificate that will help them achieve their aspirations, fit into the job market and equally support the family, (Anane, Adangabe & Inkoom, 2021). In order to achieve this, it means that a woman does not drop out of school as a result of motherhood. This obviously comes with a lot of emotional burden as the student mother has to take on their responsibility as a parent in addition to their role as a student which is not limited to academic demands. The situation becomes even worse in African societies where most of the parenting roles are borne by the mother. Anane et al. (2021) found that in the African society, reproduction is perceived as a 'mother's work. This involves becoming pregnant and giving birth, yet it seems little or no support is given to student-mothers at school. They further indicate that being a mother naturally consumes almost all of a woman's time and combining it with studying is yet another challenge.

## BACKGROUND SECTION

Cases of student mothers are very common in educational institutions so turning a deaf ear to them would only disadvantage the affected students and make the society lose on the gains on gender parity. According to Tennant & Dickson (2019), majority of women in higher education in the United Arab Emirates (UAE) are first generation college students and about over half of them are student mothers. According to the WHO (2014) Fact sheet, about half of the 14 million pregnancies occurring across Sub-Saharan Africa are among women aged 15 to 19 years. In a study conducted by Eyeberu (2022) among 43,758 teenagers aged 13–19, the overall prevalence of teenage pregnancy was 30% and Western Africa had the highest prevalence of teenage pregnancy at 33%. This clearly is too high to be ignored.

Parenting poses psychosocial implications on student mothers because they become overwhelmed with difficulties in meeting educational, physical, emotional and financial needs (Thompson, 2010). Gyan (2013) found out that teenage mothers experience more deprivation, mental health difficulties, low educational attainment, emotional tantrum and behavioural problems. Further, a study by Moreau et al. (2013) also shows that student mothers have difficulties in terms of time, financial, health and emotional problems. With the data from the aforementioned literature, the researcher was inspired to determine emotional burden that students who are also mothers face.

## EMOTIONAL BURDEN

Emotional burden are psychological problems that one may experience. The double role of being a mother and learner is a major concern that impacts on the psychological development of the learner (Yussuf, & Afolayan, 2009). Literature indicates that student mothers are not able to balance child care and education favourably (Tezza & Gulanhem, 2010; Banko, Navraga, & Obansa, 2012). They also have mix feelings about the behaviours of the people in their communities who as much as cherish children also frown on teenage mothers (Faku, & Kablavoh, 2006). This causes psychological challenges that would no doubt affect their educational lives, both socially and academically (Buku, Namale & Oppong, 2018). The next section discusses ways in which emotional burden is expressed.

## Stress

According to Feldman (2005), responses that people give to challenges are known as stressors. Exposure to stressors generates a rise in certain hormones secreted by the adrenal glands, causing an increase in heart rate and blood pressure (Affum et al., 2013). Student mothers experience added pressure and stress while pursuing their education (Dafig, 2020; Brown et al., 2012).

## Low Self-Esteem, Shame, Guilt, and Regret

Student mothers are also affected by shame, guilt, and regret. Findings of a study by Adqasuraq & Kualaga (2012) show that student mothers often reveal their emotional instability in the form of shame, guilt, anger, self-doubt and dissatisfaction with their parental role. Likewise, findings of a study by Tezza et al. (2010) show that adolescent mothers feel guilty and worried because they fear that their younger siblings might copy them. Furthermore, a study by Buku et al. (2018) found that adolescent student mothers use avoidance of contact with other students as a coping strategy due to low self-esteem, shame, regret and guilt.

## Burnout

Student mothers experience a lot of burnout due to the multiple roles they play. Findings of studies by Bosch (2013) and Ajandi (2011) indicate that student mothers have to sacrifice time spent socializing and sleeping. For example, if a student mother is unable participate in group discussions or private studies due to demands of her child during the day, she would stay up at night or dawn when the child is asleep to make up. Studies by Stringer, Saqr, Tennant (2014); Thomas, Raynor & Al Marzooqi, (2012) also show that student mothers lack quality time to spend with family as well as meet academic requirements. This will clearly lead to burnout.

## Loneliness/Isolation

Student mothers face loneliness. Findings of a study by Ogunji, Nwajiuba & Uwakwe (2019) revealed that student mothers feel excluded in the main stream of academics due to their inability to measure up with fellow students. Similarly, a study by Tauken (2014) identified challenges that student mothers face as being angry, loneliness, drowsy, restless, skipping lectures, failing some modules and failing to write examination.

## Ridicule by Classmates, Teachers, and Family Members

Student mothers have been found to be exposed to ridicule in the form of bullying. Bullying is characterized by repeated exposure to physical and/or emotional aggression including teasing, name calling, mockery, threats, harassment, taunting, hazing, social exclusion, or rumours (Srabstein & Leventhal, 2010). A study by Ansah and Tiwaah (2007) noted that teenage mothers did not see the school as a welcoming environment because their colleague students and teachers ridiculed them making them feel belittled, humiliated, and embarrassed. These challenges can be overwhelming. It is therefore necessary to look at coping strategies used by student mothers which the following section addresses.

## COPING STRATEGIES

The responsibilities of a student mother are very many and demanding. She must therefore device ways and means of handling the situation hence the need to cope, Affum et al. (2013). Coping is the method of attempting to balance the demands imposed by challenging circumstances that are deemed to be taxing or beyond the capacity of an individual's resources (Lazarus & Folkman, 1984). It describes how individuals balance external and internal demands through cognitive, emotional, and behavioral efforts (Folkman & Moskowitz, 2004). Coping has two primary functions: resolving the problem that triggered the distress (cognitive or problem-focused coping) and controlling one's emotions to mitigate the distress caused by stressors (emotion-focused coping); (Carver & Connor-Smith, 2010).

According to Anspaugh, Hamrick & Rosato (2003) issue-focused coping involves attempting to resolve or alter the source of issues by collecting information, analysing it, and making meaningful decisions on how to approach a problem, thus removing or evading the problem, or minimizing its effect if it cannot be avoided. For example, during a test, the student-mothers' primary concern may be juggling the needs of the child to study, attend group discussions, and sacrifice sleep in order to prevent failure. On the other hand, emotion-focused coping involves techniques aimed at alleviating or controlling the emotional discomfort associated with issues. For example, getting emotional support from others and books, drinking alcohol, and abusing drugs.

Another form of coping strategy employed most frequently is relaxation. This implies that the student mother going through such stressful situation of mothering and studying concurrently may either have to consult a professional who can help her overcome some of her problems (Anane, et al., 2021). Lynch (2008) posits that student-mothers cope with their conflicting identities by practicing maternal or academic invisibility. This implies that depending on the situation and priority of the student mother, she may choose to concentrate either on her academics or mothering role.

Some student mothers avoid interactions so as to cope with their situation. A study by Buku et al. (2018) found that student mothers use avoidance of contact with other students as a coping strategy. This is because they feel that other students may judge them harshly for having had babies while still in school. The following section looks into ways of helping student mothers combine the multiple roles successfully.

## WAYS OF HELPING STUDENT MOTHERS COMBINE ROLES SUCCESSFULLY

Findings of various studies show that studying while raising children involves a lot of juggling, and thus considering strategies that will help the student mother combine these roles successfully is of great benefit, Lynch (2008).

To begin with, family members could support the student mother by offering necessary assistance. A student mother could assign all or most of her mothering responsibilities to the one assisting in taking care of the child so that she gets adequate time for academic work. Results of a study by Amos, Amoako & Antwi et al. (2021) indicate that student mothers would be able to cope with challenges by receiving social and instrumental support from family members.

In order to succeed, the student mother would have to be organized and work on a strict routine so as to determine when she could focus on her studies and when to be available to her family. A study by Torres, Sangala, & Jose et al. (2020) found that to cope with these challenges, the participants relied on doing what were relevant, making things fast, multi-tasking, and dividing school and family time wisely.

Similarly, according to Ajandi (2011) and Bosch (2013), a student mother would have to miss certain social events and sacrifice sleeping time so that she can properly manage herself, academic work and child rearing responsibilities. She could also choose to defer her course to times when the child is old enough.

Psycho-education is another strategy that can help student mothers manage their multiple roles. Psycho-educational interventions are techniques that provide information about the situation, help the individual to learn and develop problem-solving techniques (Chi et al. 2015). A study by Zariatu (2018) established that young mothers need people who motivate them and let them understand that all hope is not lost and that they can make it even after having a baby. About 60% of young mothers who participated in the study said that their mothers played a significant role in their reengagement. In addition, institutions can also help the students by providing necessary support. A study by Kiburi (2022) also proposes that the student mother be provided with societal and institutional support specifically psycho-social support for the student mothers to deal with individual stigma.

Tennant & Dickson (2019) indicate that it is critical that learning institutions provide student mothers with adequate facilities and support. Ogunji et al. (2019) also recommended an inclusion approach by establishing student support centre, early childhood educational development center and counseling units in higher institutions to help address the issues.

Similarly, a study by Dafig (2020) recommended the following for learning institutions to help student mothers combine their multiple roles more successfully: offering childcare services or facilities on college campuses to allow student mothers convenient access to their babies during the early months of childhood for bonding and breastfeeding; provision of distance education or a blended teaching approach, creating more cultural awareness of the roles of student mothers among faculty to allow for greater understanding of their concerns. They should also have special counseling services and session on coping strategies, stress and time management. Moreover, financial assistance as well as a good support system that includes family members, relatives and college fraternity.

It is also in order that adolescent students in general be offered guidance on sex education and also make it known to them the negative effect their attitude would have on their colleagues who might by some circumstances become student mothers. This guidance information should be extended to parents and guardians, (Buku et al. (2018).

Encouraging student mothers to mingle with other colleagues for their social and emotional stability and academic work has also been found to help them cope. Tauken (2014) identified the need for student mothers support group on campus to alleviate isolation and stress.

## METHOD

The study adopted a qualitative approach and interpretive paradigm approach. The interpretive paradigm assumes that understanding of the social world can be deepened through conscious effort to explore the experiences, feelings, and viewpoints of respondents (White, Morrison, & Jane, 2011). This approach was adopted to enable the researchers explore and obtain first-hand information about the psychological challenges faced by student mothers. 13 participants (5 in secondary school and 8 in college/university) aged between 14-26 years were selected using purposive and snow ball sampling techniques. Student mothers who had babies below 5 years and were not married were chosen. The reason was that children under 5 years would require more attention as compared to those over 5 years. Students who had no partners were also chosen so that the researcher could get problems that cut across. A structured interview was used to collect data which was categorized and analyzed thematically. The participants were assured of confidentiality.

## FEMINIST STANDPOINT THEORY

This study was anchored on Feminist Standpoint theory as discussed by Aptheker (1989). The theory suggests that the kind of life women lead and their experiences whether personal or social contribute to their total wellbeing. Communication and friendship are also very significant in the dailies of life. Dailies are the activities being done by women that create a pattern in achieving certain goals in life. This study therefore purposed to find out emotional burden among student mothers, coping strategies they employ and ways of helping them combine the multiple roles successfully.

## RESULTS

See Table 1.

*Table 1. The following are the results of the study*

| | Theme | Sub theme |
|---|---|---|
| 1. | Emotional burden | Abandonment by boyfriends |
| | | Demands of child care |
| | | Rejection by parents and relatives/ Isolation by friends and family members |
| | | Lack of confidants they could share their problems with |
| | | Conflicts in the family particularly among parents who blamed each other for the occurrence |
| | | Backbiting by friends |
| | | Burn out |
| | | Low self esteem |
| | | Loneliness |
| | | Stress |
| | | Being regarded as bad girls/ tags |
| | | Ridicule by classmates, teachers and family members |
| | | Shame, guilt and regrets |
| 2. | Coping strategies | Asking someone to help take care of the child during class time |
| | | Planning ones' time<br>Accepting the situation |
| | | Sharing with religious leaders |
| | | Sharing with friends |
| | | Avoiding interactions |
| 3. | Strategies that can help them cope | Creating social support groups |
| | | Guidance and counselling |
| | | Sensitization of the community |
| | | Support by learning institutions |

## EMOTIONAL BURDEN OF ADOLESCENT STUDENT MOTHERS

The study revealed that student mothers suffer from emotional burden. They were depicted in the following ways;

### Abandonment by Boyfriends

Most of the student mothers indicated that their boyfriends abandoned them when they learnt they were pregnant. They therefore have to take care of the children and this was very difficult since they did not have emotional support, leave alone the financial burden. In some cases, the boyfriends denied responsibility. A student had this to say:

*The day I was sick and went to the hospital and was told I was expectant, I went to my boyfriend. I told him that and he told me I should not involve him in the issue. I have now to take care of the child alone. It would be good if he was close to me. I would feel supported.*

Yet another said:

*I wish my boyfriend could help me more so I can have some rest. It is so tiring and you feel that you are working twenty four seven. I will surely do with some help.*

### Demands of Child Care

Taking care of a child was reported to be demanding. Most of the student mothers said that they had to miss lessons when their children were ill or when they had to take them for routine clinics.

One of them recounted having had to miss exams because her child was sick:

*There is a time my son was seriously ill and was admitted. I had to stay with him in the hospital and missed exams. I could not even have concentrated even if I had a choice to do the exams. It was so difficult.*

This resonates with the findings of a study by Morandet et al. (2009) that some of the issues students with dependent children faced are time and childcare. Tauken (2014) also found out that student mothers may find themselves being angry, drowsy and restless; may skip lectures, fail some modules and even fail to write examination due to demands of child care.

### Rejection by Family, Friends, and Relatives

Rejection by family, friends and relatives was also found to cause emotional burden among student mothers. Several participants indicated that their family members did not want to associate with them. This led to the student mothers feeling lonely and isolated. Their friends did not want to associate with them.

One particular student mother recounted how she had to go and stay with the grandfather.

*When I got pregnant and got my baby, my mother said she did not want to see me because I had embarrassed her. My brothers would beat me for no reason. I got tired of this kind of treatment and decided to go to my grandfather who was staying alone since my grandmother had died.*

This finding confirms those by Teeza et al. (2010) and Banko et al. (2012) that having a baby influenced a teenage mother to feel lonely and isolated and no longer willing to interact with their peers. This situation could affect their studies since they may find it difficult to share ideas and express their opinions in any learning environment (Stephenson, 2013).

## Lack of Confidants They Could Share Their Problems With

Majority of the student mothers indicated that they lacked people they could trust with their problems which they feared could be used against them. One of them narrated how a person they had trusted betrayed them.

*There is this girl I was close to. I could tell her the problems I was facing at home. One day I heard others talking about it. I lost trust and swore never to share with any other person.*

## Conflicts in the Family, Particularly Among Parents Who Blame Each Other for the Occurrence

Some of the student mothers said that their parents had differed because of them. In many cases, the father blamed the mother for not teaching her daughter good manners.

In one instance, the father had accused the mother for trading with her daughter and this led to their separation.

*My father used to tell my mother that she was responsible for my getting a child before completing college. That she did not teach me well. They used to quarrel every day and my father could even tell my mother that she was benefitting from my boyfriend. My mother decided to leave and now I am staying with my father who is cruel to me. When I go back home, life is hard.*

## Burnout

Burnout also came up as a form of emotional burden. Most of the respondents indicated that they felt fatigued due to the many roles they had to play. The main reason for burnout was the pressures of combining academic work and parenting.

Majority of the student mothers expressed that they experienced burnout due to overworking. They could no longer socialize with their friends or even engage in recreational activities. Most of the time, they did not have enough sleep because they had to balance between taking care of the child and academic demands.

One of them said:

*I find it so exhausting having to combine academic work and taking care of my child. Sometimes I feel so bad that I lose the strength to do anything.*

Still another reiterated:

*How I wish my parents could support me. It is so overwhelming to be a mother and a student at the same time. Sometimes I feel I cannot hold it anymore.*

One of the student mothers in secondary school lamented:

*I hardly get enough sleep. When I get home, I have to fetch water, cook, feed the baby and then do homework when the baby is asleep. I feel tired all the time.*

## Low Self-Esteem

Some of the student mothers reported suffering from low self-esteem. As a result, they avoided interactions with their peers.

One of them had the following to say:

*I feel like the other students are better than me. They are better behaved because they have been able to avoid early pregnancy. I also don't like being seen with a baby in school. I'm also bigger in size and I feel I'm not as beautiful.*

This resonates with the findings of the study by Buku et al. (2018) that adolescent student mothers use avoidance of contact with other students as a coping strategy.

## Loneliness/Isolation

The student mothers also expressed feelings of loneliness. They were isolated by their friends and family members. They therefore found themselves all alone most of the time. Again because they felt inadequate, they also avoided interactions which made the situation even worse.

Some of the responses were as follows:

*Many times I keep to myself because I feel my friends and siblings would judge me for having got a baby before marriage.*

*My friends do not play with me any more so I feel really lonely.*

*I'm usually left out of family functions because my parents don't want our relatives to know I have a baby. This makes me feel so lonely.*

The findings are similar to those of a study by Ogunji et al. (2019) which revealed that student mothers feel very much excluded in the main stream of academics due to their inability to measure up with fellow students.

## Stress

Most of the respondents indicated that stress was a major emotional burden they faced. The following are the causes of stress that came out from the interviews:

*I feel so stressed because my boyfriend abandoned me.*

*The fact that my father blames my mother for my pregnancy makes me feel really sad.*

*I sometimes feel really down but I do not have anyone to tell. This really disturbs me.*

*I'm really stressed because my parents have rejected me. I was chased away from home and I have to live with my grandfather. He does not even have a way to support me financially. So life is so difficult.*

## Being Regarded as Bad Girls/ Tags

Some of the student mothers reported suffering because of being tagged as bad girls particularly by their neighbours who regarded them as bad influence to their children. As such, they avoided relating with their peers to avoid such negative comments.

One of the girls shared how their neighbor told them not to relate with his daughter.

*A neighbor told me he did not want me near his daughter because I am a bad girl. This made me feel bad.*

This study supports the view of Stephenson (2013) who states that distressed students avoid environments that make them feel more uncomfortable.

## Ridicule By Classmates, Teachers, and Family Members

The study again established that adolescent student mothers were ridiculed by their teachers and classmates. Several of those in secondary schools said they were nicknamed by their classmates, teachers and even family members. This made them feel very unsettled both at school and at home.

One of them recounted how she is called names and teased by others:

*Most of the time my classmates do not call me using my name. They call me "mother" which makes me feel really bad. Sometimes I feel I do not belong and wish I could change schools. But it is not possible because my parents won't allow it.*

Another one had this to say:

*I had to change schools because of name calling. My colleagues used to call me "mama toto" meaning mother of a child. I felt really stressed. Luckily, my mother understood and I was able to transfer to another school.*

This finding confirms a study by Ansah and Tiwaah (2007) which noted that teenage mothers did not see the school as a welcoming environment because their colleague students and teachers no longer called them by their names.

## Shame, Guilt, and Regrets

A number of the student mothers said that they felt shame, guilty and regretted their actions. This is so as they had been warned about their behaviour but they did not listen.

One had this to say:

*When I think about the life I'm leading now, I feel ashamed. I also regret and feel guilty because my parents and teacher taught me what to do but I was tough headed. I wish I listened. I feel I have failed them.*

This finding confirms a study by Tezza et al. (2010) which show that adolescent mothers felt guilty and worried because they had the conviction that their younger siblings might copy the act and become teenage mothers.

## COPING MECHANISMS EMPLOYED BY THE STUDENT MOTHERS

The second question was on coping mechanisms. The findings of the study revealed that student mothers employed the following mechanisms.

### Asking Someone to Help Take Care of the Child During Class Time

Some students reported asking someone to help them with the child as they attended lessons and did their assignments.

A form one student mother had the following to say:

*I usually have to make arrangements with my mother or sister to take care of my daughter when I go to school. I'm happy they are usually willing to do so.*

A student mother in a college said:

*I have to organize with my boyfriend who to go to class and who to remain with the baby.*

These findings are similar to those of the study by Dasig (2020) that the support of immediate surroundings like families, friends, especially partners or boyfriends was very critical for women in achieving their dreams in life particularly in finishing their education.

### Planning Ones' Time

A student at a university had this to say:

*I try as much as possible to do my academic work when the child is asleep. Otherwise, I may not be able to complete my assignments. This means I do not do any other thing.*

These findings were supported by the study of the studies by Bosch (2013) and Ajandi (2011) that the student mothers coped with the challenges by being organized with good time- management skills. A study by Torres et al. (2020) also found that to cope with these challenges, the participants relied on doing what were relevant, making things fast, multi-tasking, and dividing school and family time wisely.

## Accepting the Situation

It also came out that some of the student mothers chose to accept the situation. They felt they were already in it and needed to move on.

One of them had this to say:

*I just encourage myself that I cannot change the fact that I have a child. I just told myself to accept and move on. I'm not the only one.*

## Sharing With Religious Leaders and Friends

Other students indicated that they share their problems with their priests, pastors and friends. These were however few as many feared that their issues could become public.

One of the responses was as follows:

*I sometimes go to my priest when I am overwhelmed. He is kind and understands me. At least he gives me advice.*

## Avoiding Interactions

It came out clearly that some student mothers avoided relating with other girls or friends. This was a way of protecting themselves from hearing hurtful remarks. They felt it made them have some peace.

Some of the utterances were as follows:

*I don't like being seen breastfeeding so I rather keep to myself.*

*I just feel that I'm different from my friends. I no longer feel good when with them.*

These findings confirm those of the study by Banko et al. (2012) which also found out that adolescent student mothers use avoidance of contact with other students as a coping strategy.

## STRATEGIES THAT CAN HELP STUDENT MOTHERS HANDLE THE MULTIPLE ROLES SUCCESSFULLY

The third question was on ways of helping student mothers combine their roles. During the interviews, various strategies were suggested to be used to help student mothers handle the multiple roles successfully. The following came up.

### Creating Social Support Groups

The need to form support groups for the student mothers was identified.

One student said:

*It would really be good if I could have a group of girls with the same problem so we can share our challenges.*

Tauken (2014) also identified the need for student mothers support group on campus to alleviate isolation and some stress associated with the multiple roles.

### Sensitizing the Community Particularly Family Members About the Needs of the Student Mothers

For instance, a form two student said:

*It would really be good if my parents accepted me the way I am since it cannot be changed.*

Yet another one said:

*Sometimes my classmate makes me feel very bad and I feel like I am useless. I wish someone told them this.*

These findings resonate with those of a study by Amos et al. (2021) that student nursing mothers would be able to cope with challenges by receiving social and instrumental support from family members. Banko et al. (2012) emphasizes that student mothers should be motivated to see themselves as smart, confident and strong to help them meet the challenges of schooling.

### Support by the Learning Institutions

Most of the participants indicated that it would be good if the institutions supported them. The following are some of the responses:

*Sometimes I feel very uncomfortable because of accumulated breast milk. It would be so good if the school allowed me breaks to rush home to breastfeed the baby.*

*Oh....I would love playing with my child during breaks if we had some room of sorts to leave them when classes are on.*

*Having a baby class within the school would be great. I believe it would be cheaper than hiring a nanny.*

These results are supported by those of a study by Dafig (2020) that learning institutions should support student mothers by offering childcare services or facilities on college campuses.

## Psychosocial Support to the Student Mothers

The need for psychosocial support for the student mothers also came up.

One of the participants said:

*If the counsellors, pastors or colleagues encouraged us to move on despite the challenges, it would be lighter.*

Another one said:

*I wish I could be told what I will face and how I can behave.*

The study by Zariatu (2018) also established that young mothers need people who motivate them and let them understand that all hope is not lost and that they can make it even after having a baby. Likewise, a study by Kiburi (2022) proposes that the student mother be provided with psychosocial support to help them deal with individual stigma emanating from their peers.

# FUTURE RESEARCH DIRECTIONS

Implementation of appropriate strategies may help student mothers combine the multiple roles effectively. It is therefore recommended that ways of helping student mothers be looked into. Institutions have a key role to play in this endeavor. The study by Dafig (2020) recommended that learning institutions support student mothers by offering childcare services or facilities on college campuses, provision of distance education or a blended teaching approach, creating more cultural awareness of the roles of student mothers among faculty and having special counseling services and psychosocial support for the student mothers. In addition, they should come up with wellness programs. Banko et al. (2012) believes that adolescent student mothers should be motivated to see themselves as smart, confident and strong to help them meet the challenges of schooling. Further recommendations are for sensitization of the community to be kind to the student mothers, particularly teenage or adolescent student mothers. This is because they already have so much to handle, are already guilty (Tezza et al., 2010) and the additional stress caused by a society so harsh may break them. These would make it possible for the student mothers to achieve their potential.

## CONCLUSION

The life of student mothers is challenging and they undergo a lot of pressure in order to perform the multiple tasks. The study revealed that student mothers encounter emotional burden which include loneliness, stress, burnout, ridicule, shame, regret and guilt feeling. As they struggle to cope with the challenges the student mothers device strategies such as avoiding interactions, planning their time meticulously well, accepting the situation the way it is and seeking help from spiritual leaders and friends. The need for support from the institutions and psycho-social support arose. Based on the findings, it is recommended that learning institutions come up with ways to support the student mothers to enable them combine the multiple roles. This could be in terms of availing places on campus or school where the student mothers could have their children and be able to breastfeed or interact with them while at school and providing psycho-social support among others. There is also need for sensitization of the community about the needs of these mothers. These would improve the overall wellness of the student mothers hence a healthy society.

## REFERENCES


Adqasuraq, G., & Kualaga, O. (2012). Exploring the Role of Teachers in the Lives of Teenage Learners. *Journal of Humanities*, *37*(7), 203–211.

Affum, P. K., Kusi, H., Mensah, D. K. D., & Afful-Broni, A. (2013). “Serving ‘Two Masters’ in The Ghanaian Educational Context”: The Experiences of Working Post Graduate Students, at the Department of Psychology and Education, University of Education, Winneba, Ghana. *African Journal of Inter Disciplinary Studies.*, *6*(2), 13–22.

Aitken, M. E., Mccarthy, M. L., Slomine, B. S., Ding, R., Durbin, D. R., Jaffe, K. M., Paidas, C. N., Dorsch, A. M., Christensen, J. R., & MacKenzie, E. J. (2009). Family Burden after Traumatic Brain Injury in Children. *Pediatrics*, *123*(1), 199–206. doi:10.1542/peds.2008-0607 PMID:19117883

Ajandi, J. (2011). Single Mothers by Choice: Discourses of the Family through Social Justice Alternatives. *International Journal of Child, Youth & Family Studies : IJCYFS*, *3*(4), 410–431. doi:10.18357/ijcyfs23/420117757

Amos, P. M., Amoako, B. M., Antwi, T., & Amoah, H. (2021). Motherhood and higher education in Ghana: Experiences of student-nursing mothers. *International Journal of Didactical Studies*, *2*(1), 1–9. doi:10.33902/IJODS.2021167163

Ansah, T., & Tiwaah, W. E. (2007). Perceived Social and Psychological Challenges of Adolescent Mothers in Manso Nkwanta. *Journal of Social Sciences and Education*, *3*(7), 423–431.

Arseneault, L., Bowes, L., & Shakoor, S. (2010). Bullying Victimization in Youths and Mental Health Problems: ‘Much Ado about Nothing’? *Psychological Medicine*, *40*(5), 717–729. doi:10.1017/S0033291709991383 PMID:19785920

Banko, J., Navraga, H., & Obansa, L. K. (2012). Exploring the Academic Stress of Adolescent Mothers. *Education and Counselling*, *7*, 351–360.

Bedu-Addo, P. K. A. (2000). *Guidance and Counselling Unmasked* (3rd ed.). Type Company Ltd.

Bøe, T., Serlachius, A. S., Sivertsen, B., Petrie, K. J., & Hysing, M. (2018). Cumulative Effects of Negative Life Events and Family Stress on Children's Mental Health: The Bergen Child Study. *Social Psychiatry and Psychiatric Epidemiology*, *53*(1), 1–9. doi:10.100700127-017-1451-4 PMID:29090324

Bosch, B. (2013). Balancing the Dual Role of Post Graduate Student and Mother. Edith Cowan University: Brown, V., & Nichols, T. R. (2013). Pregnant and Parenting Students on Campus: Policy and Program Implications for a Growing Population. *Educational Policy*, *27*(3), 499–530. doi:10.1177/0895904812453995

Buku, D. K., Namale, M. K., & Oppong, R. (2018). Psychosocial Challenges of Adolescent Student Mothers in Senior High Schools: Guidance and Counselling Implications. *International Journal of Basic Education Research & Policy*, *1*(2), 10.

Chen, Z., Xiaoming, L., Yu, L., Shan, Q., Liying, Z., Yuejiao, Z., Zhiyong, S., & And Zhengzhu, T. (2016). Emotional, Physical and Financial Burdens of Stigma against People Living with HIV/AIDS in China. *AIDS Care*, *28*(1), 124–131. PMID:26886415

Chi, N. C., Demiris, G., Lewis, F. M., Walker, A. J., Langer, S. (2015). Behavioral and Educational Interventions to Support Family Caregivers in End-Of-Life Care: A Systematic Review. *Am J Hosp Palliat Care*, (7).

Coleman, M., & And Thomas, D. (2003). An Economic Model of Locus of Control and the Human Capital Investment Decision. *The Journal of Human Resources*, *38*(3), 701–721. doi:10.2307/1558773

Cooper, C. L., Hoel, H., & Faragher, B. (2004). Bullying is Detri-Mental to Health, but not Necessarily Equally Damaging. *British Journal of Guidance & Counselling*, *32*, 367–387. doi:10.1080/03069880410001723594

Copeland, W. E., Bulik, C. M., Zucker, N., Wolke, D., Lereya, S. T., & Costello, E. J. (2015, December). Does Childhood Bullying Predict Eating Disorder Symptoms? A Prospective, Longitudinal Analysis. *International Journal of Eating Disorders*, *48*(8), 1141–1149. doi:10.1002/eat.22459 PMID:26337405

Dahal, P., Joshi, S. K., & Swahnberg, K. (2022). A Qualitative Study on Gender Inequality and Gender-Based Violence in Nepal. *BMC Public Health*, *22*(1), 2005. doi:10.118612889-022-14389-x PMID:36320057

Dasig, J. P. (2020). Challenges of Student-Mothers in the Tertiary Education of University of Perpetual Help System-DALTA. [JWEEP]. *Journal of World Englishes and Educational Practices*, *2*(6), 1–33. doi:10.32996/jweep.2020.2.6.4

Eyeberu, A., Getachew, T., Sertsu, A., Sisay, M., Baye, Y., Debella, A., & Alemu, A. (2022). Teenage Pregnancy and Its Predictors in Africa: A Systematic Review and Meta-Analysis. *International Journal of Health Sciences (Qassim)*, *16*(6), 47–60. PMID:36475034

Faku, T. U., & Kablavoh. (2006). Coping Strategies for Adolescent Mothers Who Return to School after Giving Birth. *The Journal of Psychology and Measurement*, *4*, 361–372.

Holt, M. K., Vivolo-Kantor, A. M., Polanin, J. R., Holland, K. M., Degue, S., Matjasko, J. L., & Reid, G. (2015). Bullying and Suicidal Ideation and Behaviors: A Meta-Analysis. *Pediatrics, 135*(2), E496–E509. doi:10.1542/peds.2014-1864 PMID:25560447

Ingrum, A. (2006). High School Dropout Determinants: The Effect of Socioeconomic Status And Learning Disabilities. *Honors Projects, 24*.

Kiburi, R. K. (2022). *Challenges, Coping Mechanisms and the Support Accorded to Student Mothers in Academic Pursuit: A Case Study of Egerton University, Nakuru County, Kenya*. [Thesis, Egerton University].

Larson, J. S. (1996). The World Health Organization's Definition of Health: Social Versus Spiritual Health. *Social Indicators Research, 38*(2), 181–192. doi:10.1007/BF00300458

Marandet, E., & Wainwright, E. (2010). Invisible Experiences: Understanding the Choices And Needs of University Students with Dependent Children. *British Educational Research Journal, 36*(5), 787–805. doi:10.1080/01411920903165595

Moreau, M. P., & Kerner, C. (2015). Care In Academia: An Exploration of Student Parents' Experiences. *British Journal of Sociology of Education, 36*(2), 215–233. doi:10.1080/01425692.2013.814533

National Academies of Science, Engineering, and Medicine. (2016). *Preventing Bullying through Science, Policy, and Practice*. Washington, DC: The National Academies Press.

Ogunji, C. V., Nwajiuba, C. A., & Uwakwe, R. C. (2019). Student-Mothers in Higher Education: An Exploratory Study of Challenges and Support System for Inclusion. *Journal of the Nigerian Academy of Education, 15*(2), 278–294.

Srabstein, J. C., & Leventhal, B. L. (2010). Prevention of Bullying-Related Morbidity and Mortality: A Call for Public Health Policies. *Bulletin of the World Health Organization, 88*(6), 403–403. doi:10.2471/BLT.10.077123 PMID:20539848

Stancin, T., Wade, S. L., Walz, N. C., Yeates, K. O., & Taylor, H. G. (2010). Family Adaptation. 18 Months after Traumatic Brain Injury in Early Childhood. *Journal of Developmental and Behavioral Pediatrics, 31*(4), 317–325. doi:10.1097/DBP.0b013e3181dbaf32 PMID:20431399

Stephenson, B. C. (2013). Guidance and Counselling. In *Schools and Colleges*. University of London Press.

Stringer, P., Saqr, S., & Tennant, L. (2014). Challenges and Support Factors of Married Emirati Students in Teacher Education. *Journal of Research in Humanities and Social Science, 2*(8), 46–56.

Tauken, S. (2014). The Main Challenges Student Mothers Experience to Manage Their Dual Roles. [IJAP]. *International Journal of Advances in Psychology, 3*(3), 94–98. doi:10.14355/ijap.2014.0303.04

Taylor, H. G., Yeates, K. O., Wade, S. L., Drotar, D., Stancin, T., & Minich, M. (2006). A Prospective Study of Short- and Long-Term Outcomes after Traumatic Brain Injury in Children: Behavior and Achievement. *Neuropsychology, 16*(1), 15–27. doi:10.1037/0894-4105.16.1.15 PMID:11853353

Tennant, L., & Dickson, M. (2019). Challenges Facing Emirati College Student Mothers Post Childbirth. *Journal of Research on Women and Gender, 9*, 76–90.

Tennant, L., Stringer, P., & Saqr, S. (2013). Motivation and Challenges of Married Emirati Students in Teacher Education. *International Review of Contemporary Learning Research, 2*(2), 99–109. doi:10.12785/irclr/020205

Tezza, S. F., & Gulanhem, O. P. (2010). Parents' Involvement in Managing Adolescent Mothers' Psychological Stress. *The Journal of Psychology, 4*(2), 215–221.

Thomas, J., Raynor, M., & Al-Marzooqi, A. (2012). Marital Status and Gender as Predictors Of Undergraduate Academic Performance: United Arab Emirates Context. *Learning And Teaching in Higher Education: Gulf Perspectives, 9*(2).

Thompson, S. (2010). Complexities of Supporting Teenagers in Pregnancy. *The Journal of School Nursing: the Official Publication of the National Association of School Nurses, 5*(8), 388–392. doi:10.12968/bjsn.2010.5.8.78911

Torres, V. M. R., Sangala, L. J. T., Jose, A. E. S., & Mortos, A. R. (2020). Untold Stories of Student-Mothers' Academic Journey: A Phenomenology. *Journal of Studies in Social Sciences and Humanities, 6*(4), 58–169.

Vryonides, M., & Vitsilakis, C. (2008). Widening Participation in Postgraduate Studies in Greece: Mature Working Women Attending An E-Learning Programme. *Journal of Education Policy, 23*(3), 199–208. doi:10.1080/02680930801923781

White, K., Morrison, S. P., & Jane, V. V. (2011). Basics in Education Research. London: Lawrence Erlbaum Associates.

Williams, S. A. (2011). Graduate Students/Mothers Negotiating Academia and Family Life: Discourses, Experiences, and Alternatives Education, Implication, Counselling and Education. *Edo Journal of Counselling, 4*(1, 2).

World Health Organization. (2009). Promoting Gender Equality to Prevent Violence against. *Women.*

World Health Organization (2014). *Fact Sheet.* WHO. Http:Wen.Tvv.Stats. 1421ysr.Adyi/Od/

Zariatu, I. (2018). Back to School—Resilience among Student Mothers in Ghana: The case of Nkawkaw. *Scientific Research Journal (SCIRJ), 6*(11), 68.

# Chapter 8
# Mental Health Crisis at Higher Education Institutions:
## A Conceptual Review

**Anna Niitembu Hako**
https://orcid.org/0000-0001-6367-1969
*University of Namibia, Namibia*

## ABSTRACT

*Mental health of students in higher education is a public concern and its impacts have heightened awareness of this issue. A conceptual review has been carried out to address the central question of this chapter—what are the mental health disorders that affect students in higher education institutions? Improved knowledge of aspects associated with mental health crises and also those that increase the mental well-being of students can provide a foundation for designing plans and specific interventions that can prevent poor mental health and ensure targeted support is available for students at increased risk. Therefore, the chapter recommends that universities adopt a proactive approach and implement innovative programs that can preempt students' misery*

## INTRODUCTION

Concerns about the mental health of university students have spread throughout the world even before the COVID-19 pandemic. Numerous studies that looked into students' mental health found common mental disorders such as addiction and substance use disorders, attention deficit hyperactivity disorder(ADHD), anxiety disorders, bipolar disorder, eating disorders, depression, suicide, self-injury, and sleeping disorders (Liu et al., 2019; Reddy et al., 2018; Saleh et al., 2017; Pedrelli et al., 2015). Indeed, many mental health disorders, including depression and substance abuse disorder, tobacco usage, emotional abuse, unwanted sexual encounters, academic performance stress, relationships, and financial, emotional, and social issues begin during the period of transition to university. Other authors Manwell et al. (2015) and Patel et al. (2013) reported that a substantial number of students experienced negative emotions such as fear and grief as well as tension and suicidal ideation. Similarly, McPhillips (2023) confirmed that

DOI: 10.4018/979-8-3693-2833-0.ch008

mental health struggles triggered more university students to consider dropping out and terminating study programmes prematurely. The students who partake in the McPhillips study cited personal mental health as the reason for feeling overwhelmed, far more often than others like financial considerations and difficulty of coursework. The National College Health Assessment (NCHA) (2015); however, states that 18-25 ages are disproportionately affected. Barrable et al. (2018) found that 80% of respondents had experienced stress, 70% had experienced a lack of energy or motivation, and 55% reported feelings of anxiety. Causes for such negative feelings can be found mainly in academic responsibilities, such as course deadlines (65%), and exam pressures (54%). An overview of the most prevalent mental health issues among university students, including anxiety and depression, suicide, and emotional stress are provided in this chapter, with an emphasis on their effects and associated factors.The next section discusses the background of the study.

## BACKGROUND

Over the years, there has been a common agreement among scholars that there is a health crisis in university settings resulting from an increased number of students suffering from mental illness (Porru et al., 2022; Asif et al., 2020; Enwefa et al.,2020; Auerbach et al., 2018 & Larcombe et al. (2016). For this chapter, a student is defined as a person registered at a higher education (HE) institution who reports to the National Council for Higher Education (NCHE) and who follows a course that leads to the award of a qualification. From the analysis of the literature, several risk factors emerge that are involved in the development of mental problems in students. These factors are financial problems, chronic disease, severe or long-term stress, long-term physical health condition, experiencing discrimination and stigma, including racism, childhood abuse, trauma, or neglect and social relations are the main factors of mental illness (Kandasamy et al., 2020). In particular, to classify the main factors in: academic factors, social factors, psychological risk factors, lifestyle factors and physiological factors. It is further revealed that the mental health problem is not only specific to higher education students in certain countries but also a challenge to other higher education students across the globe. For instance, based on studies from countries like Australia (Baik, et al., 2019), the United States (Eisenberg et al., 2013) and the United Kingdom (Kerr, 2013), tertiary students have a higher incidence of mental health issues. Using Depression Anxiety and Stress Scales (DASA) to survey more than 5000 students at a major Australian university, Larcombe et al. (2016) found that 13% of students reported severe or extremely severe depressive symptoms and 18% reported severe or extremely severe anxiety symptoms, whereas only 5% of Australian population samples reported such levels. The studies of Auerbach et al. (2018) and Asif et al. (2020) show how common mental health issues are among university students, with depression accounting for 76% of cases, anxiety for 88.4%, stress for 84.4%, and other mental disorders for 45.5%. Further, Enwefa et al. (2020) and Porru et al. (2022) claim that approximately half of the diseases among university students are caused by mental health conditions. As a result, some university students experience increased stress and mental health issues like anxiety, depression, substance abuse, aggression, sleep problems, suicidal ideation, and other behavioural issues.

In Nigeria, Idowu's (2020) study found students more prone than the general population to feel lonely, experience anxiety, and feel depressed; whereas in Ireland, social isolation, despair, anxiety, depression and an increase in maladaptive behaviour were among the negative mental health outcomes that adolescents encountered (O'Sullivan et al., 2021). Once more, some anxiety was observed among

Italian students (Vallejo-Slocker et al., 2020). Similarly, Kons et al. (2022) study in China, the students voiced behavioural and mental suffering. In their study, the most frequent behavioural issues reported were clinginess, distraction, irritation, anxiety, sadness, sleep and food disorders, as well as impairment in social relations were also observed. The studies presented thus far provide evidence that mental health issues affect a large number of student population globally and higher education institutions can no longer ignore this problem.

Further to this, Manwell et al. (2015) expressed concern about the lack of consensus on a definition of mental health among scholars that implement research, policy and practice. Currently, the word "mental health" is frequently used as a euphemism for "mental illnesses" because there is little consensus on what it means in general (Patel et al., 2013; Bhugra et al., 2013). Barkkham et al. (2019) also argue that there is a need for greater clarity and consistency in the use of terminology and a need to distinguish well-being and mental disorders. Bhugra et al. (2013) described mental health as a state of well-being in which individuals achieve their potential and have coping mechanisms for dealing with everyday challenges. To them, a person's state of well-being also includes the biological, psychological, or social variables that affect their mental state and ability to operate in their environment. According to the World Health Organization (WHO, 2020), mental health is a condition of mental well-being that enables people to manage life's challenges, achieve their potential, learn and work effectively, and give back to their communities. Further, mental health is a crucial element of health and well-being that supports both our individual and group capacity to decide, form connections, and influence the world we live in. It is, therefore, the conceptual underpinnings of human beings' ability to process, engage with one another, work, think, and, most importantly, enjoy life depend on their mental health.

On the other hand, Enwefa et al. (2020) defined a mental health crisis as any condition in which a person's actions, feelings, and behaviour them at risk of injuring themselves or others, not being able to take care of themselves, or of not being able to function in society in a healthily. Scholarly literature identified typical mental health crisis warning indicators as poor and personal hygiene; a significant shift in sleep patterns, such as sleeping less soundly or more frequently; gaining or losing weight; a decline in professional or academic performance; noticeable mood swings including irritation, wrath, anxiety, or sadness; absence from regular activities and connections (Thompson, et al., 2022; Kim & Asbury, 2020; Reimers & Schleicher, 2020; Olingo, 2020). SAMHSA (2021) added that some instances of mental health crises include depression, trauma, eating disorders, alcohol or substance abuse, self-injury and suicidal thoughts. The same author asserts that if you believe a friend or member of your family is going through an emotional crisis your involvement and assistance can make a difference. Based on the definitions above, a mental health condition can simply be described as a persistent psychological or psychiatric disorder, an emotional condition, or a mental ailment that can have an impact on academic performance. Additionally, the U.S. Department of Health and Human Services (HHS) (2021) identified potential causes for an increase in mental health concerns among university students in the recent three years as follows: the dramatic change may be difficult to adjust due to the increasing levels of anxiety and despair in society, excessive pressure to perform well academically, the rapid advancement of technology and the overabundance of information, particularly social media, financial and economic pressure. Together, these studies provide insights into the difficulties faced by students in higher education and demonstrate the links between students' mental health issues and dropout rates, depression, and suicide ideation, as well as lower academic performance.The next section discusses theoretical framework.

## THEORETICAL FRAMEWORK

This chapter is discussed within the context of Urie Bronfenbrenner's ecological system theory (1979), which postulates that every aspect of our life is influenced by the environmental levels we grow up in. The theory went through several revisions during Bronfenbrenner's career (Eriksson et al., 2018; Tudge et al., 2009). Generally, this is a theoretical system that accentuates the significance of taking into account various settings and levels of influence that affect human development. For instance, different systems that influence the student include (micro-face-to-face interactions with the individual [e.g., university setting or home]; meso-linkages between two settings both involving the individual [university setting 'and' home]; exo-linkages between two settings one of which does not involve the individual [university setting and management]; macro- [wider culture and belief systems influencing all settings, chrono-changes and transitions that occur throughout an individual's life [historical events, societal changes, and individual transitions such as aging or major life events like transition to the university (Bronfenbrenner, 1979). Ecological systems theory suggests that if wider contextual influences on the individual over time are important (e.g., prior experiences rooted in prior education and/ or wider socio-economic conditions), then simply trying to influence the individual skills of an individual in isolation (once they have entered, Higher Education, for example) may be limited in its impact. Indeed, there is evidence to suggest that an ecological system theory that acknowledges how wider contexts may interact with individual factors might be particularly valuable in understanding young peoples' experience (Holloway & Jonas, 2016), and guiding responses to mental health problems (Eriksson et al., 2018). Adopting this broader perspective on student mental health distress may allow researchers to become more aware of other potential influences on students' well-being. Focusing specifically on the chrono-, it seems possible that relatively recent changes in wider contexts (i.e., micro-to-macro) around education such as the COVID-19 pandemic may contribute to the increasing levels of student mental health crises witnessed in higher education institutions. For this reason, it seems important not just to explore any changes that may have taken place within higher education alone but also to look further upstream to other potential factors impacting the individual student's education journey as they move throughout all education levels. The higher institution setting exposes students to diverse perspectives and cultures, promotes social justice and equity, and fosters an appreciation for global interconnectedness. Overall, applying Bronfenbrenner's Ecological Theory to the higher institution students' mental problems assists the university management and student-counsellors in creating a holistic and comprehensive approach to student development that takes into account the various ecological systems that influence their learning and growth. The next section discusses the literature review.

## LITERATURE REVIEW

### Specific Mental Health Disorders Affecting Students In Higher Education

#### Depression

Substance Abuse and Mental Health Services Administration (SAMHSA, 2021) report explains that a major depressive disorder, also known as depression, is a mood illness that is characterized by the presence of a "sad, empty, or irritable mood, accompanied by somatic and cognitive changes that significantly affect the individual's capacity to function." Major depression is the most frequent type of depression and is different from regular sadness and grief, including bereavement. Depressed mood changes in appetite, depressed mood (such as feeling sad, empty, or hopeless) most of the day, almost every day, major weight loss or gain unrelated to dieting, and significant depressive symptoms are just a few of the major depressive disorder symptoms that can range in severity from mild to severe (SAMHSA, 2021; Thanoi et al., 2023; Porru et al., 2022). Similarly, depression is a common disease in most countries around the world, with an estimated 350 million people affected, but it is a highly treatable mood disorder (Manap et al., 2018). It is different from the usual mood fluctuations and emotional responses to challenges in everyday life. Normally, depression often presents with physical symptoms, primarily fatigue, pain, sleep disturbance and inability to concentrate (O'Sullivan et al., 2021; Teh et al., 2015). To Chand and Arif (2022), depression refers to a mood disorder that causes a persistent feeling of sadness and loss of interest and impacts growth and development, school performance and peer and family relationships and it can be fatal. Other scholars Salik and Marwaha (2022) indicate that depressive disorder is one of the disposition issues and is becoming more frequent day by day. It comes with symptoms of anxiety and at its worst can lead to suicide. Manap et al. (2018) assert that identifying depression, anxiety and stress levels are considered important indicators of mental health. These three emotional disorders can lead to negative outcomes, such as impaired normal functioning, burnout, and health problems. Idowu (2020) and Ormel et al. (2019) highlight that the common features of all depressive disorders are sadness, emptiness, or irritable mood, accompanied by somatic and cognitive changes that significantly affect the individual's capacity to function. Equally, Lipson and Eisenberg (2018), Baker (2018) and Camacho (2016) concur that the important fact is that traumatic events such as the death or loss of a loved one, lack of or reduced social support, caregiver burden, financial problems, interpersonal difficulties, and conflicts are examples of stressors that can trigger depression. It is crucial to note that feelings of sadness, hopelessness, disappointment, guilt, and loss of interest in life or daily activities are depressive symptoms. According to this study, depression is an emotional condition characterized by thoughts of sadness and worthlessness, social seclusion, irregular eating and sleeping patterns, and a loss of interest in often enjoyable activities. The next sub-section discusses suicide.

## Suicide

Data from several sources have identified the increased suicide and suicide attempts in university settings associated with mental health problems (Bryan, 2021; Lipson et al., 2022; Gratz et al., 2021 & Duffy et al., 2020). It is predicted that suicide rates will increase in the future given the WHO's prediction that they will surpass 1 million in the following 15 years (Arensman, et al., 2020). As an illustration, the Centers for Disease Control and Prevention [CDC] (2022) reveals that one of the main causes of death among young adults and university students is suicide. Student suicide is defined as those who die by suicide or an event of undetermined intent before or on the end date of their studies (Levi-Belz et al., 2019). Findings from recent research have shown that most youth suicides are the result of an interaction between biological, psychological, sociocultural, and family factors (/Oaes, 2021; Wango, 2023; Zhai & Du, 2021; Dubé et al., 2021). Notably, on a university campus, Causer et al. (2021) stated that students are likely to be exposed to suicides and suicide attempts due to various factors. For instance, common factors comprise academic pressure, social and cultural issues, conflicts in relationships, a dysfunctional and unhelpful environment, conduct disorder, substance abuse, depression, psychiatric illness, previous failed attempts, and the ready availability of lethal means to commit suicide. Casey et al. (2022) claim that suicidal thoughts and actions are more likely to occur in students who are depressed or anxious. Additionally, in Oh et al. (2022) recent nationwide survey, 12% of students reported having suicidal thoughts, which suggests that university students may be more at risk for suicide than the overall population. Wango (2023) describes suicide as the taking of one's life by a definite act, such as shooting oneself. It is; however, also possible to take one's by failing to act, for instance, by not eating. Similarly, an individual can also commit suicide by allowing another person to act on his or her behalf. This occurs when an individual asks another person to kill him or her (Curtin et al., 2016). Levi-Belz et al. (2018) and Verrocchio et al. (2016) maintain that suicide can be seen as a behaviour motivated by the desire to escape from unbearable psychological pain. Among the most common methods of suicide include pesticides and other drugs, hanging, drowning, and the use of firearms Bryan (2021).

As noted by Wango (2023) and Causer et al. (2021), the intensity of the thoughts might range from a vague desire to die without any method, plan, motive, or to actively considering suicide with a specific objective. That is to say, suicide frequently happens amid a significant depressive episode, although it can also arise from drug use or another disorder. Curtin et al. (2016) state that suicide occasionally happens in the absence of any psychiatric disease, particularly in unfavourable circumstances like acute or protracted bereavement or decreasing health. In this study, suicide is conceptualised as a method of taking one's own life when faced with a perplexing circumstance and lacking the fortitude to face the next day. The next sub-section discusses anxiety.

## Anxiety

Anxiety has been identified as a primary cause of university student mental health concerns and Spielberger (2013) defined it as an unpleasant emotional state or condition characterized by subjective feelings of tension, apprehension and worry, and by activation or arousal of the autonomic nervous system. This definition is close to that of Wiedemann (2015) and Galderisi et al. (2015) who define anxiety as a state emotion, that is, affective adaptations to specific situations, genetic disposition, environmental impact on individual and acute stressors that result in adaptational changes. Based on their views, anxiety is a reaction of the human body to threat, danger or stress. Maina et al. (2016) also describe anxiety as "a state of being sad and feeling stress and disruptive mood, the anxious person feels empty and fearful all the time". Factors associated with anxiety in students are similar to those in depression, having a history of psychological or psychiatric treatment, perceived lack of psychological and poor social support (Mhata et al., 2023; Campbell et al., 2022; Ribeiro et al., 2020; Kebede et al., 2019 & Brenneisen- Mayer et al., 2016).

Anxiety is frequently accompanied by "muscle tension, vigilance in anticipation of impending danger, and cautious or avoidant behaviours (CDC, 2022). In other words, anxiety is a reaction of the human body to threat, danger or stress. Mayo Clinic (2019) identified symptoms of anxiety as nervousness, unease, a sense of impending doom or danger, sweating, trembling, an inability to maintain focus, uncontrollable worry, restlessness, fatigue, and insomnia. As stated by Lisiecka et al. (2023), additional signs and symptoms may include excessive worry, palpitations, restlessness, being easily tired, trembling, feelings of choking, sweating, chest pain, nausea, dizziness, paresthesias (numbness or tingling sensations), problems concentrating, irritability, and sleep disturbances. These symptoms are typically persistent and last for six months or longer (Enwefa et al., 2020). Therefore, feeling anxious occasionally is a normal emotion that everyone faces. However, constant anxiety will cause overwhelming worry and fear which can interfere with our daily activities. In this study, anxiety is understood as a feeling of fear, nervousness, or disquiet resulting from an uncertain situation. the next section discusses prevalence and incidence of students with mental health illnesses.

## PREVALENCE AND INCIDENCE OF STUDENTS WITH MENTAL HEALTH ILLNESSES

The number of university students reporting anxiety, stress depression and other mental health problems has been increasing for years. According to research in the literature (Mhata et al., 2023; Douwes et al., 2023; Kajjimu et al., 2021; Frajerman et al., 2019; Tam et al., 2019; Kebede et al., 2019, Haile et al., 2019; Tian-Ci Quek et al., 2019; & Rotenstein et al., 2016), students are more likely to experience depression, feelings of anxiety, psychological and emotional distress, and increased risk of burnout. Similarly, Eisenberg et al. (2013), Larcombe et al. (2016), and Orgyen (2017), maintain that university students are a "very high-risk population" for psychological distress and mental disorders. Although dealing with stress is a normal part of life, for some students it can hurt their physical, emotional, and psychological health (Barbayannis et al., 2022). This is especially true considering that the majority of mental illnesses first appear in adolescence and early adulthood (Meeus et al., 2016 & Verrocchio et al., 2016). Many students arrive on campus with a mental health issue or having gone through a significant traumatic event in their lives, which can hurt their physical, emotional, and psychological well-being. These students are in addition to those who may experience mental health challenges while enrolled in postsecondary education.

According to the Centers for Disease Control and Prevention (CDC) (2022), one of the main causes of death among university students is suicide. Casey et al. (2022) believe that suicidal thoughts and actions are more likely to occur in students who are depressed or anxious. It has been reported that the male suicide rate for higher education students was statistically significantly higher (5.6 deaths per 100,000 students; 202 suicide deaths) compared with female students at 2.5 deaths per 100,000 students (117 suicide deaths); this is in line with the trend seen in the general population where suicide rates are higher among males (CDC) (2022). Additionally, in Oh et al. (2022) recent nationwide survey, 12% of students reported having suicidal thoughts, which suggests that university students may be more at risk for suicide than the overall population. Recent figures reveal that over one million people commit suicide each year, resulting in an age-standardized annual suicide rate of 11.4 per 100,000 persons (15.0 for men and 8.0 for women) (Levi-Belz et al., 2019). In addition, Schmits et al. (2021) study revealed that 50.6% of students presented anxiety symptoms; 55.1% reported depressive symptoms; 20.8% manifested suicidal ideations; 42.4% saw their financial situation deteriorate; 39.1% felt they were dropping out of school. A recent study, Dhar et al.(2020) reports that, among university students in Bangladesh, 44.59% are suffering from severe anxiety and 48.41% are suffering from moderate anxiety. Moreover, the mean score is higher in the student sample than the Chinese national norm during COVID-19 pandemic. Another study revealed high rates of anxiety (29.5%) and depression (31.7%) among the student population.

The National College Health Assessment (NCHA) (2015) shows that traditional causes of mental health disorders among college students include separation from family, homesickness, and transitional problems, to name a few. All students, regardless of their gender, race, or ethnicity, are having these experiences. Some are discovered to be highly significant, while others are quite complex. The results of NCHA's study on college students' feelings were shocking as about 56.9% of college students indicated having anxiety. Similarly, linkage with Higher Education Statistics Authority (HESA) data identified

319 students who died by suicide between the academic year ending 2017 and the academic year ending 2020, equivalent to a rate of 3.9 deaths per 100,000 students. Of these, 202 (63.3%) were males and 117 (36.7%) were females. Over the period, the median age at death has been 22 years, which is mostly consistent over time.

Further to this, Kajjimu et al. (2021) and Haile et al. (2019) point out that several stress-related aspects have an impact on university life and, over time, may have an impact on student's academic advancement. It is a common occurrence that when students experience mental health problems, they might exhibit various academic warning signs that could hamper their ability to succeed in the university setting. As an illustration, these signs may include repeated absences from the class, missed assignments, examinations, and appointments, to name just a few. Relatedly, Kebede et al. (2019) and Tam et al. (2019) state that lecturers can observe extreme disorganisation behaviour, excessively anxious behaviours when students are called upon in class, persistent requests for additional time for deadlines, make-up exams, or even an extension on a project, and a decline in the quality of the work. Evidently, during examination time, it is common for students with mental health problems to forget crucial items at home such as student identification cards and the examination timetable that are necessary for entry into the exam room (Barkham et al., 2019; Rotenstein et al., 2016). It is therefore advisable for educators to be vigilant and identify at-risk students as early as possible for proper interventions.The next section discusses university campus-based interventions to promote mental health.

## UNIVERSITY CAMPUS-BASED INTERVENTIONS TO PROMOTE MENTAL HEALTH

Currently, there are many interventions aimed at developing and adjusting emotional and social skills in higher institutions, such as social and emotional learning (SEL) programs or positive youth development (PYD) interventions(Benoit et al., 2021). Further, universities adopt a proactive approach and implement innovative programs such as awareness creation, counselling services, student drop-in centres and the promotion of social and recreational activities to pre-empt students' misery. Auerbach et al. (2018) found that resilience training and stress management significantly increased resilience, perceived stress, anxiety, and quality of life eight weeks after the intervention.Furthermore,commonly reported preventive strategies included accessing social support, attending professional services, following a routine for taking medication, exercising and attending to personal hygiene and sleep. Yanos and Rosario (2014) study supported that preventive strategies are frequently used by members of this population, and that accessing social support and engaging in activities/hobbies are the most frequently used preventive strategies. The prevention-focused coping strategies is the best for students in higher education institutions. Care strategies must be urgently developed in response to these alarming rates. Every student should have easy access to such care, especially given that many students have witnessed a significant and stressful deterioration in their financial situation, as reported in this research. In Belgium, the authorities installed exceptional measures, such as the reimbursement of psychological help, in order to meet the needs of the population. Clearly, it is crucial to develop other forms of support for students within the educational institutions themselves (individual and group consultations, relaxation sessions, meditation, etc.). Educational institutions should understand that they ought to make a long-term investment in the well-being and positive mental health of the student community.

As previously discoursed, there has reportedly been an increase in the number of students with mental health-related ailments while enrolled in institutions of higher learning during the past three years (Aragon, 2020; Backhause et al., 2020; Dopmeijer, 2021; Baik et al., 2019). Many scholars are worried that if students' mental health disorders remain untreated their conditions might deteriorate and become a burden to society (Douwes et al., 2023; Doolan, 2021; Lipson & Eisenberg, 2018). Chipare et al. (2021) maintain that mental disorders contribute significantly to the global burden of diseases affecting about 30% of the population. This necessitates the creation of supportive physical, social, and academic environments at university campuses that promote students' mental well-being. Lisiecka et al. (2023) and Conley et al. (2015) claim that there is most compelling evidence of several programs and services aiming at the well-being and mental health of students. What is needed is that university counselling units implement a fundamental and/or integral educational approach that concentrates on academic integration, social integration, and skill-training programmes such as coping. Based on the views of (Freire et al., 2020; Yusufov et al., 2019; Houston et al., 2017; Molla-Jafar et al., 2015; Phang et al., 2015; & Regehr et al., 2013), other interventions that have been effective in improving the coping skills of college students are cognitive behavioural therapy, mindfulness mediation, and online coping tools. With this in mind, the student affairs department and counselling centre staff are expected to offer a lot of educational training, regarding stress management, self-awareness, self-compassion, yoga, diet and ergonomics, mindfulness, meditation, daring to speak, pushing behaviour or stopping postponing. They must train and educate students on how to prioritize and reduce their performance anxiety and their emotional regulation. In this way, they might assist students to work on different levels of the issues concurrently, such as the identification of stressors, maintaining a positive mind, practising good behaviours, and handling and controlling their thoughts and emotions (Garriott & Nisle, 2018). The next section discusses the significance of parental involvement in students' mental health development

## SIGNIFICANCE OF PARENTAL INVOLVEMENT IN STUDENTS' MENTAL HEALTH DEVELOPMENT

The involvement of parents in a child's life is crucial to student well-being, especially to those in higher education institutions, Normally, these students live far from their families and home backgrounds as they pursue their education in different countries or cities. It is, therefore, imperative that parents play a pivotal role in helping students maintain mental health in a new environment (Fernández-Alonso et al., 2017; Broonk, et al.,2018; & Rodríguez, 2017). Parental involvement is defined as the amount of participation in their children's schooling and academic learning (Thomas et al., 2020). The first step in parental involvement in a child's education is for parents to provide a safe and healthy environment, appropriate learning experiences, support, and a good outlook on school. As Baig et al. (2021) explained, the parents play a significant role in the overall development of an adolescent, including behaviour, physical health, and mental health outcomes. Nowadays, the majority of adolescents go to university while they are at a critical stage of development. As such, this stage of transitioning into adulthood undergoes simultaneous physical, mental, and social developmental changes that bring mental health challenges. Indeed, the mental and physical development of an adolescent is extremely susceptible and complex because this is a time when they are more inclined to experiment with psychological, physical, and social boundaries, which can have a big impact on development and maturity into adulthood.

Further to this, several parental participation variables, including parental warmth, parental support, parental encouragement, and overall parental involvement, were linked to better adolescent health outcomes (Broonk et al., 2018). Thomas et al. (2020) and Yap et al. (2014) claim that parental participation is still strongly linked to several students' health indicators, such as less risky behaviour and improved mental and physical health while schooling. Additionally, Pengpid et al. (2018) and Meeus (2016) assert that better dietary habits, personal hygiene, and exercise habits in adolescents are substantially correlated with greater parental participation.

Equally important, Baig et al. (2021) hold the view that increased parental participation is also linked to a lower risk of physical harm, bullying, using tobacco or other drugs, and poor mental health in adolescents. Consequently, higher parental involvement is perceived as an indicator of better adolescent mental and physical health (Nguyen et al., 2020; Fernández-Alonso et al., 2017). Consistently, studies from various nations, like India, revealed greater rates of poor mental health in children with less parental participation, while studies from Lebanon, Palestine, Jordan, Syria, and Vietnam revealed a link between a lack of parental comprehension and a higher prevalence of suicide ideation (Nguyen et al., 2020; Itani et al., 2017; Hasumi et al., 2014). In this study, adolescent and student terms are used interchangeably for the reason that currently, many students in higher education institutions are at the adolescent stage. The next section discusses the barriers to mental health treatment.

## BARRIERS TO MENTAL HEALTH TREATMENT

Although it has been widely reported that there has been a rise in the number of students with mental health problems, the majority of students with these problems do not receive treatment (Mhata et al., 2023; Bantjes et al.,2020; Cage et al., 2020; Busby et al., 2019; Orgyen, 2017; Larcombe et al., 2016). It is also known that university students often do not seek help or support within or outside the educational context (Broglia et al., 2021; Anderson, 2017; Kearns et al., 2015). According to Lipson et al. (2018) and O' Keeffe, (2013), a large proportion of students with mental health issues still do not seek formal treatment, and Gallagher (2012) confirms that that 87% of college students who die by suicide do not go to their local campus clinics for help. This deficient mental health treatment for depressed students evokes fear among scholars that many students might drop out of university or commit suicide. As stated by DiPlacito-DeRango, (2016), Polanczyk et al. (2015) and Duffy et al. (2020) untreated mental health issues may become more severe and lead to suicide attempts, alcohol and drug use, and other major challenges. They argued that beyond personal consequences, adolescent mental health problems may have an adverse economic impact on society.

A growing body of literature has provided vital insights into barriers that prevent students from seeking help (SAMHSA, 2021; Cage et al., 2020; Hughes & Spanner, 2019; Lipson et al., 2019; Anderson, 2017; Hartrey et al., 2017; Camacho, 2016 & O' Keeffe, 2013). Grounded on the discussed literature, the following barriers were identified: public stigma, self-stigma, lack of proper mental health support system and education, lack of representation in the psychological and counselling staff, cultural mistrust, stigma regarding mental illness, university counselling units struggling with high demand of students and a lack of qualified employees as deterrents of students from getting mental health treatment.

Similarly, the Horwitz et al. (2020) study revealed most common barriers as lack of time (66.7%), questioning seriousness of needs (65.0%), and feeling as though stress is a normal aspect of being a graduate student (57.5%). In addition, financial resources appeared to be a bigger barrier for students who identified as sexual and gender minorities, as well as Black and Hispanic students. Concerns about privacy and stigma were more prevalent among male and younger undergraduate students (Busby et al., 2019; Eagan et al., 2017). Ebert et al. (2019), who studied barriers to mental health treatment utilization among first-year college students found that only 24.6% of students reported that they would seek treatment if they had a future emotional problem, (56.4%) preferred to handle the problem alone, while (48.0%) wanting to talk with friends or relatives instead. In line with Saade et al. (2023), who studied the mental health needs of African teenagers, the three most common barriers were stigma (25%), a lack of knowledge or unfamiliarity with the mental health condition (33.33%), and a preference for traditional complementary treatments (33.33%). Given the context above, Broglia et al. (2021), Horwitz et al. (2020), Cage et al. (2020) and Lipson et al. (2019) suggest internet-based psychological treatments, which can be accessed privately and are frequently built as self-help approaches to students who report hesitation about seeking treatment than other types of treatments, given that the preference to handle problems alone and stigma appear to be critical. It is critical to encourage students to seek help as the potential long-term consequences of untreated mental health problems could lead to death and loss of life. The next section discusses the methodology.

## METHODOLOGY

This being a conceptual review chapter, it relied on a review of secondary data materials to discuss the mental health crisis at higher education institutions. The inclusion criteria for article selection included those that investigated the mental health crises of students in postsecondary education institutions. Search engines such as Google Scholar, the Educational Resources Information Center (ERIC), PubMed, the Web of Science, and Psych INFO were used to obtain secondary data. The desktop review resulted in the descriptive analysis of mental health concepts, the prevalence of mental health issues, campus-based interventions, the role of parents and barriers to mental health treatment of higher education students. The next section discusses the conclusion.

## CONCLUSION

The growing discussion of mental health in recent years has led to closer attention to the mental health issues and struggles of university students, including deaths by suicide. Anxiety, depression, mental health problems and sadness may result in several negative outcomes such as substance misuse, academic dishonesty, dropping out of university, poor self-care, and even death if not timely treated. This paper contends that the provision of information on mental illness, information on campus-based treatment opportunities and the creation of an open environment where mental illness can be discussed, are critical to the improvement of help-seeking behaviour. It is, therefore, crucial for institutions of higher education to develop proactive outreach activities with students and initiate programs to support earlier engagement with services to preempt students' mental illness. The study recommendations for a proactive approach, such as early identification and prevention measures and strategies to reduce the stigma associated with seeking help for mental health issues in higher education.

## REFERENCES

Anderson, M. S. (2017). Barriers to the Utilization of Mental Health Services on College Campuses by African-American Students1. *McNair Scholar Research Journal, 11*(3), 1–12.

Aragon, T. J. (2020.) epitools: Epidemiology tools. *R package version 0.5-10.1.* Cran. https://cran.r-project. org/web/packages/epitools/epitools.pdf.

Arensman, E., Scott, V., De Leo, D., & Pirkis, J. (2020). Suicide and suicide prevention from a global perspective. *Crisis, 41*(Supplement 1), S3–S7. doi:10.1027/0227-5910/a000664 PMID:32208759

Asif, S., Mudassar, A., Shahzad, T. Z., Raouf, M., & Pervaiz, T. (2020). Frequency of depression, anxiety and stress among university students. [CrossRef]. *Pakistan Journal of Medical Sciences, 36*(5), 971–976. doi:10.12669/pjms.36.5.1873 PMID:32704273

Auerbach, R. P., Mortier, P., Bruffaerts, R., Alonso, J., Benjet, C., Cuijpers, P., Demyttenaere, K., Ebert, D. D., Green, J. G., Hasking, P., Murray, E., Nock, M. K., Pinder-Amaker, S., Sampson, N. A., Stein, D. J., Vilagut, G., Zaslavsky, A. M., & Kessler, R. C. (2018). WHO world mental health surveys international college student project: Prevalence and distribution of mental disorders. [CrossRef]. *Journal of Abnormal Psychology, 127*(7), 623–638. doi:10.1037/abn0000362 PMID:30211576

Backhaus, I., Varela, A. R., Khoo, S., Siefken, K., Crozier, A., Begotaraj, E., Fischer, F., Wiehn, J., Lanning, B., Lin, P., Jan, S., Zaranza Monteiro, L., Al-Shamli, A., La Torre, G., & Kawachi, I. (2020). Associations between social capital and depressive symptoms among college students in 12 countries: Results of a cross-national study. *Frontiers in Psychology, 11*, 644. doi:10.3389/fpsyg.2020.00644 PMID:32411038

Baig, T., Ganesan, G. S., Ibrahim, H., Yousuf, W., & Mahfoud, Z. R. (2021). The association of parental involvement with adolescents' well-being in Oman: Evidence from the 2015 Global School Health Survey. *BMC Psychology, 9*(1), 1–9. doi:10.118640359-021-00677-5 PMID:34749828

Baik, C., Larcombe, W., & Brooker, A. (2019). How universities can enhance student mental wellbeing: The student perspective. *Higher Education Research & Development, 38*(4), 674–687. Advance online publication. doi:10.1080/07294360.2019.1576596

Baker, C. (2018). *Mental Health Statistics for England: Prevalence, Services and Funding*. House of Commons Library. http://researchbriefings.files.parliament.uk/documents/SN06988/SN06988.pd

Bantjes, J., Saal, W., Christine Lochner, C., Roos, J., Auerbach, R. P., Mortier, P., Bruffaerts, R., & Ronald, C. (2020). Inequality and mental healthcare utilisation among first-year university students in South Africa. *International Journal of Mental Health Systems, 14*(1), 5. doi:10.118613033-020-0339-y PMID:31998406

Barbayannis, G., Bandari, M., Zheng, X., Baquerizo, H., Pecor, K. W., & Ming, X. (2022). Academic Stress and Mental Well-Being in College Students: Correlations, Affected Groups, and COVID-19. *Frontiers in Psychology, 13*, 886344. doi:10.3389/fpsyg.2022.886344 PMID:35677139

Barkham, M., Broglia, E., Dufour, G., Fudge, M., Knowles, L., Percy, A., Turner, A., & Williams, C. (2019). Towards an evidence base for student wellbeing and mental health. *Counselling & Psychotherapy Research, 19*(4), 351–357. doi:10.1002/capr.12227

Barrable, A., Papadatou-Pastou, M., & Tzotzoli, P. (2018). Supporting mental health, wellbeing and study skills in Higher Education: An online intervention system. *International Journal of Mental Health Systems, 12*(1), 54. doi:10.118613033-018-0233-z PMID:30323858

Benoit, V., & Gabola, P. (2021). Effects of Positive Psychology Interventions on the Well-Being of Young Children: A Systematic Literature Review. *International Journal of Environmental Research and Public Health, 18*(22), 12065. doi:10.3390/ijerph182212065 PMID:34831827

Bhatia, D., Roerig, M., Marani, H., King, M., Morales-Vstressedazquez, M., & Allin, S. (2020). Supporting Mental Health and Wellbeing Among Students in Higher Education. Toronto: North American Observatory on Health Systems and Policies. *Rapid Review*, (24).

Bhugra, D., Till, A., & Sartorius, N. (2013). What is mental health? *The International Journal of Social Psychiatry, 1*(1), 3–4. doi:10.1177/0020764012463315 PMID:23349505

Brenneisen Mayer, F., Souza Santos, I., Silveira, P. S. P., Itaqui Lopes, M. H., de Souza, A. R. N. D., Campos, E. P., de Abreu, B. A. L., Hoffman, I. II, Magalhães, C. R., Lima, M. C. P., Almeida, R., Spinardi, M., & Tempski, P. (2016). Factors associated to depression and anxiety in medical students: A multicenter study. *BMC Medical Education, 16*(1), 282. doi:10.118612909-016-0791-1 PMID:27784316

Broglia, E., Millings, A., & Barkham, M. (2021). Student mental health profiles and barriers to help-seeking: When and why students seek help for a mental health concern. *Counselling and Psychotherapy Research, 21*(4), 816-826.

Bronfenbrenner, U. (1979). *The ecology of human development: Experiments by nature and design.* Harvard University Press. https://www.hup.harvard.edu/catalog.php?isbn=9780674224575

Broonk, L., Gijselaers, H. J. M., Ritzen, H., & Brand-Gruwel, S. (2018). A review of the relationship between parental involvement indicators and academic achievement. *Educational Research Review, 24*, 10–30. doi:10.1016/j.edurev.2018.02.001

Bryan, C. J. (2021). *Rethinking Suicide: Why Prevention Fails, and How We Can Do Better.* Oxford University Press. https://www.amazon.com/Rethinking-Suicide-Prevention-Fails-Better/dp/0190050632 doi:10.1093/med-psych/9780190050634.001.0001

Busby, D. R., Zheng, K., Eisenberg, D., Albucher, R. C., Favorite, T., Coryell, W., & King, C. A. (2019). Black college students at elevated risk for suicide: Barriers to mental health service utilization. *Journal of American College Health*, 1–7. PMID:31662044

Cage, E., Stock, M., Sharpington, A., Pitman, E., & Batchelor, E. (2020). Barriers to accessing support for mental health issues at university. *Studies in Higher Education, 45*(8), 1637–1649. doi:10.1080/03075079.2018.1544237

Camacho, E. (2016). Minority student perceptions of mental health. *Journal of Undergraduate Research (Gainesville, Fla.), 14*, 35–54. http://openprairie.sdstate. edu/jur/vol14/iss1/6

Campbell, F., Blank, L., Cantrell, A., Baxter, S., Blackmore, C., Dixon, J., & Goyde, E. (2022). Factors that influence the mental health of university and college students in the UK: A systematic review. *BMC Public Health, 22*(1), 1778. doi:10.118612889-022-13943-x PMID:36123714

Casey, S. M., Varela, A., Marriott, J. P., Coleman, C. M., & Harlow, B. L. (2022). The influence of diagnosed mental health conditions and symptoms of depression and/or anxiety on suicide ideation, plan, and attempt among college students: Findings from the healthy minds study, 2018-2019. *Journal of Affective Disorders, 298*, 464–471. doi:10.1016/j.jad.2021.11.006 PMID:34774646

Causer, H., Bradley, E., Muse, K., & Smith, J. (2021). Bearing Witness: A grounded theory of the experiences of staff at two United Kingdom Higher Education Institutions following a student death by suicide. *PLoS One*, *16*(5), e0251369. doi:10.1371/journal.pone.0251369 PMID:33979333

Chand, S. P., & Arif, H. (2022). *Depression*. StatPearls Publishing. https://www.ncbi.nlm.nih.gov/books/NBK430847/

Chipare, M. A., Mupazvihwo, T., Tapera, R., & January, J. (2021). Mental Health Research in Namibia: A Scoping Review of Literature. *Medical Journal of Zambia*, *48*(2), 119–124. doi:10.55320/mjz.48.2.39

Conley, C. S., Shapiro, J. B., Kirsch, A. C., & Durlak, J. A. (2017). A meta-analysis of indicated mental health prevention programs for at-risk higher education students. *Journal of Counseling Psychology, 64*(2), 121–140. doi:10.1037/cou0000190 PMID:28277730

Curtin, S. C., Warner, M., & Hedegaard, H. (2016). Increase in suicide in the United States, 1999–2014. *NCHS Data Brief, 241*, 1–8. PMID:27111185

Dhar, B. K., Ayittey, F. K., & Sarkar, S. M. (2020). Impact of COVID-19 on Psychology among the University Students. [CrossRef]. *Global Challenges (Hoboken, NJ), 4*(11), 2000038. doi:10.1002/gch2.202000038 PMID:33042575

DiPlacito-DeRango, M. L. (2016). Acknowledge the Barriers to Better the Practices: Support for Student Mental Health in Higher Education. *The Canadian Journal for the Scholarship of Teaching and Learning*, *7*(2), 2. https://ir.lib.uwo.ca/cjsotl_rcacea/vol7/iss2/2. doi:10.5206/cjsotl-rcacea.2016.2.2

Doolan, K. (2021). *Student life during the COVID-19 pandemic lockdown: Europe-wide insights*. European Students' Union.

Dopmeijer, J. M. (2021). *Running on empty. The impact of challenging student life on well-being and academic performance.* [Doctoral dissertation, University of Amsterdam]. Digital Academic Repository.

Douwes, R., Metselaar, J., Gerdina, H. Pijnenborg, M., & Boonstra, N. (2023). The well-being of students in higher education: The importance of a student perspective, *Cogent Education,* 10:1, 2190697, DOI: . doi:10.1080/2331186X.2023.2190697

Dubé, J. P., Smith, M. M., Sherry, S. B., Hewitt, P. L., & Stewart, S. H. (2021). Suicide behaviours during the COVID-19 pandemic: A meta-analysis of 54 studies. *Psychiatry Research, 301*, 113998. doi:10.1016/j.psychres.2021.113998 PMID:34022657

Duffy, A., Keown-Stoneman, C., Goodday, S., Horrocks, J., Lowe, M., King, N., Pickett, W., McNevin, S. H., Cunningham, S., Rivera, D., Bisdounis, L., Bowie, C. R., Harkness, K., & Saunders, K. E. (2020). Predictors of mental health and academic outcomes in first-year university students: Identifying prevention and early-intervention targets. *BJPsych Open*, *6*(3), e46. doi:10.1192/bjo.2020.24 PMID:32381150

Durkheim, E. (1951). *Suicide: a study in sociology [1897]*. The Free Press.

Eagan, M. K., Stoltenberg, E. B., Zimmerman, H. B., Aragon, M. C., Whang Sayson, H., & Rios-Aguilar, C. (2017). The American freshman: National norms fall. *Higher Education Research Institute*. UCLA. https://www.heri.ucla.edu/monographs/ TheAmericanFreshman2016.pdf

Ebert, D. D., Mortier, P., Kaehlke, F., Bruffaerts, R., Baumeister, H., Auerbach, R. P., Alonso, J., Vilagut, G., Martínez, K. U., Lochner, C., Cuijpers, P., Kuechler, A.-M., Green, J., Hasking, P., Lapsley, C., Sampson, N. A., & Kessler, R. C. (2019). WHO World Mental Health-International College Student Initiative collaborators. Barriers of mental health treatment utilization among first-year college students: First cross-national results from the WHO World Mental Health International College Student Initiative. *International Journal of Methods in Psychiatric Research*, *28*(2), e1782. doi:10.1002/mpr.1782 PMID:31069905

Eisenberg, D., Hunt, J., Speer, M.D., & Nicole, M.S. (2013). Mental Health in American Colleges and Universities: Variation Across Student Subgroups and Across Campuses. *The Journal of Nervous and Mental Disease, 201*(1), 60-67. . doi:10.1097/NMD.0b013e31827ab077

Enwefa, R., Enwefa, S., & Fagbeyiro, G. (2020). The Epidemic of Mental Health in Higher Education and Its Impact on Students' Academic Success. [IJTIE]. *International Journal of Technology and Inclusive Education*, *1*(9), 1500–1504. doi:10.20533/ijtie.2047.0533.2020.0184

Eriksson, M., Ghazinour, M., & Hammarstrom, A. (2018). Different uses of Bronfenbrenner's ecological theory in public mental health research: What is their value for guiding public mental health policy and practice? *Social Theory & Health*, *16*(4), 414–433. doi:10.105741285-018-0065-6

Fernández-Alonso, R., & Álvarez-Díaz, M. Woitschach, Pamela., Suárez-Álvarez, J., & Cuesta, M. (2017). Parental involvement and academic performance: Less control and more communication. Psicothema, 29(4), 453-461 doi:10.7334/psicothema2017.181

Frajerman, A., Morvan, Y., Krebs, M. O., Gorwood, P., & Chaumette, B. (2019). Burnout in medical students before residency: A systematic review and meta-analysis. *European Psychiatry*, *5*, 36–42. doi:10.1016/j.eurpsy.2018.08.006 PMID:30384110

Freire, C., Ferradás, M., Regueiro, B., Rodríguez, S., Valle, A., & Núñez, J. C. (2020). Coping strategies and self-efficacy in university students: A person-centered approach. *Frontiers in Psychology*, *11*, 841. doi:10.3389/fpsyg.2020.00841 PMID:32508707

Galderisi, S., Heinz, A., Kastrup, M., Beezhold, J., & Sartorius, N. (2015). Toward a new definition of mental health. *World Psychiatry; Official Journal of the World Psychiatric Association (WPA)*, *14*(2), 231–233. doi:10.1002/wps.20231 PMID:26043341

Gallagher, S. (2012). Multiple aspects in the sense of agency. *New Ideas in Psychology*, *30*(1), 15–31. doi:10.1016/j.newideapsych.2010.03.003

Garriott, P. O., & Nisle, S. (2018). Stress, coping, and perceived academic goal progress in first-generation college students: The role of institutional supports. *Journal of Diversity in Higher Education, 11*(4), 436–450. doi:10.1037/dhe0000068

Gratz, K. L., Mann, A. J. D., & Tull, M. T. (2021). Suicidal ideation among university students during the COVID-19 pandemic: Identifying at-risk subgroups. *Psychiatry Research, 302*, 114034. doi:10.1016/j.psychres.2021.114034 PMID:34098158

Haile, Y. G., Senkute, A. L., Alemu, B. T., Bedane, D. M., & Kebede, K. B. (2019). Prevalence and associated factors of burnout among Debre Berhan University medical students: A cross-sectional study. *BMC Medical Education, 19*(1), 1–11. doi:10.118612909-019-1864-8 PMID:31703674

Hartrey, L., Denieffe, S., & Wells, J. S. (2017). A systematic review of barriers and supports to the participation of students with mental health difficulties in higher education. *Mental Health & Prevention, 6*, 26–43. doi:10.1016/j.mhp.2017.03.002

He, F. X., Turnbull, B., Kirshbaum, M. N., Phillips, B., & Klainin-Yobas, P. (2018). Assessing Stress, Protective Factors and Psychological Well-Being among Undergraduate Nursing Students. [CrossRef]. *Nurse Education Today, 68*, 4–12. doi:10.1016/j.nedt.2018.05.013 PMID:29870871

Holloway, S. D., & Jonas, M. (2016). Families, culture, and schooling: A critical review of theory and research. In K. R. Wentzel & G. B. Ramani (Eds.), *Handbook of social influences in school contexts: Socio-emotional, motivation, cognitive outcomes* (pp. 258–272). Taylor & Francis.

Horwitz, A. G., McGuire, T., Busby, D. R., Eisenberg, D., Zheng, K., Pistorello, J., & King, C. A. (2020). Sociodemographic differences in barriers to mental health care among college students at elevated suicide risk. *Journal of Affective Disorders, 271*, 123–130. doi:10.1016/j.jad.2020.03.115 PMID:32479307

Houston, J. B., First, J., Spialek, M. L., Sorenson, M. E., Mills-Sandoval, T., Lockett, M. K., First, N. L., Nitiéma, P., Allen, S. F., & Pfefferbaum, B. (2017). Randomized controlled trial of the Resilience and Coping Intervention (RCI) with undergraduate university students. *Journal of American College Health, 65*(1), 1–9. doi:10.1080/07448481.2016.1227826 PMID:27559857

Hughes, G., & Spanner, L. (2019). The University Mental Health Charter. *Student Minds*. https://www.studentminds.org.uk/uploads/3/7/8/4/37845 84/191208_umhc_artwo rk.pdf

Idowu, A., Olawuyi, D. A., & Nwadioke, C. O. (2020). Impacts of the COVID-19 pandemic on the psychological well-being of students in a Nigerian university. *Journal of Medical and Surgical Research, 7*, 798–806. doi:10.46327/msrjg.1.000000000000173

Itani, T., Jacobsen, K.H., & Kraemer, A. (2017). Suicidal ideation and planning among Palestinian middle school students living in Gaza Strip, West Bank, and United Nations Relief and Works Agency (UNRWA) camps. *Int J Pediatr Adolesc Med. 4*(2), 54–60. https://doi.org/. 003. doi:10.1016/j.ijpam.2017.03

Kajjimu, J., Kaggwa, M. M., & Bongomin, F. (2021, January). Burnout and associated factors among medical students in a Public University in Uganda: A cross-sectional study. *Advances in Medical Education and Practice, 12*, 63–75. doi:10.2147/AMEP.S287928 PMID:33531852

Kandasamy, N., Indraah, K., Tukiman, N. A., Khalil Kusairi, F. W. K., Amir Sjarif, S. I., & Shahrul Nizar, M. S. S. (2020). Factors That Influence Mental Illness Among Students in Public Universities. *Journal of Business and Economic Analysis, 3*(1), 77–90. doi:10.1142/j_10.36924sbe.2020.3106

Kearns, M., Muldoon, O. T., Msetfi, R. M., & Surgenor, P. W. G. (2015). Understanding help-seeking amongst university students: The role of group identity, stigma, and exposure to suicide and help-seeking. *Frontiers in Psychology, 6*, 6. doi:10.3389/fpsyg.2015.01462 PMID:26483722

Kebede, M. A., Anbessie, B., & Ayano, G. (2019). Prevalence and predictors of depression and anxiety among medical students in Addis Ababa, Ethiopia. *International Journal of Mental Health Systems, 13*(1), 30. doi:10.118613033-019-0287-6 PMID:31080499

Kerr, H. (2013). *Mental distress survey overview*. MRS Evidence Matters: United Kingdom. https://www.nus.org.uk/Global/Campaigns/20130517%20Mental%20Distress%20Survey%20%20Overview.pdf.

Kons, K., Biney, A. A., & Sznajder, K. (2022). Factors associated with adolescent pregnancy in sub-Saharan Africa during the COVID-19 pandemic: A review of socioeconomic influences and essential interventions. *International Journal of Sexual Health, 34*(3), 386–396. doi:10.1080/19317611.2022.2084199

Larcombe, W., Finch, S., Sore, R., Murray, C. M., Kentish, S., Mulder, R. A., & Williams, D. (2016). Prevalence and socio-demographic correlates of psychological distress among students at an Australian university. *Studies in Higher Education, 41*(6), 1074–1091. doi:10.1080/03075079.2014.966072

Levi-Belz, Y., Gvion, Y., & Apter, A. (2019). The psychology of suicide: From research understandings to intervention and treatment. *Frontiers in Psychiatry, 10*, 214. doi:10.3389/fpsyt.2019.00214 PMID:31019475

Levi-Belz, Y., Gvion, Y., Grisaru, S., & Apter, A. (2018). When the pain becomes unbearable: A case-control study of mental pain characteristics among medically serious suicide attempters. *Archives of Suicide Research, 22*(3), 380–393. doi:10.1080/13811118.2017.1355288 PMID:28786756

Lipson, S. K., & Eisenberg, D. (2018). Mental health and academic attitudes and expectations in university populations: Results from the healthy minds study. *Journal of Mental Health (Abingdon, England), 27*(3), 205–213. doi:10.1080/09638237.2017.1417567 PMID:29265935

Lipson, S. K., Lattie, E. G., & Eisenberg, D. (2019). Increased rates of mental health service utilization by US college students: 10-year population-level trends (2007–2017). *Psychiatric Services (Washington, D.C.), 70*(1), 60–63. doi:10.1176/appi.ps.201800332 PMID:30394183

Lipson, S. K., Zhou, S., Abelson, S., Heinze, J., Jirsa, M., Morigney, J., Patterson, A., & Eisenberg, D. (2022). Trends in college student mental health and help-seeking by race/ethnicity: Findings from the National Healthy Minds study, 2013–2021. *Journal of Affective Disorders, 306*, 138–147. doi:10.1016/j.jad.2022.03.038 PMID:35307411

Lisiecka, A., Chimicz, D., & Lewicka-Zelent, A. (2023). Mental Health Support in Higher Education during the COVID-19 Pandemic: A Case Study and Recommendations for Practice. *International Journal of Environmental Research and Public Health, 20*(6), 4969. doi:10.3390/ijerph20064969 PMID:36981877

Liu, C. H., Stevens, C., Wong, S., Yasui, M., & Chen, J. A. (2019). The prevalence and predictors of mental health diagnoses and suicide among U.S. college students: Implications for addressing disparities in service use. *Depression and Anxiety*, *36*(1), 8–17. doi:10.1002/da.22830 PMID:30188598

Maina, G., Mauri, M., & Rossi, A. (2016). Anxiety and depression. *Journal of Psychopathology*, (22), 236–250.

Manap, R., Hamid, S. A., & Ghani, M. A. (2018). Depression, anxiety and stress among undergraduate students. *Journal of Social Sciences and Humanities*, *16*(2), 1–7.

Manwell, L. A., Barbic, S. P., Roberts, K., Durisko, Z., Lee, C., Ware, E., & McKenzie, K. (2015). What is mental health? Evidence towards a new definition from a mixed methods multidisciplinary international survey. *BMJ Open*, *007079*(6), e007079. doi:10.1136/bmjopen-2014-007079 PMID:26038353

Mayo Clinic. (2019). *Anxiety disorders-Symptoms and causes*. Mayo Clinic. www.mayoclinic.org/diseases-conditions/ anxiety/symptoms-causes/sync-20350961

McPhillips, D. (2023). *Mental health struggles are driving more college students to consider dropping out, survey.* Finds Edition. finds.edition.cnn.com/2023/03/23/health/mental-health-college-dropout-survey-wellness/index.html

Meeus, W. (2016). Adolescent psychosocial development: A review of longitudinal models and research. *Developmental Psychology*, *52*(12), 1969–1993. doi:10.1037/dev0000243 PMID:27893243

Mhata, N.T., Ntlantsana, V., Tomita, A.M., Mwambene, K., & Saloojee, S. (2023). Prevalence of depression, anxiety and burnout in medical students at the University of Namibia. *S Afr J Psychiatr, 31*(29), 2044. doi: . v29i0.2044. PMID: 37292521; PMCID: PMC10244924. doi:10.4102/sajpsychiatry

Molla- Jafar, H., Salabifard, S., Mousavi, S. M., and Sobhani, Z. (2015). The effectiveness of group training of CBT-based stress management on anxiety, psychological hardiness and general self-efficacy among university students. *Glob. J. Health Sci.* 8, 47–54. doi: . v8n6p47. doi:10.5539/gjhs

National College Health Assessment. (2015). *Annual Report sponsored by the American College Health Assessment.* ACHA-NCHA.

National Institute of Mental Health (NIMH). (n.d.). *Suicide. Bethesda, MD.* NIMH. https://www.nimh.nih.gov/ health/statistics/suicide.shtml

Nguyen, H. T. L., Nakamura, K., Seino, K., & Vo, V. T. (2020). Relationships among cyberbullying, parental attitudes, self-harm and suicidal behaviour among adolescents: Results from a school-based survey in Vietnam. *BMC Public Health*, *20*(1), 476. doi:10.118612889-020-08500-3 PMID:32276608

O'Keeffe, P. (2013). Mental Illness within Higher Education: Risk Factors, Barriers to Help Seeking and Pressures on Counselling Centres. *JANZSSA. Journal of the Australian and New Zealand Student Services Association*, 1–12.

O'Sullivan, K., Clark, S., McGrane, A., Rock, N., Burke, L., Boyle, N., Joksimovic, N., & Marshall, K. (2021). A qualitative study of child and adolescent mental health during the COVID-19 pandemic in Ireland. *International Journal of Environmental Research and Public Health*, *18*(3), 1062. doi:10.3390/ijerph18031062 PMID:33504101

Oaes, J. (2023). Namibia. Mental Health Conversation-Stress and Depression among Children and Adolescents is Real. *New Era*, *21*(May), 1–3.

Oh, H., Marinovich, C., Jay, S., Marsh, J., Zhou, S., & DeVylder, J. E. (2022). COVID-19 factors and self-injurious behaviors among us college students: Findings from the healthy minds study 2020. *Journal of American College Health*, 1–5. doi:10.1080/07448481.2022.2081059 PMID:35728007

Olingo, A. (2020 April 29th). The economy hit hard as services slow down. *Daily Nation P.2*. Nation Media Group: Nairobi, Kenya.

Ormel, J., Kessler, R. C., & Schoevers, R. (2019). Depression: more treatment but no drop in prevalence: How effective is the treatment? And can we do better? *Current Opinion in Psychiatry*, *32*(4), 348–354. doi:10.1097/YCO.0000000000000505 PMID:30855297

Orygen. ((2017)). *Under the radar.* The mental health of Australian university students. Melbourne: Orygen, The National Centre of Excellence in Youth Mental Health.

Patel, V., Belkin, G. S., & Chockalingham, A. (2013). Grand challenges; integrating mental health services into priority care platforms. *PLoS Medicine*, *10*(5), e1001448. doi:10.1371/journal.pmed.1001448 PMID:23737736

Pedrelli, P., Nyer, M., Yeung, A., Zulauf, C., & Wilens, T. (2015). College students: Mental health problems and treatment considerations. *Academic Psychiatry*, *39*(5), 503–511. doi:10.100740596-014-0205-9 PMID:25142250

Pengpid, S., & Peltzer, K. (2018). Parental involvement and health risk behaviours among school-going adolescents in six African countries. *Journal of Psychology in Africa*, *28*(3), 212–217. doi:10.1080/14330237.2017.1409481

Phang, C. K., Mukhtar, F., Ibrahim, N., & Keng, S. L., & Mohd- Sidik, S. (2015). Effects of a brief mindfulness-based intervention program for stress management among medical students: The Mindful-Gym randomized controlled study. *Advances in Health Sciences Education : Theory and Practice*, *20*, 1115–1134. doi:10.100710459-015-9591-3 PMID:25697124

Polanczyk, G.V., Salum, G.A., Sugaya, L.S., Caye, A., Rohde, L.A. (2015). Annual research review: a meta-analysis of the worldwide prevalence of mental disorders in children and adolescents. *J Child Psychol Psychiatry, 56*(3), 345–65.

Porru, F., Schuring, M., Bultmann, U., Portoghese, I., Busdorf, A., & Robroek, S. J. N. (2022). Associations of university student life challenges with mental health and self-rated health: A longitudinal study with 6 months follow-up. [CrossRef]. *Journal of Affective Disorders*, *296*, 250–257. doi:10.1016/j.jad.2021.09.057 PMID:34624809

Reddy, K. J., Menon, K. R., & Thattil, A. (2018). Academic stress and its sources among university students. *Biomedical & Pharmacology Journal*, *11*(1), 1. doi:10.13005/bpj/1404

Regehr, C., Glancy, D., & Pitts, A. (2013). Interventions to reduce stress in university students: A review and meta-analysis. *Journal of Affective Disorders*, *148*(1), 1–11. doi:10.1016/j.jad.2012.11.026 PMID:23246209

Reimers, F., Schleicher, A., Saavedra, J., & Tuominen, S. (2020). Supporting the continuation of teaching and learning during the COVID-19 Pandemic. *Oecd, 1*(1), 1–38.

Ribeiro, I. J. S., Freire, I. V., & de Araújo, T. M. (2020). Are stress management interventions effective in reducing stress, anxiety, and depression in college students? *Clinical Psychology : a Publication of the Division of Clinical Psychology of the American Psychological Association.* doi:10.1111/cpsp.12385

Rodríguez, S., Piñeiro, I., Gómez-Taibo, M. L., Regueiro, B., Estévez, I., & Valle, A. (2017). An explanatory model of maths achievement: Perceived parental involvement and academic motivation. *Psicothema, 29*(2), 184–190. 10.7334 PMID:28438240

Rotenstein, L. S., Ramos, M. A., Torre, M., Segal, J. B., Peluso, M. J., Guille, C., Sen, S., & Mata, D. A. (2016). Prevalence of depression, depressive symptoms, and suicidal ideation among medical students: A systematic review and meta-analysis. *Journal of the American Medical Association, 316*(21), 2214–2236. doi:10.1001/jama.2016.17324 PMID:27923088

Saade, S., Lamarche, A. P., Khalaf, T., Makke, S., & Legg, A. (2023). What barriers could impede access to mental health services for children and adolescents in Africa? A scoping review. *BMC Health Services Research, 23*(1), 348. doi:10.118612913-023-09294-x PMID:37024835

Saleh, D., Camart, N., & Romo, L. (2017). Predictors of stress in college students. *Frontiers in Psychology, 8*, 19. doi:10.3389/fpsyg.2017.00019 PMID:28179889

Salik, I., & Marwaha, R. (2022*). Electroconvulsive Therapy*. StatPearls Publishing. https://www.ncbi.nlm.nih.gov/books/NBK538266/

Schmits, E., Dekeyser, S., Klein, O., Luminet, O., Yzerbyt, V., & Glowacz, F. (2021). Psychological Distress among Students in Higher Education: One Year after the Beginning of the COVID-19 Pandemic. *International Journal of Environmental Research and Public Health, 18*(14), 7445. doi:10.3390/ijerph18147445 PMID:34299896

Spielberger, C. D. (2013). *Anxiety: Current trends in theory and research.* Elsevier.

Substance Abuse and Mental Health Services Administration (SAMHSA). (2021). *Prevention and Treatment of Anxiety, Depression, and Suicidal Thoughts and Behaviors Among College Students.* SAMHSA Publication No. PEP21-06-05-002. Rockville, MD: National Mental Health and Substance Use Policy Laboratory.

Tam, W., Lo, K., & Pacheco, J. (2019). Prevalence of depressive symptoms among medical students: Overview of systematic reviews. Med Educ. *Medical Education, 53*(4), 345–354. doi:10.1111/medu.13770 PMID:30474128

Teh, C. K., Ngo, C. W., Binti Zulkifli, R. A., Vellasamy, R., & Suresh, K. (2015). Depression, anxiety and stress among undergraduate students: A cross-sectional study. [Crossref]. *Open Journal of Epidemiology, 5*(04), 260–268. doi:10.4236/ojepi.2015.54030

Thanoi, W., Vongsirimas, N., Sitthimongkol, Y., & Klainin-Yobas, P. (2023). Examining Predictors of Psychological Well-Being among University Students: A Descriptive Comparative Study across Thailand and Singapore. *International Journal of Environmental Research and Public Health, 20*(3), 1875. doi:10.3390/ijerph20031875 PMID:36767238

Thomas, V., Muls, J., De Backer, F., & Lombaerts, K. (2020). Middle school student and parent perceptions of parental involvement: Unravelling the associations with school achievement and wellbeing. *Educational Studies, 46*(4), 404–421. doi:10.1080/03055698.2019.1590182

Tian-Ci Quek, T., & Wai-San Tam, W. (2019). The global prevalence of anxiety among medical students: A meta-analysis. *Int J Environ Res Public Health, 16*(15), 2735. 10.3390/ijerph16152735

Tudge, J. R. H., Mokrova, I., Hatfield, B. E., & Karnik, R. B. (2009). Uses and Misuses of Bronfenbrenner's Bioecological Theory of Human Development. *Journal of Family Theory & Review, 1*(4), 198–210. doi:10.1111/j.1756-2589.2009.00026.x

Vallejo- Slocker, L., Fresneda- Sánchez, F. J., & Vallejo -Pareja, M. Á. (2020). Psychological well-being of vulnerable children during the COVID-19 pandemic. *Psicothema.*

Verrocchio, M. C., Carrozzino, D., Marchetti, D., Andreasson, K., Fulcheri, M., & Bech, P. (2016). Mental pain and suicide: A systematic review of the literature. *Frontiers in Psychiatry, 7*, 108. doi:10.3389/fpsyt.2016.00108 PMID:27378956

Wango, G. (2023). Psychological Health. Counselling Diary. University of Nairobi: Kenya.

Wiedemann, K. (2015). Anxiety and anxiety disorders. International Encyclopedia of the Social & Behavioral Sciences, (2nd ed) 804-810.

World Health Organization. (2020). *Mental Health and Substance Use.* Geneva: WHO https://www.who.int/teams/mental-health-and-substance-use/overview

Yanos, P. T., & Rosario, A. (2014). Preventive coping among people with severe mental illness in daily life: Strategies used and associations with mood. *The International Journal of Social Psychiatry, 60*(5), 489–491. doi:10.1177/0020764013501291 PMID:24004616

Yap, M.B.H., Pilkington, P.D., Ryan, S.M., Jorm, A.F. (2014). Parental factors associated with depression and anxiety in young people: a systematic review and meta-analysis. *J Affect Disord. 156*(8), 23. https://doi.org/. jad.2013.11.007. doi:10.1016/j

Yusufov, M., Nicoloro-SantaBarbara, J., Grey, N. E., Moyer, A., & Lobel, M. (2019). A meta-analytic evaluation of stress reduction interventions for undergraduate and graduate students. *International Journal of Stress Management, 26*(2), 132–145. doi:10.1037tr0000099

Zhai, Y., & Du, X. (2023). Trends and prevalence of suicide 2017–2021 and its association with COVID-19: Interrupted time series analysis of a national sample of college students in the United States. *Psychiatry Research*, 1–7. www.elsevier.com/locate/psychres PMID:35987067

# Chapter 9
# Mental Health Challenges in HigherEd Students:
## Framework and Implications for Institutions

**Vivek Ahuja**
https://orcid.org/0000-0001-5073-4342
*FLAME University, India*

## ABSTRACT

*This chapter explores challenges faced by higher education students related to adjustment, stress, and mental health. It focuses on stress's impact on students' well-being and academic, physical, social, and psychological aspects during their university journey. The transitional phase from secondary school to higher education is examined, shedding light on unique challenges. Additionally, a conceptual framework is introduced, offering structured insights into these challenges within the higher education context. Implications for institutions, management, students, and parents are discussed. This chapter aims to comprehensively analyze stress and mental health challenges among higher education students, raising awareness and promoting strategies for a supportive environment, guided by the presented conceptual framework.*

## INTRODUCTION

Higher education institutions play a pivotal role in shaping the future of students, offering them opportunities for personal and academic growth. However, this journey is not without its challenges. Students entering higher education often face adjustment issues, academic stressors, and mental health concerns that can significantly impact their overall well-being and success in their academic pursuits. Understanding the complex interplay between these challenges and students' mental health is crucial for providing effective support and promoting an environment where students can thrive (Ross, 1999; Ong and Cheong, 2009).

DOI: 10.4018/979-8-3693-2833-0.ch009

## Significance of Understanding the Impact of Stress and Mental Health

The significance of understanding the impact of stress and mental health on higher education students cannot be overstated. Research has shown that students' mental health is closely linked to their academic performance, physical health, and social relationships (Fletcher et al., 2009; Lipson & Eisenberg, 2018). Moreover, the well-being of students is intertwined with their overall success in higher education. Recognizing the multifaceted nature of these challenges and their effects on students' lives is a critical step in addressing their needs.

This chapter aims to explore the challenges faced by students in higher education institutions related to adjustment, stress, and mental health. It seeks to shed light on the intricate relationships between these challenges and students' overall well-being. Additionally, this chapter outlines a conceptual framework developed to understand the interplay between mental health and various aspects of students' lives in higher education (Priestley et al., 2022). This chapter sets the stage for continued research, awareness, and action to support higher education students' well-being by examining the existing research and proposing a structured framework.

### Conceptual Framework

The conceptual framework presented herein provides a structured guide to understanding how mental health influences different dimensions of the student experience within higher education. This framework identifies key factors, including academic performance, physical health, social relationships, and overall well-being, and illustrates how they are interconnected with students' mental health. It also suggests propositions for future research and strategies to support students' mental health, emphasizing the need for a holistic approach to address the challenges they encounter (Priestley et al., 2022).

With these objectives and the conceptual framework as a backdrop, this chapter discusses the complexities of students' experiences in higher education and offers insights into how institutions can create an environment that prioritizes student mental health and facilitates their success.

## CHALLENGES ENCOUNTERED BY STUDENTS DURING THE TRANSITION FROM SECONDARY SCHOOL TO HIGHER EDUCATION

Students often experience difficulty in transitioning from secondary school to higher education. This transition can be marked by differences in curricula, teaching methods, and expectations between secondary schools and universities, leading to an *academic shock* (Briggs, Clark, and Hall, 2012). Academic shock refers to the significant and sometimes overwhelming challenges that students may encounter when they enter a higher education environment. These challenges often arise due to the differences in teaching methods, curricula, expectations, and the overall academic demands between secondary school and university or college. They are suddenly exposed to a more independent and rigorous learning environment. This can include larger class sizes, more complex course materials, higher expectations for self-directed learning, and greater academic responsibility. As a result, students might struggle initially to adapt to these new academic demands, which can lead to stress, anxiety, and difficulties in their academic performance. Fook and Sidhu's (2015) research explores a range of learning challenges encountered by students in higher education, shedding light on the multifaceted nature of these obstacles. Their findings reveal that students grapple with various *cognitive challenges*, which may involve adapting to higher levels of complexity and critical thinking expected in college or university-level coursework. These challenges often require students to develop advanced problem-solving skills and analytical thinking. Furthermore, the difficulty in becoming active learners suggests that students may initially struggle with the transition from passive learning in secondary school to the more self-directed and participatory learning environment of higher education. This shift necessitates greater autonomy in seeking out resources, asking questions, and engaging actively in class discussions and projects.

Abbott-Chapman's (2011) work highlights that *disadvantaged students* face unique challenges during this transition. These challenges are multifaceted and can encompass various factors such as hailing from a low socio-economic background, residing in rural areas with limited access to educational resources, or being mature-age students who are returning to education after a hiatus. These students often encounter challenges of financial barriers, lack of academic preparation, and a sense of isolation during this transition.

Students with *learning disabilities* face unique obstacles as they navigate the transition from secondary school to higher education, a challenge highlighted by Brinckerhoff (1996). Learning disabilities, such as dyslexia, ADHD, or autism, can significantly impact a student's ability to process information and learn using conventional methods. They may struggle to cope with the increased academic demands and complex coursework, which can be particularly challenging for them given their learning differences. Additionally, the need for specialized support and accommodations, such as extended time for exams or assistive technology, may not always be readily available or well-understood in higher education settings. This lack of understanding or accessibility can create barriers to their learning and hinder their academic progress. Moreover, the students themselves may face self-esteem issues and confidence challenges, making it harder for them to advocate for the support they need. Therefore, the difficulties lie in both the academic demands and the need for a supportive and inclusive learning environment.

Evans (2000) emphasizes the significant negative outcomes associated with *insufficient planning for students' transition* to higher education. When students face difficulties in adjusting to the rigorous demands of higher education, it can lead to both social and economic inefficiencies. They may end up discontinuing their studies, failing to attain their degrees, or encountering challenges that impede their academic and personal growth. In situations where educational institutions fail to adequately prepare students for this transition, they may encounter hardships in adapting to the academic requirements and other complexities of higher education. Consequently, this can result in adverse consequences, including dropout rates, incomplete degrees, and obstacles affecting both their educational progress and personal development. In essence, the challenge lies in students successfully navigating this critical phase without the essential guidance, support, and resources.

## IMPACT OF STRESS ON STUDENTS' MENTAL HEALTH AND OVERALL WELL-BEING

The impact of stress on students' mental health and overall well-being is profound and multifaceted. Elevated stress levels can lead to a range of adverse outcomes, including increased feelings of anxiety and depression, reduced emotional well-being, and diminished overall psychological health. Additionally, stress can manifest in physical symptoms, exacerbating the toll it takes on students' well-being. Furthermore, academic-related stressors, such as the burden of coursework and the pressure to perform, can contribute to feelings of overwhelm and burnout. These effects can ripple into various aspects of students' lives, affecting their motivation, engagement in learning, and even their decision to persist in their educational journey. Recognizing and addressing the impact of stress on students' mental health is important for creating a supportive and conducive learning environment that leads not only to academic success but also the holistic well-being of students in higher education.

Several researchers have investigated the impact of stress on students' mental health and overall well-being, shedding light on various facets of this complex relationship. Yusof et al. (2019) conducted a study investigating the profound influence of stress and depression on the psychological well-being of university students. This research brought to the forefront that elevated levels of stress and depression can significantly impact the emotional and mental health of students during their academic journey. Consequently, this highlights the critical need for interventions and support mechanisms to address these mental health challenges among university students.

Building upon this exploration, Pascoe, Hetrick, and Parker (2020) ventured into the realm of academic-related stress and its far-reaching ramifications. This study uncovered that academic stress not only obstructs academic achievements but also diminishes motivation and raises the risk of school dropout. These findings underscore the importance of proactive efforts to mitigate academic stress, including the provision of counseling services and stress management programs, aiming to bolster academic performance and promote student retention.

Moving into a specialized domain, Backović et al. (2013) extended this inquiry to the context of medical students. The study illuminated the substantial impact of academic stress on the mental health of medical students. These findings advocate for targeted mental health support within the medical education framework to ensure the well-being of future healthcare professionals.

Shankar and Park (2016) contributed to the comprehensive understanding of stress's multifaceted influence on students' lives by providing a conceptual overview of the intricate pathways involved. This work elucidated the direct and indirect connections between stress, physical health, mental health, and academic success. Such a holistic perspective underscores the need for integrated interventions that address these interconnected dimensions of students' well-being.

Additionally, Suldo, Shaunessy, and Hardesty (2008) explored the experiences of high-achieving high school students, revealing that they often grapple with heightened levels of stress compared to their peers. Moreover, their study identified various coping styles that relate to distinct mental health outcomes, emphasizing the importance of equipping high-achieving students with effective coping strategies to mitigate the negative effects of stress.

Pluut, Curşeu, and Ilies (2015) examined the impact of study-related stressors on academic performance and study-leisure conflicts. This investigation unveiled that such stressors can detrimentally affect academic outcomes and lead to conflicts between academic responsibilities and leisure activities. Consequently, this highlights the importance of promoting a balanced approach to academics and leisure, as well as developing strategies to manage study-related stress effectively.

In summary, the collective body of research explains the critical role that stress, particularly academic-related stress, plays in shaping the psychological well-being, academic achievements, and overall success of students in higher education. These findings (see Table 1 below) emphasize the necessity for comprehensive support systems, mental health interventions, and effective stress management strategies to foster positive outcomes for students in the academic realm.

*Table 1. Impacts of stress and related factors on students*

| Impact Categories | Key Findings |
|---|---|
| Psychological Well-being (Yusof et al., 2019) | Elevated stress and depression negatively affect psychological well-being. |
| | Emotional and mental health may be compromised during the academic journey. |
| Academic Achievement and Retention (Pascoe, Hetrick, & Parker, 2020) | Academic-related stress can lead to reduced academic performance. |
| | Decreased motivation and a higher risk of school dropout are associated with academic stress. |
| Mental Health of Specific Student Groups (Backović et al., 2013) | In the context of medical education, academic stress significantly impacts the mental health of medical students. |
| | There is a need for targeted mental health support within specialized academic programs. |
| Complex Pathways of Stress (Shankar & Park, 2016) | Stress influences physical health, mental health, and academic success through direct and indirect pathways. |
| | Understanding these interconnected dimensions of stress is crucial for holistic student support. |
| High-Achieving Students (Suldo, Shaunessy, & Hardesty, 2008) | High-achieving high school students may experience heightened levels of stress. |
| | The choice of coping strategies is related to distinct mental health outcomes among high-achieving students. |
| Study-Related Stressors (Pluut, Curşeu, & Ilies, 2015) | Study-related stressors can negatively impact academic performance. |
| | Conflict between study and leisure activities arises, affecting academic satisfaction and performance. |

## UNIQUE STRESSORS AND OBSTACLES FACED BY STUDENTS IN HIGHER EDUCATION

Higher education is a pivotal phase in a student's life, marked by a unique set of stressors and obstacles that can significantly impact their academic journey and overall well-being. These challenges encompass a wide range of academic and non-academic factors, which have been extensively explored in research.

### Academic Stressors

Ross et al. (1999) found that academic requirements, such as earning good grades and completing assignments, were major sources of stress for college students. Ong and Cheong (2009) further emphasized the burden of an excessive workload, exams, grades, and unclear course objectives as significant academic stressors. These findings align with the academic rigor experienced by students, which often entails navigating complex subject matter and maintaining high-grade point averages. The pressure to excel academically can indeed be a significant source of stress in higher education.

### Non-Academic Stressors

Beyond academics, students grapple with a multitude of non-academic stressors. Aselton (2012) identified a range of stressors, including roommate issues, academic problems, financial and career concerns, and pressure from family. These non-academic stressors intertwine with the academic challenges, creating a complex landscape for students to navigate. Financial concerns, in particular, loom large, impacting students' ability to focus on their studies and contributing to anxiety.

### Diversity and Inclusion

Inclusive and diverse campus environments are essential considerations in the higher education landscape. Students from various backgrounds may face unique challenges related to discrimination, prejudice, or feelings of exclusion. Abbott-Chapman (2011) and Brinckerhoff (1996), as mentioned earlier, have addressed this issue and concern for creating inclusive and supportive campus environments crucial for addressing diversity-related stressors.

### Mental Health and Well-Being

Saleh (2017) delved into the predictors of stress in college students, revealing psychological distress, anxiety, depressive symptoms, low self-esteem, little optimism, and low sense of self-efficacy as contributors to stress. These mental health challenges are increasingly prevalent among students and are exacerbated by the demands of higher education. Balancing academic responsibilities with extracurricular activities, part-time jobs, or internships often results in time management difficulties, potentially leading to stress and burnout.

In sum, the journey through higher education is marked by a myriad of academic and non-academic stressors. These stressors include academic rigor, financial concerns, social adjustments, time management, career decisions, diversity and inclusion considerations, and mental health challenges. Recognizing and addressing these stressors is vital in ensuring that students not only succeed academically but also thrive emotionally and socially during their higher education experience. This comprehensive understanding of stressors is essential for institutions to develop effective support mechanisms and interventions to promote students' well-being and success in higher education.

## ROLE OF MENTAL HEALTH IN STUDENTS' ACADEMIC PERFORMANCE, PHYSICAL HEALTH, SOCIAL RELATIONSHIPS, AND PSYCHOLOGICAL WELL-BEING

The mental health of students in higher education is a topic of great significance, and its importance reverberates through every facet of their academic journey and overall well-being. The profound interplay between mental health and students' academic performance, physical health, social relationships, and psychological well-being cannot be overstated. Within the dynamic environment of higher education, understanding the pivotal role of mental health is essential for institutions, educators, and policymakers. Prioritizing students' mental health is not merely an option but a necessity for their success and holistic development. In this exploration, we delve into the multifaceted relationship between mental health and the various dimensions of students' lives in higher education, underscoring the significance of fostering a mentally healthy campus environment.

## Academic Performance

Mental health significantly influences students' academic journeys and overall well-being, as evidenced by several studies (Fletcher et al., 2009; Lipson & Eisenberg, 2018; Bostani et al., 2014; Mohammad et al., 2015). Fletcher et al. (2009) found that depression is a significant predictor of lower GPAs and a higher probability of dropping out among college students. Lipson and Eisenberg (2018) expanded on this theme, demonstrating that mental health problems, such as depression and anxiety, serve as significant predictors of academic dissatisfaction and intentions to drop out, while positive mental health is linked to increased satisfaction and persistence (Fletcher et al., 2009; Lipson & Eisenberg, 2018).

Furthermore, Bostani, Nadri, and Nasab (2014) delved into the specific dimensions of mental health, highlighting the relationship between depression, anxiety, and educational performance (Bostani et al., 2014). Their findings underscored how internal factors related to mental well-being can significantly impact students' academic potential. Mohammad et al. (2015) provided a comprehensive view of the ripple effect of mental health on students' motivation and academic performance, emphasizing the intricate interplay between mental well-being, motivation, and academic outcomes (Mohammad et al., 2015).

## Physical Health

The intricate relationship between students' mental and physical health is a subject of extensive research, with findings from Tyson et al. (2010), Roberts et al. (2000), Miller, Gilman, and Martens (2008), and Jeoung, Hong, and Lee (2013) collectively demonstrating the interdependence of these two aspects. Tyson et al. (2010) uncovered a positive correlation between physical activity and mental health, indicating that students who engage in more physical activity tend to have better mental well-being. This explains the role of exercise as a valuable tool in enhancing students' psychological health. On the other hand, Roberts et al. (2000) explored the impact of financial difficulties on students' mental and physical health. Their research revealed that financial stress was associated with poorer mental and physical health among students, emphasizing the far-reaching consequences of economic challenges on overall well-being. Miller, Gilman, and Martens (2008) contributed to this discourse by highlighting the reciprocal relationship between mental and physical health. They advocate the potential for promoting both aspects to positively affect students' overall well-being, emphasizing the interconnected nature of mental and physical health. Furthermore, Jeoung, Hong, and Lee (2013) established a correlation between mental health and health-related physical fitness in university students, highlighting the importance of considering mental well-being alongside physical fitness initiatives.

## Social Relationships

Mental health indeed plays a pivotal role in shaping students' social relationships, with several studies providing valuable insights into this relationship. For instance, Khodabakhsh, Kiani, and Ahmedbookani (2014) found a significant link between parenting styles and students' mental health. This connection suggests that the emotional well-being fostered by positive parenting can contribute to students' ability to form and maintain healthy social relationships. When students grow up in supportive and emotionally nurturing environments, they tend to develop better emotional regulation skills, which are essential for fostering positive interactions and resolving conflicts within their social circles.

Additionally, Kotera, Green, and Sheffield's (2019) research explores the mental health of therapeutic students and its associations with attitudes, self-criticism/self-reassurance, and self-compassion. This study sheds light on how students' internal attitudes and self-perceptions, influenced by their mental health, can impact their social interactions. Students with better mental health tend to exhibit more self-compassion and self-assuredness, which can enhance their communication skills, making their expressions more honest and effective in social contexts. Furthermore, the concept of resilience is important when considering the role of mental health in students' social relationships. The research by Hefner and Eisenberg (2009) emphasizes that students with strong social support networks are better equipped to navigate mental health challenges, suggesting that good mental health not only directly influences students' social interactions but also indirectly bolsters their resilience in the face of social setbacks or conflicts. Resilient individuals can maintain healthier relationships by effectively coping with stressors and maintaining a positive outlook.

### Psychological Well-Being

Mental health and psychological well-being share a complex and interdependent relationship. Mental health encompasses emotional, psychological, and social well-being, representing a broader concept. Research conducted by Khodabakhsh, Kiani, and Ahmedbookani (2014) reveals a significant connection between psychological well-being and parenting styles, illustrating how these elements are intertwined with students' mental health.

Psychological well-being, on the other hand, refers to an individual's subjective evaluation of their emotional and psychological state. This subjective assessment encompasses various facets of one's life satisfaction, positive emotions, and overall sense of purpose and fulfillment. Research by Kotera, Green, and Sheffield (2019) delves into the mental health of therapeutic students, investigating its associations with attitudes, self-criticism/self-reassurance, and self-compassion, providing insights into the complex factors influencing students' psychological well-being.

Generally, a positive mental health status is closely linked to higher levels of psychological well-being, indicating that individuals experiencing good mental health are more inclined to report greater life satisfaction and a more positive emotional state. In contrast, mental health challenges can hinder psychological well-being, potentially leading to feelings of distress, anxiety, and a diminished overall sense of life satisfaction. This intricate relationship is further highlighted by Roberts et al. (2000), who explored the repercussions of students' financial circumstances on their mental and physical health, underscoring the potential adverse effects of financial stress on students' holistic well-being.

## DEVELOPMENT OF A CONCEPTUAL FRAMEWORK ON INTERPLAY BETWEEN MENTAL HEALTH AND STUDENTS' LIVES IN HIGHER EDUCATION

An intricately designed and comprehensive model (ref Figure 1) has been crafted to shed light on the complex interconnections between mental health and the various facets of students' lives in the higher education setting. This model is grounded in the insights and research discoveries amassed through a thorough examination of numerous studies conducted in this field and discussed above. The overarching aim of this framework is to provide a unified perspective, serving the dual purpose of unveiling the multifaceted associations between mental health and different dimensions of the student experience, while also articulating propositions that can serve as guiding principles for future research initiatives.

This framework is an endeavor to provide a holistic understanding of how mental health influences the academic performance, social interactions, and overall quality of life of students in higher education. It acknowledges that mental health is not isolated but intricately connected to these diverse facets of the student journey. Through this framework, the author aims to offer a structured approach for institutions, researchers, and policymakers to better comprehend and address the pivotal role of mental health in the higher education landscape.

## Proposition 1: Mental Health and Academic Performance

**Proposition 1a:** Good mental health positively impacts academic performance by enhancing cognitive abilities, concentration, and motivation (Fletcher et al., 2009; Mohammad et al., 2015).

**Proposition 1b:** Mental health challenges, such as stress and depression, can negatively affect academic performance by impairing students' ability to focus and meet academic demands (Lipson & Eisenberg, 2018; Evans, 2000).

## Proposition 2: Mental Health and Social Relationships

**Proposition 2a:** Positive mental health facilitates healthy social interactions, leading to the formation of meaningful friendships and supportive social networks (Priestley et al., 2022; Alsubaie et al., 2019).

**Proposition 2b:** Poor mental health can lead to social withdrawal, isolation, and strained relationships due to symptoms like mood disturbances and social anxiety (Suldo, 2008; Pachucki et al., 2015).

## Proposition 3: Mental Health and Overall Quality of Life

**Proposition 3a:** Positive mental health contributes to students' overall quality of life by enhancing well-being, life satisfaction, and a positive outlook on the future (Tyson et al., 2010; Saleh, 2017).

**Proposition 3b:** Poor mental health diminishes students' overall quality of life, leading to reduced life satisfaction, feelings of distress, and a decreased sense of fulfillment (Backović, 2013; Kotera, Green, & Sheffield, 2019).

## Proposition 4: Intervention and Support

**Proposition 4a:** Early intervention and support programs aimed at addressing mental health challenges can have a positive impact on academic performance (Abbott-Chapman, 2011; Brinckerhoff, 1996).

**Proposition 4b:** Creating a supportive and inclusive learning environment that promotes positive mental health can lead to stronger social relationships (Briggs, Clark, & Hall, 2012; Hefner & Eisenberg, 2009).

**Proposition 4c:** Early intervention and support programs aimed at addressing mental health challenges can have a positive impact on overall well-being (Abbott-Chapman, 2011; Brinckerhoff, 1996).

This framework and its associated propositions provide a structured understanding of how mental health influences various aspects of students' lives in higher education. It also highlights the importance of proactive interventions and support systems to enhance students' mental health and, subsequently, their academic success, social connections, and overall quality of life.

*Figure 1.*

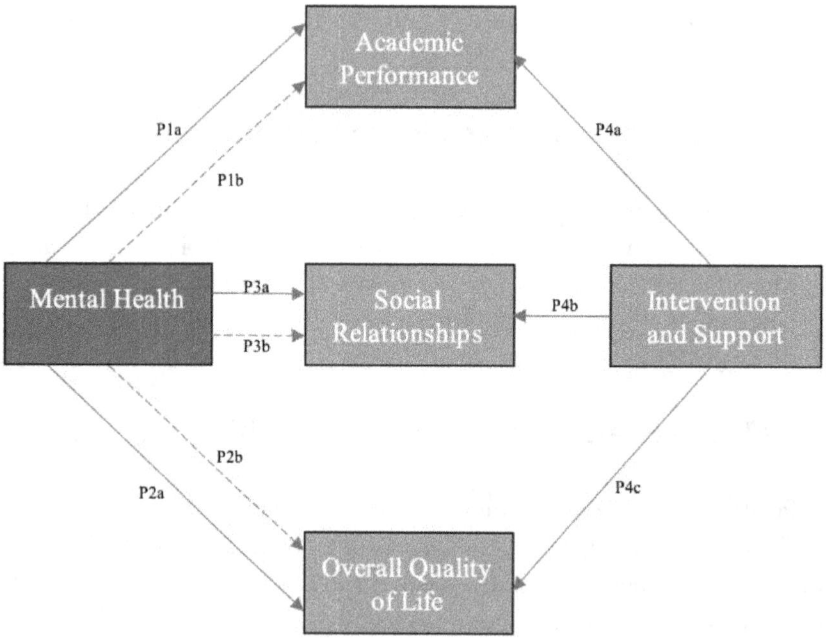


## IMPLICATIONS OF STRESS AND MENTAL HEALTH CHALLENGES FOR HIGHER EDUCATION INSTITUTIONS

The implications of stress and mental health challenges for higher education institutions are multifaceted and demand careful consideration. Research and studies have shed light on several key implications that institutions must address to ensure the well-being and success of their students.

First and foremost, the academic consequences of stress and mental health challenges cannot be overlooked. As highlighted by studies like Eisenberg, Golberstein, and Hunt (2009), students grappling with mental health issues are at a higher risk of lower GPAs and dropping out. Consequently, institutions must recognize that students' mental well-being directly impacts their academic performance. To mitigate these academic consequences, universities should invest in mental health support services, including counseling and intervention programs.

Furthermore, the broader campus community must be aware of the prevalence and impact of mental health challenges among students. Creating a stigma-free environment where students feel comfortable seeking help is essential. Studies such as Nami, Nami, and Eishani (2014) emphasize the importance of mental health education on campuses, and institutions should take steps to promote awareness and destigmatize mental health issues.

In terms of resources, Martineau, Beauchamp, and Marcotte (2017) suggest that implementing supervised mental health prevention strategies can significantly reduce mental health problems among students. This implies that institutions should consider the allocation of resources to proactive mental health programs and interventions.

Lastly, a campus-wide commitment to mental health, as advocated by Leshner (2021), is vital. Coordinated action plans involving faculty, staff, and administration are essential to create a holistic support system for students. This not only ensures that students have access to the necessary resources but also fosters a culture of well-being within the institution.

The implications of stress and mental health challenges for higher education institutions are far-reaching. They necessitate a proactive and comprehensive approach that encompasses academic support, awareness, resource allocation, and a campus-wide commitment to student well-being. Redressal of these implications can help institutions to better support their students and create an environment conducive to both academic success and personal growth.

## ROLE OF STAKEHOLDERS IN PROMOTING MENTAL HEALTH IN HIGHER EDUCATION

Promoting mental health in higher education is a collective effort involving faculty, staff, and students, and each group plays a crucial role. Faculty members, as highlighted by Kalkbrenner (2019), can contribute significantly by recognizing signs of mental distress in students and referring them to appropriate resources. However, Ramluggun's findings in 2022 indicate that faculty and staff may encounter uncertainties in providing support, emphasizing the need for clearly defined roles and responsibilities in supporting students with mental health needs.

Staff members, as revealed by Payne (2022), should undergo training in mental health literacy to effectively support students. This training, especially in pastoral care and pedagogy on health professional programs, is crucial in equipping staff with the skills to address mental health concerns.

Furthermore, students themselves, as active participants in the campus community, have a vital role to play. Creating a culture of openness and support, as advocated by Ramluggun (2022), involves students providing emotional support to their peers and engaging in mental health awareness campaigns and support groups.

These research findings collectively underscore the importance of collaboration and support from all stakeholders, including faculty, staff, and students, in promoting mental health in higher education. To effectively implement these strategies, institutions should establish clear policies and comprehensive training programs to ensure that everyone involved is equipped to contribute to the mental well-being of students on campus.

### Importance of Creating a Supportive and Nurturing Environment for Students in Higher Education

Promoting positive teacher-student relationships and reducing the emphasis on standardized assessments within classrooms holds great importance in cultivating student creativity. This approach creates a secure and motivational environment where students can freely express their ideas, alleviating stress and pressure, encouraging divergent thinking, and granting them the freedom to explore and experiment. As a result, it facilitates the development of imaginative thinking and problem-solving skills, as observed by Cole, Sugioka, and Yamagata-Lynch (1999).

Turner et al. (2015) note the value of knowledge acquired within one's home community and offers guidance on establishing environments conducive to knowledge cultivation for others. This perspective emphasizes the significance of recognizing and appreciating the cultural wisdom and insights individuals gain from their own communities. It stresses that local knowledge, deeply rooted in tradition and communal practices, holds great significance. Furthermore, it advocates for the creation of inclusive spaces where individuals can nurture and share this knowledge, creating settings that honor diverse perspectives and experiences. These inclusive environments can be found in educational institutions, workplaces, or community organizations, where local knowledge is celebrated and embraced.

The importance of student support services in higher education institutions (HEIs), particularly in developing countries, cannot be overstated. These services play a pivotal role in addressing the unique challenges faced by HEIs in such regions. To effectively address these challenges, it becomes imperative to allocate adequate resources and reconfigure the support system, as emphasized by Jumani, Bhatti, and Malik (2013). The significance of these student support services lies in their ability to address the challenges confronted by HEIs. Through the reallocation of resources and restructuring of support mechanisms, HEIs can provide tailored assistance that enhances student success, addresses issues related to access and retention, and cultivates a conducive learning environment. This transformation enables HEIs in developing countries to better fulfill their educational objectives and make substantial contributions to the overall progress and advancement of their societies.

Efficient student services, offering crucial academic support while concurrently nurturing personal, social, cultural, and cognitive development, are imperative in addressing the complexities brought about by multicultural academic diversity. These services ensure that students of diverse backgrounds receive tailored assistance for academic success and, at the same time, create opportunities for comprehensive growth. This encompasses improving personal well-being, cultivating social connections, respecting and celebrating diverse cultures, and advancing cognitive development within a diverse and inclusive learning environment. Ciobanu (2013) contends that such student services are essential for effectively meeting the challenges posed by multicultural academic diversity.

## Practical Approaches and Initiatives That Institutions Can Adopt to Address Stress and Promote Mental Health

Over the years, research has proposed several methods that educational institutions can implement to address the mental health needs of students. The subsequent sections outline these approaches in detail.

### Effective Interventions for Student Stress Reduction

Cognitive, behavioral, and mindfulness interventions have consistently demonstrated their effectiveness in mitigating stress among university students. These approaches encompass a range of methods: cognitive interventions assist students in reframing negative thought patterns, behavioral strategies equip them with coping mechanisms, and mindfulness practices promote relaxation and emotional regulation. As supported by Regehr, Glancy, and Pitts (2013), the empirical evidence reinforces that these interventions not only reduce stress levels but also contribute positively to students' overall well-being, academic achievements, and mental health. This empirical foundation equips universities with valuable tools to assist their students in stress management and cultivate a more nurturing campus environment. Some illustrative examples are as follows:

- **Mindfulness-Based Stress Reduction (MBSR) Programs:** Many universities have implemented MBSR programs that teach students mindfulness and meditation techniques to reduce stress and improve well-being. Research has shown that these programs can lead to significant reductions in stress levels among students (Deshpande et al., 2023).
- **Cognitive-Behavioral Therapy (CBT) Workshops:** Some institutions offer CBT workshops or counseling services to help students reframe negative thought patterns and develop coping strategies. These programs have been successful in improving students' mental health and resilience (Hamdan-Mansour, Puskar, and Bandak, 2009) .
- **Online Mental Health Resources:** Several universities provide online resources and apps that offer stress management tools, relaxation exercises, and mental health support. These digital platforms have made it easier for students to access help and guidance (Gong et al., 2023).

## A Holistic Approach to Student Mental Health

In the context of student mental health within educational institutions, adopting a nested approach places the individual as the central focus, encircled by concentric spheres representing the influence of family and, subsequently, society at large, all with the shared aim of promoting mental health. This holistic perspective acknowledges that a student's mental well-being is intricately shaped by their immediate family environment and further influenced by broader societal factors. As proposed by Kalra et al. (2012), this nested framework focuses on the centrality of the student while recognizing the vital roles played by family dynamics and societal support structures in nurturing mental health. It advocates for collaborative efforts across these interconnected layers to establish a comprehensive framework for advancing mental health within educational institutions. Some illustrative ways are as follows:

- **Comprehensive Campus Mental Health Centers:** Some universities have established comprehensive mental health centers that not only offer individual counseling but also focus on creating a supportive campus culture. These centers may host events, courses, and workshops, facilitating a holistic approach to mental well-being (Rowe, 2015).
- **Community Engagement Programs:** Educational institutions have initiated programs that encourage community engagement and service-learning opportunities. These initiatives promote social connections and a sense of belonging among students, positively impacting their mental health (Wilczenski and Cook, 2009).
- **Peer Support Networks:** Universities often establish peer support networks where students can connect with one another for emotional support. These networks create a sense of community and help combat feelings of isolation (Brar et al., 2012).

### Primary Health Care: Bridging the Gap in Student Mental Health Initiatives

In addressing the need for mental health promotion initiatives within educational institutions, primary health care emerges as a potent solution. Integrating mental health support into primary care settings can help students gain enhanced access to mental health services and resources within the academic environment. This approach, as advocated by Barkway (2006), not only destigmatizes discussions surrounding mental well-being but also firmly establishes mental health as an integral facet of students' overall well-being. Leveraging the established infrastructure of primary care, it offers preventive measures, early intervention, and holistic support, ultimately crafting a comprehensive system for promoting mental health within educational institutions. Primary health care's patient-centered and community-oriented approach harmonizes with the multifaceted nature of mental well-being, making it a potent strategy to bridge existing gaps in student mental health initiatives and foster a healthier and more supportive educational environment. Some illustrative ways are as follows:

- **Integrated Health Clinics:** Some educational institutions have integrated mental health services into their primary health care clinics. This approach ensures that mental health is treated with the same importance as physical health, reducing stigma and improving accessibility (Lai et al., 2016).
- **Mental Health Screening Programs:** Universities have implemented mental health screening programs during routine medical check-ups. This proactive approach helps identify mental health concerns early and provides timely intervention (Kim, Kim, and Kamphaus, 2022).
- **Mental Health Awareness Campaigns:** Educational institutions often run awareness campaigns that educate students and staff about mental health issues, reducing misconceptions and encouraging individuals to seek help when needed (Giroux and Geiss, 2019).

## Collaborative Efforts Between Institutions, Students, and Parents to Foster a Culture of Well-Being

Promoting a culture of well-being within the academic community requires collaborative efforts between educational institutions, students, and parents. Recognizing that the well-being of students is a collective responsibility, these stakeholders can actively contribute to creating an environment that supports and nurtures well-being. A cohesive approach that integrates insights from various studies into these collaborative efforts is given below.

### Institutional Support and Student Engagement

Collaborative planning between institutions, students, and parents is vital to enhancing student well-being. As suggested by Amaya et al. (2019), institutions should seize the opportunity to cultivate campus cultures that prioritize health and well-being. One effective strategy is the provision of comprehensive mental health services, including counseling and support groups. Active involvement of students and parents may help the institutions in ensuring that these services address the diverse needs of the student body.

Moreover, as highlighted by Wessels and Wood (2019), participatory action learning and action research approaches can empower teachers to enhance their own well-being. When institutions collaborate with educators, students, and parents in the design and implementation of wellness programs, it promotes a holistic approach to well-being. These programs can encompass physical, emotional, and social aspects of health, resonating more profoundly with the academic community.

### Student-Led Initiatives and Peer Support

To encourage student engagement and ownership, institutions, in line with the insights of Graham, Powell, and Truscott (2016), should empower students to lead well-being initiatives. When students take the lead, they become advocates for their peers' mental health. Collaborative support from institutions and parents provides the necessary resources and guidance for these initiatives to thrive.

Peer support networks, as recommended by Zheng (2022), offer a supportive space for discussing mental health challenges. Collaboration among institutions, parents, and students ensures these networks are well-promoted and receive the necessary backing to flourish. Moreover, establishing feedback mechanisms, as Graham's recognition theory suggests, allows students to voice concerns and ideas collaboratively. Institutions and parents can work together to address these issues, thereby enhancing the overall well-being of the student body.

### Parental Involvement and Advocacy

Parental involvement is crucial, as emphasized by Keeling (2014), in ensuring students' well-being. Collaborative educational programs can educate parents about recognizing signs of stress or mental health issues in their children. Institutions can work alongside parents to provide these resources, fostering a supportive home environment where mental health discussions are encouraged.

Furthermore, parents can play a significant role in advocating for improved mental health services within educational institutions. Parent-teacher associations and similar groups can engage in collaborative advocacy efforts with institutions, resulting in policy changes and increased funding for mental health initiatives.

## CONCLUSION

In this chapter, a comprehensive exploration of various crucial aspects related to the well-being of higher education students has taken place. The chapter has thoroughly examined the challenges and stressors commonly encountered by students during their academic journeys, including academic pressures, workloads, financial concerns, social relationships, and the overall transition to college life. Throughout this analysis, it has become increasingly evident that these challenges significantly impact the mental health and overall well-being of students.

The paramount importance of mental health in the lives of students has been emphasized. Mental health is not limited to the absence of mental illness; rather, it includes emotional, psychological, and social well-being. The intricate interplay between mental health and students' academic performance, physical health, social relationships, and overall life satisfaction stresses on the need for a holistic approach to well-being.

Moreover, the chapter has explored various interventions that have demonstrated their effectiveness in mitigating stress and promoting well-being among higher education students. These interventions, including cognitive, behavioral, and mindfulness approaches, provide students with the tools to reframe negative thought patterns, develop coping strategies, and engage in relaxation and emotional regulation practices.

The discussion has also highlighted the importance of a nested approach, underscoring the interconnectedness between an individual's mental well-being, their family environment, and the broader societal context. This perspective acknowledges that students' mental health is influenced by various factors, such as family dynamics, cultural background, and the support structures available within their communities.

Collaborative efforts have emerged as a pivotal aspect of encouraging a culture of well-being within the academic community. When educational institutions, students, and parents collaborate, they can collectively address mental health challenges more effectively. These collaborative efforts encompass a range of initiatives, including the provision of mental health services, the promotion of wellness programs, the engagement of students in peer support networks, and the establishment of feedback mechanisms.

Finally, the chapter emphasized upon the ongoing need for research, awareness, and action to support the well-being of higher education students. Research plays a crucial role in enhancing the understanding of the evolving challenges faced by students, while awareness campaigns ensure that students, parents, educators, and institutions are well-informed about mental health issues. Taking action involves translating this knowledge into tangible steps, such as improving mental health services, implementing wellness programs, and fostering a supportive academic environment.

In conclusion, this chapter focuses on the complexity of higher education students' well-being and the multifaceted approach required to address it effectively. A conducive environment that prioritizes student well-being and enhances their chances of success in higher education can be created by acknowledging the significance of mental health, implementing evidence-based interventions, and fostering collaborative efforts.

## REFERENCES

Abbott-chapman, J. (2011). Making the most of the mosaic: Facilitating post-school transitions to higher education of disadvantaged students. *Australian Educational Researcher*, *38*(1), 57–71. doi:10.100713384-010-0001-9

Alsubaie, M. M., Stain, H. J., Webster, L. A., & Wadman, R. (2019). The role of sources of social support on depression and quality of life for university students. *International Journal of Adolescence and Youth*, *24*(4), 484–496. doi:10.1080/02673843.2019.1568887

Amaya, M., Donegan, T.E., Conner, D.R., Edwards, J., & Gipson, C.S. (2019). Creating a Culture of Wellness: A Call to Action for Higher Education, Igniting Change in Academic Institutions. *Building Healthy Academic Communities Journal.*

Aselton, P. (2012). Sources of stress and coping in American college students who have been diagnosed with depression. *Journal of child and adolescent psychiatric nursing: Official publication of the Association of Child and Adolescent Psychiatric Nurses*, *25*(3), 119–123.

Backović, D. V., Maksimovic, M. Z., Davidovic, D., Živojinović, J., & Stevanović, D. (2013). Stress and mental health among medical students. *Srpski Arhiv za Celokupno Lekarstvo*, *141*(11-12), 11–12, 780–784. doi:10.2298/SARH1312780B

Baik, C., Larcombe, W., & Brooker, A. (2019). How universities can enhance student mental wellbeing: The student perspective. *Higher Education Research & Development*, *38*(4), 674–687. doi:10.1080/07294360.2019.1576596

Barkway, P. M. (2006). Creating supportive environments for mental health promotion in the workplace. *Contemporary Nurse*, *21*(1), 131–141. doi:10.5172/conu.2006.21.1.131 PMID:16594890

Bostani, M., Nadri, A., & Nasab, A. R. (2014). A Study of the Relation between Mental health and Academic Performance of Students of the Islamic Azad University Ahvaz Branch. *Procedia: Social and Behavioral Sciences*, *116*, 163–165. doi:10.1016/j.sbspro.2014.01.186

Brar, I.K., Ryu, J., Shaikh, K., Altman, A., & Ng, J.Y. (2012). University Campus Peer Support Centres: Benefits for Student Emotional and Mental Well-Being. *The Meducator*, 1.

Briggs, A. R., Clark, J., & Hall, I. (2012). Building bridges: Understanding student transition to university. *Quality in Higher Education*, *18*(1), 21–23. doi:10.1080/13538322.2011.614468

Brinckerhoff, L. C. (1996). Making the Transition to Higher Education. *Journal of Learning Disabilities*, *29*(2), 118–136. doi:10.1177/002221949602900202 PMID:8820197

Ciobanu, A. M. (2013). The Role of Student Services in the Improving of Student Experience in Higher Education. *Procedia: Social and Behavioral Sciences*, *92*, 169–173. doi:10.1016/j.sbspro.2013.08.654

Cole, D., Sugioka, H. L., & Yamagata-Lynch, L. C. (1999). Supportive Classroom Environments For Creativity in Higher Education. *The Journal of Creative Behavior*, *33*(4), 277–293. doi:10.1002/j.2162-6057.1999.tb01407.x

Deshpande, A.G., Johnson, J.R., Casta, A.M., Marien, M.S., & Reiff, M. (2023). The impact of a mindfulness-based stress reduction program on university students' mental health: A mixed-methods evaluation. *Journal of American college health*, 1-11.

Eisenberg, D., Golberstein, E., & Hunt, J. B. (2009). Mental Health and Academic Success in College. *The B.E. Journal of Economic Analysis & Policy*, *9*(1), 9. doi:10.2202/1935-1682.2191

Evans, M.G. (2000). *Planning for the transition to tertiary study: A literature review.*

Fletcher, J.M., Frank, R.G., Mcguire, T., Meara, E., Stange, K.C., & Vigdor, J.L. (2009). *Mental health and academic success in college.*

Fook, C. Y., & Sidhu, G. K. (2015). Investigating Learning Challenges Faced by Students in Higher Education. *Procedia: Social and Behavioral Sciences*, *186*, 604–612. doi:10.1016/j.sbspro.2015.04.001

Giroux, D., & Geiss, E. G. (2019). Evaluating a Student-Led Mental Health Awareness Campaign. *Psi Chi Journal of Psychological Research*, *24*(1), 61–66. doi:10.24839/2325-7342.JN24.1.61

Gong, X., Wang, L., Rong, G., Zhang, D., Zhang, A. Y., & Liu, C. (2023). Effects of online mindfulness-based interventions on the mental health of university students: A systematic review and meta-analysis. *Frontiers in Psychology*, *14*, 14. doi:10.3389/fpsyg.2023.1073647 PMID:36844353

Graham, A., Powell, M. A., & Truscott, J. (2016). Facilitating student well-being: Relationships do matter. *Educational Research*, *58*(4), 366–383. doi:10.1080/00131881.2016.1228841

Hamdan-Mansour, A. M., Puskar, K., & Bandak, A. G. (2009). Effectiveness of Cognitive-Behavioral Therapy on Depressive Symptomatology, Stress and Coping Strategies among Jordanian University Students. *Issues in Mental Health Nursing, 30*(3), 188–196. doi:10.1080/01612840802694577 PMID:19291496

Hefner, J. L., & Eisenberg, D. (2009). Social support and mental health among college students. *The American Journal of Orthopsychiatry, 79*(4), 491–499. doi:10.1037/a0016918 PMID:20099940

Jeoung, B., Hong, M., & Lee, Y. C. (2013). The relationship between mental health and health-related physical fitness of university students. *Journal of Exercise Rehabilitation, 9*(6), 544–548. doi:10.12965/jer.130082 PMID:24409433

Jumani, N. B., Bhatti, A. J., & Malik, S. (2013). Student Support in Higher Education: Lessons Learnt and Challenges Ahead. *International Journal of Technology and Educational Marketing, 3*(1), 77–88. doi:10.4018/ijtem.2013010106

Kalkbrenner, M. T., Jolley, A. L., & Hays, D. G. (2019). Faculty Views on College Student Mental Health: Implications for Retention and Student Success. *Journal of College Student Retention, 23*(3), 636–658. doi:10.1177/1521025119867639

Kalra, G., Christodoulou, G. N., Jenkins, R., Tsipas, V., Christodoulou, N., Lečić-Toševski, D., Mezzich, J. E., & Bhugra, D. (2012). Mental health promotion: Guidance and strategies. *European Psychiatry, 27*(2), 81–86. doi:10.1016/j.eurpsy.2011.10.001 PMID:22197146

Keeling, R. P. (2014). An Ethic of Care in Higher Education: Well-Being and Learning. *Journal of College and Character, 15*(3), 141–148. doi:10.1515/jcc-2014-0018

Khodabakhsh, M., Kiani, F. K., & Ahmedbookani, S. (2014). Psychological Well-being and Parenting Styles as Predictors of Mental Health among Students: Implication for Health Promotion. *International Journal of Pediatrics, 2*, 39–46.

Kim, J., Kim, D., & Kamphaus, R. W. (2022). *Early Detection of Mental Health Through Universal Screening at Schools*. Georgia Educational Researcher. doi:10.20429/ger.2022.190104

Kotera, Y., Green, P., & Sheffield, D. (2019). Mental health of therapeutic students: Relationships with attitudes, self-criticism, self-compassion, and caregiver identity. *British Journal of Guidance & Counselling, 49*(5), 701–712. doi:10.1080/03069885.2019.1704683

Lai, K., Guo, S., Ijadi-Maghsoodi, R., Puffer, M., & Kataoka, S. (2016). Bringing Wellness to Schools: Opportunities for and Challenges to Mental Health Integration in School-Based Health Centers. *Psychiatric Services (Washington, D.C.), 67*(12), 1328–1333. doi:10.1176/appi.ps.201500401 PMID:27417895

Leshner, A. (2021). Target student mental well-being. *Science, 371*(6527), 325–325. doi:10.1126cience.abg5770 PMID:33479127

Lipson, S. K., & Eisenberg, D. (2018). Mental health and academic attitudes and expectations in university populations: Results from the healthy minds study. *Journal of Mental Health (Abingdon, England), 27*(3), 205–213. doi:10.1080/09638237.2017.1417567 PMID:29265935

Martineau, M., Beauchamp, G., & Marcotte, D. (2017). Efficacité des interventions en prévention et en promotion de la santé mentale dans les établissements d'enseignement postsecondaire. *Sante Mentale au Quebec*, *42*(1), 165–182. doi:10.7202/1040249ar PMID:28792567

Miller, D. N., Gilman, R., & Martens, M. P. (2008). Wellness promotion in the schools: Enhancing students' mental and physical health. *Psychology in the Schools*, *45*(1), 5–15. doi:10.1002/pits.20274

Mohammad, M.S., Kobra, K., Ebrahim, M., & Farhad, F.A. (2015). *The Role of Mental Health on Academic Performance of University Students with the Meditation of Academic Achievement Motivation.*

Nami, Y., Nami, M. S., & Eishani, K. A. (2014). The Students' Mental Health Status. *Procedia: Social and Behavioral Sciences*, *114*, 840–844. doi:10.1016/j.sbspro.2013.12.794

Ong, B., & Cheong, K. C. (2009). Sources of Stress among College Students—The Case of a Credit Transfer Program. *College Student Journal*, *43*, 1279–1286.

Pachucki, M. C., Ozer, E. J., Barrat, A., & Cattuto, C. (2015). Mental health and social networks in early adolescence: A dynamic study of objectively-measured social interaction behaviors. *Social Science & Medicine*, *125*, 40–50. doi:10.1016/j.socscimed.2014.04.015 PMID:24797692

Pascoe, M. C., Hetrick, S. E., & Parker, A. G. (2020). The impact of stress on students in secondary school and higher education. *International Journal of Adolescence and Youth*, *25*(1), 104–112. doi:10.1080/02673843.2019.1596823

Payne, H. (2022). Teaching Staff and Student Perceptions of Staff Support for Student Mental Health: A University Case Study. *Education Sciences*, *12*(4), 237. doi:10.3390/educsci12040237

Pluut, H., Curşeu, P. L., & Ilies, R. (2015). Social and study related stressors and resources among university entrants: Effects on well-being and academic performance. *Learning and Individual Differences*, *37*, 262–268. doi:10.1016/j.lindif.2014.11.018

Priestley, M., Hall, A., Wilbraham, S. J., Mistry, V., Hughes, G., & Spanner, L. (2022). Student perceptions and proposals for promoting wellbeing through social relationships at university. *Journal of Further and Higher Education*, *46*(9), 1243–1256. doi:10.1080/0309877X.2022.2061844

Ramluggun, P., Kozlowska, O., Mansbridge, S., Rioga, M., & Anjoyeb, M. (2022). Mental health in higher education: Faculty staff survey on supporting students with mental health needs. *Health Education*, *122*(6), 601–616. doi:10.1108/HE-02-2022-0011

Regehr, C., Glancy, D., & Pitts, A. (2013). Interventions to reduce stress in university students: A review and meta-analysis. *Journal of Affective Disorders*, *148*(1), 1–11. doi:10.1016/j.jad.2012.11.026 PMID:23246209

Roberts, R., Golding, J. F., Towell, T., Reid, S., Woodford, S., Vetere, A. L., & Weinreb, I. (2000). Mental and physical health in students: The role of economic circumstances. *British Journal of Health Psychology*, *5*(3), 289–297. doi:10.1348/135910700168928

Roberts, R., Golding, J. F., Towell, T., Reid, S., Woodford, S., Vetere, A. L., & Weinreb, I. (2000). Mental and physical health in students: The role of economic circumstances. *British Journal of Health Psychology*, *5*(3), 289–297. doi:10.1348/135910700168928

Ross, S. E., Niebling, B. C., & Heckert, T. M. (1999). Sources of stress among college students. *College Student Journal, 33*, 312–317.

Rowe, N. (2015). *Creating a Healing Campus: A Partnership between a University and a Provider of Mental Health Services.*

Saleh, D., Camart, N., & Romo, L. (2017). Predictors of Stress in College Students. *Frontiers in Psychology*, 8. PMID:28179889

Shankar, N. L., & Park, C. (2016). Effects of stress on students' physical and mental health and academic success. *International Journal of School & Educational Psychology*, *4*(1), 5–9. doi:10.1080/21683603.2016.1130532

Suldo, S. M., Shaunessy, E., & Hardesty, R. B. (2008). Relationships among Stress, Coping, and Mental Health in High-Achieving High School Students. *Psychology in the Schools*, *45*(4), 273–290. doi:10.1002/pits.20300

Turner, C.S., Ro, H.K., Loya, K.I., Rhoads, R.A., Camacho, M.S., Toven-Lindsey, B., Lozano, J.B., Cowan, J., Goldhaber, D., Lopez, H.D., Ream, T.C., Hurst, A.L., Crisp, G., Curette, A., Hansen, T.I., & Nehls, K. (2015). Lessons from the Field: Cultivating Nurturing Environments in Higher Education. *The Review of Higher Education.*

Tyson, P. J., Wilson, K. L., Crone, D. M., Brailsford, R., & Laws, K. R. (2010). Physical activity and mental health in a student population. *Journal of Mental Health (Abingdon, England)*, *19*(6), 492–499. doi:10.3109/09638230902968308 PMID:20812852

Wessels, E., & Wood, L. (2019). Fostering teachers' experiences of well-being: A participatory action learning and action research approach. *South African Journal of Education*, *39*(1), 1–10. doi:10.15700aje.v39n1a1619

Wilczenski, F. L., & Cook, A. L. (2009). How service learning addresses the mental health needs of students in urban school. *Journal of School Counseling*, *7*, 1–20.

Yusof, H. M., Rahman, R. H., Noordin, N. F., Patah, S. A., Yunus, W. M., & Fei, G. C. (2019). Does University Students' Stress Have an Impact on their Psychological Well-Being? *Indian Journal of Public Health Research & Development*, *10*(6), 1290. doi:10.5958/0976-5506.2019.01473.6


## KEY TERMS AND DEFINITIONS

**Academic Performance:** The level of achievement and success in educational pursuits, typically measured through grades, test scores, and coursework completion.

**Inclusive Learning Environment:** A setting that values and accommodates diverse perspectives, backgrounds, and needs, promoting equal opportunities and participation for all students.

**Intervention:** Purposeful actions, programs, or strategies designed to address and mitigate mental health challenges, such as counseling, therapy, or support services.

**Mental Health:** The state of emotional, psychological, and social well-being in which an individual can effectively cope with stress, work productively, and contribute to their community.

**Quality of Life:** A subjective assessment of an individual's overall life satisfaction, happiness, and fulfillment in various life domains, including physical, emotional, and social well-being.

**Resilience:** The capacity to adapt, bounce back from adversity, and maintain mental well-being in the face of challenges or setbacks.

**Social Relationships:** Interactions and connections between individuals, encompassing friendships, family ties, and other forms of social engagement.

**Stress:** A physiological and psychological response to external pressures or challenges, which can have both positive (eustress) and negative (distress) effects on an individual's well-being.

**Support Systems:** Formal or informal networks and resources that provide assistance and encouragement to individuals facing mental health issues or other challenges.

**Well-Being:** A holistic concept encompassing physical, mental, and social health, reflecting the overall quality of life and satisfaction with one's circumstances.

# Chapter 10
# First-Aid Mental Health for the Pre-Medical Student

**Robert Lubin**
https://orcid.org/0000-0002-7325-3469
*Touro University Worldwide, USA*

**Benjamin Katz**
*University of Southern California, USA*

**Michelle Marants**
*Queen's University, USA*

**Mia Medney**
*Florida State University, USA*

**Charles Rosin**
*Rutgers University, USA*

**Dean Sandler**
*Southern Methodist University, USA*

**Sophie Schonberger**
*Yale University, USA*

**Jamie R. Sharabani**
*University of Miami, USA*

**Jacqueline Sherry**
*University of Delaware, USA*

**Gary Shteyman**
*Syracuse University, USA*

**Theodore Tran**
https://orcid.org/0000-0002-3590-3862
*California University of Science and Medicine, USA*

**Elana Weiss**
*Hunter College, USA*

**Edward Zeltner**
*Cornell University, USA*

**Matthew Zisu**
*McGill University, Canada*

## ABSTRACT

*College is intended to prepare students to become successful members of society. However, the academic demands of college can trigger stress and mental health problems. College students are in a unique position where they have to juggle academics, a social life, and, often, part-time jobs. As a result, college students are a particularly vulnerable group when it comes to stress and mental health issues. One subset of students facing the struggles of college achievements are pre-med students. Pre-med students face numerous challenges that can negatively impact their mental health. The academic pressures, financial stress, lack of social support, and relationship challenges, among others, can increase the risk of depression, anxiety, and other mental health disorders. The team of contributing authors on this chapter will address mental health in the higher education environment. This chapter will present a program for educators, peer students, and staff to provide mental health assistance for the premedical student.*

DOI: 10.4018/979-8-3693-2833-0.ch010

## INTRODUCTION

Healthcare workers worldwide are subject to increasing pressures resulting from rapid escalation of change, growing economic pressures, technological advances and increasing patient expectations. Some believe many physicians suffer from a highly demanding work environment combined with lower levels of control, according to Karasek's model of demand-control imbalance, or from an effort-reward imbalance, according to Siegrist (Riley, 2004). A Medscape report indicated that 59% of doctors cited bureaucratic tasks as a leading contributor to burnout, 34% cited long hours, and 70% cited healthcare information-technology or electronic health records (Patientpop, 2019). Stress experienced by working physicians and medical students is inordinately high relative to the general population, leading to higher rates of anxiety, depression, thoughts of suicide, and burnout. We propose that this situation exists before the student even enters medical school. The experience of the pre-medical undergraduate student foreshadows the issues later experienced by the medical student and practicing physician.

A recent survey of freshmen (Stolzenberg et al., 2020) listed "premed" as the most desired choice of study consistently for the past 5 years. Nevertheless, the stress that pre-medical undergraduate students face is not always a priority within the education system. The issue should be addressed, being that there have been significant negative results of the effect this has on students' mental health. Particularly, the stress resulting from the competitive pre-med culture, familial pressure and responsibilities, and a students' personal circumstances substantially contributes to a student's academic performance and ambition to achieve. Starting from the first semester, the expectations for pre-medical include perfect grades, a high MCAT score, competitive clinical and research experience, and impressive volunteering and extracurricular activities. Ludmerer (1999) stated that a "student's success at learning medicine depended heavily on the aptitude, characteristics, and educational background that person brought to medical school in the first place" (p. 59) highlighting that the process of becoming a physician starts long before the first day of medical school.

As a result, students deal with stress that they have never experienced. This change can drastically harm their mental health, since too much stress on a person can lead to anxiety and depression (Sawatzky et al., 2012). As a result, students can experience difficulty concentrating and trouble retaining the proper amount of sleep (Mindell et al., 2011; Misra & McKean, 2000). Furthermore, students that struggle with mental health issues prior to joining a pre-med track during their undergraduate education often find it more difficult to manage. A study focusing on the anxiety of students in an introductory level biology course found that students with previous general anxiety disorders tend to perform poorly and change their major or career path as a result (England et al., 2017). In addition, students with depression were shown to correlate with a decrease in interest in becoming a doctor (Grace, 2018). Additional studies have found that there is a close relationship between depression and burnout in premedical undergraduate students. (Fang et al., 2012)

The competitive nature of pre-medical education, formulated by the high expectations and low acceptance rates of medical school, perpetuates an unhealthy culture that is psychologically detrimental to the students within. Ahmed (2019) discussed this culture in "The Real Core Competencies in PreMed Culture," specifically noting how the pressure of medical school replaces requirements like orientation towards service and curiosity for science with a focus on grades and resumes. He acknowledged the palpable tension in an organic chemistry class and the number of students who hold research positions they despise simply to check the box on their medical school admissions checklist. This culture is improperly setting up students for a future in medicine, as their priorities are imbalanced, with a stronger focus on grades than on the actual learning and an aspiration of prestige and success rather than healing and discovery of science.

## STRENGTH IN COMMUNITY?

It is commonly believed that having a community of pre-medical peers for social support is beneficial to a student's mental health; however, a study found that for those who experience significant academic stress, being surrounded by peers of similar situations increases the effects of their stress (Grace, 2021). This has been supported by the lack of effectiveness shown in certain peer group programs (Lilienfeld, 2007). When a student is seeking support and aid, a fellow student who is similarly in search of support can be more draining than helpful. According to surveys, students do not feel like they can turn to their peers due to the consequences of comparison. Anticipatory stress and pressure to succeed are highly influenced by factors like race, ethnicity, and socio-economic status (Grace, 2021). Having access to peers should be more helpful as they understand the social sacrifices and mental strength required to complete the courses and battle the fear of failure.

### Strength in Family

The role of familial stress in education, and in particular pre-medical and medical education, cannot be overstated. A survey of 278 undergraduate medical students from MES Medical College in Kerala, India found that 80.9% of participants cited parental expectations as a major stress factor (Salgar, 2014). The exact mechanism behind this stressor, however, remains multi-faceted. Yussof et al. (2013) suggested that parental education has a significant correlation with the self-reported anxiety score of medical students. According to their findings, students who have a parent who has completed secondary or tertiary education report lower anxiety scores. The explanation they provide for this finding is that more educated parents are able to provide more effective support networks for their children. This hypothesis holds weight in more anecdotal sources as well; interviews conducted by Barnett (2004) of 50 African American students at an Ivy League university found that 84% of students had at least one parent with post-high-school education. Quotes from interviewed students also show that these family members were instrumental in getting them into the educational position they were in, whether through financial means, emotional means, or both.

Ding and Rubie-Davies (2019) discuss the theory that parental expectations can directly interfere with students' self-expectations, which could impact both their academic performance and stress. When putting this theory to the test, Zheng et al. (2023) found that academic stress and parental expectation actually had a significant negative correlation. The answer might lie in the duality of the human stress response. In short doses, stress is how our body improves performance and keeps us focused on our goals (Dhabar, 2018). It is only when stress is chronic that it leads to severe health complications. Applying this to family dynamics, students might find parental expectations stressful in the short-term, but in the long-term they provide a means of moral support and self-elevation.

Although there are a variety of personal factors which can determine a students' performance, ones' academic self-efficacy, organizational skills, study methods, time management skills, external stress factors, social factors, and personal motivation are among the most outstanding personal factors that affect college student success (Newton et al., 2008). Research has shown that students with exceptional time management skills tend to perform better and experience less burnout than their peers. In an observation of the performance of pre-medical students, it was seen that students who study and practice together outperform their peers who study alone (Tolsgaard, 2013).

## Toxic Pre-Med Culture

According to Conrad, a professor at Brandeis University, toxic pre-med culture and cutthroat stereotypes are rooted in the competitiveness of medical school admission (Conrad, 1986). Statistics from American Medical Colleges show that there has been a 30% increase in medical school applicants in the past years (Pacifici et al., 2011). However, in comparison, the number of medical school matriculates has only seen a modest rise of 11.5% (Pacifici et al., 2011). These figures highlight the growing interest in pursuing a medical career and the challenges those who embark on this honorable path face. Unfortunately, despite this significant increase in medical school applicants, many schools still limit their class sizes to 100-200 (Pacifici et al., 2011). High admission stats, including competitive GPA requirements and standardized test scores, significantly contribute to toxic pre-med culture. McGill's latest admission statistics further exemplify this: an average GPA of 3.88 for Quebec residents and 3.90 for non-Quebec residents (McGill, 2023). These high admission stats contribute to the intense competition and pressures pre-med students face, exacerbating the challenges in creating a supportive and inclusive learning environment for aspiring healthcare professionals.

Conrad underscores the toxic environment fostered by medical school competition, where an "every man for himself" mentality prevails (Conrad, 1986). Furthermore, a study done at Yale concluded that pre-med students were given the most negative rating of all majors (Conrad, 1986). Hackman suggests pre-med students are perceived as grade-conscious, selfish, less friendly than others, and primarily interested in esteem (Conrad, 1986). Toxic pre-med culture has undeniably impacted how other undergraduate students perceive those aspiring for a career in medicine.

The competitive nature of the pre-med track has fostered an atmosphere of cutthroat rivalry among students on campus. The situation has forced students to resort to deceitful tactics to secure a place in medical school (Conrad, 1986). Ultimately, competition remains an inevitable aspect of the medical journey, yet it is crucial to confront and address it. Halting this toxic pre-med culture cycle holds paramount importance in preserving aspiring health professionals' mental and physical well-being.

## Positive Interventions for Pre-Med Students' Mental Health

When medical schools assess the suitability of applicants, they seek individuals who possess the intellectual capacity and character traits necessary to thrive as competent and compassionate doctors. At the same time, aspiring medical students are confronted with the challenging responsibility of effectively presenting themselves to admissions committees in a manner that grabs their attention and highlights their potential. As students continue through their undergraduate years, they must acquire the skills to efficiently manage both the academic and non-academic aspects of their resumes. This section of the chapter explores positive interventions to support pre-med students' mental health by investigating four categories: the utilization of counseling centers, the benefits of upper-class mentorship, the impact of exercise, and the significance of extracurricular activities. Examining these interventions better provides helpful insights into creating well-rounded and resilient pre-medical students, and in the end contributes to the development of successful future physicians.

## Counseling Centers

Counseling centers are an important tool in supporting the mental health of pre-med students. A study conducted by Hinderaker (2013) showed a high prevalence of mental health issues among college students. Some factors included academic stress, social pressures, and life transitions. However, several barriers hinder students from seeking help. These include the stigma associated with mental health, lack of knowledge about available services, concerns about confidentiality, and limited time due to academic and personal commitments. These findings showed how effective the promotion of counseling centers can be to the overall well-being of pre-med students and addressing their mental health concerns. Levitt (2007) highlighted the importance of identifying mental health issues in schools and discussed different instruments used in schools to assess mental health problems among students, such as screening tools, self-report questionnaires, and behavior rating scales.

## Mentors

When comparing college students with peer mentors to college students without peer mentors, research found that mentees with peer mentors had better grades, less failure, and stronger retention (Yomtov et al., 2015). A study in the UK looked at undergraduate students with and without peer mentors, comparing them at week 1 and at week 10 within the same university. The study found that students without a peer mentor were four times more likely to seriously consider leaving their university compared to those with a peer mentor (Sheldon, et al., 2021). Mentees find a friend and role model in an older peer because they have persevered through similar temptations and social hurdles. Peer mentor programs serve as a buffer to unavoidable circumstances. In the same UK study, students without peer mentors showed significant decreases in self-esteem and social support after week 10. Nearly one-third of those students reported feeling homesick. They also had higher levels of psychological disturbances and cognitive failure (Sheldon, et al., 2021). Students with peer mentors showed little or no change. In general, they are better able to adapt to higher education (Collier, 2017).

The similarity-attraction paradigm is the notion that people are drawn to and experience greater effects from those who they perceive to be like themselves (Liviatan, Trope, & Liberman, 2008). On the first day of higher education, students explore the campus and connect with peers, asking questions like "What's your major?" or "Where are you from?" If students are from the same place or have the same major, an immediate link is established. Similarities foster an intrinsic desire from the mentor to help the mentee. A study showed that perceived similarity from mentors to mentees was significantly related to higher quality mentorships and learning (Allen & Eby, 2003). Peer mentors who work with first-year students see reflections of their freshman selves in the mentee.

Upperclassman mentorship programs offer a valuable positive intervention for pre-med students. This tool helps provide guidance, support, and resources to navigate the challenges of the pre-medical track. Wallick's (2023) pre-med mentorship program proposal at Boise State University outlined the key elements of such a program. His program is designed to have mentor selection and training, matching process, regular meetings and communication, resources and workshops, and program evaluation.

## Physical Activity

Physical activity serves as a positive intervention for the mental health of pre-med students, as it plays a significant role in preventing non-communicable diseases and promoting overall well-being. According to a study conducted by Rao et al. (2012), non-communicable diseases (NCDs) are projected to account for 73% of deaths and 60% of the global disease burden by 2020. These diseases, including cardiovascular disease, cancer, and diabetes, are strongly associated with unhealthy lifestyle habits such as lack of exercise. In the 20th century, there was a shift in the primary causes of death from infectious diseases to chronic illnesses, mainly due to factors like improper nutrition, sedentary lifestyles, and other unhealthy habits.

## Extracurricular Activities

Engaging in extracurricular activities acts as a beneficial intervention for the mental well-being of pre-med students, offering opportunities for development and personal growth. Gross et al., (2008) focused on the content of coursework in premedical education. They emphasized the need to recognize the "hidden premedical curriculum," which includes the social and noncurricular demands placed on premedical students (p. 516). As the authors stated, "The hidden premedical curriculum shapes not only what students know, but also how they know, and thus, who they are" (Gross et al., 2008, p. 516). The authors came to the conclusion that the pre-medical years are often perceived by students as a competitive journey rather than a self-discovery process. The advice provided by advisors typically focuses on meeting admission requirements and building a competitive application, overlooking the importance of character development.

To address this gap, Gross et al., (2008) advocated for a reevaluation of pre-medical education and proposed a comprehensive approach that combines the necessary coursework with opportunities for students to reflect on the positive and negative effects of the premedical years. Academic stress plays a large role in the mental health of first-year students. Students who can manage their studies may have better coping strategies for the overall transition to higher education (Brougham et al., 2009). The study found that American culture views the college experience as a chance for youth to learn adult responsibilities and understand their more mature roles. Learning coping strategies to handle academic stress can help in the transition into adulthood. Some students found that extracurricular events mitigate academic stress and provide gratification that is lacking in the academic realm.

## Missing Aspects of Intervention

Pursuing a medical career can be a challenging path that places immense pressure on pre-medical students. Institutions have implemented positive interventions to support their academic needs and mental health; however, crucial aspects still require attention to adequately address their needs and ensure the success of these students in their journey to becoming healthcare professionals. This section explores critical areas currently lacking in mental health support for pre-med students despite the aforementioned positive interventions already in place.

## Structured Guidance

One crucial aspect lacking in the support system for pre-med students is allocating dedicated time for academic advisors to provide comprehensive guidance. This process entails offering guidance on course selection, career planning, and strategies to balance academic and personal responsibilities effectively. Studies have shown that pre-medical students with continued guidance, in many cases from parents who are physicians or family members in the healthcare field, are often higher-achieving students than those without (Foong et al., 2021). Additionally, pre-medical students likely have a more extensive course workload and added pressures of acquiring clinical and research hours during their undergraduate degree (Zhang et al., 2020). These heavy demands often discourage pre-medical studies, especially when the proper guidance is unavailable. When beginning the path as a pre-medical student, there are already defining factors that could put one student ahead or behind another, such as socioeconomic status, high school GPA, and SAT scores (Zhang et al., 2020). However, suppose students had full access and structured guidance as pre-medical students. In that case, they might have an easier time reaching the milestones needed to finish pre-med requisites (Zhang et al., 2020). Universities should establish specialized academic support services tailored to pre-med students' unique challenges to equip them with the best strategies for navigating the demanding path into medical school.

## Mental Health Follow-Ups and Support Systems

Establishing a system that ensures regular mental health follow-ups with pre-med students is imperative throughout their undergraduate degree. While counseling centers are beneficial, they often do not give the full service that students, especially pre-medical students, would need to function properly. This approach would enable professionals to monitor their mental well-being, identify signs of distress, and provide appropriate interventions. Pre-medical students tend to have a greater intensity of depression and a higher likelihood of the onset of major depressive disorder (MDD) than non-pre-medical students (Fang et al., 2009). The lack of mental health follow-ups leaves pre-med students without the tools to combat the extrinsic and intrinsic pressures beyond the usual pressures of the college experience (Fang et al., 2009). In a study assessing the mental state of pre-med students, researchers showed that there is a strong connection between alexithymia (difficulty determining or expressing emotions), locus of control (the degree to which people feel control over their actions and the outcomes), and feelings of burnout (Lang, 2019). The same study has shown that if a professor or professional is supportive, or if there is at least a perception of support for the student, there is a significant decrease in at least one aspect of burnout (Lang, 2019). Without any sense of consistent mental support from their surrounding professionals, pre-med students feel overwhelmed and overworked, making it difficult to succeed in their careers without burning out or falling into a depressive state (Dou et al., 2021). A recent study from the American Sociological Association showed that pre-medical students with a more extensive support system of professionals and other students tended to experience fewer depressive symptoms, especially when feeling like the medical administration was failing them (Grace, 2020). By proactively addressing potential mental health concerns, such as burnout, anxiety, and depression, these follow-ups can mitigate the negative impact on pre-med students' overall well-being and academic performance.

## Study Techniques

Pre-med students face rigorous academic demands that necessitate effective study techniques and learning strategies that often need to be provided. Resources and workshops tailored to the demanding pre-med curriculum can empower students to optimize their academic performance while managing stress. While counseling centers and pre-medical advisors exist, students need more foundation in study techniques and habits to get them through their pre-medical courses (Grace, 2020). Following an analysis of the study habits of students at the Royal College of Surgeons in Ireland, a study course was created to help pre-medical students develop study habits that would help them succeed in their prerequisite classes. The study proved that those who took the class reported more positive study habits and better course outcomes than those who did not take the course (Schreiber and Cunningham, 2015). These initiatives should focus on teaching evidence-based study techniques, time management skills, and stress reduction strategies. The initiatives could come from upper-class pre-medical students, given that students find comfort in the support of their peers (Grace, 2020). Educational institutions can alleviate the pressure of demanding coursework by equipping students with effective study habits.

## Training Pre-Medical Students

In recent years, mental health issues among college students have gained increasing attention, prompting educators to address these concerns more effectively. Pre-healthcare professional students, in particular, face unique challenges due to the demanding nature of their academic programs. The highly competitive environment, demanding coursework, and societal expectations place immense pressure on these students, increasing their vulnerability to mental health issues such as burnout, anxiety, and depression. According to the World Health Organization (WHO), burnout is defined as "feelings of energy depletion or exhaustion, increased mental distance from one's job, feelings of negativism or cynicism related to one's job, and reduced professional efficacy (WHO, 2019). Fang et al., (2012) explored burnout among pre-med students. Burnout, a syndrome characterized by emotional exhaustion, depersonalization, and decreased personal accomplishment, has become a growing concern in the field of medicine. Burnout is a psychological syndrome leading to a worker's erosion of engagement with their job due to long-term exposure to emotionally demanding work (Hinami and Wetterneck, 2017). It is a condition observed predominantly among those in the helping professions, like health and social services where direct, frequent, and intense interactions with people are common and where the outcomes of work are not fully dependent on worker actions.

Lang (2019) revealed a significant association between burnout and career calling, suggesting that as burnout levels increased, career calling decreased. This finding supports the notion that burnout and career calling are inversely related, meaning that high levels of burnout can lead to a diminished sense of purpose and motivation in ones chosen career path. Furthermore, higher levels of burnout were associated with lower GPAs, higher levels of stress, and lower levels of perceived social support. The study suggests that interventions aimed at reducing burnout and enhancing career calling in undergraduate pre-medical students may have a positive impact on students' well-being and career trajectories.

The research highlights the demanding nature of a pre-medical curriculum. Pre-medical students are often required to balance a heavy workload consisting of challenging science courses, extracurricular activities, research experience, and volunteer work. This intense pressure and high level of expectations can contribute to the development of burnout among these students. The Lang (2019) study revealed that a significant number of pre-medical students experience burnout, with a large portion reporting moderate to high levels of emotional exhaustion and depersonalization. The study suggested that burnout has a negative impact on academic performance and students experiencing burnout reported lower GPA scores and higher rates of academic probation or dismissal. Burnout also affects students' mental well-being, with higher levels of stress, anxiety, and depression observed in those experiencing burnout.

Sevlever and Rice (2010) found a significant positive correlation between socially prescribed perfectionism and depression, meaning that students who felt pressured to meet certain societal standards of perfection were more likely to experience symptoms of depression. Additionally, socially prescribed perfectionism was negatively associated with academic performance, indicating that students who felt this external pressure had lower GPA. Additionally, self-oriented perfectionism was positively associated with anxiety symptoms, suggesting that students who set high standards for themselves might experience higher levels of anxiety. The competition to earn acceptance to medical school is extremely fierce and takes a significant toll on the undergraduate experience of pre-med students. There is often an unspoken competitive and cutthroat culture between pre-medical students which promotes the idea that in order to succeed another must fail (Denslow, 2023). This has a significant effect on the well-being of pre-med students and may deter them from pursuing medicine. Furthermore, the schedule of a pre-medical student includes rigorous STEM coursework. These classes are challenging enough without the toxic comparison between classmates. Given the high achieving nature of pre-med students, many associate their self-worth with academic accomplishments. This works against students' best interests when many experience the typical GPA plummet in difficult courses such as organic chemistry. This strain on students' self-esteem and overall mental health must be addressed and prevented.

Physicians can experience high levels of stress and burnout related to their jobs. They can deal with intense and emotional situations, confrontational patients, difficult colleagues, long hours, fear of making mistakes, and feelings of loneliness and isolation (Riley et al., 2018). Physician burnout is a systemic problem and contributes to medical errors, higher costs, and lower quality of care (Yates, 2019). Since the evidence is alarming for physicians, it is even more concerning that the knowledge and awareness gap exists at the pre-medical stage. Recognizing the signs and symptoms of mental health challenges among pre-healthcare professional students is crucial for early intervention and support yet remains a cryptic discussion across campuses. Though universities are increasingly providing resources for pre-health students, there is a lack of emphasis on student mental health, thus leaving room for formalized protocols that could help students at high risk for depression (Grace, 2018). Furthermore, the implications of mental health issues in the pre-healthcare professional student population extend beyond individual well-being. Recognizing the broader implications of these mental health challenges emphasizes the urgency of implementing effective support systems within the higher education system (Lattie, Lipson, & Eisenberg, 2019).

## Mental Health Stigma

Mental health "is a state of well-being that allows individuals to enjoy and maintain relationships as well as handle stress in a healthy manner without compromising on productivity" (Nair et al. 2021, p. 1). Teenagers oftentimes ignore their mental health problems not realizing the detrimental effects this has on their mental and physical wellbeing. There are three main types of stigmas, and all three can be observed in colleges across America: public stigma, self-stigma, and institutional stigma. Public stigma refers to how one's peers view mental illness. This is very apparent during the college transition because if a student's new friend does not support them seeking help, they will most likely decide not to do so. Self-stigma occurs when an individual does not see the benefit of speaking to a licensed professional about their problems and thinks they will eventually be resolved with no help (Borenstein, 2020).

The third type of stigma is institutional stigma. Institutional stigma refers to the intentional or unintentional barriers that institutions place on seeking mental health support. A research study performed at Boston University "found that the mental health of college students across the United States has been on a consistent decline for all eight years of data analyzed, with an overall 135 percent increase in depression and 110 percent increase in anxiety from 2013 to 2021" (Colarossi, 2022, p. 2). Many colleges advertise their mental health clinics to the students during orientation, but the culture of America has led these students to only view these resources as detrimental.

A range of mindsets (mental filters through which students view themselves and their environment) appear prevalent in the medical education community. Viewing performance as identity appears widespread and pre-medical students can experience it in the following way: "I am my MCAT score" rather than "I got this score on my MCAT." Given the relentless measuring and ranking within the educational continuum, comparison to peers is inevitable. Additionally, mental health history can also have an impact on mental health in the pre-med curriculum. We expect our physicians to deal effectively with emotions—their patients' and their own—so we need to provide the training and support to preserve pre-med students across the education continuum.

Addressing mental health concerns among pre-healthcare professional students requires a comprehensive approach that combines awareness, prevention, and support. Educational programs tailored to this student population can be pivotal in promoting mental well-being, reducing stigma, and encouraging help-seeking behavior. By integrating mental health education into the curriculum, providing accessible resources, and equipping faculty and staff with the necessary training, colleges and universities can create an environment conducive to positive mental health outcomes for the pre-health community. A program that encourages students to prioritize their mental health just as much as their physical health and academic progress can aid in the prevention of burnout and lost interest in medicine (Lattie, Lipson, & Eisenberg, 2019). Effectively responding to the mental health needs of pre-med students will aid the prevention of burnout and lost interest in medicine (Goel, 2020).

## Focus on the Individual

Considerable evidence supports the fact that organizational and job factors play a greater role in burnout than individual worker characteristics (Laschinger & Leiter, 2006). The goal should be to balance the demands of the academic curriculum with the control, reward, and support needs of the student. Pre-medical students are also social creatures, thus focusing on relationships is important. Fostering a mutually supportive culture focused on common goals, mutual respect, and implementing systems to facilitate rewarding interpersonal interactions are likely to minimize burnout. Students who feel they are working as part of a cohesive team, who are supported and appreciated by those around them, and who feel positively recognized will have less burn out.

Individuals can do more than simply cope with adverse conditions. Resilience is a trait that enables individuals or organizations to persevere or even thrive in the face of threats. Organizational scholars Sutcliffe and Vogus (2003) defined resilience as the ability to flourish or thrive amid adverse conditions when rigidity might be expected. Resilience results when systems retain resources in a form that is sufficiently flexible to cope positively with the unexpected. They must be prepared for developing resilience and adaptability can help navigate the uncertainty of the academic and admissions to medical school process (Van Der Feltz-Cornelis et al., 2020).

Slavin et al., (2014) emphasized the importance of addressing the mental health challenges faced by medical students and the negative impacts on their well-being and academic performance. They proposed a three-dimensional approach to improve student wellness through curricular changes. First, they suggested enhancing awareness and destigmatizing mental health by integrating mental health education and resources into the curriculum. Lastly, Slavin et al. emphasized the importance of self-care and resilience-building activities incorporated into the curriculum. They suggested incorporating mindfulness, exercise, and reflective practices to help students develop coping mechanisms and improve their overall well-being.

We present a similar paradigm for the pre-medical community. We emphasize the need for a comprehensive approach that addresses mental health at all levels of pre-medical education to ensure the well-being and success of future healthcare professionals. As part of our curriculum initiative, we present several case studies to help the pre-med student learn to be aware of mental health issues and build resiliency. These cases can be discussed by faculty, staff, and peers to bring awareness and build resilience among the pre-medical community.

## PROBLEM-BASED LEARNING (PBL)

Problem-based learning (PBL) is an essential skill for undergraduate students intending to attend medical school to understand and utilize. PBL is an innovative method of teaching where the role of the teacher is switched to the student by five stages: (1) determining the research question, (2) finding relevant studies, (3) selecting studies, (4) data charting, and (5) results (Trullas et al., 2022). PBL is effective at developing skills such as emotional intelligence, tolerance for uncertainty, conceptual understanding, independent working, and the application, performance, and retention of content knowledge (Nilson, 2010). Skills developed through the practice of PBL can help students become more self-aware. Thus, PBL is a helpful tool that aids in giving and receiving help from peers and mentors.

PBL can help with mental health awareness and ensure that pre-med students can efficiently get the help they need. PBL allows students to be more self-aware through self-learning by acquiring knowledge and competencies needed for their future medical profession (Trullas et al., 2022). Mental health issues often present a lot of ambiguity, a challenge for pre-med students as they are in the habit of learning how to problem-solve and memorize. With the help of PBL, we can teach pre-med students direct strategies for helping one another with their mental health. The first step would be to have each individual reflect on what mental health is for them and their peers around them; this is a useful technique as the act of someone carrying out the activity they strive to learn, the better they comprehend it and are able to apply what they learned (Trullas et al., 2022). We propose the use of case studies (as shown below) to provide examples of how a PBL-based curriculum would be developed.

### Case Study for Depression

A 20-year-old first-year medical student is coming to the department of student health with complaints of feeling fatigued on a daily basis; during the day, she is sleepy and sometimes she cannot keep her eyes open during lectures which is starting to affect her medical school grades. She says that although she is very sleepy and tired, she feels very anxious at night with racing thoughts of doom, and these thoughts keep her awake until late. She says that she stays up until three or four a.m. each night with a pile of books to read and endless work; however, even though she sits and studies for hours, she cannot concentrate, putting her even further behind on work as her grades plummet. She thinks about all the upcoming reading and tests in her classes, especially the anatomy class, and she bursts into tears.

She is having difficulty concentrating and just prefers to sleep much of the day. She does not even go to the cafeteria to eat as she feels she has lost all interest in food and subsequently has lost over 15 pounds since she started medical school 4 months ago. Before starting school, she used to go out with her friends. Now, she has no energy to brush her hair, do her laundry, or clean her dorm room and appears slightly disheveled and unkempt. She misses her family, as she says she is very close to her mother; however, she has not told her family how she is feeling for fear of disappointing them or being judged. Her mother keeps asking her what is wrong and she says that everything is fine but is secretly worried that she looks skinny and pale.

Prior to medical school, she had a complete physical examination required for entry, and this included labs: CBC, chemistries, and a TSH (thyroid test). Blood pressure, cardiac, pulmonary, and other systems examination appeared unremarkable, as did her labs. The physical examination was normal and the doctor wrote that she is healthy, an athlete, and has no prior or current medical issues. She never had a history of any psychiatric diagnosis and did not use any substances or illicit drugs; she never smoked or drank alcohol.

The patient admitted that sometimes she had thoughts of just ending it all, which would stop the stress, pain, loneliness, and embarrassment, but she would never have the courage to do something like that.

## What Is the Diagnosis?

The diagnosis, according to the fifth edition of the *Diagnostic and Statistical Manual of Mental Disorders* Published by the American Psychiatric Association (*DSM-5*), is Major Depressive Disorder with anxious distress. The case meets the following diagnosis criteria:

**A1:** Depressed mood as indicated by the patient and observed by others.
**A2:** She has lost interest or pleasure in almost all activities.
**A3:** Significant (more than 5 percent) unintentional weight loss and decreased appetite (Some people can gain weight).
**A4:** Sleep disturbances (insomnia or hypersomnia).
**A5:** Tiredness, fatigue, low energy, and decreased efficiency with which routine tasks are completed (as she is failing tests and has low power to do daily tasks).
**A6:** Sense of worthlessness or excessive inappropriate or delusional guilt.
**A7:** Impaired ability to think, concentrate, or make decisions indicated by subjective report or observation by others.
**A8:** Recurrent thoughts of death or suicidal ideation (here she has no attempts).

The *DSM-V* notes that “these symptoms cause clinically significant distress or impairment of social, occupational, or other important areas of functioning” (p. 148). These symptoms are not due to the direct physiological effects of substances or medical conditions (she does not take drugs or have hypothyroidism).

There has never been a manic or hypomanic episode. Symptoms are not accounted for by bereavement and are longer than two months, characterized by marked functional impairment, morbid preoccupation with worthlessness, and suicidal ideation.

Mirza et al. (2021) mentioned that medical students have about a 30.6% rate of major depression compared to the general population. The prevalence in females is higher than in males, yet both have a higher-than-average prevalence than the general population. Mirza et al. (2021) mentioned the "lifestyle, financial stressors, family relationships, and academic worries" prevalent in this population. The research highlighted a Pakistani study which showed that first-year students had a 28.4% rate, and third-year students had a 39% rate of depression.

## What Is the Best Treatment?

Treatment can include psychotherapy and possible pharmacotherapy. According to Rush (2022), the United Kingdom's National Institute for Health and Care Excellence recommends using psychotherapy if the condition is mild and then adding pharmacotherapy if needed.

There are many treatment options, and the selection depends on the severity of the depression after having a thorough evaluation, usually by a qualified medical professional and a psychiatrist. According to the Mayo Clinic, many antidepressant medication options are available to patients, such as serotonin reuptake inhibitors (SSRIs) like Citalopram, fluoxetine (Prozac), paroxetine (Paxil), sertraline (Zoloft), and many others.

There are also serotonin norepinephrine reuptake inhibitors (SNRIs) like venlafaxine (Effexor) and others, as well as atypical antidepressants and tricyclic depressants like amitriptyline. Psychotherapy is also an option, with medication or alone, and includes cognitive therapy or interpersonal therapy to cope better. Those were superior to pharmacotherapy alone (Rush, 2022). For very severe cases, there are other treatments such as hospitalization, electroconvulsive therapy, and transcranial magnetic stimulation (TMS). However, with the patient above, psychotherapy, counseling, ways of coping with stress, stress reduction, and lifestyle modifications, with or without medication would be the best option.

## Discussion Points

- As many as 50% of depressed patients seem unaware of or deny depression and thus are said to have "masked depression."
- Patients with masked depression often visit their doctors complaining of vague physical symptoms.

## Signs to Look For

Depressed mood is the most characteristic symptom, occurring in over 90% of patients. The patients usually describe themselves as feeling sad, low, empty, hopeless, gloomy, or down in the dumps. The quality of mood is likely to be portrayed as different from a normal sense of sadness or grief. Outward observations can be seen in changes in posture, speech, a melancholic expression, dress, and grooming issues. Many depressed patients state that they are unable to cry, whereas others report frequent weeping spells that occur without significant precipitants (Loosen & Shelton, 2019).

It is important for educators, faculty and staff to be aware of these issues and discuss depression with the pre-medical community.

## Case Study for Uncertainty

Pre-med students are faced with a lot of uncertainty surrounding their future that can lead to self-doubt and be extremely detrimental to students' mental health and outlook. The main reason pre-med students deal with uncertainty is due to the competitive nature of the pre-medical track with a lack of formal support. Pre-med classes are some of the most difficult classes offered at universities. On top of the difficulty of these classes is the strong emphasis placed on grading and the need for pre-med students to achieve certain grades in order to get into medical schools. Pre-med classes are rarely designed for students to succeed. Many of the introductory classes are termed "weeder classes" as they "weed out" students not fit for medical school and a career in medicine (Barr et al., 2008). Many pre-med classes also have a skewed grading system. Professors give exams that are intentionally too difficult such that the mean score falls around 50% and adjust students' grades to fit a bell curve. Intentionally difficult classes and the threat of being "weeded out" breeds uncertainty, and consistently receiving grades that reflect knowing less than half the material on the exam—even when the final grade is curved—leads to feelings of self-doubt and worthlessness.

Very few schools offer a pre-med major meaning that each students' path is unique. Each school offers different classes and though there are some classes that everyone completes, since they are required by all medical schools, there is no standardization of other classes students should take once they have completed their introductory required courses. In addition, the pre-med advising at most schools is severely lacking with advisors rarely accessible to students who are embarking on a long and difficult academic journey.

### Example

A pre-med student is in their second year of study. So far, they have been getting decent grades and feel that they are understanding the material well. However, every time they take a test in one of their pre-med classes, they get a grade in the 50s. Since the class is curved, they end up maintaining a fairly good final grade in the course, but despite that, the student becomes consistently discouraged by the fact that exam scores reflect them only knowing half of the material. This student begins to both fear their preparedness for future pre-medical courses, as so much of the material is cumulative, and experience feelings of worthlessness.

### Discussion Points

- What are some of the ways that faculty and fellow students could support this student mentally and/or academically?
- Is the student experiencing depression?
- What can be done to move the student to engage in pleasurable activities?
- What type of support can be helpful?
- How can we help the student derive alternative interpretations to the situation?

### Cognitive Therapy

Corey (2012) outlines the cognitive–behavioral model of depression developed by Aaron Beck. He suggests that depression develops when the patient cognitively misinterprets life events. The conceptual core of this model consists of the cognitive triad of depression: (1) a negative self-view (i.e., "things are bad because I am bad"), (2) a negative interpretation of experience (i.e., "everything has always been bad"), and (3) a negative view of the future (i.e., "everything will always be bad"). It is a basic tenet of this theory that a depressed person interprets the world through depressive schemata that distort experiences in a negative direction.

### Possible Solutions for Discussion

It can be helpful for pre-med students to form study groups both to help each other prepare for assessments and to provide comradery and peer support. Having comradery can help this student feel less alone in what they are going through and as a result more confident in their abilities.

It could also be helpful for professors to be more transparent with their students about their grading systems and reasoning behind the difficulty of their exams. This could help students feel better about their results and more confident despite their low scores.

## Case Study for Test Anxiety

Many students suffer from testing anxiety making it hard for them to perform to their ability on tests and exams. The competitive nature of pre-med classes and the need to achieve certain grades to get into medical school causes inherent stress which can be exacerbated by students who suffer from test anxiety. Testing anxiety harms students not only because the extreme stress is detrimental to overall mental health, but also because it prevents students from demonstrating their true knowledge as it causes them to underperform.

### Example

A pre-med student is in their first year of college. The high school that they went to was small and had a relaxed atmosphere. Though they took many tests and quizzes in high school they were never required to take tests in the type of conditions that are administered in college (a lecture hall with hundreds of people taking an exam for many hours straight). When they took their first college exams, they found themselves overwhelmed by the testing conditions. Despite feeling confident in the material that they learned in class and consistently scoring highly on self-administered practice tests in relaxed conditions, they consistently underperform on exams. This student has expressed that under standardized testing conditions they experience a racing heart, difficulty breathing, and sweating.

### Discussion Points

- In anxiety, the individual is frightened but the source of danger is not known, not recognized, or inadequate to account for the symptoms (Fadem, 2014).
- Is the anxiety a manifestation of a larger issue?
- Has it developed into a phobia? What is acute stress disorder?
- Individuals with generalized anxiety disorder (GAD) have persistent, excessive, and/or unrealistic worry associated with muscle tension, impaired concentration, autonomic arousal, feeling "on edge" or restless, and insomnia.

- What are all the characteristics of this case?
- What are some of the ways that faculty and fellow students could support this student mentally and/or academically?

### Possible Solutions for Discussion

This student might benefit from a diagnosis of anxiety along with some form of psychotherapy and/or medication. It could also be helpful for them to receive accommodations allowing them to take their exams in a less triggering environment and with extended time to help relieve some of the pressure that they feel while taking exams.

## CONCLUSION

This chapter focused on the experience of the pre-med student. The pre-medical student faces numerous challenges that can negatively impact their mental health. Academic pressures, financial stress, lack of social support, and relationship challenges, among others factors, can increase the risk of depression, anxiety, and other mental health disorders. It is essential that colleges develop and implement interventions aimed at helping students manage stress, build resilience, and foster positive mental health outcomes. In addition to highlighting the need to implement college-wide programs, this chapter emphasized the need to create a comprehensive curriculum to address mental health for the pre-medical community.

## REFERENCES

Ahmed, A. M. (2019). The real core competencies in premed culture. *Academic Medicine*, *94*(5), 611. doi:10.1097/ACM.0000000000002616 PMID:31021862

Allen, T. D., & Eby, L. T. (2003). Relationship effectiveness for mentors: Factors associated with learning and quality. *Journal of Management*, *29*(4), 469–486. doi:10.1016/S0149-2063(03)00021-7

American Psychiatric Association. (2013). *Diagnostic and statistical manual of mental disorders* (5th ed.). APA. doi:10.1176/appi.books.9780890425596

Barnett, M. (2004). A qualitative analysis of family support and interaction among Black college students at an ivy league university. *The Journal of Negro Education*, *73*(1), 53–68. doi:10.2307/3211259

Barr, D. A., Gonzalez, M. E., & Wanat, S. F. (2008). The leaky pipeline: Factors associated with early decline in interest in premedical studies among underrepresented minority undergraduate students. *Academic Medicine*, *83*(5), 503–511. doi:10.1097/ACM.0b013e31816bda16 PMID:18448909

Borenstein, J. (2020, August). *Stigma, prejudice and discrimination against people with mental illness.* American Psychiatric Association. https://www.psychiatry.org/patients-families/stigma-and-discrimination

Brougham, R. R., Zail, C. M., Mendoza, C. M., & Miller, J. R. (2009). Stress, sex differences, and coping strategies among college students. *Current Psychology (New Brunswick, N.J.)*, *28*(2), 85–97. doi:10.100712144-009-9047-0

Colarossi, J. (2022, April 21). *Mental health of college students is getting worse*. The Brink: Pioneering Research from Boston University. https://www.bu.edu/articles/2022/mental-health-of-college-students-is-getting-worse/

Collier, P. (2017). Why peer mentoring is an effective approach for promoting college student success. *Metropolitan Universities*, *28*(3), 9–19. doi:10.18060/21539

Conrad, P. (1986). The myth of cut-throats among premedical students: On the role of stereotypes in justifying failure and success. *Journal of Health and Social Behavior*, *27*(2), 150–160. doi:10.2307/2136313 PMID:3734381

Corey, G. (2012). *Theory and practice of counseling and psychotherapy*. Cengage learning.

Denslow, C. (2023, February 12). Pre-med students need our support. The high suicide rates tell as much. *The Daily Orange*. https://dailyorange.com/2023/02/pre-med-students-need-support-high-suicide-rates-tells-as-much/#google_vignette

*Depression*. (2022, October 14). Mayo Clinic. www.mayoclinic.org/diseases-conditions/depression/diagnosis-treatment/drc-20356013

Dhabhar, F. S. (2018). The short-term stress response - Mother nature's mechanism for enhancing protection and performance under conditions of threat, challenge, and opportunity. *Frontiers in Neuroendocrinology*, *49*, 175–192. doi:10.1016/j.yfrne.2018.03.004 PMID:29596867

Ding, H., & Rubie-Davies, C. M. (2019). Teacher expectation intervention: Is it effective for all students? *Learning and Individual Differences*, *74*, 101751. doi:10.1016/j.lindif.2019.06.005

Dou, R., Cian, H., & Espinosa-Suarez, V. (2021). Undergraduate STEM majors on and off the pre-med/health track: A STEM identity perspective. *CBE Life Sciences Education*, *20*(2), ar24. doi:10.1187/cbe.20-12-0281 PMID:33856900

England, B. J., Brigati, J. R., & Schussler, E. E. (2017). Student anxiety in introductory biology classrooms: Perceptions about active learning and persistence in the major. *PLoS One*, *12*(8), e0182506. doi:10.1371/journal.pone.0182506 PMID:28771564

Fadem, B. (2012). *Behavioral science in medicine*. Lippincott Williams & Wilkins.

Fang, D. Z., Young, C. B., Golshan, S., Fellows, I., Moutier, C., & Zisook, S. (2010). Depression in premedical undergraduates: A cross-sectional survey. *Primary Care Companion to the Journal of Clinical Psychiatry*, *12*(6), e1–e6. doi:10.4088/PCC.10m00958blu PMID:21494338

Fang, D. Z., Young, C. B., Golshan, S., Moutier, C., & Zisook, S. (2012). Burnout in premedical undergraduate students. *Academic Psychiatry*, *36*(1), 11–16. doi:10.1176/appi.ap.10080125 PMID:22362430

Foong, C. C., Bashir Ghouse, N. L., Lye, A. J., Pallath, V., Hong, H., & Vadivelu, J. (2021). Differences between high- and low-achieving pre-clinical medical students: A qualitative instrumental case study from a theory of action perspective. *Annals of Medicine*, *54*(1), 195–210. doi:10.1080/07853890.2021.1967440 PMID:35019800

Goel, D. (2020, May 26). Premed burnout and medical education. *Journal of Young Investigators*. www.jyi.org/blog/2020/5/26/premed-burnout-and-medical-education

Grace, M. K. (2018). Depressive symptoms, burnout, and declining medical career interest among undergraduate pre-medical students. *International Journal of Medical Education*, *9*, 302–308. doi:10.5116/ijme.5be5.8131 PMID:30481160

Grace, M. K. (2020). "They understand what you're going through": Experientially similar others, anticipatory stress, and depressive symptoms. *Society and Mental Health*, *11*(1), 20–37. doi:10.1177/2156869320910773

Gross, J. P., Mommaerts, C. D., Earl, D., & De Vries, R. G. (2008). Perspective: After a century of criticizing premedical education, are we missing the point? *Academic Medicine*, *83*(5), 516–520. doi:10.1097/ACM.0b013e31816bdb58 PMID:18448911

Hinami, K., & Wetterneck, T. B. (2017). For individuals and practices: Career sustainability and avoiding burnout. In McKean S.C., & Ross J.J., & Dressler D.D., & Scheurer D.B.(Eds.), Principles and Practice of Hospital Medicine (2nd ed.). McGraw Hill.

Hinderaker, D. J. (2013). *Counseling center college student mental health and use of counseling center services*. St. Catherine University Repository. https://sophia.stkate.edu/cgi/viewcontent.cgi?article=1191&context=msw_papers

Lang, A. (2019). Analysis of burnout and career calling in undergraduate pre-medical students. *Journal of Interdisciplinary Undergraduate Research*, *11*(1), 1.

Laschinger, H. K. S., & Leiter, M. P. (2006). The impact of nursing work environments on patient safety outcomes: The mediating role of burnout engagement. *The Journal of Nursing Administration*, *36*(5), 259–267. doi:10.1097/00005110-200605000-00019 PMID:16705307

Lattie, E. G., Lipson, S. K., & Eisenberg, D. (2019). Technology and college student mental health: Challenges and opportunities. *Frontiers in Psychiatry*, *10*(15), 246. doi:10.3389/fpsyt.2019.00246 PMID:31037061

Levitt, J. M., Saka, N., Romanelli, L. H., & Hoagwood, K. E. (2007). Early identification of mental health problems in schools: The status of instrumentation. *Journal of School Psychology*, *45*(2), 163–191. doi:10.1016/j.jsp.2006.11.005

Lilienfeld, S. O. (2007). Psychological treatments that cause harm. *Perspectives on Psychological Science*, *2*(1), 53–70. doi:10.1111/j.1745-6916.2007.00029.x PMID:26151919

Liviatan, I., Trope, Y., & Liberman, N. (2008). Interpersonal similarity as a social distance dimension: Implications for perception of others' actions. *Journal of Experimental Social Psychology*, *44*(5), 1256–1269. doi:10.1016/j.jesp.2008.04.007 PMID:19352440

Loosen, P. T., & Shelton, R. C. (2019). Mood disorders. In M. H. Ebert, J. F. Leckman, & I. L. Petrakis (Eds.), *Current Diagnosis & Treatment: Psychiatry* (3rd ed.). McGraw Hill.

Ludmerer, K. M. (1999). *Time to heal: American medical education from the turn of the century to the era of managed care*. Oxford University Press.

McGill. (2023). *Current applicant statistics.* Undergraduate Medical Admissions. https://www.mcgill.ca/medadmissions/after-youve-applied/currentapplicantstats

Minasi, P., Jr. (2022, January 24). *Reflecting on the Kaplan med school admissions officers survey*. Med Educators Blog. https://www.kaptest.com/blogs/med-educators/author/petros-minasi

Mindell, J. A., Bartle, A., Abd Wahab, N., Ahn, Y., Ramamurthy, M. B., Huong, H. T. D., Kohyama, J., Ruangdaraganon, N., Sekartini, R., Teng, A., & Goh, D. Y. (2011). Sleep education in medical school curriculum: A glimpse across countries. *Sleep Medicine*, *12*(9), 928–931. doi:10.1016/j.sleep.2011.07.001 PMID:21924951

Mirza, A. A., Baig, M., Beyari, G. M., Halawani, M. A., & Mirza, A. A. (2021). Depression and anxiety among medical students: A brief overview. *Advances in Medical Education and Practice*, *12*, 393–398. doi:10.2147/AMEP.S302897 PMID:33911913

Misra, R., & McKean, M. (2000). College students' academic stress and its relation to their anxiety, time management, and leisure satisfaction. *American Journal of Health Studies*, *16*(1), 41–51.

Murphy, B. (2021). *How the pandemic has spiked stress for many med school applicants.* American Medical Association. https://www.ama-assn.org/medical-students/preparing-medical-school/how-pandemic-has-spiked-stress-many-med-school-applicants

Nair, B., & Otaki, F. (2021). Promoting university students' mental health: A systematic literature review introducing the 4M-model of individual-level interventions. *Frontiers in Public Health, 9.* httpss://doi:10.3389/fpubh.2021.699030

Nilson, L. B. (2010). *Teaching at its best: A research-based resource for college instructors* (2nd ed.). Jossey-Bass.

Pacifici, L. B., & Thomson, N. (2011). Undergraduate science research: A comparison of influences and experiences between premed and non-premed students. *CBE Life Sciences Education*, *10*(2), 199–208. doi:10.1187/cbe.11-01-0005 PMID:21633068

PatientPop. (2019, April 16). *Why doctors are stressed and how to lower stress at your practice*. PatientPop. https://www.patientpop.com/blog/lessen-stress-and-physician-burnout/

Rao, C. R., Darshan, B. B., Das, N., Rajan, V., Bhogun, M., & Gupta, A. (2012). Practice of physical activity among future doctors: A cross-sectional analysis. *International Journal of Preventive Medicine*, *3*(5), 365–369. PMID:22708033

Riley, R., Spiers, J., Buszewicz, M., Taylor, A., Thorton, G., & Chew-Graham, C. (2018). What are the sources of stress and distress for general practitioners working in England? A qualitative study. *BMJ Open*, *8*(1), e017361. doi:10.1136/bmjopen-2017-017361 PMID:29326181

Riley, (2004), Understanding the stresses and strains of being a doctor, *MJA, 181*(7). doi:10.5694/j.1326-5377.2004.tb06322.x

Rush, A. J. (2022, November 28). Unipolar major depression in adults: Choosing initial treatment. *Up to Date.* https://www.uptodate.com/contents/unipolar-major-depression-in-adults-choosing-initial-treatment

Salgar, S. (2014). Stress in first year medical students. *International Journal of Biomedical and Advance Research*, *5*(1), 1. doi:10.7439/ijbar.v5i1.580

Sawatzky, R. G., Ratner, P. A., Richardson, C. G., Washburn, C., Sudmant, W., & Mirwaldt, P. (2012). Stress and depression in students: The mediating role of stress management self-efficacy. *Nursing Research*, *61*(1), 13–21. doi:10.1097/NNR.0b013e31823b1440 PMID:22166906

Schreiber, K. R., & Cunningham, F. O. (2016). Nutrition education in the medical school curriculum: A review of the course content at the Royal College of Surgeons in Ireland-Bahrain. *Irish Journal of Medical Science*, *185*(4), 853–856. doi:10.100711845-015-1380-8 PMID:26563109

Sevlever, M., & Rice, K. G. (2010). Perfectionism, depression, anxiety, and academic performance in premedical students. *Canadian Medical Education Journal*, *1*(2), e96–e104. doi:10.36834/cmej.36537

Sheldon, E., Simmonds-Buckley, M., Bone, C., Mascarenhas, T., Chan, N., Wincott, M., Gleeson, K., Sow, D., Hind, M., & Barkham, M. (2021). Prevalence and risk factors for mental health problems in university undergraduate students: A systematic review with meta-analysis. *Journal of Affective Disorders*, *287*, 282–292. doi:10.1016/j.jad.2021.03.054 PMID:33812241

Slavin, S. J., Schindler, D. L., & Chibnall, J. T. (2014). Medical student mental health 3.0: Improving student wellness through curricular changes. *Academic Medicine*, *89*(4), 573–577. doi:10.1097/ACM.0000000000000166 PMID:24556765

Stolzenberg, E. B., Aragon, M. C., Romo, E., Couch, V., McLennan, D., Eagan, M. K., & Kang, N. (2019). The American freshman: National norms fall 2018. *Higher Education Research Institute, UCLA*. https://www.pushkin.fm/wp-content/uploads/imported-files/TheAmericanFreshman2018.pdf

Sutcliffe, K. M., & Vogus, T. (2003). Organizing for resilience. In K. S. Cameron, J. E. Dutton, & R. E. Quinn (Eds.), *Positive organizational scholarship: Foundations of a new discipline*. Berrett-Koehler Press.

Tolsgaard, M. G. (2013). Clinical skills training in undergraduate medical education using a student-centered approach. *Danish Medical Journal*, *60*(8), B4690. PMID:23905573

Trullàs, J. C., Blay, C., Sarri, E., & Pujol, R. (2022). Effectiveness of problem-based learning methodology in undergraduate medical education: A scoping review. *BMC Medical Education*, *22*(1), 104. doi:10.118612909-022-03154-8 PMID:35177063

Van Der Feltz-Cornelis, C. M., Varley, D., Allgar, V. L., & De Beurs, E. (2020). Workplace stress, presenteeism, absenteeism, and resilience amongst university staff and students in the COVID-19 lockdown. *Frontiers in Psychiatry*, *11*, 588803. doi:10.3389/fpsyt.2020.588803 PMID:33329135

Wallick, W. T. (2023). *Pre-med mentorship program proposal*. Boise State University. https://scholarworks.boisestate.edu/cgi/viewcontent.cgi?article=1220&context=mds495_proj

WHO. (2019 May 28). *Burn-out an "occupational phenomenon": International classification of diseases*. World Health Organization. https://www.who.int/news/item/28-05-2019-burn-out-an-occupational-phenomenon-international-classification-of-diseases

Yates, S. (2019). Physician stress and burnout. *The American Journal of Medicine*, *133*(2), 160–164. doi:10.1016/j.amjmed.2019.08.034 PMID:31520624

Yomtov, D., Plunkett, S. W., Efrat, R., & Marin, A. G. (2015). Can peer mentors improve first-year experiences of university students? *Journal of College Student Retention*, *19*(1), 25–44. doi:10.1177/1521025115611398

Yusoff, M. S. B., Mat Pa, M. N., Esa, A. R., & Abdul Rahim, A. F. (2013). Mental health of medical students before and during medical education: A prospective study. *Journal of Taibah University Medical Sciences*, *8*(2), 86–92. doi:10.1016/j.jtumed.2013.03.004

Zhang, C., Kuncel, N. R., & Sackett, P. R. (2020). The process of attrition in pre-medical studies: A large-scale analysis across 102 schools. *PLoS One*, *15*(12), e0243546. doi:10.1371/journal.pone.0243546 PMID:33370336

Zheng, G., Zhang, Q., & Ran, G. (2023). The association between academic stress and test anxiety in college students: The mediating role of regulatory emotional self-efficacy and the moderating role of parental expectations. *Frontiers in Psychology*, *14*, 1008679. Advance online publication. doi:10.3389/fpsyg.2023.1008679 PMID:36824305

## KEY TERMS AND DEFINITIONS

**Burnout:** It is an internal psychological experience involving feelings, attitudes, motives, and distress. It is perceived by the individual as a negative experience.

**Hidden Curriculum:** Unintended but essential learning objectives.

**Mental Health:** A person's condition with regard to their psychological and emotional well-being.

**Mentors:** An advisor who leads through guidance.

**Problem Based Learning:** A pedagogical approach used to develop critical thinking skills.

**Stigma:** Expectations from others.

**Stress:** The concept of stress was borrowed by physiology where it generally refers to a force acting against some resistance.

# Chapter 11
# Teaching Students to Harness Their Anxiety and Maintain Well-Being in the Period Leading to and During Important Exams:
## Using Well-Being and Neuroscience Findings for the Appropriate Mental Preparation

**Ingrid R. C. Delange**
*École Internationale de Mondorf-les-Bains, Luxembourg*

## ABSTRACT

*Standard-based tests are a common form of final assessment in secondary education worldwide, but they pose many challenges for students. They require not only academic competence, but also mental resilience, which is rarely instructed in school. This chapter argues for the inclusion of strong mental training during revision. for this, it will review the history and rationale of standard-based assessments, and how they relate to the political and social aspects of different countries. It will also examine the controversies and criticisms of this form of evaluation, and how it affects the students' emotions and perspectives. The chapter will then suggest some practical strategies that teachers can use in the classroom to foster a holistic approach to learning. These strategies include mindfulness exercises, collaboration activities, feedback mechanisms, and the facilitation of healthy habits.*

DOI: 10.4018/979-8-3693-2833-0.ch011

## INTRODUCTION

Standard-based tests are a prevalent form of final assessment in secondary education around the world, but they also entail many challenges for students who need to show not only their academic competence, but also their mental strengths. These tests demand both a good command of the knowledge and skills taught during the lessons and also a strong mental resilience that is often not addressed in school. This paper will advocate for the inclusion of such practice in the general education context.

The paper will draw on the recent progress in brain imagery that has enabled scientists to make significant advances in understanding how the brain functions and how we can control our emotions. These findings have had a remarkable impact on various domains, including some unexpected ones. In areas such as sports, public speaking, performing arts, etc., athletes, politicians, and performers have adopted the use of mental coaches as part of their training and have improved their results considerably (Svoboda, 2021). It is now widely acknowledged that practice alone is not enough to achieve success; one also needs to comprehend their mental processes and train them to respond appropriately under any situation, even the most stressful ones. As TED-Ed (2018a) puts it, one needs to prevent "choking in the critical moment". This paper will suggest applying similar techniques to the educational setting, especially during the exam preparation and delivery phases.

To support this claim, the paper will first review the history and rationale of standard-based assessments, and how they are related to the political and social aspects of different countries. It will also examine the controversies and criticisms that surround this form of evaluation, and how it affects the students' perspectives and emotions. The paper will then propose some practical strategies that teachers can implement in the classroom and during exam preparation to foster a holistic approach to learning. These strategies include mindfulness exercises, collaboration activities, feedback mechanisms, and healthy habits. These techniques should help students identify their emotions and their readiness for exams, lower their anxiety and increase their motivation, distinguish the elements that trigger their stress, and find time to keep a healthy life and brain efficiency. The paper will argue that these strategies should help students develop the mental strength needed to overcome the fear generated by high-stakes exams and keep their stress and anxiety under control throughout the period.

The paper will conclude by discussing the implications and limitations of these strategies, and suggesting some directions for future research.

## EXAMINING THE SOURCES AND EFFECTS OF STRESS

### Eustress as a Positive Outcome of Standard-Based Testing and a Facilitator of Student Social Integration

#### Stress as a Catalyst: The Role of Stress in Building a Better Society

Harari (2018) divided the life of older generations into three stages. The first stage was the education period, where people "accumulated information, developed skills, constructed a world view, and built a stable identity". This period prepared them for the second stage, where they "relied on (their) accumulated skills to navigate the world, earn a living, and contribute to society…". High-stakes, standardized, and end-of-cycle tests have been essential components of this societal structure. They were based on the "collective myths" or "fictions" that exams measured intelligence, revealed high potentials, and enabled a fair selection of candidates (Harari, 2016). Exams were used for various purposes, such as identifying the best-qualified candidate for a position, holding educators and students accountable for their achievements, or increasing student learning incentive (Jones & Ennes, 2018). Exams were integrated into people's lives as meaningful and worthwhile. The stress associated with them was considered normal and beneficial for developing focus and resilience. Supporters of standard-based and high-stakes testing emphasize its potential to enhance learning outcomes. Data analysis of results allows stakeholders to identify strengths and weaknesses and offer an opportunity for adjustments. The emotions involved in the process help students get motivated, learn from their mistakes and achieve the required knowledge and skills. They are also socially beneficial emotions as they promote the egalitarian idea that hard work, a good memory, and the ability to fit the required mold are enough to pass or be accepted in a field. Tests measuring consistent standards for all students regardless of their location, gender, ethnicity, or socioeconomic background are not only regarded as fair (JCTP, n.d.) and they also aim at developing a society where everyone has equal opportunity to succeed and contribute to the common good. They appear to wisely address the country human capital in supporting the creation of a well-balanced high-quality workforce only regulated according to competence and skills as exemplified by the article from Chen, L., Duan, J., & Lu, M. (2019) on the Gaokao. In this setting, stress is eustress, a positive feeling that helps students stay motivated, energized, and excited to learn.

### Stress and the Elite: A Price Worth Paying

In the western world, more selective schools or university paths such as medical, law, or business courses took this idea further with the use of numerus clausus, a harsh and impersonal selection of students uniquely based on their academic performance and potential. This competitive system also helped the government precisely forecast quantities and quality in its future workforce (OECD, 2016). It, however, also forces students to cope with high levels of stress and pressure. To counterbalance all the psychological sacrifice to make, students focus their vision on the spirit of meritocracy and the unique opportunity to belong to an elite. Dealing with stress is harsh but is the inevitable price of pursuing excellence. Candidates who aspire to be part of the crème de la crème know that they need to excel not only in their academic skills, but also in their mental mastery during adversity. Stress and exam help them surpass themselves in driving them to go beyond their absolute performance to reach the highest ranking of their group.(Sommet et al., 2013). In this view, they seem to go hand in hand to serve social cohesion and the fair construct of the society. This view has been gradually described as untrue or unfit for 21st-century society.

## The Fall of Meritocracy: The Emotional Tall of Disillusionment, Social Collapse, and Tyranny of Conformity

### How Educational Systems Fail to Deliver on Their Promise

Research has shown that meritocracy is mostly an unfulfilled promise in education and that social inequalities persist despite efforts to create a meritocratic system. Governments have failed their mission to level the playing field in both rich (Ikeda, M. 2022) or emerging countries (EducationWorld, 2021) …... They have not secured that that all students have equal starting lines, not developed standardized tests based on a"fair" judgment. Mijs (2018) goes further in his studies on education systems in the United States and concludes that it is an « unfulfillable promise ». His argument can be summarized in three points: « educational institutions in practice significantly distort the ideal meritocratic process », «opportunities for merit are themselves determined by nonmeritocratic factors », « any definition of merit must favor some groups in society while putting others at a disadvantage. ». Skepticism also spread in the general population. A 2021 survey conducted by Boston Consulting Group/ IPSOS (2021) in France, the UK, Germany, Italy, Poland, the US, Argentina, Turkey, Australia, and Japan reveals that an average of 49% of the population thinks that meritocracy is not supported effectively. The consequences of this disillusionment are huge for the approach to exams. If careers are not open to talents, if educational opportunities do not support talented students sufficiently, if rewards do not correlate with merit, and if the 'one size fits all' approach marginalizes students with neurodiversity and socioeconomic differences, then the whole philosophy behind the assessment system collapses. This creates a split among the students: some still hold on to a faint hope of achieving success through effort and merit, while others simply resign themselves. The feelings that both groups experience are intense, and demand different approaches to deal with them.

## Focus on Confucian Countries

Some Asian countries, despite their traditional emphasis on high academic performance and achievement, have also witnessed this phenomenon of educational disillusionment. The phenomenon of Hikikomori, which refers to the social withdrawal of young people who isolate themselves from society, started in Japan in the 1990s and has since affected an estimated 1.5 million people, especially those aged 15 to 39 (Yeung & Karasawa, 2023). The willingness of these youngsters to leave as recluses can be explained by multiple factors, two of them however stand out: the anxiety of not coping with the highly competitive education system and the pressures of conforming to societal norms. Similarly, in Singapore and China, where students face severe stress to meet the expectations of their families and communities, the gap between meritocracy dream and reality is widening. Suicide is the leading cause of death for Singaporeans aged 10 to 29 (SOS Samaritans of Singapore., n.d.) and the trend is increasing. China is also facing similar issue (Cheng et al., 2020). Its "ultra-competitive system, which once propelled the country's economic rise, has now reached its inherent limits" (Gao, 2021). The uncertainty of a better future and the increasing demand to work harder and outperform peers have become unbearable (Siqi & Siqi, 2023). Young generations, especially new graduates, question the value and meaning of their studies and existence. They protest by joining the "Tang ping" movement or "lying flat", which means doing the minimum to survive and not striving for anything more than what is necessary. This way of living contradicts the deep-rooted Confucianist culture, which has valued hard work and merit-based selection for over a thousand years to select candidates for the state bureaucracy. It has become such a concern that recently, XingJing Ping reminded his people that "A happy life is achieved through struggle" (Bram, 2022.). However, this message did not resonate with the same intensity as it would have during the revolutionary fervor of the Mao era. For most Chinese, competitions, titles, and awards have become toxic educational rat races that students cannot escape without facing moral disgrace (Qianni and Shifan, 2020). Yet these are the only things that offer them a chance of not falling behind and having a possibility of a decent future where unemployment is rising.

### The Almightiness of the Few and the Trap for the Many

Meritocracy is not just a victim of socio-economic problems. Its own essence holds its downfall. By creating the false impression of « fair chance » and « manageable success », meritocracy breeds unfair discrimination and emotional resentment. In his book « The Tyranny of Merit », Sandel (2021) argues that meritocracy "invites the winners to consider their success their own doing and the losers to feel that those on top look down on them with disdain." This deepens the emotional gap between those who strive for exams and those who fall behind. Markovits (2019), in his book "The Meritocracy Trap", also warns about this harmful trend where being « the best » becomes more important than being « good enough » as this morally justifies the exclusion of non-specialists, individuals with hands-on skills, or people with different learning styles. Moreover, as achievement-based society becomes more competitive and exclusive, it also becomes more corrupt and rigged, favoring those who have the resources and connections to gain an edge over others. This not only harms those at the bottom of the meritocratic ladder, but also the elite themselves, as they become trapped in a relentless competition that erodes their well-being and happiness.

## Dejection Caused by Education Systems' Failure to Adapt to the Changing World

### Outdated and Out of Touch Education Systems Leave Students Demotivated

The assessment backbone of numerous educational system lead students feel that their progress and their worth is based on their grades (Family Central, 2021). When faced with the difficulty of responding to questions, student usually don't question the assessment itself but blame themselves (Wiederkehr et al., 2015). Their failure to comply doom their future. Their self-esteem spirals down while their anxiety levels spiral up. Exam questions and criteria however with their fit all approach is however often non fully relevant to their life. The last 50 years have seen unprecedented changes that have broken the myth of conformity. The overwhelming presence of the digital world, the emergence of Artificial intelligence, as well as the transformation of the cultural mosaics of numerous countries, and the rising trend of migration of various socio-educational groups have raised questions about the nature of academic basic knowledge and skills needed for future generations. In his book Out of Our Minds: Learning to be Creative, Ken Robinson (2017) examines the origins and shortcomings of contemporary educational systems. Although he mainly focuses on the American program, many of his conclusions are relevant to various education systems around the world. Created in the middle of the 19th century to serve the needs of the Industrial Revolution, national teaching and learning frameworks and pedagogies have not evolved as fast as the rest of the society. It still aims to perpetuate the functioning of society (Social Efficiency Ideology in Educationl ipl.org, n.d.), creating a good match between the supply and demand of the expected workforce, with the curriculum playing a central point as the « instrument that prepares students to be contributing members of society. » but the perpetual recreation as well as the technology requires has presented economical and philosophical issues to government and exam boards. How to equip the future generation with a solid understanding of basic academic knowledge and skills they will need when the speed of the innovation is so fast? How government can carry on fostering cultural norms and ideologies when the nature of their population is evolving constantly? (ARTE, 2018). Should government give up on their agenda of social and ideological conformity?

## The Impact of Cultural Hegemonies on Multicultural Student Bodies

In the United States, scholars, educators, and students led resounding pledges for the end of the hegemony of the white culture in programs and textbooks (LEA, V., & SIMS, E. J., 2008). Various European educational programs have also faced this criticism. In the UK the Museum of British Colonialism has emphasized the importance of "decolonizing the curriculum" in schools to raise attainment and a sense of belonging. (The Museum of British Colonialism, 2023) In France, the idea of the school promoting « republican assimilation » has been criticized for reinforcing a narrow definition of French identity and struggling to incorporate immigrants and minorities. (Safran,1990). More recently the incoming number of migrant children in Germany posed major challenges for many mainstream schools (Terhart & Von Dewitz, 2017). The OECD (2015) concluded that second-generation immigrant students in Denmark, France, and Mexico feel most alienated in their schools and have less of a sense of belonging. When first-generation immigrant students have stronger ties to their language, cultural heritage, and community, second-generation may feel caught between two disconnected cultures and struggle to find a sense of identity. Herzog-Punzenberger et al. (2020) conducted a study on how teachers in four countries (Austria, Ireland, Norway and Turkey) support students from diverse backgrounds to demonstrate their competencies and achieve success. They found that the main factor that affects how teachers perceive diversity in classrooms is the 'proficiency in the language of instruction'. They also noted that 'cultural differences' were less frequently mentioned by teachers, and that the responses to this aspect were often individual and not systematic "rather than organized by the school or regional education authorities". Moreover, those responses "were also strongly influenced and at times, limited by government-mandated assessment regimes that exist in each country". Creating an inclusive program that respects and values diversity is not easy to build, especially content-based instruction is dominant because such initiative will either cause alienation due to the multiplicity of cultures to include or raise opposition from the population who regard themselves as the original or dominant culture. This leaves a complex situation in multicultural or muti ethnical countries. Either a fair number of students of sit culturally non resonant and/or linguistically challenging exams or they have to rely on teachers who take it upon themselves to make their lessons and assessment more inclusive. They are however then at the risk of being treated with a deficit view and not having recognize their cultural and linguistic resources recognized either. (Koehler & Schneider, 2019) The emotional toll of blending and focusing mostly on achieving good grades rather than gaining meaningful learning is generating a high rise in students' emotional frustration and stress.

## The Gap Between the Digital World and the Educational System

The internet and artificial intelligence (AI) have transformed the world and challenged the validity of many educational programs. Students today are hyperconnected and have access to information that was previously unavailable. However, education systems have often lagged behind in adapting to these changes and adopting innovative ideas or technologies. For example, it took decades for calculators to be allowed in mainstream exams, leaving students with poor numeracy skills develop a fear of mathematics. How long will it take for AI to support students in their assessments?

Very few programs offer exams in the form of computer-based assessments, and even fewer have moved beyond traditional multiple-choice questions to more interactive formats that integrate simulation, digital graphing packages or interactive media. Yet, most jobs in the modern world do not require people to research, investigate, write, display datas, or produce reports without any digital tools. In the early 2010s, two prominent educators from Newcastle University and Harvard and, S. Mitra (2013) and E. Mazur (Paton, G. 2014), advocated for allowing the internet in exams. They envisioned a new form of assessment that would replace regurgitating knowledge with collaboration and problem solving. Some schools in Denmark (Hobson, 2009) took the lead in this innovative view of assessing, but were not followed by any other country, according to my research. Instead many countries take great pride in ranking high in outdated assessment leagues, such as PISA, that still "squeeze" skills that are becoming obsolete in the digital age. (Coulter et al., 2022) Some countries are even going backward. In France, the education minister suggested that French pupils who make spelling mistakes should have marks deducted from their school-leaving examination (Chazan, 2023), instead of encouraging them to improve their communication skills using spelling check programs. Economic factors (World Bank Group, 2022), tradition and culture (Mission Laïque Française, 2020), or political agendas often prevent the educational system from making radical changes. This has a negative impact on students' morale and readiness to succeed. According to a survey run by UNICEF (2020), one-third of the youth worldwide worry that their education is not preparing them with the skills to get jobs.

### In Conclusion

Skepticism toward the form and the purpose of exams is growing worldwide. Many students have lost trust in traditional institutions such as education and prefer to pursue "the universal purpose of life of being happy and feeling good about oneself." (Closson, n.d.) They do not see the value of acquiring knowledge or skills, but rather feel trapped in a rigid and stressful system of academic achievement. Educators have also expressed their concerns. In France, Celine Alvarez criticizes the fact that « We try to bring out intelligence at the same time as we stubbornly damage life » (Demain, L'école (2/2) - Les Innovations Dans Le Monde - Regarder Le Documentaire Complet | ARTE 2022, n.d.). In the US, Robinson and Aronica (2015) compare education to « Abattoirs ». Despite their flaws and limitations, standardized tests are still a reality that students have to face and prepare for. Therefore, exam revision needs to be reimagined as a meaningful holistic learning process, not just a means to an end. In the following section, we will explore this holistic approach to exam preparation, drawing on findings from well-being and mental preparation research and neuroscience discoveries.

## TEACHING REVISION STRATEGIES FOR EXAMS WITH A HOLISTIC MINDSET: IMPLICATIONS AND RECOMMENDATIONS

### Beyond Memorization: How to Coach Students Emotionally and Cognitively for Exams

#### The Importance of Balancing Academic and Emotional Demands in Exam Periods

With exams approaching, students feel the pressure mounting. They are required to memorize and understand a lot of information at the same time and a stronger focus on work need to be balanced with self-care and well-being strategies. Research shows that emotional competencies can affect exam performance, and that lack of them can lead to depression, anxiety, or stress. (Shrivastava, A., & Rajan, D., 2019). Moreover, students may face the risk of "choking" under pressure (TED-Ed, 2018), which is when they experience a mental blank at the most critical moments. This phenomenon can haunts anyone who has to perform in high-stakes situations, such as athletes, public speakers, or performers. Teachers have a role to play in supporting their students' mental health, but they often lack the official guidance and resources to do so. They have to rely on external sources to find advice on how to coach their students emotionally and prepare them for exams in a holistic way.

## Transitioning From GI Joe Fallacies to Effective Nudges

Don't stress out", "Make sure that you revise", "Give yourself some short breaks", "You'll be fine", "You can do it!", "You shouldn't worry" … Although encouraging and soothing, those sentences often heard during revision or exam time are hardly efficient. As Laurie Santos (2018) Associate Professor of Psychology at Yale explained in her Science of Wellbeing course: knowing about one's cognitive biases is not enough to overcome them. New routines need to be actively built and patiently nurtured to become automatisms when the time comes. The Nudge Theory (Thaler and Sunstein, 2008) could play a key role. Teachers may shape the classroom environment so that it "nudged" their classes to adopt new habits. By transforming their surroundings with visual and aural cues, teachers can boost student mental and physical readiness. Research on neuroscience shows that simple changes can have a powerful impact (Robson, 2022). For example, teachers can use nudges such as:

- Decorating the desks, floor, or table dividers with quotes inviting students to adopt a more relaxed and mindful approach (Thaler and Sunstein, 2008);
- Playing a relaxing music (De Witte et al., 2020);
- Providing them with material to doodle or color in while waiting for their papers (Harvard Health Publishing, 2018); and
- Having soft natural light (Garone, 2020).

A crafted calming environment will indirectly lead them to break their routine and shift their mindset toward becoming quieter, more attentive, and more focused. Teachers can also model stress relief behaviors such as:

- Slowing down (Toni Bernhard, 2011);
- Closing eyes for a couple of minutes to remove external stimulation (Aaron, 1996);
- Breathing deeply (Seppälä, 2021); and
- Trying a mindfulness exercise such as taking a few minutes to enjoy something (Santos, 2018).

The whole process should be approached as an invitation to grow and be detached from an authoritarian approach to prevent resentment. By influencing the likelihood that healthier habits are chosen over others, while maintaining freedom of choice, the teacher instills a sense of responsibility and self-awareness. Students are then more likely to evaluate what works best for them and make sustainable changes.

## Integrating a Range of Stress Relief Techniques Into Class Routines

The Harvard Health newsletter (Godman, 2022) lists some tips to ward off stress, such as relaxation exercises, stretching muscles, brisk walks, laughter, soothing music, positive self-talk, and reaching out for help. Teachers should introduce some of these techniques to students and include them in class routine. Even though revision times are often busy with academic work, these short techniques can be incorporated as breaks, intermissions, or transitions between tasks. For example, students can be reminded to stretch their back or legs, slow down their breathing, or look out of the window to activate their senses and detach themselves from their reality. This gives their brain space for daydreaming or idling, which can boost motivation (Henry, 2016). Students can also practice guided imagery by closing their eyes and visualizing a soothing image, which can help them calm themselves and find serenity in any setting (West, 2022). Closing the eyes can also improve memory recall (Brokaw et al., 2016).Including ritual breaks can make revision more efficient and send a strong message that self-care is a priority even when time is limited. Students might be reluctant or nonreceptive at first, as Boyce (2022) explains: "It takes a tremendous amount of work to bring someone to a level of competency in transmitting mindfulness." Mindfulness sessions are not a panacea, and it takes effort and practice for the effects to become visible. However, the conscious decision to rest the brain can prevent their concentration span from reaching its limit. It can also help improve focus, comprehension, accuracy, creativity, perspective, and memory. "Rest is (…) not idleness, nor is it a wasted opportunity for productivity," (Immordino-Yang et al., 2012). Encouraging routine breaks is essential as it enables the brain to sort information and recharge. (Brooks et al., 2016)

## Practicing Putting Things in Perspective Under Stress

Some stress-relieving activities, such as listening to soothing music or practicing positive self-talk, may face some cultural barriers, but putting things in perspective is a routine that can be easily adopted by any community. Students around the world often experience intense anxiety when they encounter an unexpected question in an exam. This triggers a panic response that prevents them from regaining focus on the rest of the paper. This happens because the brain perceives the question as a threat and releases a stress hormone called cortisol, which impairs rational thinking and activates the fight-or-flight response. This causes cloudy thinking to enable the brain to focus on fleeing from harm (Echouffo-Tcheugui et al., 2018). When students feel unprepared for the exam, they cannot run away, instead, they get stuck in a improvised chain of illogical reasoning that focuses on the minor issue instead of the big picture. Even though they know they are wasting time, their panic stops them from moving on. This inconsistency creates a mental dichotomy that makes them incapable of processing information rationally and lowers their confidence. To help them overcome this issue, it is essential to provide in-class opportunities to train their brain to adopt a new sequence of responses (Kahneman, 2011) to unexpected events.Psychologists believes that the brain can be reprogrammed by rehearsing a chosen sequence of responses under stressful conditions. This is a common practice in athletes' training (Arte, 2021). It can be applied in a class by including a few harder or even off-topic questions in revision tests. The stress induced by these questions will allow students to reflect on how they cope with difficulties and practice better strategies. Teachers' presence and guidance when students struggle is crucial, as it can calm their anxiety and remind them to take a step back and look at the bigger picture. By developing this mindful approach, students also become aware that their brain tends to focus on the harder questions due to a cognitive bias. Adopting a non-judgmental attitude will help them lower their tension and find a solution.

## Helping Students to Be Aware and Manage Their Stress Response

Lazarus & Folkman (2013) argue that stress is not a uniform phenomenon, and that the effectiveness of coping mechanisms depends on its source, people's personality, and their perception of the stressor. Some students may not recognize their stress or may resort to quick-relief stress tools, such as medicine and massage chairs, as a last resort (Davis & Olpin, 2021). This denial or lack of awareness can lead them to develop unhealthy habits that increase their anxiety (Conley et al., 2013). Therefore, it is important to help students become aware of their own patterns and attitudes and help them use their stress response as an ally, not an enemy.To help students with this task, King and Nicolson (2019) suggest a questionnaire and some research activities on how famous people cope with stress. This student-centered approach may work well for students who are willing to change, but it may also become a superficial exercise for others. Teachers' supervision should support the process. Observing students' reactions during exam practice and recording their signs of nervousness, distraction, or coping mechanisms can be more effective with the most closeminded students as the paper tracking give them the data to reflect on their stressors and response mechanism.

The timing of their reaction provides students with evidence to analyze their difficulties and improve their own stress-coping techniques. They may need to improve their revision skills, adopt a more confident posture, pace themselves better, or use more mindfulness breaks... This exercise also provides them with the opportunities to verbalize their apprehension and be more accepting of their weakness. Stress is often a mental response to people's unrealistic expectations of perfection (Suh et al., 2022). Harsh self-judgment and the fear of losing face can lead to low self-esteem and lack of self-trust (ARTE, 2022). Practicing catharsis has been proven to reduce rumination, increase self-compassion, and boost confidence (Yu, 2015).

## Implementing the Premortem or WOOP Techniques as Rituals for Exam Preparation

Listening to one's needs, learning to let it go, or aiming for the bigger picture goal are complex processes to teach. There is no one-size-fits-all solution for these challenges. Students need to find their own approach, playing with their own mental strengths and weaknesses. One technique that can help students cope with difficulties is the premortem technique, suggested by psychologist Gary Klein (2014) for business it can be adapted to schooling. It involves looking ahead and trying to figure out all the things that could go wrong, and then planning how to prevent them to happen or minimize their effect. A more student-friendly version of this technique is called WOOP. Developed by Gabriele Oettingen (2014), WOOP provides a scaffolded meditation routine with teaching resources and videos. Students learn to single out their true wish, through a thorough analysis of its outcome and consequences. They then list all the possible obstacles, visualize themselves in the difficult situation, and plan and practice possible solutions. This technique goes beyond the "think positively" meditation exercises. It engages students in a real growth mindset reflection and helps them develop their inner strength to reach their ideal self. Through regular practice, students grow a better grasp of their capacity, befriend themselves, and reduce their stress levels. Saddawi-Konefka et al. (2017) found that WOOP was efficient and increased the time students spent studying toward their goals, compared to setting goals alone.

## Students' Confidence and Success on Exam Day

### Minimizing the Impact of External Stressors

Stress is not a curse and can be an ally: time pressure helps memorize a list faster; finish an essay on time (Cox, 2018); or accomplish tasks faster than one could have imagined. However, for this students need to enter their personal bubble and be protected from external stressors. Unfortunately, some, such as family issues, insecurity, or living in an urban life with no green space (Beyer et al., 2014), are difficult to soften. In contrast, some factors that are known to influence students' stress levels and ability to concentrate can be controlled. These include:

- Sleep deprivation (American Psychological Association. 2013)
- Lack of exercise (Environment et al., 2013)
- Unhealthy food (ARTE-2)
- Hyper-connectivity and digital addiction (Worland, 2014)
- Feeling of disorganization or lateness on revision schedule (Harvard Health, 2021)

In this section, we will explore how to support students against them.

### Early Exam Practice: A Strategy for Creating a Deja Vu Effect

To perform well on exams, students need to be familiar with the format, structure, wording, and requirements of the test, such as the number of questions, the time limit, the marking scheme, or the use of calculators. This may reduce the novelty and uncertainty that could cause stress and anxiety. Therefore, it is essential that students practice the exam process until it becomes fully internalized (Busch, 2017). Teachers can help students by providing them with resources and opportunities to practice in realistic conditions. Exam centers usually offer a range of resources, such as past papers, marking schemes, and examiners' reports, that can help students prepare for exams. Practice testing enhances the long-term retention of material by promoting the retrieval of information from memory. It also assist students in identify their strengths and weaknesses and focus their study efforts accordingly. Rehearsing exam questions develops automaticity and confidence in their skills. Research in Taiwan has shown that attending cram schools results in a positive effect on students' analytical ability and mathematical results (Liu, 2012), as cramming helps the brain focus on the performance. Teachers should also simulate the exam environment by asking students to line up in the corridor, wait silently for the teacher to collect the papers, and follow the exam instructions. This will create a sense of familiarity and deja vu on the exam day. Finally, it is important to note that while practice testing can help students develop metacognitive skills, such as self-monitoring and self-regulation, it is paramount to remind students that it should not compromise their sleep quality, as sleep deprivation has negative consequences on thinking skills and memory (UCLA, 2012).

### Using Self-Marking, Feedback, and Self-Affirmation to Boost Students' Confidence and Performance in Exams

Exam practice can have some drawbacks, especially for students who lack confidence or motivation or who underperform under pressure. They may develop self-blaming or avoidance patterns that hinder their learning and progress and increase their anxiety. Wright (2013) suggests that these students need a teacher who acts as a mental coach to help them stay geared towards a growth mindset. They need support to believe that they can improve through effort and feedback. One possible solution is to make students take ownership of their learning and have them mark their own papers. This technique helps them save face and forces them to analyze their mistakes or speak to the teacher or their peers to clarify doubts. Dunlosky et al. (2013) argue that "students who are actively involved in the learning process retain more information and perform better than those who are passive recipients of information". However, self-marking is not an easy process. Students may not be able to assess their own work accurately or be tempted to cheat. To remediate from this, it is important to create a safe and trusting atmosphere. In such context, students view teachers and classmates as facilitators of knowledge and skills, not as judges or critics. With the solution, communication and in particular feedback is essential. It should be well thought and phrased in a way that guides and supports students in their development, rather than undermining their confidence. Peer feedback possess tremendous strength. Simonsmeier et al. (2020) conclude without doubt that it is "an effective strategy to improve academic achievement." In an article from the Harvard Graduate School of Education, L. Shaffer (2017) offers some strategies to build an efficient culture of feedback and highlights how it boosts the whole community's personal development including teachers. Feedback helps each member to connect on a human level. Lazarus (1985) explains how an imbalance between the demands placed on the individual and the individual's resources to cope leads to stress and can undermine their self-esteem. Personalizing our wording by considering students' cognitive appraisal styles, paying attention to choose non-threatening or negative terminology, and opening the dialogue demonstrates remarkable effectiveness as recipient fully listened to the message and taken into consideration. When it is close to exam time, communication should be honest, but students' feelings should be preserved and focus needs to stay on the positive. Godman (2022) in his studies about the importance of staying positive showed that practicing self-affirmation and countering negative thoughts favorably affect students' performance. It would be interesting to study how much turning teachers' feedback into mantras leads students from cultures geared towards critical thoughts into developing a more positive outlook. Scaffolding such practice can be as simple as introducing the new ritual of thinking about at least one student's strength and practicing self-affirmation while papers are given out.

## Developing Effective Study Habits and Self-Regulation Skills During the Final Weeks

Another critical factor in preparing for exams is developing effective study habits. Interactive study resources that can be personalized to individual needs with the help of artificial intelligence enable students to develop meaningful revision plans. Students often feel stressed about timing. Breaking down the workload into manageable recommended 45-minute to 60-minute chunks of various topics (NHS, 2023) helps with speed, as each break and switch prevent mental fatigue and boredom of working only on one subject. They also offer a refreshed view and attention on following topic (Jones, 2012). Practicing the planification of revision as a class activity, helps students reflect on their way of learning, routine and efficiency. This also should prevent the rise of unnecessary distractions and consequent feeling of remorse and anxiety. Imagining a dynamic schedule conveys a pace in the day and provides a good visual progression where leisure time to balance study is included. It also requires for them to practice their skills in organization, prioritization, and monitoring. Students' self-regulatory ability however vary greatly. Differentiation and a la carte response need to be set to help students hit their targets. Teachers' rapport with their classes is the key to efficiently balancing compassion and pressure. This is not an easy task especially when it comes to procrastinators. They need more scaffolding, shorter chunks, and regular prompts to reflect on their time management and progress. Kindness and empathy are the way forward, to avoid lowering their self-esteem, reinforcing their feeling of shame (TEd-Ed., 2022), and making them think they will never be sufficiently prepared for the day of the exam. Relying on study groups with a timekeeper, has been shown to be effective (UNC-Chapel Hill Learning Center, 2022). Pear pressure is a good strategy to motivate students to keep a healthy pace.

## Balancing Life and Boosting Performance for D-Days

Many students and their families believe that focusing on revision is the key to success in exams. However, this can be counterproductive if it leads to neglecting other aspects of a balanced life, such as physical and mental health. In fact, research shows that students who maintain a healthy lifestyle tend to perform better academically and experience less stress than those who do not (UCLA, 2012.). Physical activity is beneficial for both the body and the brain. It helps students clear their minds, boost their energy levels, improve their mood, and socialize with others. Some innovative schools include physical activity in their exam revision schedule, such as walking, running, or playing games during breaks but no research have been formally done to analyse the outcome. Doing sports however offers a perfect opportunity to laugh, which enhances confidence and happiness. Another major aspect of life which is neglected often during exam is sleep. Sleep is however crucial for academic success. It enhances memory and cognitive functioning, which are essential for exam performance. Research suggests that students who get enough sleep for at least a week before the exam, follow a regular sleep schedule, and have a cool, dark, and quiet sleeping environment tend to have better results than those who do not (Scullin et al., 2019; Ryan & Ryan, 2022). If students are too behind to have long night sleep, taking the form of short naps (less than an hour), improve alertness, creativity, productivity, and mood, and decrease stress (Klein, 2014). Finally, nutrition is another important factor in exam preparation. Students often rely on junk food, caffeine, and sugar to boost their energy levels, but these can have negative effects on their concentration, mood, and health. Nutritional therapist O'Shaughnessy (O'Mahony, 2017) said "While caffeine may make you more alert, individuals can build up a tolerance meaning this is short-lived. Caffeine can also increase blood sugar and eventually lead to dips, causing a lack of focus and energy." Instead, students should eat healthy food that supports their brain function, such as fruits, vegetables, nuts, seeds, eggs, fish, and yogurt (Richardson, 2019; QS International, 2021). They should also drink plenty of water, as it improves attention and hydration (O'Mahony, 2017). On the day of the exam, having breakfast or lunch, even if they feel nauseous is paramount. It is recommended to eat protein-filled food up to two hours before taking the exam, as it helps keep the same energy level during the whole session. They should however avoid caffeine (Frothingham, 2023) and energy drinks (Kaur et al., 2020), as they can increase anxiety and jitteriness.

In conclusion, this paper has explored the challenges and opportunities that students face in the period leading to and during important exams. We have argued that students should harness their anxiety and maintain well-being for their academic and emotional success. We have also explored how stress, both positive and negative, affects students' performance. We analyzed how educational systems fail to deliver on their promise and foster a fractured society between elites and disillusioned. We have highlighted the gap between the educational system and the current multicultural and digital world, and the impact of cultural hegemonies on some students. We have concluded the importance of rethinking assessment format to make them relevant to the new generation. Until this is achieved, we have underlined the importance of teachers in developing a holistic approach to exam preparation. This preparation will have to use their creativity and bond with the students to keep them motivated and mentally healthy and fulfill their true potential on exam days. The second half of the paper suggests some coaching strategies for teachers and students to prepare for exams with a holistic mindset. They draw on the latest results in neuropsychology and their applications in business, public speaking or athlete performances. They involve putting things in perspective, applying the premortem or WOOP techniques, practicing self-marking, feedback, and self-affirmation. Closer to the day of the exams research also shows the importance of keeping a healthy active lifestyle by developing effective study habits and self-regulation skills. By following these recommendations, students have increased their confidence and success on exam day and beyond. Further testing nonetheless should be performed to quantify the impact of successfully implementing the coaching strategies and exercising efficient organizational and health-promoting skills.

## REFERENCES

American Psychological Association. (2013, January 1). *Stress and sleep*. APA. https://www.apa.org. https://www.apa.org/news/press/releases/stress/2013/sleep

Aron, E. N. (1996). *The highly sensitive person: How to thrive when the world overwhelms you*. Perpus. https://perpus.univpancasila.ac.id/index.php?p=show_detail&id=124394

ARTE. (2018). *Demain, l'école (2/2) - Les innovations dans le monde* [Video]. Youtube. https://www.youtube.com/watch?v=9POzTRzuQnw

ARTE. (2021). *Dans la tête des champions* [Video]. ARTE Boutique. https://boutique.arte.tv/detail/dans-la-tete-des-champions

ARTE. (2022, September 17). *Peut-on se fier à soi-même? | 42, la réponse à presque tout.* [Video]. YouTube. https://www.youtube.com/watch?v=jeAfbTKmZng

Beyer, K., Kaltenbach, A., Szabo, A., Bogar, S., Nieto, F. J., & Malecki, K. (2014). Exposure to Neighborhood Green Space and Mental Health: Evidence from the Survey of the Health of Wisconsin. *International Journal of Environmental Research and Public Health, 11*(3), 3453–3472. doi:10.3390/ijerph110303453 PMID:24662966

Boston consulting group/ IPSOS. (2021, December 3). *Les paradoxes et illusions perdues de la méritocratie en France*. IPSOS. https://www.ipsos.com/. https://www.ipsos.com/sites/default/files/ct/news/documents/2021-12/IpsosxBCG%20-%20Enquete%20meritocratie.pdf

Bram, B. (2022, November). *Involution: the generation turning inward and away from Xi's Chinese dream.* Asia Society. https://asiasociety.org/policy-institute/involution-generation-turning-inward-and-away-xis-chinese-dream

Brokaw, K., Tishler, W., Manceor, S., Hamilton, K., Gaulden, A. D., Parr, E., & Wamsley, E. J. (2016). Resting state EEG correlates with memory consolidation. *Neurobiology of Learning and Memory, 130*, 17–25. doi:10.1016/j.nlm.2016.01.008 PMID:26802698

Brooks, A. W., Schroeder, J., Risen, J. L., Gino, F., Galinsky, A. D., Norton, M. I., & Schweitzer, M. E. (2016). Don't stop believing: Rituals improve performance by decreasing anxiety. *Organizational Behavior and Human Decision Processes, 137*, 71–85. doi:10.1016/j.obhdp.2016.07.004

Busch, B. (2017, August 17). Practice makes perfect: why mock exams are great for students' brains. *The Guardian*. https://www.theguardian.com/teacher-network/2015/dec/03/practice-makes-perfect-why-mock-exams-students-brains

Chazan, D. (2023, July 13). Mark pupils down for poor French spelling, says education MP. *Times*. https://www.thetimes.co.uk/article/mark-pupils-down-for-poor-french-spelling-says-education-mp-6q86h82ls

Chen, L., Duan, J., & Lu, M. (2019). The Gaokao: A decisive filter for human capital allocation in China. *China Economic Review, 58*, 101341.

Cheng, Y., Zhang, X. M., Ye, S. Y., Jin, H., & Yang, X. H. (2020). Suicide in Chinese graduate students: A review from 2000 to 2019. *Frontiers in Psychiatry, 11*, 579745. doi:10.3389/fpsyt.2020.579745 PMID:33424658

Closson, M. C. D. (n.d.). *New Barna's research reveals the extent of America's loss of faith*. FRC. https://www.frc.org/blog/2021/06/new-barna-research-reveals-extent-americas-loss-faith

Conley, C. S., Travers, L. V., & Bryant, F. B. (2013). Promoting Psychosocial Adjustment and Stress Management in First-Year College Students: The Benefits of Engagement in a Psychosocial Wellness Seminar. *Journal of American College Health, 61*(2), 75–86. doi:10.1080/07448481.2012.754757 PMID:23409857

Coulter, S., Iosad, A., & Scales, J. (2022, August 23). *Ending the big squeeze on skills: How to Futureproof education in England*. Global Institute. https://www.institute.global/insights/public-services/ending-big-squeeze-skills-how-futureproof-education-england

Cox, E. (2018). *The surprising link between stress and memory* [Video]. TED Talks. https://www.ted.com/talks/elizabeth_cox_the_surprising_link_between_stress_and_memory/transcript.%22%20n.d.%20The%20surprising%20link%20between%20stress%20and%20memory

Davis, R. R., & Olpin, M. (2021). The Effects of Stress Relief Tools and Interventions on Student Well-Being. *ResearchGate*. https://www.researchgate.net/publication/351424377_The_Effects_of_Stress_Relief_Tools_and_Interventions_on_Student_Well-Being

De Witte, M., Da Silva Pinho, A., Stams, G. J., Moonen, X., Bos, A. E. R., & Van Hooren, S. (2020). Music therapy for stress reduction: A systematic review and meta-analysis. *Health Psychology Review, 16*(1), 134–159. doi:10.1080/17437199.2020.1846580 PMID:33176590

Dunlosky, J., Rawson, K. A., Marsh, E. J., Nathan, M. J., & Willingham, D. T. (2013). *Improving students' learning with effective learning techniques: Promising directions from Cognitive and Educational Psychology*. Association for Psychological Science-APS. https://www.psychologicalscience.org/publications/journals/pspi/learning-techniques.html

Echouffo-Tcheugui, J. B., Conner, S. C., Himali, J. J., Maillard, P., DeCarli, C., Beiser, A. S., Vasan, R. S., & Seshadri, S. (2018). Circulating cortisol and cognitive and structural brain measures. *Neurology, 91*(21), e1961–e1970. doi:10.1212/WNL.0000000000006549 PMID:30355700

EducationWorld. (2021). *Towards a level playing field in K-12 education.* Education World. https://www.educationworld.in/towards-a-level-playing-field-in-k-12-education/

Family Central. (2021). *Children - so much more than just grades.* Family Central. https://www.family-central.sg/news-articles/children-more-than-grades/

Frothingham, S. (2023, March 29). *Does caffeine cause anxiety?* Healthline. https://www.healthline.com/health/caffeine-and-anxiety%23caffeine-and-anxiety

Gao, H. (2021). Beijing is worried young Chinese are embracing nihilism. *Foreign Policy.* https://foreignpolicy.com/2021/10/23/china-meritocracy-youth-burned-out/

Garone, S. (2020, August 11). *The health benefits of natural light (and 7 ways to get more of it).* Healthline. https://www.healthline.com/health/natural-light-benefits#benefits

Godman, H. (2022). Top ways to reduce daily stress. *Harvard Health.* https://www.health.harvard.edu/staying-healthy/top-ways-to-reduce-daily-stress

Harari, Y. N. (2016). *Sapiens: A Brief History of Humankind.* Signal.

Harari, Y. N. (2018). Yuval Noah Harari on what 2050 has in store for humankind. *WIRED UK.* https://www.wired.co.uk/article/yuval-noah-harari-extract-21-lessons-for-the-21st-century

Harvard Health. (2021). *Protect your brain from stress.* https://www.health.harvard.edu/mind-and-mood/protect-your-brain-from-stress

Henry, A. (2016, August 11). Why we should all spend more time staring out of the window. *Lifehacker.* https://lifehacker.com/why-we-should-all-spend-more-time-staring-out-of-the-wi-1784903049

Herzog-Punzenberger, B., Altrichter, H., Brown, M., Burns, D., Nortvedt, G. A., Skedsmo, G., Wiese, E. F., Nayır, F., Fellner, M., McNamara, G., & O'Hara, J. (2020). Teachers responding to cultural diversity: Case studies on assessment practices, challenges and experiences in secondary schools in Austria, Ireland, Norway and Turkey. *Educational Assessment, Evaluation and Accountability, 32*(3), 395–424. doi:10.100711092-020-09330-y

Hobson, J. (2009, November 4). *Danish pupils use web in exams.* BBC. http://news.bbc.co.uk/2/hi/uk_news/education/8341886.stm

Ikeda, M. (2022). What can we do to ensure a level playing field for all students? In *PISA in Focus, No. 117.* OECD Publishing. doi:10.1787/e297c355-

Immordino-Yang, M. H., Christodoulou, J. A., & Singh, V. (2012). Rest is not idleness. *Perspectives on Psychological Science, 7*(4), 352–364. doi:10.1177/1745691612447308 PMID:26168472

International, Q. S. (2021). Brain food: What to eat when revising. *Top Universities.* https://www.topuniversities.com/blog/brain-food-what-eat-when-revising

JCTP. (n.d.). *Code of FairTesting Practices in Education*. APA. https://www.apa.org/science/programs/testing/fair-testing.pdf

Jones, G. A. (2012). Why Chunking Should be Considered as an Explanation for Developmental Change before Short-Term Memory Capacity and Processing Speed. *Frontiers in Psychology, 3*. doi:10.3389/fpsyg.2012.00167 PMID:22715331

Jones, M. G., & Ennes, M. (2018). *High-stakes testing* [Dataset]. doi:10.1093/obo/9780199756810-0200

Kahneman, D. (2011). *Thinking, fast and slow*. NII. http://ci.nii.ac.jp/ncid/BB2184891X

Kaur, S., Christian, H., Cooper, M. N., Francis, J., Allen, K. L., & Trapp, G. (2020). Consumption of energy drinks is associated with depression, anxiety, and stress in young adult males: Evidence from a longitudinal cohort study. *Depression and Anxiety, 37*(11), 1089–1098. doi:10.1002/da.23090 PMID:32845046

King, L., & Nicolson, M. (2019). *DP ATL Skills Student Workbook: DP ATL Skills. 3i Deal effectively with pressure, stress and anxiety.*

Klein, G. (2014). Performing a project premortem. *Harvard Business Review*. https://hbr.org/2007/09/performing-a-project-premortem

Koehler, C., & Schneider, J. (2019). Young refugees in education: The particular challenges of school systems in Europe. *Comparative Migration Studies, 7*(1), 28. doi:10.118640878-019-0129-3

Lazarus, R. S. (1985). The Psychology of stress and coping. *Issues in Mental Health Nursing, 7*(1–4), 399–418. doi:10.3109/01612848509009463 PMID:3854019

Lazarus, R. S., & Folkman, S. (2013). Stress: appraisal and coping. In Springer eBooks (pp. 1913–1915). doi:10.1007/978-1-4419-1005-9_215

Lea, V., & Sims, E. J. (2008). Imaging Whiteness Hegemony in the Classroom: Undoing Oppressive Practice and Inspiring Social Justice Activism. *Counterpoints, 321,* 185–202. https://www.jstor.org/stable/42979967

Liu, J. (2012). Does cram schooling matter? Who goes to cram schools? Evidence from Taiwan. *International Journal of Educational Development, 32*(1), 46–52. doi:10.1016/j.ijedudev.2011.01.014

Markovits, D. (2019). The Meritocracy Trap: How America's foundational myth feeds inequality, dismantles the middle class, and devours the elite. https://openlibrary.org/books/OL28209037M/The_Meritocracy_Trap

MijsJ. J. B. (2018). The Unfulfillable Promise of Meritocracy: Three Lessons and their Implications for Justice in Education. SocArXiv *Papers*. https://doi.org/ doi:10.31235/osf.io/6w9rg

*Mission Laïque Française, (*2020, May 17). *Réinventer l'éducation, une nécessité - Mission laïque française*. Mission Laïque Française. https://www.mlfmonde.org/tribunes/reinventer-leducation-une-necessite/

Mitra, S. (2013). Should students be allowed to use the internet in exams? The Guardian. https://www.theguardian.com/teacher-network/teacher-blog/2013/jun/17/ipads-exams-teaching-test-schools

Mollah Jérusalem. (2019, September 20). *Comment notre alimentation influence notre santé mentale | ARTE* [Video]. YouTube. https://www.youtube.com/watch?v=IM-YhqnybJM

NHS. (2023). *Tips on preparing for exams.* nhs.uk. https://www.nhs.uk/mental-health/children-and-young-adults/help-for-teenagers-young-adults-and-students/tips-on-preparing-for-exams/

O'Mahony, H. (2017). The revision diet: what's the best food and drink to help students focus? *The Guardian*. https://www.theguardian.com/education/2017/may/29/the-revision-diet-whats-the-best-food-and-drink-to-help-students-focus

OECD. (2015). *Helping immigrant students to succeed at school – and beyond.* OECD. https://www.oecd.org/education/Helping-immigrant-students-to-succeed-at-school-and-beyond.pdf

OECD. (2016). Education and training for doctors and nurses: What's happening with numerus clausus policies? In *Health Workforce Policies in OECD Countries: Right Jobs, Right Skills, Right Places*. OECD Publishing. doi:10.1787/9789264239517-6-

Oettingen, G. (2014). *Rethinking Positive Thinking: Inside the New Science of Motivation*. Penguin.

Paton, G. (2014). Allow pupils to use Google in GCSE exams, says academic. *The Telegraph*. https://www.telegraph.co.uk/education/educationnews/11275200/Allow-pupils-to-use-Google-in-GCSE-exams-says-academic.html

Richardson, A. (2019). Can food improve your exam performance? *BBC Food*. https://www.bbc.co.uk/food/articles/food_exam_performance

Robinson, K. (2017). *Out of our minds: The Power of Being Creative*. John Wiley & Sons.

Robinson, K., & Aronica, L. (2015). How schools kill creativity: Forget standardized tests, here's how we really engage our kids. *Salon*. https://www.salon.com/2015/04/26 how_schools_kill_creativity_forget_standardized_tests_heres_how_we_really_engage_our_kids/)

Robson, D. (2022). How interior design choices can boost your mental and physical health. *New Scientist*. https://www.newscientist.com/article/mg25433823-000-how-interior-design-choices-can-boost-your-mental-and-physical-health/

Ryan, T., & Ryan, T. (2022). A Study Guide To Getting Sleep During Final Exams. *Sleep Foundation*. https://www.sleepfoundation.org/school-and-sleep/final-exams-and-sleep

Safran, W. (1990). Review: The French and Their National Identity: The Quest for an Elusive Substance? on JSTOR. Vol. 8, No. 1 (Winter 1990), pp. 56-67 (12 pages). https://doi.org/ doi:10.2307/42844146

Sandel, M. J. (2021). *The tyranny of merit: Can We Find the Common Good?* Picador.

Scullin, M. K., MacGregor, J., & King, E. (2019). 0096 Sleep in college students during final exams week: The Eight Hour challenge. *Sleep*, *42*(Supplement_1), A39–A40. Advance online publication. doi:10.1093leep/zsz067.095

Seppälä, E. (2021). Research: Why Breathing Is So Effective at Reducing Stress. *Harvard Business Review*. https://hbr.org/2020/09/research-why-breathing-is-so-effective-at-reducing-stress

Shafer, L. (2017). *Making student feedback work*. Harvard Graduate School of Education. https://www.gse.harvard.edu/ideas/usable-knowledge/17/11/making-student-feedback-work

Shrivastava, A., & Rajan, D. (2019). Assessmen Competitive Exams. *International Journal of Healthcare Sciences*, 2348-5728. doi:10.13140/RG.2.2.10711.42406

Simonsmeier, B. A., Peiffer, H., Flaig, M., & Schneider, M. (2020). Peer Feedback Improves Students' Academic Self-Concept in Higher Education. *Research in Higher Education, 61*(6), 706–724. doi:10.100711162-020-09591-y

Siqi, J., & Siqi, J. (2023b). What is 'lying flat', and why are Chinese officials standing up to it? *South China Morning Post*. https://www.scmp.com/economy/china-economy/article/3153362/what-lying-flat-and-why-are-chinese-officials-standing-it

Sommet, N., Pulfrey, C., & Butera, F. (2013). Did my M.D. really go to university to learn? Detrimental Effects of Numerus Clausus on Self-Efficacy, Mastery Goals and learning. *PLoS One*, *8*(12), e84178. doi:10.1371/journal.pone.0084178 PMID:24376794

SOS Samaritans of Singapore. (n.d.). *Suicide facts and figures*. SOS. https://www.sos.org.sg/learn-about-suicide/quick-facts

Suh, H., Liou, P., Jeong, J., & Kim, S. Y. (2022). Perfectionism, Prolonged stress reactivity, and Depression: A Two-Wave Cross-Lagged Analysis. *Journal of Rational-Emotive & Cognitive-Behavior Therapy*. doi:10.100710942-022-00483-x PMID:36406657

Svoboda, E. (2021, August 9). What is mental skills coaching? *The New York Times*. https: www.nytimes.com/2021/08/05/well/move/mental-skills-coaching-olympics.html

TED-Ed. (2018a, May 21). *How to stay calm under pressure - Noa Kageyama and Pen-Pen Chen* [Video]. YouTube. https://www.youtube.com/watch?v=CqgmozFr_GM

TEd-Ed. (2022). *Why you procrastinate even when it feels bad* [Video]. TED Talks. https://www.ted.com/talks/ted_ed_why_you_procrastinate_even_when_it_feels_bad/comments/transcript

Terhart, H., & Von Dewitz, N. (2017). Newly arrived migrant students in German schools: Exclusive and inclusive structures and practices. *European Educational Research Journal, 17*(2), 290–304. doi:10.1177/1474904117722623

The Museum of British Colonialism. (2023, April 10). *Education*. MBC. https://museumofbritishcolonialism.org/education/

Tone, S. (2020, November 5). *How one obscure word captures urban China's unhappiness*. #SixthTone. https://www.sixthtone.com/news/1006391/how-one-obscure-word-captures-urban-chinas-unhappiness

Toni Bernhard, J. D. (2011, September 11). 4 Tips for Slowing Down to Reduce Stress. *psychologytoday.com*. https://www.psychologytoday.com/us/blog/turning-straw-gold/201109/4-tips-slowing-down-reduce-stress

UCLA. (2012). Cramming for a test? Don't do it, say UCLA researchers. *UCLA Health*. https://www.uclahealth.org/news/cramming-for-a-test-dont-do-it-say-ucla-researchers

UNC-Chapel Hill Learning Center. (2022, July 12). *Study Groups – Learning Center*. Learning Center. https://learningcenter.unc.edu/tips-and-tools/study-partners/

UNICEF. (2020, March 10). *A third of youth surveyed globally by UNICEF say their education is not preparing them with the skills to get jobs*. aunicef.org. https://aunicef.org/press-releases/third-youth-surveyed-globally-unicef-say-their-education-not-preparing-them-skills

West, M. (2022, April 21). *What to know about guided imagery*. https://www.medicalnewstoday.com/articles/guided-imagery#techniques

Wiederkehr, V., Bonnot, V., Krauth-Gruber, S., & Darnon, C. (2015). Belief in school meritocracy as a system-justifying tool for low-status students. *Frontiers in Psychology*, *6*. doi:10.3389/fpsyg.2015.01053 PMID:26283991

Worland, J. (2014, December 4). How your cell phone distracts you even when you're not using it. *Time*. https://time.com/3616383/cell-phone-distraction/

World Bank Group. (2022, July 14). Financing for Education Stagnant or Declining Despite Chronic Learning Needs Post-COVID-19. *World Bank*. https://www.worldbank.org/en/news/press-release/2022/06/28/financing-for-education-stagnant-or-declining-despite-chronic-learning-needs-post-covid-19

Wright, C. N. (2013, August 29). *Examining the silence of academic disappointment: A typology of students' reasons for not discussing disappointing grades with instructors*. ScholarWorks. https://scholarworks.iu.edu/journals/index.php/josotl/article/view/3513

Yeung, J., & Karasawa, M. (2023, April 7). *Japan was already grappling with isolation and loneliness. The pandemic made it worse*. CNN. https://edition.cnn.com/2023/04/06/asia/japan-hikikomori-study-covid-intl-hnk/index.html

Yu, R. (2015). Choking under pressure: The neuropsychological mechanisms of incentive-induced performance decrements. *Frontiers in Behavioral Neuroscience*, *9*. doi:10.3389/fnbeh.2015.00019 PMID:25713517

# Chapter 12
# Gender Differences in Stress Among Students of Higher Education During the COVID-19 Pandemic: A Textual Narrative Meta-Synthesis

**Nestor Tomas**
https://orcid.org/0000-0002-4769-2724
*University of Namibia, Namibia*

**Atanasia Nangula Awala-Nashima**
*University of Namibia, Namibia*

**Theolinda Nuugwanga Tomas**
*Hangana Sea Food Clinic, Namibia*

## ABSTRACT

*The impact of the stress during COVID-19 pandemic among students of different genders is clear. However, there is lack of review on the extent of how students of various genders were affected, and the strategies used during COVID-19 pandemic within higher education setting. Using a textual narrative synthesis, this chapter searched databases for primary articles to explore the extent to which students of different genders were affected and the strategies used to cope during COVID-19 pandemic. The review used a priori tool for inclusion and exclusion criteria. Out of the total of 16,308 citations, 11 were identified from six different countries in the final review.*

DOI: 10.4018/979-8-3693-2833-0.ch012

## INTRODUCTION

Mental well-being is increasingly receiving researchers' attention, with a wide range of studies claiming that higher education students are suffering from stress and other mental health conditions (Gao et al., 2020; Johnson, & Lester, 2022). The COVID-19 pandemic has had a significant impact on the mental health of university students, who generally fall within the age range of 18 to 25 and are considered young or emerging adults. These students are experiencing increased levels of psychological distress, poor sleep quality, post-traumatic stress disorder (PTSD), depression and anxiety when compared to older individuals (Findlay & Arim, 2020; Casagrande et al., 2020). The sudden closure of universities introduced a sense of uncertainty and worry among students, as they faced challenges regarding their academic prospects, social isolation, and the absence of support systems. This situation contributed to heightened levels of stress, anxiety and depression due to the demanding nature of academic pursuits, the need to navigate through social interactions, and the personal pressures associated with higher education (Prowse et al., 2021).

## LITERATURE REVIEW

The examination of psychological distress in relation to gender has been a prominent area of research for quite some time. Previous epidemiological studies have consistently indicated that, in general, females experience a higher prevalence of mental health issues compared to males (Gao et al., 2020). This disparity can be attributed to two primary factors, the first one being the inherent physiological distinctions between females and males, such as genetic vulnerability and variations in cortisol hormonal levels, which may manifest as emotional and behavioural challenges. The second factor is the attitudes and behaviours towards life experiences, as influenced by individuals' self-perceptions of traditional masculinity and femininity (Berke et al., 2021; McCreary, 2021).

The stressors among students come from various sources, including academic pressure, feelings of isolation, the search for employment opportunities, familial obligations, aspirations in life, societal expectations, and physiological factors (Karaman, et al., 2019). Research has shown that students were susceptible to mental health issues even before the onset of the pandemic as a result of academic difficulties and diverse personal and psychosocial stressors (Auerbach et al., 2018). These stressors encompass factors such as transitioning away from the family home, establishing new social connections, effectively managing their time and juggling multiple responsibilities, adapting to unfamiliar social and geographic surroundings, and seeking appropriate financial resources (Jehi et al., 2022). Conversely, the levels of academic stress among students are also influenced by cognitive and biological factors, wherein female students tend to experience higher levels of both academic and general stress in comparison to their male counterparts (Hyde & Mezulis, 2020).

Initial findings suggest that remote learning had an adverse effect on students' overall well-being, with them reporting higher levels of stress, feelings of isolation, and a negative mood during online learning in comparison to the traditional face-to-face format (Hassan, et al., 2022). Some university students were reported as becoming dependent on substance use in an effort to cope with their social and academic stress (American College Health Association, 2019), however other students employed various strategies to effectively manage their stress levels. Some studies found that females' prolonged use of social media as a means of coping led to heightened perceptions of negative consequences regarding their academic performance and stress levels, surpassing the effects observed in males (Oberst et al., 2017; Alabri, 2022). The use of social media included engaging in activities such as listening to music, exercising, getting enough sleep, and spending time alone (Rogowska et al., 2020; Yasmin et al., 2020; Vidas et al., 2021). Furthermore, research has indicated that regular yoga practices can mitigate the adverse effects of depression in young individuals (Dalpati et al., 2022; Chang et al., 2022). Additionally, some students utilise coping mechanisms such as disengaging from stressful situations, embracing religious beliefs, distracting themselves, seeking support from others, planning ahead, and accepting their circumstances (Guszkowska, & Dąbrowska-Zimakowska, 2022; Mishra et al., 2023).

According to a recent meta-analysis conducted by Pankowski et al. (2023), there is a statistically significant relationship between religious coping and flourishing in a stressful environment. The overall correlation values were determined to be 0.35 [0.30; 0.40], indicating a moderate positive association between these two variables. This research suggests that individuals who engage in religious coping mechanisms may experience higher levels of flourishing, highlighting the potential benefits of incorporating religious practices and beliefs into one's life. However, further studies need to investigate the use of religious coping strategies among students of different genders. Moreover, individuals can experience positive outcomes by incorporating relaxation techniques into their routine, dispelling misconceptions, effectively managing their time, asserting themselves, maintaining a nutritious diet, engaging in physical exercise, diversifying their daily activities, and participating in leisure pursuits. Furthermore, various studies have found that college students who have meaningful connections with their families and friends tend to report higher levels of life satisfaction overall (Babicka-Wirkus, et al., 2021; Alsubaie et al., 2019).

The review found that both males and females face similar mental health repercussions as a result of frequent social media use. Although both male and female students reported resorting to substances as a coping mechanism, the use of cannabis among males was linked to more significant adverse effects on academic achievements, stress levels, and overall mental well-being compared to females (Prowse et al., 2021). In contrast, other studies have asserted that male students have a higher propensity for experiencing depressive disorders compared to their female counterparts. These findings align with the notion that femininity seems to serve as a protective factor against depressive symptoms among individual students (Gao et al., 2020; Vloo et al., 2021), yet several other studies (Cao et al., 2020; Mamun et al., 2019), have reported no significant gender-related impacts on individuals' mental health conditions. This chapter will explicitly highlight the extent to which higher education students of different genders were affected by COVID-19, as well as the strategies they used to cope with the resulting stress.

## RESEARCH QUESTION

- What is the gender differences in stress and their coping strategies among higher education students during COVID-19 pandemic?

## OBJECTIVES

The objectives of this review were to:

- Compare the stress levels between higher education students of different genders during the COVID-19 pandemic; and
- Describe the associated factors and coping strategies used by higher education students of different genders to cope with stress during the COVID-19 pandemic.

## Methods

### Search Strategy and Inclusion Criteria

A systematic review of the scientific literature was conducted using the Preferred Reporting Items for Systematic Review and Meta-analysis (PRISMA) guidelines. Various databases, including PUBMED, MEDLINE, Google Scholar, ScienceDirect, Scopus and Embase, were thoroughly searched to identify pertinent studies. The search encompassed the period from March 2020, which marked the initiation of the COVID-19 lockdown, to June 2022. MeSH terms (Supplementary 1 table) were utilised to compile a list of relevant articles. The key phrases employed were ((((Gender differences) AND (coping)) AND (stress)) OR (university students)) AND (COVID-19). To be eligible for inclusion in this review, the studies had to meet the following criteria: (i) publication in open access peer-reviewed journals, (ii) written in English, (iii) involving students from higher education institutions, (iv) examining factors contributing to stress, and (v) exploring coping strategies during the Covid-19 pandemic. Studies that did not involve higher education students or assess gender-specific stress factors were not included, and nor were pre-pandemic studies, commentaries, editorials, letters, and review studies. Additionally, non-English publications, book chapters, theses and dissertations were not considered for this review.

### Screening and Data Extraction

As shown in the flowchart (Figure 1), the initial screening process for articles that examine the prevalence of anxiety among students yielded a total of 16,308 articles, including citations. After eliminating duplicates, 15,700 articles were excluded, leaving 608 abstracts for further evaluation. Among these abstracts, 530 were excluded due to reasons such as incomplete texts. The remaining 88 articles, which had full texts available, underwent a thorough eligibility screening. Ultimately, 77 articles were excluded based on the predetermined inclusion and exclusion criteria. Consequently, only 6 articles met the criteria and were considered for inclusion in the final review process.

The data extracted from these selected articles encompassed various aspects, including authorship, publication year, students' majors or fields of study, date of data collection, country of origin, sample size, assessment tools employed to measure anxiety, and key findings. The findings of the screening encompassed an analysis of the impact of different factors on stress levels among students of different genders during the COVID-19 pandemic and the extent to which various coping strategies were implemented.

*Figure 1. Screening process for studies on gender differences in stress and coping strategies in higher education during the COVID-19 pandemic*

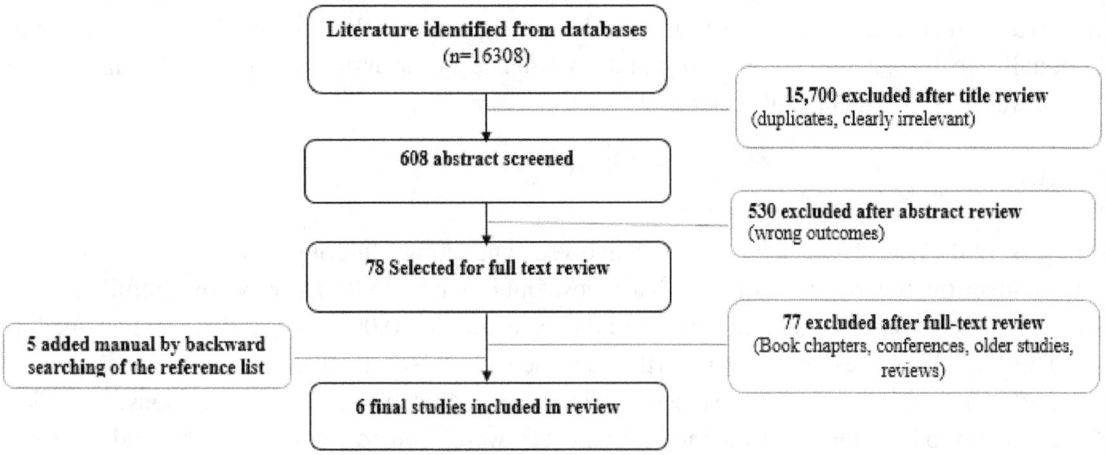


## Data Synthesis

The textual narrative synthesis approach was employed in this study, following the guidelines proposed by Barnett-Page and Thomas (2009). Narrative synthesis is widely recognised as an effective method for integrating diverse quantitative data, allowing for the synthesis of heterogeneous evidence (Campbell et al., 2019; Jameson et al., 2022). The studies' characteristics, contexts, similarities and differences were carefully documented and compared. Furthermore, structured summaries were developed to provide a comprehensive understanding of the extracted data within their appropriate contexts (Thomas & Harden, 2008). This methodology ensured transparency in addressing heterogeneity among the studies. To evaluate the reliability of the qualitative review findings, an assessment was conducted using the JBI Critical Appraisal Checklist for analytical cross-sectional studies (Joanna Briggs Institute, 2017; Paque et al., 2019). This process aimed to determine the level of confidence that could be attributed to each finding.

# QUALITY APPRAISAL

The JBI Critical Appraisal Checklist for analytical cross-sectional studies was determined to be the most suitable and comprehensive tool for evaluating the selected studies (Joanna Briggs Institute, 2017; Paque et al., 2019). The present study employed Rayyan software to conduct a qualitative meta-analysis review. Two independent reviewers (NT & TNT) carried out blind assessments to determine the eligibility of the studies. In the event of any disagreements, a third reviewer (ANA) would have acted as an arbitrator, although no instances of such disagreements were reported between the two reviewers. Data extraction was performed by one reviewer and verified by the others. All six final articles were evaluated based on the clarity of their research aims, methodology and design, data collection methods, findings, and overall research value. A scale ranging from 0 to 10 was used to assign total scores for the assessment of the studies' overall quality. Each study was then categorised as high-quality (scoring between 9 and 10), medium-quality (scoring between 6 and 8), or low-quality (scoring 5 or less). Consensus was reached among the three reviewers, who unanimously agreed that all the studies met the criteria for inclusion in the review. Inter-rater reliability was ensured by adding together the percent of observed agreement. Additionally, to further ensure reliability and confidence in the individual review findings, Rayyan software was used (Ouzzani et al., 2016).

## Results

The process of the qualitative meta-synthesis involved conducting a thorough search of databases, resulting in the identification of a total of 16,308 articles. Out of these, 15,700 titles were carefully reviewed, leading to the removal of 4,700 duplicates and the exclusion of 10,000 articles that were deemed irrelevant. This left 608 articles, which were further assessed through abstract reading and screening. Among the 608 articles subjected to abstract screening, 530 were excluded due to various reasons. Specifically, 416 were found to have incorrect outcomes, while 114 were deemed irrelevant to the study. To ensure comprehensiveness, ten additional articles were manually included by conducting backward referencing searches. Consequently, 88 articles remained for full-text reading. During this stage, 77 articles were excluded as they primarily focused on reviews rather than original research articles. As a result, the final review process involved assessing articles from six different countries that fulfilled the study's inclusion criteria. For reference and transparency, the PRISMA flow diagram and Table 1 provide an overview of the final articles that underwent review (Prowse et al., 2021; Adasi et al., 2020; Graves et al., 2021; Rogowska et al., 2020; Sheroun et al., 2020; Savitsky et al., 2020). Based on the quality appraisal, the majority of included articles were of good quality.

The purpose of this review was to examine the gender differences and coping strategies employed by higher education students in response to stress during the COVID-19 pandemic. Through a textual narrative synthesis, the researchers analysed various factors and coping strategies. Using textual narrative synthesis, this study investigated the gender differences and coping strategies employed by higher education students in response to stress during the COVID-19 pandemic. An analysis revealed that different genders exhibited significant but varying levels of stress when exposed to different factors, leading to the adoption of distinct coping strategies based on gender preferences. Notable factors affecting both females and males included social isolation, academic pressure, self-rated health, gender-related challenges, insufficient access to Personal Protective Equipment (PPE), and fear of infection (Prowse et al., 2021; Graves et al., 2021; Adasi et al., 2020; Rogowska et al., 2020; Savitsky et al., 2020). The following factors and coping strategies are outlined and organised below.

# STRESSORS AND COPING STRATEGIES AMONG STUDENTS OF DIFFERENT GENDERS

Out of the six studies reviewed, four (n=4) indicated that female students are more susceptible to stress (Prowse et al., 2021; Graves et al., 2021; Adasi et al., 2020; Rogowska et al., 2020; Savitsky et al., 2020). In a Canadian context (Prowse et al., 2021), a cross-sectional study involving 366 students from various disciplines revealed that when faced with social isolation and academic pressure, female students tend to experience higher levels of stress compared to their male counterparts. Similarly, a study conducted in the United States (US) with 448 participants, who were majoring in Exercise Science and Health Promotion, Yoga, Pilates, or Health Fitness for Life, found that female students also exhibited elevated levels of stress relative to their male peers (Graves et al., 2021).

In Canada, it was observed that females were more inclined to utilise social media as a coping mechanism, whereas males tended to resort to cannabis use. Both male and female students, however, commonly turned to substance use as a means of dealing with stress (Prowse et al., 2021). Conversely, in the US, female students were found to prefer using emotion-focused coping strategies such as self-distraction, instrumental support, emotional support and venting, while the male participants favoured different approaches (Graves et al., 2021). Interestingly, a study conducted in Ghana involving 270 students demonstrated insignificant differences between males and females in terms of stress levels when confronted with academic demands and health-related stressors. This suggests that both genders in that country experience comparable levels of stress in such circumstances. Furthermore, it was observed that both male and female students engaged in self-distracting activities and utilised prayer or meditation as coping mechanisms. Females tended to adopt adaptive coping strategies, however, whereas males exhibited a preference for maladaptive and avoidance coping strategies (Adasi et al., 2020).

In an online survey in Poland with 914 students from different field of studies, female students were 60% more prone to experiencing stress compared to their male counterparts. This increase in stress levels was attributed to the students' self-rated health during the COVID-19 pandemic. Both male and female students reported frequently resorting to coping mechanisms such as emotion-oriented, avoidance, and task-oriented approaches (Rogowska et al., 2020). In Israel, a study involving 244 nursing students (Savitsky et al., 2020) revealed that 14.9% of female nursing students experienced severe stress, while no males reported such levels of stress. These high level of stress clearly highlights the influence of fear of infection on stress levels, and the lack of personal protective equipment (PPE). Participants in the survey also emphasised the role of resilience and a strong sense of humour in reducing stress levels (Savitsky et al., 2020).

## DISCUSSION

The comprehensive meta-synthesis of textual narratives revealed that there are distinct differences in the ways male and female students respond to stress, with female students exhibiting a higher susceptibility to stress compared to their male counterparts. The primary stressors identified include social isolation, academic pressure, health-related concerns, the use of Personal Protective Equipment (PPE) and fear of contracting infections (Karaman, et al., 2019; Prowse et al., 2021; Adasi et al., 2020; Rogowska et al., 2020; Savitsky et al., 2020). However, it was observed that several other factors, such as a lack of sense of control, online learning, challenging learning tasks and a lack of knowledge about COVID-19 also significantly contributed to students' stress levels (Livana et al., 2020; Xiong et al., 2021; Abdelwahed et al., 2022). The discovery that females are more prone to experiencing stress compared to their male counterparts aligns with several studies (Kowal, et al., 2020; Gao et al., 2020; Graves et al., 2021) that have documented the same findings, however it is important to note that contrary to our findings, some studies did not find significant gender differences ($p > 0.05$) in stress levels among students (Cao et al., 2020; Mamun et al., 2019). The inconsistency observed may stem from variances in cross-cultural dynamics and physiological factors influencing hormonal levels, which subsequently impact female

*Table 1. Summary of findings regarding gender differences and coping strategies to combat stress among higher education students during the COVID-19 pandemic*

| Author (year) | Study design | Methods of data collection | Population | Country | Date of collection | Sample size | Key findings |
|---|---|---|---|---|---|---|---|
| Prowse et al., (2021) | Cross-sectional | Questionnaire | Different fields | Canada | May 2020 | 366 | Females were affected by social isolation, and academics, compared to their male counterparts. Significance level was not indicated. Females tend to use social media as a coping mechanism compared to the use of cannabis by males. Both male and female students tend to use substances to cope with stress. |
| Adasi et al., (2020) | Cross-sectional survey | Self-administered questionnaire | Undergraduate teacher education students | Ghana | 2018–2019 | 270 | Insignificant (p = ’0.05), high stress levels between females and males. Factor include academic activities and health stressors. Coping strategies include self-distracting activities and praying or meditating. Females prefer using adaptive coping strategies whilst males prefer maladaptive and avoidance coping strategies. |
| Graves et al., (2021) | Cross-sectional survey | Self-administered questionnaire | Department of Exercise Science and Health Promotion, Yoga, Pilates or Health Fitness for Life. | USA | 2020 | 448 | Females possessed higher levels of stress compared to the male students. Significant difference in stress levels existed between males and females (p = <0.05). Females prefer utilising the emotion-focused coping strategies, i.e., self-distraction, instrumental support, emotional support and venting than male participants |
| Rogowska et al., (2020) | Cross-sectional survey | Online survey | Different fields | Poland | March to April 2020 | 914 | Female are 60% more likely to be stressed than males. Significant differences exist (p = <0.05) Other factors include self-rated health and being female. Participants frequently use emotion-oriented, avoidance and task-oriented coping styles. |
| Sheroun et al., (2020) | Cross sectional Descriptive study | Online Questionnaire | BSc Nursing Students | India | May 2020 | 427 | Male students had a higher perceived stress score (22.73) than female students (21.86). Significance level not indicated. Coping included maladaptive coping such substance abuse. |
| Savitsky et al., (2020) | Cross-sectional study | Online questionnaire | Nursing students | Israel | 2019 | 244 | More females (14.9%) compared to 0% males presented with severe anxiety/stress level among female and females. Significant differences exist between gender (p = <0.05). Gender, lack of PPE, and fear of infection influenced stress level. Resilience and humour was found to lower stress. |

behaviour and emotional responses. Women generally exhibit higher emotional sensitivity and empathy, thus leading to a greater susceptibility to negative emotions and experiences such as anxiety and depression during challenging circumstances (Rogowska et al., 2020). These findings are concerning and highlight the need for gender-specific approaches to stress management and support.

Students have the responsibility of adopting mitigating measures in order to succeed in their studies. This synthesis of research reveals that different coping mechanisms are employed by individuals of different genders in response to stress. Notably, female students commonly utilise problem-focused strategies and emotional/adaptive coping strategies (Prowse et al., 2021; Adasi et al., 2020; Graves et al., 2021). Our findings indicate that female students tend to employ self-distraction and venting, as well as seeking instrumental and emotional support, more frequently than their male counterparts (Graves et al., 2021). Literature suggests that problem-focused and emotional strategies are two broad coping strategies, with the former seeking action-oriented solutions to problems and the latter involving motivation for behaviour change and the development of specific strategies to manage stressful situations (Gustems-Carnicer et al., 2019; Huang et al., 2020). Kwaah and Essilfie (2017) found that self-distracting activities such as listening to music, working out, cooking, watching television, and praying or meditating are useful strategies for coping with stress. Therefore, emotion-focused strategies are considered adaptive and include behaviours like active planning and positive reframing, which have shown positive outcomes (Gloria & Steinhardt, 2016). Dealing with stress during the COVID-19 pandemic required students to be mindful in order to cope effectively with various factors. In essence, female students were found to exhibit mindfulness, which involved awareness, prevention of negative emotions, and distraction. Mindfulness is widely recognised as an effective treatment for psychological and somatic symptoms (Xiong et al., 2021).

Conversely, the review revealed that male students also tend to adopt maladaptive and avoidance coping strategies like denial and venting, which can lead to unfavourable consequences (LeSueur, 2019; Prowse et al., 2021; Adasi et al., 2020). Maladaptive coping strategies encompass behaviours such as substance abuse and mental disengagement (Kamaludin et al., 2020; Eisenbarth, 2019), while avoidance coping strategies include cognitive avoidance and emotional discharge such as fear and feeling of hurt (Gustems-Carnicer et al., 2019). Research has shown that relying on avoidance strategies centred around emotions can lead to an increased dependence on substances such as tobacco and cannabis (Gustems-Carnicer et al., 2019; Tavolacci et al., 2021). The use of maladaptive coping strategies dated back to before COVID-19, as men have long tended to utilise strategies centred around escape and avoidance. These strategies are often characterised by an excessive use of substances like drugs or alcohol in order to numb emotional distress. Additionally, men may focus excessively on their work as a way to divert their attention from mental health challenges. They may also make efforts to hide or downplay symptoms by withdrawing socially, disengaging from relationships and being suicidal (Wilson et al., 2022). Since the outbreak of COVID-19, the widespread psychological distress caused by the pandemic has been well-documented, encompassing feelings of sadness, depression, anxiety, fear, anger, annoyance, frustration, guilt, hopelessness, boredom, panic, and even suicidal ideation (Martínez-Líbano & Yeomans Cabrera, 2021; Tasnim et al., 2020). The varying frequencies of suicidal tendencies and suicide attempts can be attributed to heightened exposure to distressing circumstances, significantly amplifying the probability of suicidal thoughts. Research indicates that rates of contemplating suicide and making attempts at self-harm are notably higher among male students (Zhou et al., 2021; Chen et al., 2021; van Hooijdonk et al., 2022) and individuals of mixed race and Asian descent compared to their White counterparts (Seehuus et al., 2021). Women often develop brief, task-oriented friendships, whereas men typically form enduring friendships centred around common interests and activities. These friendships are often characterised by engaging in activities together or having a "shoulder-to-shoulder" approach (Teichman, 2020). This pattern is believed to be influenced by masculine ideals of self-reliance and emotional resilience, where engaging in open and vulnerable communication may be seen as uncomfortable or shameful due to feelings of dependency and vulnerability (Oliffe et al., 2022). Moreover, the inadequate methods of managing stress in males may be linked to their outlook and actions in response to life events, which are shaped by their personal perceptions of conventional masculinity and femininity (Berke et al., 2021; McCreary, 2021).

The review demonstrated a clear disparity in stress levels between female and male students, with females experiencing higher levels of stress. Identifying the specific factors that contribute to stress in each gender proved challenging, nevertheless it was apparent that female students tend to employ problem-focused and emotional strategies to cope, whereas male students lean towards maladaptive and avoidance strategies. Higher education institutions may find it beneficial to take these strategies into account when designing teaching plans.

## STRENGTH AND LIMITATIONS

This review presents a narrative analysis of students' stress levels and the coping strategies they employ when faced with various factors. It aimed to provide insight into these aspects using quantitative data, as meta-analysis was not deemed suitable for this purpose. This review used rigorous criteria during the final selection of eligible articles in order to maintain the standards of systematic reviews. One of the reviewers followed a predetermined protocol to conduct data extraction, data analysis, and quality assessment of the methods utilised in the systematic reviews and meta-analyses included in the study, while the remaining reviewers verified the accuracy and correctness of these procedures. These findings could be advantageous for higher education institutions when devising educational curricula during and after a crisis.

This narrative synthesis is subject to certain limitations, as it did not encompass 'gray' literature and the scope of the search was restricted to journal articles exclusively published in English. Additionally, given the inherit poorly reporting transparency in textual narrative synthesis. While the review offers valuable information regarding stress levels, related factors, and methods of dealing with stress, the use of quantitative findings makes it challenging to present a comprehensive textual narrative meta-analysis. Consequently, it becomes less effective in identifying commonalities between male and female students.

In light of the fact that the reviewed studies were conducted amidst the pandemic, it is imperative for governments and higher education institutions to focus their attention on developing effective strategies to address the mental and emotional stress experienced by students of varying genders in the aftermath of COVID-19.

## CONCLUSION

The review clearly indicates a significant disparity between female and male students, with female students exhibiting a higher level of stress when confronted with social isolation, health concerns, academic pressure, personal protective equipment (PPE), and the fear of contracting infections. Surprisingly, male students resorted to maladaptive strategies such as substance abuse, while female students employed problem-focused and emotion-focused techniques. These findings suggest that COVID-19 has had a detrimental impact on the lives of students who already faced high academic demands, resulting in increased stress levels among them. It is noteworthy that while female students had a higher susceptibility to stress in comparison to their male peers, they utilised the most efficient strategies for dealing with stress. It is therefore important that both the government and higher education institutions prioritise implementing comprehensive student support services throughout their university life by employing gender-informed interventions as a means to effectively mitigate the repercussions of the COVID-19 pandemic.

## REFERENCES

Abdelwahed, N. A. A., Aldoghan, M. A., Moustafa, M. A., & Soomro, B. A. (2022). Factors affecting online learning, stress and anxiety during the COVID-19 pandemic in Saudi Arabia. *International Journal of Human Rights in Healthcare*. doi:10.1108/IJHRH-03-2022-0012

Adasi, G. S., Amponsah, K. D., Mohammed, S. M., Yeboah, R., & Mintah, P. C. (2020). Gender differences in stressors and coping strategies among teacher education students at University of Ghana. *Journal of Education and Learning*, *9*(2), 123–133. doi:10.5539/jel.v9n2p123

Alabri, A. (2022). Fear of missing out (FOMO): The effects of the need to belong, perceived centrality, and fear of social exclusion. *Human Behavior and Emerging Technologies*, *2022*, 1–12. doi:10.1155/2022/4824256

Alsubaie, M. M., Stain, H. J., Webster, L. A. D., & Wadman, R. (2019). The role of sources of social support on depression and quality of life for university students. *International Journal of Adolescence and Youth*, *24*(4), 484–496. doi:10.1080/02673843.2019.1568887

American College Health Association. (2019). *American College Health Association-national College Health Assessment II: Canadian consortium executive summary*. ACHA.

Auerbach, R. P., Mortier, P., Bruffaerts, R., Alonso, J., Benjet, C., Cuijpers, P., Demyttenaere, K., Ebert, D. D., Green, J. G., Hasking, P., Murray, E., Nock, M. K., Pinder-Amaker, S., Sampson, N. A., Stein, D. J., Vilagut, G., Zaslavsky, A. M., & Kessler, R. C. (2018). WHO world mental health surveys international college student project: Prevalence and distribution of mental disorders. *Journal of Abnormal Psychology*, *127*(7), 623–638. doi:10.1037/abn0000362 PMID:30211576

Babicka-Wirkus, A., Wirkus, L., Stasiak, K., & Kozłowski, P. (2021). University students' strategies of coping with stress during the coronavirus pandemic: Data from Poland. *PLoS One*, *16*(7), e0255041. doi:10.1371/journal.pone.0255041 PMID:34310649

Barnett-Page, E., & Thomas, J. (2009). Methods for the synthesis of qualitative research: A critical review. *BMC Medical Research Methodology*, *9*(1), 1–11. doi:10.1186/1471-2288-9-59 PMID:19671152

Berke, D. S., Leone, R. M., Hyatt, C. S., Zeichner, A., & Parrott, D. J. (2021). Correlates of men's bystander intervention to prevent sexual and relationship violence: The role of masculine discrepancy stress. *Journal of Interpersonal Violence*, *36*(21-22), 9877–9903. doi:10.1177/0886260519880999 PMID:31608781

Campbell, M., Katikireddi, S. V., Sowden, A., & Thomson, H. (2019). Lack of transparency in reporting narrative synthesis of quantitative data: A methodological assessment of systematic reviews. *Journal of Clinical Epidemiology*, *105*, 1–9. doi:10.1016/j.jclinepi.2018.08.019 PMID:30196129

Cao, W., Fang, Z., Hou, G., Han, M., Xu, X., Dong, J., & Zheng, J. (2020). The psychological impact of the COVID-19 epidemic on college students in China. *Psychiatry Research*, *287*, 112934. doi:10.1016/j.psychres.2020.112934 PMID:32229390

Casagrande, M., Favieri, F., Tambelli, R., & Forte, G. (2020). The enemy who sealed the world: Effects quarantine due to the COVID-19 on sleep quality, anxiety, and psychological distress in the Italian population. *Sleep Medicine*, *75*, 12–20. doi:10.1016/j.sleep.2020.05.011 PMID:32853913

Chang, T. F., Ley, B. L., Ramburn, T. T., Srinivasan, S., Hariri, S., Purandare, P., & Subramaniam, B. (2022). Online isha upa yoga for student mental health and well-being during COVID-19: A randomized control trial. *Applied Psychology. Health and Well-Being*, *14*(4), 1408–1428. doi:10.1111/aphw.12341 PMID:35064741

Chen, Y., Zhu, L. J., Fang, Z. M., Wu, N., Du, M. X., Jiang, M. M., Wang, J., Yao, Y., & Zhou, C. C. (2021). The association of suicidal ideation with family characteristics and social support of the first batch of students returning to a college during the COVID-19 epidemic period: A cross sectional study in China. *Frontiers in Psychiatry*, *12*, 653245. doi:10.3389/fpsyt.2021.653245 PMID:34262488

Dalpati, N., Jena, S., Jain, S., & Sarangi, P. P. (2022). Yoga and meditation, an essential tool to alleviate stress and enhance immunity to emerging infections: A perspective on the effect of COVID-19 pandemic on students. *Brain, Behavior, & Immunity - Health*, *20*, 100420. doi:10.1016/j.bbih.2022.100420 PMID:35072120

Eisenbarth, C. A. (2019). Coping with stress: Gender differences among college students. *College Student Journal*, *53*(2), 151–162.

Findlay, L., & Arim, R. (2020). *Canadians Report Lower Self-Perceived Mental Health During The COVID-19 Pandemic.* Statistics Canada. https://www150.statcan.gc.ca/n1/pub/45-28-0001/2020001/article/00003-eng.htm

Gao, W., Ping, S., & Liu, X. (2020). Gender differences in depression, anxiety, and stress among college students: A longitudinal study from China. *Journal of Affective Disorders*, *263*, 292–300. doi:10.1016/j.jad.2019.11.121 PMID:31818792

Gloria, C. T., & Steinhardt, M. A. (2016). Relationships among positive emotions, coping, resilience and mental health. *Stress and Health*, *32*(2), 145–156. doi:10.1002mi.2589 PMID:24962138

Graves, B. S., Hall, M. E., Dias-Karch, C., Haischer, M. H., & Apter, C. (2021). Gender differences in perceived stress and coping among college students. *PLoS One*, *16*(8), e0255634. doi:10.1371/journal.pone.0255634 PMID:34383790

Gustems-Carnicer, J., Calderón, C., & Calderón-Garrido, D. (2019). Stress, coping strategies and academic achievement in teacher education students. *European Journal of Teacher Education*, *42*(3), 375–390. doi:10.1080/02619768.2019.1576629

Guszkowska, M., & Dąbrowska-Zimakowska, A. (2022). Coping with stress during the second wave of the COVID-19 pandemic by Polish university students: Strategies, structure, and relation to psychological well-being. *Psychology Research and Behavior Management, 15*, 339–352. doi:10.2147/PRBM.S345648 PMID:35210882

Hassan, S. U. N., Algahtani, F. D., Atteya, M. R., Almishaal, A. A., Ahmed, A. A., Obeidat, S. T., Kamel, R. M., & Mohamed, R. F. (2022). The impact of extended E-Learning on the emotional well-being of students during the COVID-19 pandemic in Saudi Arabia. *Children (Basel, Switzerland), 9*(1), 13. doi:10.3390/children9010013 PMID:35053638

Huang, L., Xu, F., & Liu, H. (2020). Emotional responses and coping strategies of nurses and nursing college students during the COVID-19 outbreak. MedRxiv, 2020-03. doi:10.1101/2020.03.05.20031898

Hyde, J. S., & Mezulis, A. H. (2020). Gender differences in depression: Biological, affective, cognitive, and sociocultural factors. *Harvard Review of Psychiatry, 28*(1), 4–13. doi:10.1097/HRP.0000000000000230 PMID:31913978

Jameson, J., Rumyantseva, N., Cai, M., Markowski, M., Essex, R., & McNay, I. (2022). A systematic review, textual narrative synthesis and framework for digital leadership research maturity in Higher Education. *Computers and Education Open, 100115*. Advance online publication. doi:10.1080/03075079.2022.2145278

Jehi, T., Khan, R., Dos Santos, H., & Majzoub, N. (2022). Effect of COVID-19 outbreak on anxiety among students of higher education; A review of literature. *Current Psychology (New Brunswick, N.J.)*, 1–15. doi:10.100712144-021-02587-6 PMID:35018081

Joanna Briggs Institute. (2017). JBI critical appraisal checklist for analytical cross sectional studies. 2017. *Diakses Pada, 22*, 2019–05.

Johnson, A. P., & Lester, R. J. (2022). Mental health in academia: Hacks for cultivating and sustaining wellbeing. *American Journal of Human Biology, 34*(S1), e23664. doi:10.1002/ajhb.23664 PMID:34357661

Kamaludin, K., Chinna, K., Sundarasen, S., Khoshaim, H. B., Nurunnabi, M., Baloch, G. M., Sukayt, A., & Hossain, S. F. A. (2020). Coping with COVID-19 and movement control order (MCO): Experiences of university students in Malaysia. *Heliyon, 6*(11), e05339. doi:10.1016/j.heliyon.2020.e05339 PMID:33134570

Karaman, M. A., Lerma, E., Vela, J. C., & Watson, J. C. (2019). Predictors of academic stress among college students. *Journal of College Counseling, 22*(1), 41–55. doi:10.1002/jocc.12113

Kowal, M., Coll-Martín, T., Ikizer, G., Rasmussen, J., Eichel, K., Studzińska, A., Koszałkowska, K., Karwowski, M., Najmussaqib, A., Pankowski, D., Lieberoth, A., & Ahmed, O. (2020). Who is the most stressed during the COVID-19 pandemic? Data from 26 countries and areas. *Applied Psychology. Health and Well-Being, 12*(4), 946–966. doi:10.1111/aphw.12234 PMID:32996217

Kwaah, C. Y., & Essilfie, G. (2017). Stress and coping strategies among distance education students at the University of Cape Coast, Ghana. *Turkish Online Journal of Distance Education, 18*(3), 120-134. doi:10.17718/tojde.328942

LeSueur, I. (2019). An investigation of existential and positive psychological resources in college students. City: Seton Hall University.

Livana, P. H., Mubin, M. F., & Basthomi, Y. (2020). "Learning Task" Attributable to Students' Stress During the Pandemic Covid-19. *Jurnal Ilmu Keperawatan Jiwa*, *3*(2), 203–208. doi:10.32584/jikj.v3i2.590

Mamun, M. A., Hossain, M. S., & Griffiths, M. D. (2019). Mental health problems and associated predictors among Bangladeshi students. *International Journal of Mental Health and Addiction*, 1–15. doi:10.100711469-019-00144-8

Martínez-Líbano, J., & Yeomans Cabrera, M. M. (2021). Suicidal ideation and suicidal thoughts in university students during the COVID-19 pandemic. *Systematic Reviews*, *XXX*(2), 390–405. doi:10.24205/03276716.2020.4038

McCreary, D. R. (2021). Psychology of Men and Masculinities: Implications for Men's Experiences of Posttraumatic Stress Disorder. In authors Handbook of Posttraumatic Stress (pp. 177-197). Routledge.

Mishra, J., Samanta, P., Panigrahi, A., Dash, K., Behera, M. R., & Das, R. (2023). Mental health status, coping strategies during Covid-19 pandemic among undergraduate students of healthcare profession. *International Journal of Mental Health and Addiction*, *21*(1), 562–574. doi:10.100711469-021-00611-1 PMID:34393684

Oberst, U., Wegmann, E., Stodt, B., Brand, M., & Chamarro, A. (2017). Negative consequences from heavy social networking in adolescents: The mediating role of fear of missing out. *Journal of Adolescence*, *55*(1), 51–60. doi:10.1016/j.adolescence.2016.12.008 PMID:28033503

Oliffe, J. L., Kelly, M. T., Montaner, G. G., Seidler, Z. E., Ogrodniczuk, J. S., & Rice, S. M. (2022). Masculinity and mental illness in and after men's intimate partner relationships. *SSM. Qualitative Research in Health*, *2*, 100039. doi:10.1016/j.ssmqr.2022.100039

Ouzzani, M., Hammady, H., Fedorowicz, Z., & Elmagarmid, A. (2016). Rayyan—A web and mobile app for systematic reviews. *Systematic Reviews*, *5*(1), 1–10. doi:10.118613643-016-0384-4 PMID:27919275

Pankowski, D., & Wytrychiewicz-Pankowska, K. (2023). Turning to religion during COVID-19 (Part I): A systematic review, meta-analysis and meta-regression of studies on the relationship between religious coping and mental health throughout COVID-19. *Journal of Religion and Health*, *62*(1), 510–543. doi:10.100710943-022-01703-5 PMID:36592322

Paque, K., Vander Stichele, R., Elseviers, M., Pardon, K., Dilles, T., Deliens, L., & Christiaens, T. (2019). Barriers and enablers to deprescribing in people with a life-limiting disease: A systematic review. *Palliative Medicine*, *33*(1), 37–48. doi:10.1177/0269216318801124 PMID:30229704

Prowse, R., Sherratt, F., Abizaid, A., Gabrys, R. L., Hellemans, K. G., Patterson, Z. R., & McQuaid, R. J. (2021). Coping with the COVID-19 pandemic: Examining gender differences in stress and mental health among university students. *Frontiers in Psychiatry*, *12*, 650759. doi:10.3389/fpsyt.2021.650759 PMID:33897499

Rogowska, A. M., Kuśnierz, C., & Bokszczanin, A. (2020). Examining anxiety, life satisfaction, general health, stress and coping styles during COVID-19 pandemic in Polish sample of university students. *Psychology Research and Behavior Management*, *13*, 797–811. doi:10.2147/PRBM.S266511 PMID:33061695

Rutkowska, A., Liska, D., Cieślik, B., Wrzeciono, A., Broďáni, J., Barcalová, M., Gurín, D., & Rutkowski, S. (2021). Stress levels and mental well-being among Slovak students during e-learning in the COVID-19 pandemic. *Health Care*, *9*(10), 1356. doi:10.3390/healthcare9101356 PMID:34683036

Savitsky, B., Findling, Y., Ereli, A., & Hendel, T. (2020). Anxiety and coping strategies among nursing students during the covid-19 pandemic. *Nurse Education in Practice*, *46*, 102809. doi:10.1016/j.nepr.2020.102809 PMID:32679465

Seehuus, M., Moeller, R. W., & Peisch, V. (2021). Gender effects on mental health symptoms and treatment in college students. *Journal of American College Health*, *69*(1), 95–102. doi:10.1080/07448481.2019.1656217 PMID:31513464

Sheroun, D., Wankhar, D. D., Devrani, A., Lissamma, P. V., & Chatterjee, K. (2020). A study to assess the perceived stress and coping strategies among B. Sc. nursing students of selected colleges in Pune during COVID-19 pandemic lockdown. *International Journal of Science and Healthcare Research*, *5*(2), 280–288.

Tasnim, R., Islam, M. S., Sujan, M. S. H., Sikder, M. T., & Potenza, M. N. (2020). Suicidal ideation among Bangladeshi university students early during the COVID-19 pandemic: Prevalence estimates and correlates. *Children and Youth Services Review*, *119*, 105703. doi:10.1016/j.childyouth.2020.105703 PMID:33204046

Tavolacci, M. P., Wouters, E., Van de Velde, S., Buffel, V., Déchelotte, P., Van Hal, G., & Ladner, J. (2021). The impact of COVID-19 lockdown on health behaviors among students of a French university. *International Journal of Environmental Research and Public Health*, *18*(8), 4346. doi:10.3390/ijerph18084346 PMID:33923943

Thomas, J., & Harden, A. (2008). Methods for the thematic synthesis of qualitative research in systematic reviews. *BMC Medical Research Methodology*, *8*(1), 1–10. doi:10.1186/1471-2288-8-45 PMID:18616818

van Hooijdonk, K. J., Rubio, M., Simons, S. S., van Noorden, T. H., Luijten, M., Geurts, S. A., & Vink, J. M. (2022). Student-, Study-and COVID-19-Related Predictors of Students' Smoking, Binge Drinking and Cannabis Use before and during the Initial COVID-19 Lockdown in The Netherlands. *International Journal of Environmental Research and Public Health*, *19*(2), 812. doi:10.3390/ijerph19020812 PMID:35055634

Vidas, D., Larwood, J. L., Nelson, N. L., & Dingle, G. A. (2021). Music listening as a strategy for managing COVID-19 stress in first-year university students. *Frontiers in Psychology*, *12*, 647065. doi:10.3389/fpsyg.2021.647065 PMID:33868120

Vloo, A., Alessie, R. J. M., Mierau, J. O., Boezen, M. H., Mierau, J. O., Franke, L., Dekens, J., Deelen, P., Lanting, P., Vonk, J. M., Nolte, I., Ori, A. P. S., Claringbould, A., Boulogne, F., Dijkema, M. X. L., Wiersma, H. H., Warmerdam, R., & Jankipersadsing, S. A. (2021). Gender differences in the mental health impact of the COVID-19 lockdown: Longitudinal evidence from the Netherlands. *SSM - Population Health*, *15*, 100878. doi:10.1016/j.ssmph.2021.100878 PMID:34471666

Wilson, M. J., Seidler, Z. E., Oliffe, J. L., Toogood, N., Kealy, D., Ogrodniczuk, J. S., Walther, A., & Rice, S. M. (2022). "Appreciate the little things": A qualitative survey of men's coping strategies and mental health impacts during the COVID-19 pandemic. *American Journal of Men's Health*, *16*(3), 15579883221099794. doi:10.1177/15579883221099794 PMID:35608377

Winkle-Wagner, R., McCallum, C. M., Luedke, C., & Ota-Malloy, B. (2019). Instrumental or meaningful friendships: Black alumnae perspectives on peer relationships during college. *Journal of Women and Gender in Higher Education, 12*(3), 283–298. doi:10.1080/19407882.2019.1593201

Xiong, P., Ming, W. K., Zhang, C., Bai, J., Luo, C., Cao, W., Zhang, F., & Tao, Q. (2021). Factors influencing mental health among Chinese medical and non-medical students in the early stage of the COVID-19 pandemic. *Frontiers in Public Health, 9*, 603331. doi:10.3389/fpubh.2021.603331 PMID:34095044

Yasmin, H., Khalil, S., & Mazhar, R. (2020). COVID 19: Stress management among students and its impact on their effective learning. *International Technology and Education Journal, 4*(2), 65–74.

Zhou, S. J., Wang, L. L., Qi, M., Yang, X. J., Gao, L., Zhang, S. Y., Zhang, L.-G., Yang, R., & Chen, J. X. (2021). Depression, anxiety, and suicidal ideation in Chinese university students during the COVID-19 pandemic. *Frontiers in Psychology, 12*, 669833. doi:10.3389/fpsyg.2021.669833 PMID:34421725

# APPENDIX

## Search Terms Used in Gender Differences in Stress Among Students of Higher Education During COVID-19 Pandemic: A Textual Narrative Meta-Synthesis

**Search:** ((((Gender differences) AND (coping)) AND (stress)) OR (university students)) AND (COVID-19)
**Data base:** Pubmed, MEDLINE, Google Scholar, ScienceDirect, Scopus, and Embase

*Table 2. Search terms*

| **Search terms** |
|---|
| (((“sex characteristics”[MeSH Terms] OR (“sex”[All Fields] AND “characteristics”[All Fields]) OR “sex characteristics”[All Fields] OR (“gender”[All Fields] AND “differences”[All Fields]) OR “gender differences”[All Fields]) AND (“adaptation, psychological”[MeSH Terms] OR (“adaptation”[All Fields] AND “psychological”[All Fields]) OR “psychological adaptation”[All Fields] OR “coping”[All Fields] OR “coped”[All Fields] OR “copes”[All Fields] OR “copings”[All Fields]) AND (“stress”[All Fields] OR “stressed”[All Fields] OR “stresses”[All Fields] OR “stressful”[All Fields] OR “stressfulness”[All Fields] OR “stressing”[All Fields])) OR ((“universiti”[All Fields] OR “universities”[MeSH Terms] OR “universities”[All Fields] OR “university”[All Fields] OR “university s”[All Fields]) AND (“student s”[All Fields] OR “students”[MeSH Terms] OR “students”[All Fields] OR “student”[All Fields] OR “students s”[All Fields]))) AND (“covid 19”[All Fields] OR “covid 19”[MeSH Terms] OR “covid 19 vaccines”[All Fields] OR “covid 19 vaccines”[MeSH Terms] OR “covid 19 serotherapy”[All Fields] OR “covid 19 nucleic acid testing”[All Fields] OR “covid 19 nucleic acid testing”[MeSH Terms] OR “covid 19 serological testing”[All Fields] OR “covid 19 serological testing”[MeSH Terms] OR “covid 19 testing”[All Fields] OR “covid 19 testing”[MeSH Terms] OR “sars cov 2”[All Fields] OR “sars cov 2”[MeSH Terms] OR “severe acute respiratory syndrome coronavirus 2”[All Fields] OR “ncov”[All Fields] OR “2019 ncov”[All Fields] OR ((“coronavirus”[MeSH Terms] OR “coronavirus”[All Fields] OR “cov”[All Fields]) AND 2019/11/01:3000/12/31[Date - Publication])) |
| **Translations** |
| **Gender differences:** “sex characteristics”[MeSH Terms] OR (“sex”[All Fields] AND “characteristics”[All Fields]) OR “sex characteristics”[All Fields] OR (“gender”[All Fields] AND “differences”[All Fields]) OR “gender differences”[All Fields] |
| **coping:** “adaptation, psychological”[MeSH Terms] OR (“adaptation”[All Fields] AND “psychological”[All Fields]) OR “psychological adaptation”[All Fields] OR “coping”[All Fields] OR “coped”[All Fields] OR “copes”[All Fields] OR “copings”[All Fields] |
| **stress:** “stress”[All Fields] OR “stressed”[All Fields] OR “stresses”[All Fields] OR “stressful”[All Fields] OR “stressfulness”[All Fields] OR “stressing”[All Fields] |
| **university:** “universiti”[All Fields] OR “universities”[MeSH Terms] OR “universities”[All Fields] OR “university”[All Fields] OR “university’s”[All Fields] |
| **students:** “student’s”[All Fields] OR “students”[MeSH Terms] OR “students”[All Fields] OR “student”[All Fields] OR “students’s”[All Fields] |
| **COVID-19:** (“COVID-19” OR “COVID-19”[MeSH Terms] OR “COVID-19 Vaccines” OR “COVID-19 Vaccines”[MeSH Terms] OR “COVID-19 serotherapy” OR “COVID-19 serotherapy”[Supplementary Concept] OR “COVID-19 Nucleic Acid Testing” OR “covid-19 nucleic acid testing”[MeSH Terms] OR “COVID-19 Serological Testing” OR “covid-19 serological testing”[MeSH Terms] OR “COVID-19 Testing” OR “covid-19 testing”[MeSH Terms] OR “SARS-CoV-2” OR “sars-cov-2”[MeSH Terms] OR “Severe Acute Respiratory Syndrome Coronavirus 2” OR “NCOV” OR “2019 NCOV” OR ((“coronavirus”[MeSH Terms] OR “coronavirus” OR “COV”) AND 2019/11/01[PDAT]: 3000/12/31[PDAT])) |

# Chapter 13
# Psychological Well-Being of Students in Higher Education Institutions:
## A Theoretical Review

**Anna Niitembu Hako**
https://orcid.org/0000-0001-6367-1969
*University of Namibia, Namibia*

**Emilia Ndapandula Mbongo**
https://orcid.org/0000-0001-6560-8664
*University of Namibia, Namibia*

## ABSTRACT

*Psychological well-being is a multifaceted and multidimensional concept. It includes essential elements such as happy emotions, autonomy, satisfying relationships, little negative emotion, a sense of meaning in life, and personal development. Psychological well-being is essential for overall health and happiness and has been associated with greater physical and mental health as well as a longer life span. This study attempts to gain theoretical knowledge about psychological well-being and knowledge of the various studies conducted in the area of psychological well-being. To alleviate stress and enhance students' psychological well-being, higher institutions of learning must prioritize proactive, resilience-focused, and mental health promotion efforts to assist students.*

## INTRODUCTION

Health is considered the greatest wealth and people are expected to maintain the highest possible level of health. Psychological well-being is an integral part of life. As stated by Tang et al. (2019), psychological well-being is a key component of mental health that can be described as resilience, coping, emotion control, problem-solving, enjoyment, pleasure, fulfilment, and happiness. It is beneficial for the higher

DOI: 10.4018/979-8-3693-2833-0.ch013

institution management to comprehend the underlying mechanisms linked to this construct to create specialised university training programs that would increase psychological well-being among students. According to research, self-compassion is closely linked to psychological health, including higher levels of enjoyment, optimism, initiative, and connection as well as lower levels of anxiety, depressive disorders, neurotic perfectionism, and ruminating (Neff & Dahm, 2015). Self-compassion is thought to offer similar psychological advantages to self-esteem but fewer drawbacks like egotism or narcissism. This chapter looked at the aspects of students' well-being, particularly, the psychological well-being of students in higher institutions of learning. Institutions of higher learning should find appropriate strategies to maximise the psychological well-being of their students, achieve healthy self-actualization, and develop strong future generations capable of meeting life's adversities. The next section discusses th background of the study.

## BACKGROUND

The prevalence of psychological problems among university students is extremely high, with depression (76%), anxiety (88.4%), stress (84.4%), and other mental disorders (45.5%) leading (Asif et al., 2020; Lipson et al., 2019; & Auerbach et al., 2018). Teh et al. (2015) claim that such problems affect students' psychological well-being (PWB). In the literature, psychological well-being has been defined in two different ways: (a) subjective well-being that includes happiness, positive affect, and life satisfaction (Thanoi et al., 2023; Sharma & Shara, 2018; He et al., 2018) and (b) eudaemonic well-being, including autonomy, self-acceptance, purpose in life, personal growth, positive relations with others, and environmental mastery (Ryff, 2018).

Ryff had introduced six core dimensions of PWB, specifically:

1. Self-acceptance (state of having positive thoughts and feelings about oneself);
2. Positive relations with others (ability to engage in a warm and trusting relationship with others);
3. Autonomy (ability to be independent and cope with social pressure);
4. Environmental mastery (ability to adapt, change, or create one's environment according to one's needs through physical and mental activities);
5. Purpose in life (state of having objectives and goals in life and working toward achieving goal-oriented);
6. Personal growth (continuously growing and developing as oneself) (Sharma et al., 2022, p.47).

As public knowledge and understanding have increased over the past few decades, it is now known that psychological well-being and the absence of mental illness are both components of mental health. A complex concept, psychological well-being refers to the best possible psychological experience and functioning (Christner et al., 2021). In addition to resilience coping, emotion regulation and healthy problem solving, Community Translational Science Team (CTST) (2016), NIH Report (2018) and Tang (2021) added that it may be defined as enjoyment, pleasure, fulfilment and happiness.

In light of the above, other scholars have also conceptualised PWB, for instance, White (2004) and Diener et al. (2010) define psychological well-being as a subjective evaluation of one's life or a healthy emotion based on high self-esteem and positive relationships with others, less anxiety, less depression and less delinquent. This definition encompasses a broad range of positive experiences, including happiness, satisfaction, and a sense of fulfilment. Similar to this, Seligman (2002, cited in Dhanabhakyam

& Sarath, 2023) put out the idea of "positive psychology," which sees psychological well-being as a confluence of fulfilment and enjoyment. The definition acknowledges that happiness is characterised by positive emotions, pleasure, and a sense of meaning and purpose in life rather than just the absence of unpleasant feelings or events. In addition, Roslan et al. (2017) conceptualise psychological well-being as a state that emerges from a feeling of satisfaction with one's close interpersonal relationships and with one's occupation and financial situation whereas Sharma and Shara (2018) view it as the ability to develop, maintain, and appropriately modify interdependent relationships with others to succeed in achieving goals. In the same vein, Sharma et al. (2022) described psychological well-being as a multidimensional psychological state with positive functioning, contentment, and absence of mental illnesses while Morales-Rodríguez et al. (2020) view psychological well-being as the result of a life well-lived and is an important factor in students successfully adapting to university life. Indeed, this construct usually includes dimensions such as self-acceptance, positive relationships, autonomy, environmental mastery, personal growth and purpose in life.

Furthermore, Yurayat and Seechaliao (2021) believe that psychological well-being is a continuous psychological state, in which an individual has the vitality of life, positive inner experience, good social adaptation, and can effectively exert one's physical and mental potential and positive social ability. The above definitions are in line with the definition by the World Health Organization (WHO, 2021) in which psychological well-being refers to healthy and mentally healthy individuals who are capable of maintaining harmonious relationships with others, engaging in community activities and being able to provide contributions to society. This definition highlights the multidimensional nature of psychological well-being, with the presence of affirmative emotions, psychological functioning, and a sense of purpose and significance in life. In this study, PWB is defined as a mixture of contentment, life fulfilment and despair.

On a similar note, several studies have linked psychological well-being with positive psychology (Thanoi et al., 2023; He et al., 2018; Klainin-Yobas et al., 2016; Malkoc et al., 2015). Positive psychology suggests that an individual should respect the environment, accept oneself both now and in the past, have life objectives, work to achieve them, and be able to make their own decisions. For this reason, it is more crucial for students, especially, those in higher education institutions to focus on developing positive attributes than it is to try to stop or diminish negative ones, like depression, when they have already occurred. According to positive psychology, happiness encourages achievement in several areas of human functioning and this can be beneficial to students who aim to pursue career goals at higher institutions. Equally, mindfulness, resilience, self-efficacy, and social support are perceived to have a positive influence on the psychological well-being of students and at the same time can contribute to both personal development and academic achievement (Thanoi et al., 2023; Priesack et al., 2015). Emotional intelligence, self-efficacy, and psychological well-being such as happiness, and life satisfaction are important resources for enhancing students' learning, success and quality in education (Sampath et al., 2019; Vongsirimas et al., 2017). Puma and Malavinya (2015) state that happiness is an emotional state whereas life satisfaction addresses a more global cognitive evaluation of one's life. Moreover, Haleh-Heizomi et al. (2018) reported that psychological well-being (PWB) correlated positively with life satisfaction, happiness, hope and self-efficacy, and it was negatively correlated with self-perceived stress. They believe that higher levels of happiness and self-efficacy are associated with lower levels of stress. Shah et al. (2020) findings show that three main themes encompass six dimensions that are environmental control, personal growth, purpose of life, self-acceptance, autonomy, and positive relationships with others. Further to this, the same study found psychological well-being as a vital aspect of life that every university student wants to achieve. Looking at the results of current studies, scholars still emphasize the same dimensions of well-being as those described by Ryff (1989) three decades ago such as mastery of the environment, personal growth, purpose of life, self-acceptance, autonomy, and positive relationships with others. In other words, Ryff (1989) identified six characteristics of psychological well-being: self-acceptance, autonomy, environmental mastery, personal progress, and pleasant connections. These characteristics are a person's sense of self-determination, control over their surroundings, capacity for personal development, ability to form satisfying relationships, and sense of purpose in life. Each of these dimensions is evidenced by the statements of the study subjects from their respective perspectives on psychological well-being. This group of students proved that while their lives are filled with a variety of activities based on their focus, it has a positive impact on achieving psychological well-being so that their lives on campus are filled with wonderful memories and are not focused solely on academic aspects. This is evident that engaging students in a variety of activities on campus facilitates students' pursuit of psychological well-being through these six dimensions.

Correspondingly, Siddiqui and Khan (2016) attest that the growth of psychological well-being is fundamentally influenced by emotional support and supportive social relationships. It is clear from the literature that a student's overall psychological well-being increases with their social skills level. Siddiqui and Khan concluded that having more supportive connections in one's surroundings or context resulted in higher resilience or adaptability. Panahi (2016) also confirms that a person with a high level of psychological well-being will lead a joyful and contented life with a capable and well-supported professional and personal life. On ethical grounds alone, universities have a responsibility to support and ensure the safety and well-being of all students. Indeed, supporting student well-being is also essential for fulfilling universities' core mission of providing high-quality educational experiences and positive graduate outcomes.

Additionally, the psychological well-being of university students is poorer in research (Diaz et al., 2006; García et al., 2013; Sandoval et al., 2017). A study by Sandoval et al. (2017) found that a high proportion of university students displayed a medium level of psychological well-being, suggesting that it is a sign of how well they have adjusted to their environment. Further, self-concept was found to be one of the indicators of life happiness in Fonseca-Pedrero's (2012) study. It has been discovered that emotional self-concept is inversely related to four aspects of psychological well-being such as self-acceptance, autonomy, environmental mastery, and personal growth.

On a different note, whereas psychological well-being, happiness and life satisfaction are positive effects, depression is a negative effect. Both effects tell us about the well-being of the individual. At present much more is known about the negative effects of depression on student success than about the benefits of psychological well-being, happiness and life satisfaction (Franzen et al., 2021). For example, depression is negatively related to student's success, academic performance and less time spent on homework (Duncan et al., 2021; Cooper et al., 2021; Bitew &Birhan, 2021). A study by Shahira et al. (2018) in Malaysia on stress and psychological well-being found that depression, anxiety, and stress among UniSZA students were 42.2%, 73.7%, and 34.8% respectively. Findings revealed that students who faced psychological distress levels possessed a relatively high tendency for depression, stress, and anxiety. As such, psychological distress poses negative impacts on the physical, mental and academic performance of students. What is more worrying is that students who face this kind of problem do not seek help or treatment because of the public stigma against mental illness (Mhata et al., 2023; Cage et al., 2020; Busby et al., 2019). Findings from the study of Arslan (2023) show that young people with internalizing and externalizing problems report fewer positive psychological states compared to those without such problems. This highlights the importance of understanding well-being domains, such as respect and loneliness, in addressing mental health difficulties among young people. These results can help mental health professionals create interventions to improve students' psychosocial adjustment by giving them tools to promote mental health and well-being. Therefore, the issue of students' well-being and especially the psychological well-being of those in higher education institutions should be given the due attention it deserves. The following section deals with a theoretical framework on which this study underpins.

## THEORETICAL FRAMEWORK

This chapter is based on the positive psychology theory of Seligman and Csikszentmihaly (2008). The theory posits that success is promoted by happiness in a variety of spheres of human functioning. Erez and Isen (2002) claim that elevating people's emotional states encourages adaptable, successful problem-solving, decision-making, and event appraisal. Positive emotions therefore have the potential to be adaptive and interactive, and they may be able to control the association between stress or depression and successful college behaviour and attitude. According to positive psychology, it is more crucial to concentrate on cultivating good traits rather than trying to prevent or lessen negative ones, like depression, once they have already happened. Based on this theory, a person's psychological health is based on how well they perform in various facets of life (Udhayakumar & Illango, 2018). The theory suggests that an individual should respect the environment, accept oneself both now and in the past, have life objectives, work to achieve them, and be able to make their own decisions (Siddiqui & Khan, 2016). Within the above context, this theory is deemed fit for this chapter as students' psychological well-being is developed when one maintains a positive mindset, exercises resilience and self-control, and aims to achieve self-actualization. The theory helps authors understand that high self-esteem, self-efficacy, self-awareness and autonomy not only elevate students' independent and critical thinking capacity but also increase acceptance and self-love. When students can regulate and direct their own lives, that means they have the power to think independently and can boldly handle and face any situation they find themselves in. The following section deals with the methodology followed to obtain data for this chapter. The next section discusses the literature review.

## LITERATURE REVIEW

### Psychological Well-Being Dimensions

The components of psychological well-being include life satisfaction, positive emotions, low levels of negative emotions, autonomy, positive relationships, purpose in life, and personal growth. These components are interdependent and can impact each other, leading to improved overall well-being. The other psychological well-being aspects such as mindfulness, resilience, social support, and self-efficacy and the specifics are discussed in detail below. The next sub-section discusses mindfulness.

## Mindfulness

Mindfulness is awareness of one's internal states and surroundings (Stuart-Edwards et al., 2021). Stated differently, it refers to the fundamental human capacity to be present, cognizant of our surroundings and our actions, and not unduly affected or overwhelmed by them. All people naturally possess mindfulness. By teaching students to observe their thoughts, feelings, and other in-the-moment sensations without passing judgment or responding automatically, mindfulness can help them avoid harmful or automatic behaviours and responses. Within the mindfulness concept, there are three components such as:

1. **Intention:** Deciding to develop your consciousness.
2. **Attention:** To the here and now, feelings, and ideas.
3. **Attitude:** Showing compassion, curiosity, and lack of judgment.

A growing body of research has explored the effects of mindfulness-based practices, such as meditation and yoga, on psychological well-being. These studies have demonstrated that these practices can have positive effects on mood, stress levels, and overall well-being (Dhanabhakyam & Sarath, 2023). Cognitive-behavioural therapies, such as cognitive behavioural therapy (CBT), have also been found to be effective in promoting well-being, particularly for individuals with depression and anxiety (Harding et al., 2019). According to Stuart-Edwards et al. (2021) mindfulness, mostly used as a therapeutic technique, is a mental state achieved by focusing on one's awareness of the present moment, while calmly acknowledging and accepting one's feelings, thoughts and bodily sensations. In other words, mindfulness implies maintaining our thoughts, feelings, bodily sensations and immediate environment on a moment-by-moment basis. Self-compassion's key ingredient, mindfulness, entails "being aware of one's present moment experience of suffering with clarity and balance, neither ignoring nor ruminating on negative aspects of oneself or one's life experience" (Neff & Costigan, 2014, p. 114). Family experiences are important for cultivating mindfulness, and parent-child connections have an impact on people's mindfulness (Neff & McGehee, 2010). Acceptance is also a component of mindfulness that infers to paying attention to our thoughts and feelings without passing judgment on them. For instance, by accepting ourselves and the way things are in our lives at the moment, we refrain from thinking that there is a "right or wrong" way to think or feel at any given time. Thus, by engaging in mindfulness exercises, we train our minds to focus on the present moment rather than the past or the future. It is imperative to focus on the present as we cannot reverse the past and the future is unknown. Further, mindfulness, also called "cautious attention", refers to individuals' ability to self-regulate attention to the present moment and to orientate toward acceptance, openness, and curiosity (Harley, 2018). Despite having Buddhist meditation as its foundation, secular mindfulness has recently become more popular in America and many institutions have adopted the Mindfulness-Based Stress Reduction (MBSR) program in their settings (e.g., schools, universities and hospitals) due to the positive effects on one's physical and mental health.

Additionally, numerous studies (e.g., Harrington & Dunne, (2015)., Gámez-Guadix & Calvete, 2016) showed a link between mindfulness and various mental health and wellbeing outcomes. According to Wang et al. (2017), mindfulness is a potent source of wellness that promotes people's mental health and good growth. According to studies by Bluth and Blanton (2014) and Demir (2015), people with higher levels of mindfulness reported lower levels of mental health outcomes, such as depression, anxiety, negative affect, anger, and loneliness, as well as higher levels of wellbeing indicators, such as life satisfaction, higher self-esteem, and positive affect. For instance, Barnett et al. (2021) discussed the impact of mindfulness on mental health issues and wellbeing. They found that an increase in mindfulness was a significant predictor of adults' psychological well-being, perceived stress, and psychological and physical consequences.

Another study examined the impact of a mindfulness-based program on the psychological symptoms of sexually abused adults. Depression, post-traumatic stress disorder, and anxiety were found to be significantly reduced in these adult survivors of sexual abuse (Kimbrough et al., 2010). Additionally, because people with higher levels of mindfulness use more adaptive coping strategies than maladaptive ones when dealing with stress, this ability helps these people change their relationships with negative thoughts by focusing on the present moment and, as a result, may improve a person's coping ability with stressful events (Kimbrough et al., 2010). In other words, mindfulness facilitates positive adaptation by mediating adolescent development. The relationship between transitions to higher institutions and psychological unstable might be mitigated through mindfulness, according to the literature and theoretical framework.

In Luo's (2022) study, mindfulness was a favourable means to improve psychological well-being, while rumination was an unfavourable factor affecting psychological well-being. Indeed, there is a certain relationship between the two in terms of their connotations as mindfulness can play a certain role in intervening in rumination.

Several studies involving university students have investigated mindfulness and psychological well-being and suggested that interventions like mindfulness training can improve students' psychological well-being (Goyal et al.,2014; Kong et al.,2016; & Feller et al.,2018). Similarly, integrative body-mind training (IBMT), which shares essential elements with other types of mindfulness training, has also received particular attention (Tang et al., 2016; Tang, 2017). IBMT involves systematic training of attention and self-control with an attitude of acceptance and openness to the present experiences. Halland et al. (2015) results of a randomized controlled experiment among Norwegian psychology and medical students indicated that mindfulness training could enhance problem-focused coping. This training intervention reduced avoidance-focused coping and increased social support-seeking behaviours in those with higher neuroticism scores, which was beneficial for them. Similar results were found in a second Norwegian study, which showed that mindfulness training might reduce neuroticism in medical and psychology students over a startlingly long six-year follow-up period (Hanley et al., 2019). In Spain, mindfulness exercises were found to help lower stress and anxiety generated by exams in Bachelor of Education students, demonstrating the direct influence of mindfulness-based practice on students' mental health. Nguyen-Feng et al. (2017) and Gallego et al. (2014) concluded that even when offered via an online platform, such mindfulness training may reduce stress, anxiety, and depression. The next sub-section discusses resilience.

## Resilience

Resilience has no single definition, according to Simons et al. (2018), but defined it as "the process of adapting well in the face of adversity, trauma, tragedy, threats, or significant sources of stress such as family and relationship problems, serious health problems, or workplace and financial stressors." Hence, current research still lacks an agreed operational definition for resilience, but it has been suggested that resilience consists of both behavioural characteristics, for example, maintaining effectiveness and resisting destructive behaviours (Robertson & Cooper, 2013), and psychological characteristics, such as the ability to maintain good mental health after adversity (Bonanno, 2004). Within an educational context, resilience has come to be recognised as a necessary skill for a student to fully thrive in a higher education setting. For example, in an educational framework, resilience is defined as a collection of attitudes and actions that are linked to a student's capacity to bounce back from adversity and actively adapt to it (Fuller, et al., 2016). Resilience is viewed as essential to helping students manage academic demands to enable positive progress and cope with the pressure of study, work, and life (Caruana et al., 2011). In Durso et al. (2021) research, the term "resilient student" refers to a person who, despite significant stress and/or difficulty, completes their undergraduate degree with satisfaction and/or commitment to their chosen field of study. Using the Academic Resilience Model (ARM), Durso et al. (2021), identified abilities for flexibility, self-control, personal organization, positive interactions with faculty, peer integration, and family support as main protective mechanisms or factors of resilience.

Another study by Robbins et al. (2018) examined the predicting effect on resilience, stress, mindfulness, and self-efficacy in PWB among undergraduate students and found resilience to be the strongest predictor. Notably, resilience, when coping with stress, can protect against serious negative life outcomes and lead to greater lifetime satisfaction. The literature suggests that there are internal factors that may moderate the development of resilience. For instance, whereas Johnson (2008) identified 'internal' factors such as optimism, self-efficacy, and psychological wellbeing as the being most important to the development of resilience in young people, others academics suggest that resilience can be predicted by protective characteristics such as levels of self-esteem (Robbins et al., 2018; Grills-Taquechel et al.,2010), exposure to stressful events, attachment avoidance and anxiety in parental relationships (Robbins et al., 2018; Brewer et al.,2019), positive thinking, personal organisation, problem-solving skills and support of family and friends and the availability of professors (Gallego et al., 2014) self-efficacy (Caprara et al., 2013), self-and attachment-security (Black-Hughes, 2013). Having a secure attachment status, which is thought to be constant through maturity, can promote resilient long-term effects. According to Black-Hughes (2013), secure attachment is linked to protective resilience against the risk of substance misuse and criminal behaviour in adults. Additional study indicates that attachment security is a source of resilience against the consequences of educational disadvantage in the workplace for adults, which in turn supports improved adult health behaviours through effective coping mechanisms and ultimately, better long-term health (Bartley et al., 2007; Harding et al., 2019). It is crucial that institutions of higher education initiate programmes with individual students and/or use small groups to help students develop resilience skills as literature confirmed to have robust effects on improving self-esteem (Fennell, 2016; Longworth et al., 2016). The next sub-section disussses social support.

## Social Support

Social support has been described as support accessible to an individual through social ties to other individuals, groups, and the larger community (Klainin-Yobas et al., 2016). The National Cancer Institute's Dictionary of Cancer Terms defines social support as "a network of family, friends, neighbours, and community members that is available in times of need to give psychological, physical, and financial help" Further, social support, an external protective factor, is defined as individuals' perception of adequate and valuable support influencing adjustment (Panani et al. (2016). Numerous studies indicate that social support is essential for maintaining physical and psychological health (Cho & Yu, 2015; Panani et al., 2016; Bartholomeus et al., 2016; Klainin-Yobas et al., 2016).

Panani et al. (2016) and Bartholomeus et al. (2016) believe that social support is one of the most important factors in determining the psychological well-being of students. Overall, it appears that positive social support of high quality can enhance resilience to stress, help protect against developing trauma-related psychopathology, decrease the functional consequences of trauma-induced disorders, such as posttraumatic stress disorder (PTSD), and reduce medical morbidity and mortality. However, Ryff (2023) is of the view that despite strong evidence demonstrating the beneficial effects of social support on medical and psychological well-being, the field of psychiatry has contributed relatively little to developing, testing, and implementing effective evidence-based interventions aimed at increasing social support for patients and at-risk population. Lessard et al. (2014) have strongly argued that organisational support is a critical factor that significantly influences a variety of members' cognitive and emotional outcomes, such as job satisfaction. The university setting can serve as an organisational support for students by providing services that increase students' psychological well-being and life satisfaction. The social support literature suggests that supportive social connections and strong social networks with close friends offer therapeutic benefits to students at higher education institutions mental health (Cho & Yu, 2015). Students can receive social support from significant others, such as family members, friends, and lecturers (Tang et al., 2019). In the Philippines, Klainin-Yobas et al. (2016) examined PWB's predicting factors among university students and found that social support from family and friends significantly predicted positive individual PWB. It has been argued that rich social networks may reduce the rate at which individuals engage in risky behaviours, prevent negative conduct, and increase obedience behaviour.

In light of the above, the two critical dimensions conferred below are significant in theoretical models of social support: (1) a structural dimension that takes network size and social interaction frequency into account; (2) a functional dimension that incorporates emotional elements (like receiving love and empathy) and instrumental (like getting financial gifts or help with child care). Although both the structural and functional dimensions of relationships are significant, most studies have indicated that the functional dimension, the quality of connections, is a greater predictor of good health. It should, however, be emphasized that the best social support may depend on the stage of development of the individual receiving it. For instance, early adolescence appears to be when parental support is most beneficial compared to late adolescence. It has been demonstrated that in older persons, the impression of social support is related to the level of social engagement, while in younger adults, it is related to instrumental assistance. Additionally, the nature of social support appears to have a role in promoting stress resilience. As a whole, it seems that high-quality positive social support can increase resiliency to stress, aid in preventing the emergence of trauma-related psychopathology, enhance coping skills and normalise the adjustment process. Therefore, student counsellors at the university can assist students in developing their coping abilities by teaching them to recognise and utilise social supports and create networks of beneficial interactions that ease the coping process. The next sub-section disussses self-efficacy.

## Self-Efficacy

Self-efficacy is defined as individuals' beliefs in their capabilities to produce designated levels of performance that exercise influence over events that affect their lives (Błachnio et al., 2013). In other words, self-efficacy is the belief we have in our abilities, specifically our ability to meet the challenges ahead of us and complete a task successfully. Generally, self-efficacy refers to our overall belief in our ability to succeed, but there are many more specific forms of self-efficacy as well (e.g., academic, parenting, sports). As emphasised by Fatima et al. (2018), self-efficacy aims at a broad and stable sense of personal competence to deal effectively with a variety of stressful situations. It is believed that for an individual who has low happiness and life satisfaction and high depression, having high self-efficacy will help him or her display appropriate behaviours and positive attitudes as regards his or her academic work and life in general. As a result, it is anticipated that self-efficacy will moderate the relationship between psychological factors and students' behaviours and attitudes in higher education. Students may feel vulnerable and powerless in their academic lives while attending higher education institutions, which might lower their self-efficacy. Generally, the association between self-efficacy and academic success, behaviours, attitudes, and general psychological well-being, however, has previously been established by earlier studies. For instance, studies by (Andretta et al., 2020; Fatima et al., 2018; Tommasi et al., 2018; De Caroli & Sagone, 2014) have revealed that self-efficacy is positively related to PWB, which implies the absence of psychological problems. Findings from Naeemi and Tamam (2017) show that emotional reliance on Facebook has a detrimental effect on a variety of psychological well-being factors, including autonomy, good relationships with others, and a sense of purpose in life. Furthermore, the findings show that even very high levels of self-efficacy do not mitigate the detrimental consequences of Facebook addiction on teenagers' general psychological well-being. Further to this, the results of the multimediation analyses of Fatima et al. (2018) demonstrated that the relationships between the two religiousness coping strategies and religious practices and six PWB outcomes were mediated by self-efficacy in the presence of perceived social support. Only autonomy and self-acceptance served as the mediators of these relationships in the presence of perceived social support and self-efficacy. Furthermore, the results showed that despite similar patterns of mediation effects explaining the independent effects of both, religious coping was a greater predictor of all PWB outcomes than religious behaviours.

Maddux (2016) found that students who had high self-efficacy, high emotional intelligence and who were happy were motivated to participate in relevant academic activities and developed positive attitudes that led to success in college. Evidence has revealed that happy students with high satisfaction scores were found to be flexible and efficient in problem-solving and were more committed to their academic goals and pursued success rather than focus on avoiding failure (De Caroli & Sagone, 2014); Demirtaş, 2020; Greenleaf et al., 2014). These students were more intrinsically motivated to learn, had more self-control over studying and had more respect for and appreciation for their peers and lecturers. Further to this, Greenleaf et al. (2014) self-efficacy study measured academic, social and emotional and the main variable of interest was mental well-being, while the bivariate analyses suggested that emotional self-efficacy was important. It is vital to note that self-efficacy determines an individual's resiliency to adversity and his or her vulnerability to stress and depression. The next section disussses psychological well-being and physical health.

## PSYCHOLOGICAL WELL-BEING AND PHYSICAL HEALTH

Recent years have witnessed an increased interest in the relationship between positive psychological well-being and physical health (Denollet & Brutsaert, 2018; Sin et al., 2015; Huffman et al., 2014; Hoogwegt et al., 2013). Emerging evidence suggests that psychological well-being such as positive emotions, satisfaction with life, and optimism have been linked to lower incidence of coronary heart disease, superior biological function, and longevity, independent of the effects of negative psychological states (Hoogwegt et al., 2013; DuBois et al., 2012; Boehm et al., 2012). The literature revealed that psychological and behavioural factors are important in the development and progression of diseases. For instance, Sin et al. (2015) found that positive affect was associated with 52% greater odds of being physically active, 24% greater odds of having good sleep quality, 46% greater odds of being adherent to medications, and 29% greater odds of being a non-smoker with coronary heart disease. Campbell et al. (2022) also affirmed that psychological well-being promotes well-being through the active recommendation of healthier habits linked to physical well-being, such as better sleep, physical exercise and healthy eating, as well as activities that have been associated with better psychological and subjective well-being. Other authors acknowledged that Individuals with higher well-being may be more motivated and persistent in engaging in healthy behaviours, have greater self-efficacy (Hoen et al.,2013), show more attention to and careful processing of health risk information, and are better able to adjust health-relevant goals. Indeed, increasing evidence indicates that health behaviours, namely, physical activity may be the underlying mechanisms linking positive psychological states to physical health status, reduced risk of incident coronary heart disease (Sin et al., 2015), and survival (Hoogwegt et al., 2013). Research has also shown that physical activity is positively associated with psychological well-being (Dhanabhakyam & Sarath, 2023). Physical activity has been shown to reduce stress, improve mood, and increase feelings of self-esteem and confidence. Exercise has also been found to be effective in the treatment of depression, with studies demonstrating its efficacy comparable to that of medication and psychotherapy (Dhanabhakyam & Sarath, 2023).

Additionally, practising gratitude, socialising, and helping others have all been found to increase well-being in non-clinical samples (Barrable et al., 2018). On the other hand, using a descriptive study to examine the distance learning university students in Colombia, regarding the psychological well-being area as a basic dimension of human beings, Otálora and Barros (2014) results show that only 17% of students are worried about their health and physical development, while 83% of them are not. They do not agree partially or totally or they do not show agreement or disagreement with the statements under health and physical development.The next section discusses the role of body and mind in promoting psychological well-being

## THE ROLE OF BODY AND MIND IN PROMOTING PSYCHOLOGICAL WELL-BEING

Cooperation between the body and mind is stressed in Integrative Body-Mind Training (IBMT) practice to facilitate and achieve a meditation state. Thus, Tang et al. (2019) proposed that the interplay of the central nervous system (CNS, brain) and the autonomic nervous system (ANS, body) is a crucial mechanism of IBMT. In their study, the IBMT group demonstrated lower heart rate, SCR, chest respiratory rate, and belly respiratory amplitude than the RT control both during and after the 5-session training, indicating stronger parasympathetic regulation of ANS. For institutions of higher learning management, it is essential to comprehend how mindfulness training, like IBMT, functions to create interventions that promote psychological well-being in institutions of higher learning. Earlier research has demonstrated that self-control networks are becoming more functionally and structurally flexible; the ACC/prefrontal cortex (PFC) and striatum support IBMT effects (Tang et al., 2016). Similar to this, according to Gong and Jiang (2018), the practice of Transcendental Meditation (TM) dates back thousands of years. Anyone over the age of ten can engage in this straightforward type of meditation, which is practised by millions of people worldwide. The next section discusses the methodology.

## METHODOLOGY

The systematic review was used as a research methodology to analyse secondary sources. Search engines such as Google Scholar, Educational Resources Information Center (ERIC), Web of Science, Psych INFO, Science Direct, Academic Search Elite/EBSCO, PubMed and JSTOR were used to obtain secondary data. Two reviewers independently extracted data on study characteristics, quality, and estimates of associations. The inclusion criteria for articles selected included those that investigated the psychological well-being of students in higher education institutions. Data were analysed qualitatively by using content analysis where only the main ideas of the key findings were considered focusing on the most relevant literature. The next section discusses the conclusion.

## CONCLUSION

The chapter addressed psychological core dimensions and the link between emotional self-concept and self-acceptance, autonomy, environmental mastery and personal growth. Psychological well-being is an important aspect of mental and emotional health that requires ongoing attention and care. Students can promote their psychological well-being by engaging in activities that promote personal growth, maintain positive relationships, and provide a sense of purpose and meaning in life. Additionally, students can seek support from mental health professionals if they experience difficulties with their psychological well-being. By taking a holistic approach to promoting mental and emotional health, students can enhance their overall well-being and lead a fulfilling life. Fact Because psychological well-being is a strong predictor of students' behaviours and attitudes, the demands of higher education institutions to address the underlying factors that can enhance students' satisfaction with their studies in addition to ensuring their timely access to relevant psychosocial services to mitigate mental distress cannot be overemphasised. It is, therefore, essential that university student counsellors design intervention programmes and use them to foster psychological well-being, good behaviours and attitudes of students thereby improving the quality of their lives. Evidence has revealed that a sense of belonging and a supportive social network are critical elements for building strong psychological well-being in students of higher education institutions. Hence, students' active participation in various social activities on campus is encouraged as that can enhance their general well-being. Additionally, university management, counselling centres, and other relevant authorities' prioritisation of students' psychological well-being and provision of appropriate mental health services for the betterment of holistic well-being development is highly recommended.

## REFERENCES

Andretta, J. R., & McKay, M. T. (2020). Self-efficacy and well-being in adolescents: A comparative study using variable and person-centered analyses. *Children and Youth Services Review*, *118*, 105374. doi:10.1016/j.childyouth.2020.105374

Arslan, G. (2023). Psychological Well-Being and Mental Health in Youth: Technical Adequacy of the Comprehensive Inventory of Thriving. *Children (Basel, Switzerland)*, *10*(7), 1269. doi:10.3390/children10071269 PMID:37508766

Asif, S., Mudassar, A., Shahzad, T. Z., Raouf, M., & Pervaiz, T. (2020). Frequency of depression, anxiety and stress among university students. [CrossRef]. *Pakistan Journal of Medical Sciences*, *36*(5), 971–976. doi:10.12669/pjms.36.5.1873 PMID:32704273

Auerbach, R. P., Mortier, P., Bruffaerts, R., Alonso, J., Benjet, C., Cuijpers, P., Demyttenaere, K., Ebert, D. D., Green, J. G., Hasking, P., Murray, E., Nock, M. K., Pinder-Amaker, S., Sampson, N. A., Stein, D. J., Vilagut, G., Zaslavsky, A. M., & Kessler, R. C. (2018). WHO world mental health surveys international college student project: Prevalence and distribution of mental disorders. [CrossRef]. *Journal of Abnormal Psychology*, *127*(7), 623–638. doi:10.1037/abn0000362 PMID:30211576

Barnard, L. K., & Curry, J. F. (2011). Self-compassion: Conceptualizations, correlates, & interventions. *Review of General Psychology*, *15*(4), 289–303. doi:10.1037/a0025754

Barnett, P., Arundell, L., Saunders, R., Matthews, H., & Pilling, S. (2021). The efficacy of psychological interventions for the prevention and treatment of mental health disorders in university students: A systematic review and meta-analysis. *Journal of Affective Disorders*, *280*, 381–406. doi:10.1016/j.jad.2020.10.060 PMID:33227669

Barrable, A., Papadatou-Pastou, M., & Tzotzoli, P. (2018). Supporting mental health, wellbeing and study skills in Higher Education: An online intervention system. *International Journal of Mental Health Systems*, *12*(1), 54. doi:10.118613033-018-0233-z PMID:30323858

Bartholomew, T. T. (2016). Mental Health in Namibia. *Psychology and Developing Societies*, *28*(1), 101–125. Advance online publication. doi:10.1177/0971333615622909

Bartley, M., Head, J., & Stansfeld, S. (2007). Is attachment style a source of resilience against health inequalities at work? *Social Science & Medicine*, *64*(4), 765–775. doi:10.1016/j.socscimed.2006.09.033 PMID:17129652

Bitew, T., & Birhan, W. (2021). The potential effect of depression on academic outcomes of students in higher educational institutions of northwest Ethiopia: A cross-sectional study. *Educational Research Review*, *16*(1), 9–15. doi:10.5897/ERR2020.4055

Błachnio, A., Przepiórka, A., & Rudnicka, P. (2013). Psychological determinants of using Facebook: A research review. *International Journal of Human-Computer Interaction*, *29*(11), 775–787. doi:10.1080/10447318.2013.780868

Black-Hughes, C., & Stacy, P. (2013). Early childhood attachment and its impact on later life resilience: A comparison of resilient and no resilient female siblings. *Journal of Evidence-Based Social Work*, *10*(5), 410–420. doi:10.1080/15433714.2012.759456 PMID:24066631

Bluth, K., & Blanton, P. W. (2014). Mindfulness and self-compassion: Exploring pathways to adolescent emotional well-being. *Journal of Child and Family Studies*, *23*(7), 1298–1309. doi:10.100710826-013-9830-2 PMID:25328369

Boehm, J. K., Vie, L. L., & Kubzansky, L. D. (2012). The promise of well-being interventions for improving health risk behaviours. *Current Cardiovascular Risk Reports*, *6*(6), 511–519. doi:10.100712170-012-0273-x

Bonanno, G. A. (2004). Loss, trauma, and human resilience: Have we underestimated the Human capacity to thrive after extremely aversive events? *The American Psychologist, 59*(1), 20–28. doi:10.1037/0003-066X.59.1.20 PMID:14736317

Brewer, M., van Kessel, G., Sanderson, B., Naumann, F., Lane, M., Reubenson, A., & Carter, A. (2019). Resilience in higher education students: *A scoping review. Higher Education Research & Development, 38*(6), 1105–1120. doi:10.1080/07294360.2019.1626810

Brown, K. W., Goodman, R. J., & Inzlicht, M. (2013). Dispositional *mindfulness and the attenuation of neural responses to emotional stimuli. Social Cognitive and Affective Neuroscience, 8*(1), 93–99. doi:10.1093can/nss004 PMID:22253259

Busby, D. R., Zheng, K., Eisenberg, D., Albucher, R. C., Favorite, T., Coryell, W., & King, C. A. (2019). Black college students at elevated risk for suicide: Barriers to mental health service utilization. *Journal of American College Health*, 1–7. PMID:31662044

Cage, E., Stock, M., Sharpington, A., Pitman, E., & Batchelor, E. (2020). Barriers to accessing support for mental health issues at university. *Studies in Higher Education, 45*(8), 1637–1649. doi:10.1080/03075079.2018.1544237

Campbell, F., Blank, L., Cantrell, A., Baxter, S., Blackmore, C., Dixon, J., & Goyder, E. (2022). Factors that influence the mental health of university and college students in the UK: A systematic review. *BMC Public Health, 22*(1), 1778. doi:10.118612889-022-13943-x PMID:36123714

Caprara, G. V., Alessandri, G., Barbaranelli, C., & Vecchione, M. (2013). The longitudinal relations between self-esteem and affective self-regulatory efficacy. *Journal of Research in Personality, 47*(6), 859–870. doi:10.1016/j.jrp.2013.08.011

Caruana, V., Clegg, S., & Ploner, J. (2011). *Promoting students' 'resilient thinking' in diverse higher education learning environments*. HE Academy Subject Centre for Sociology, Anthropology and Politics.

Cho, J., & Yu, H. (2015). Roles of University Support for International Students in the United States: Analysis of a Systematic Model of University Identification, University Support, and Psychological Well-Being. *Journal of Studies in International Education, 19*(1), 11–27. doi:10.1177/1028315314533606

Christner, N., Essler, S., Hazzam, A., & Paulus, M. (2021). Children's psychological well-being and problem behaviour during the COVID-19 pandemic: An online study during the lockdown period in Germany. [PMCID.]. *PLoS One, 16*(6), e0253473. doi:10.1371/journal.pone.0253473 PMID:34161376

Community Translational Science Team (CTST). (2016). *Policy Report: Building A Public Health Model for Promoting Emotional Well-Being*. University of California.

Cooper, K. M., Gin, L. E., Barnes, M. E., Sara, E., & Brownell, S. E. (2020). Exploratory Study of Students with Depression in Undergraduate Research Experiences. *CBE Life Sciences Education, 19*(2), ar19. doi:10.1187/cbe.19-11-0217 PMID:32412838

Cooper, S., & Nicholas, L. (2013). Counselling and psychotherapy in South Africa: Responding to post-apartheid counselling needs. In R. Moodley, U. P. Gielen, & R. Wu (Eds.), *Handbook of counselling and psychotherapy in an international context* (pp. 61–71). Routledge.

De Caroli, M. E., & Sagone, E. (2014). Generalized self-efficacy and well-being in adolescents with high vs. low scholastic self-efficacy. *Procedia: Social and Behavioral Sciences*, *141*, 867–874. doi:10.1016/j.sbspro.2014.05.152

Demirtaş, A. S. (2020). Cognitive flexibility and mental well-being in Turkish adolescents: The mediating role of academic, social and emotional self-efficacy. *Anales de psicología/annals of Psychology, 36*(1), 111-121.

Denollet, J., & Brutsaert, D. L. (2018). Reducing emotional distress improves prognosis in coronary heart disease: 9-year mortality in a clinical trial of rehabilitation. [PubMed: 11673339]. *Circulation, 104*(17), 23. PMID:11673339

Dhanabhakyam, M. & Sarath, M. (2023). Psychological Wellbeing: A Systematic Literature Review. *International Journal of Advanced Research in Science Communication and Technology*. . doi:10.48175/IJARSCT-8345

Díaz, D., Rodríguez-Carvajal, R., Blanco, A., Moreno-Jiménez, B., Gallardo, I., & Valle, C. (2006). The Psychological Well-Being Scales (PWBS)]. [PubMed]. *Psicothema, 18*, 572–577. PMID:17296089

Diener, E., Lucas, R. E., Schimmack, U., & Helliwell, J. (2010). *Well-being for public policy*. Oxford University Press.

DuBois, C. M., Beach, S. R., Kashdan, T. B., Nyer, M. B., Park, E. R., Celano, C. M., & Huffman, J. C. (2012). Positive psychological attributes and cardiac outcomes: Associations, mechanisms, and interventions. *Psychosomatics*, *53*(4), 303–318. doi:10.1016/j.psym.2012.04.004 PMID:22748749

Durso, S. de O., Afonso, L. E., & Beltman, S. (2021). Resilience in higher education: A conceptual model and its empirical analysis. *Education Policy Analysis Archives*, *29*(August - December), 156. doi:10.14507/epaa.29.6054

Erez, A., & Isen, A. M. (2002). The influence of positive affect on the components of expectancy motivation. *The Journal of Applied Psychology*, *87*(6), 1055–1067. doi:10.1037/0021-9010.87.6.1055 PMID:12558213

Fatima, S., Sharif, S., & Khalid, I. (2018). How does religiosity enhance psychological well-being? Roles of self-efficacy and perceived social support. *Psychology of Religion and Spirituality*, *10*(2), 119–127. doi:10.1037/rel0000168

Feller, S. C., Castillo, E. G., Greenberg, J. M., Abascal, P., Van Horn, R., & Wells, K. B. (2018). Emotional well-being and public health: Proposal for a model national initiative. *Public Health Reports (Washington, D.C.)*, *133*(2), 136–141. doi:10.1177/0033354918754540 PMID:29448872

Fennell, M. (2016). Overcoming low self-esteem: A self-help guide using cognitive behavioural techniques. Hachette UK.

Fonseca-Pedrero, E., Paino, M., Sierra-Baigrie, S., Lemos-Giráldez, S., & Muñiz, J. (2012). Psychometric Properties of the "State-Trait Anxiety Questionnaire". *Behav. Psychol. Psicol. Conduct.*, *20*, 547–561.

Franzen, J., Jermann, F., Ghisletta, P., Rudaz, S., Bondolfi, G., & Tran, N. T. (2021). Psychological Distress and Well-Being among Students of Health Disciplines: The Importance of Academic Satisfaction. *International Journal of Environmental Research and Public Health, 18*(4), 2151. doi:10.3390/ijerph18042151 PMID:33672097

Gallego, J., Aguilar-Parra, J. M., Cangas, A. J., Langer, Á. I., & Mañas, I. (2014). Effect of a Mindfulness Program on Stress, Anxiety and Depression in University Students. [CrossRef] [PubMed]. *The Spanish Journal of Psychology, 17*, 17. doi:10.1017jp.2014.102 PMID:26055051

Gámez-Guadix, M., & Calvete, E. (2016). Assessing the relationship between mindful awareness and problematic Internet use among adolescents. *Mindfulness, 7*(6), 1281–1288. doi:10.100712671-016-0566-0

García, F., & Musitu, G. (2014). *AF5: Autoconcepto Forma 5* [AF5: Form 5 Self-Concept]. TEA Ediciones.

Gong, H., & Jiang, J. (2018). The Psychological Health Promotion and Intervention Strategies of College Teachers from the Perspective of Positive Psychology. *Theor. Pract. Innov. Entrep., 10*, 27–33.

Goyal, M., Singh, S., Sibinga, E. M., Gould, N. F., Rowland-Seymour, A., Sharma, R., Berger, Z., Sleicher, D., Maron, D. D., Shihab, H. M., Ranasinghe, P. D., Linn, S., Saha, S., Bass, E. B., & Haythornthwaite, J. A. (2014). Meditation programs for psychological stress and well-being: A systematic review and meta-analysis. *JAMA Internal Medicine, 174*(3), 357–368. doi:10.1001/jamainternmed.2013.13018 PMID:24395196

Greenleaf, C., Petrie, T. A., & Martin, S. B. (2014). Relationship of weight-based teasing and adolescents' psychological well-being and physical health. *The Journal of School Health, 84*(1), 49–55. doi:10.1111/josh.12118 PMID:24320152

Grills-Taquechel, A. E., Norton, P., & Ollendick, T. H. (2010). A longitudinal examination of factors predicting anxiety during the transition to middle school. *Anxiety, Stress, and Coping, 23*(5), 493–513. doi:10.1080/10615800903494127 PMID:20711893

Haleh-Heizomi, H., Allahverdipour, H., Hejazi, S. B., Jafarabadi, M. A., & Shirazi', A. (2018). Factors Associating Perceived Stress and Psychological Well-being among Iranian Female Adolescents. *Int J Depress Anxiety, 1*(1), 1–6.

Halland, E., De Vibe, M., Solhaug, I., Friborg, O., Rosenvinge, J., Tyssen, R., Sørlie, T., & Bjørndal, A. (2015). Mindfulness training improves problem-focused coping in psychology and medical students: Results from a randomized controlled trial. *College Student Journal*, (49), 387–398.

Hamad, E. O. (2022). Psychological well-being among Saudi adults during the context of COVID-19 lockdown: A psychometric analysis of the 12-item General Health Questionnaire. *BMC Psychology, 10*(1), 319. doi:10.118640359-022-01030-0 PMID:36572926

Hanley, A. W., de Vibe, M., Solhaug, I., Gonzalez-Pons, K., & Garland, E. L. (2019). Mindfulness training reduces neuroticism over a 6-year longitudinal randomized control trial in Norwegian medical and psychology students. [CrossRef]. *Journal of Research in Personality, 82*, 103859. doi:10.1016/j.jrp.2019.103859

Harding, T., Lopez, V., & Klainin-Yobas, P. (2019). Predictors of Psychological Well-Being among Higher Education Students. *Psychology (Irvine, Calif.)*, *10*(10), 578–594. doi:10.4236/psych.2019.104037

Harrington, A., & Dunne, J. D. (2015). When mindfulness is therapy: Ethical qualms, historical perspectives. *The American Psychologist*, *70*(7), 621–631. doi:10.1037/a0039460 PMID:26436312

He, F. X., Turnbull, B., Kirshbaum, M. N., Phillips, B., & Klainin-Yobas, P. (2018). Assessing Stress, Protective Factors and Psychological Well-Being among Undergraduate Nursing Students. [CrossRef]. *Nurse Education Today*, *68*, 4–12. doi:10.1016/j.nedt.2018.05.013 PMID:29870871

Hoen, P. W., Denollet, J., de Jonge, P., & Whooley, M. A. (2013). Positive affect and survival in patients with stable coronary heart disease: Findings from the Heart and Soul Study. [PubMed: 23945449]. *The Journal of Clinical Psychiatry*, *74*(7), 716–722. doi:10.4088/JCP.12m08022 PMID:23945449

Hofmann, S. G., Grossman, P., & Hinton, D. E. (2011). Loving-kindness and compassion meditation: Potential for psychological interventions. *Clinical Psychology Review*, *31*(7), 1126–1132. doi:10.1016/j.cpr.2011.07.003 PMID:21840289

Hoogwegt, M. T., Versteeg, H., Hansen, T. B., Thygesen, L. C., Pedersen, S. S., & Zwisler, A.-D. (2013). Exercise mediates the association between positive affect and 5-year mortality in patients with ischemic heart disease. [PubMed: 24021694]. *Circulation: Cardiovascular Quality and Outcomes*, *6*(5), 559–566. doi:10.1161/CIRCOUTCOMES.113.000158 PMID:24021694

Huffman, J. C., DuBois, C. M., Mastomauro, C. A., Moore, S. V., Suarez, L., & Park, E. R. (2014). Positive psychological states and health behaviours in acute coronary syndrome patients: A qualitative study. *Journal of Health Psychology*. PMID:25114026

Hutcherson, C. A., Seppala, E. M., & Gross, J. J. (2008). Lovingkindness meditation increases social connectedness. *Emotion (Washington, D.C.)*, *8*(5), 720–724. doi:10.1037/a0013237 PMID:18837623

Hutcherson, C. A., Seppala, E. M., & Gross, J. J. (2008). Lovingkindness meditation increases social connectedness. *Emotion (Washington, D.C.)*, *8*(5), 720–724. doi:10.1037/a0013237 PMID:18837623

Kimbrough, E., Magyari, T., Langenberg, P., Chesney, M., & Berman, B. (2010). Mindfulness intervention for child abuse survivors. *Journal of Clinical Psychology*, *66*(1), 17–33. doi:10.1002/jclp.20624 PMID:19998425

Klainin-Yobas, P., Ramirez, D., Fernandez, Z., Sarmiento, J., Thanoi, W., Ignacio, J., & Lau, Y. (2016). Examining the Predicting Effect of Mindfulness on Psychological Well-Being among Undergraduate Students: A Structural Equation Modelling Approach. Personal. *Individ.* [CrossRef]. *Personality and Individual Differences*, *91*, 63–68. doi:10.1016/j.paid.2015.11.034

Kong, F., Wang, X., Song, Y., & Liu, J. (2016). Brain regions involved in dispositional mindfulness during resting state and their relation with well-being. *Social Neuroscience*, *11*(4), 331–343. doi:10.1080/17470919.2015.1092469 PMID:26360907

Koopmans, T. A., Geleijnse, J. M., Zitman, F. G., & Giltay, E. J. (2010). Effects of happiness on all-cause mortality during 15 years of follow-up: The Arnhem Elderly Study. *Journal of Happiness Studies*, *11*(1), 113–124. doi:10.100710902-008-9127-0

Lessard, A., Fortin, L., Butler-Kisber, L., & Marcotte, D. (2014). Analysing the discourse of dropouts and resilient students. *The Journal of Educational Research, 107*(2), 103–110. doi:10.1080/00220671.2012.753857

Lipson, S. K., Lattie, E. G., & Eisenberg, D. (2019). Increased rates of mental health service utilization by US college students: 10-year population-level trends (2007–2017). [CrossRef]. *Psychiatric Services (Washington, D.C.), 70*(1), 60–63. doi:10.1176/appi.ps.201800332 PMID:30394183

Longworth, C., Deakins, J., Rose, D., & Gracey, F. (2016). The nature of self-esteem and its relationship to anxiety and depression in adult acquired brain injury. *Neuropsychological Rehabilitation*, 1–17. PMID:27580356

Luo, L. (2022). The practice of psychological well-being education model for poor university students from the perspective of positive psychology. *Frontiers in Psychology, 13*, 951668. doi:10.3389/fpsyg.2022.951668 PMID:35978785

Maddux, J. E. (2016). Self-efficacy. In *Interpersonal and intrapersonal expectancies* (pp. 41–46). Routledge. doi:10.4324/9781315652535-5

Malkoc, A., & Yalcin, I. (2015). Relationships among Resilience, Social Support, Coping, and Psychological Well-Being among University Students. *Turk. Psychol. Couns. Guid. J., 5*, 35–43.

Mhata, N.T., Ntlantsana, V., Tomita, A.M., Mwambene, K., Saloojee, S. (2023). Prevalence of depression, anxiety and burnout in medical students at the University of Namibia. *S Afr J Psychiatr, 31*(29), 2044. doi:.v29i0.2044. PMID:37292521; PMCID: PMC10244924. doi:10.4102/sajpsychiatry

Morales-Rodríguez, F. M., Espigares-López, I., Brown, T., & Pérez-Mármol, J. M. (2020). The Relationship between Psychological Well-Being and Psychosocial Factors in University Students. *International Journal of Environmental Research and Public Health, 17*(13), 4778. doi:10.3390/ijerph17134778 PMID:32630816

Naeemi, S., & Tamam, E. (2017). The relationship between emotional dependence on Facebook and psychological well-being in adolescents aged 13–16. *Child Indicators Research, 10*(4), 1095–1106. doi:10.100712187-016-9438-3

Neff, K. D., & Costigan, A. P. (2014). Self-compassion, well-being, and happiness. *Psychologie in Österreich, 2*(3), 114–119.

Neff, K. D., & Dahm, K. A. (2015). Self-compassion: What it is, what it does, and how it relates to mindfulness. Handbook of mindfulness and self-regulation, 121-137.

Nguyen-Feng, V.N., Greer, C.S., & Frazier, P. (2017). Using online interventions to deliver college student mental health resources: Evidence from randomized clinical trials. *Psychol. Serv, 14*, 481.

Otálora, A. R., & Barros, A. S. S. (2014). Psychological well-being (PWB) and personal problems (PP) in university students: A descriptive study in a distance learning context, preliminary results. *Procedia: Social and Behavioral Sciences, 132*, 427–433. doi:10.1016/j.sbspro.2014.04.332

Panahi, S., Yunus, A. S. M., Roslan, S., Jaafar, R. A. K., Jaafar, W. M. W., & Panahi, M. S. (2016). Predictors of Psychological Well-being among Malaysian Graduates. *The European Journal of Social and Behavioural Sciences*, *16*(2), 2067–2083. doi:10.15405/ejsbs.186

Porru, F., Schuring, M., Bultmann, U., Portoghese, I., Busdorf, A., & Robroek, S. J. N. (2022). Associations of university student life challenges with mental health and self-rated health: A longitudinal study with 6 months follow-up. [CrossRef]. *Journal of Affective Disorders*, *296*, 250–257. doi:10.1016/j.jad.2021.09.057 PMID:34624809

Priesack, A., & Alcock, J. (2015). Well-Being and Self-Efficacy in a Sample of Undergraduate Nurse Students: A Small Survey Study. [CrossRef]. *Nurse Education Today*, *35*(5), e16–e20. doi:10.1016/j.nedt.2015.01.022 PMID:25702848

Report, N. I. H. (2018). Emotional Well-Being: Emerging Insights and Questions for Future Research. Bethesda, MD.

Robbins, A., Kaye, E., & Catling, J. C. (2018). Predictors of student resilience in higher education. *Psychology Teaching Review*, *24*(1), 44–52. doi:10.53841/bpsptr.2018.24.1.44

Robertson, I., & Cooper, C. L. (2013). Resilience. *Stress and Health*, *29*(3), 175–176. doi:10.1002mi.2512 PMID:23913839

Ryff, C. (1989). Happiness is Everything, or Is It? Exploration of the Meaning of Psychological Well-Being. *Journal of Personality and Social Psychology*, *57*(2), 1069–1081. doi:10.1037/0022-3514.57.6.1069

Ryff, C. D. (2023). A new direction in mental health: Purposeful life engagement. Encyclopedia of Mental Health (3rd ed.). Science Direct. doi:10.1016/B978-0-323-91497-0.00096-5

Salois, D. J. M. (2021). Promoting well-being among college students: the effects of a positive psychology course. *Graduate student theses, dissertations, & professional papers*. Https://scholarworks.umt.edu/etd/1179

Sampath, H., Biswas, A. G., Soohinda, G., & Dutta, S. (2019). Mindfulness and Its Role in Psychological Well-Being among Medical College Students. *Open Journal of Psychiatry & Allied Sciences*, *10*(1), 52. doi:10.5958/2394-2061.2019.00013.2

Sandoval, S., Dorner, A., & Véliz, A. (2017). Psychological well-being of students taking health degree courses]. *Investigación en Educación Médica*, *6*, 260–266.

Seligman, M. E. P., & Csikszentinihalyi, M. (2000). Positive psychology: An introduction. *The American Psychologist*, *55*(1), 5–14. doi:10.1037/0003-066X.55.1.5 PMID:11392865

Shah, K. M. D., Padli, J., Talib, J. A., & Mukhta, F. (2020). The Psychological Well-Being from The University Students' Perspective and Culture– Palarch's. *Journal of Archaeology of Egypt/Egyptology* *17*(2), 1- 11.

Shahira, M. N., Hanisshya, H., Lukman, Z. M., Normala, R., Azlini, C., & Kamal, M. Y. (2018). Psychological Well-Being among University Students in Malaysia. *International Journal of Research and Innovation in Social Science*, (2), 133–137.

Sharma, A., & Sharma, R. (2018). Internet addiction and psychological well-being among college students: A cross-sectional study from Central India. *Journal of Family Medicine and Primary Care*, *7*(1), 147–151. doi:10.4103/jfmpc.jfmpc_189_17 PMID:29915749

Sharma, A., Singh, T. P., Sharma, R., Dhakar, J. S., & Bharti, A. (2022). Psychological well-being among college students: A study from Central India. *Asian Journal of Medical Sciences*, *13*(1), 46–51. doi:10.3126/ajms.v13i1.39350

Siddiqui, Z. U., & Khan, M. I. (2016). Psychological Well-Being among University Students. *International Journal of Indian Psychology*, *3*(4), 114–118.

Simons, J., Beaumont, K., & Holland, L. (2018). What factors promote student resilience on a level 1 distance learning module? *Open Learning*, *33*(1), 4–17. doi:10.1080/02680513.2017.1415140

Sin, N. L., Moskowitz, J. T., & Whooley, M. A. (2015). Positive Affect and Health Behaviors across Five Years in Patients with Coronary Heart Disease: The Heart and Soul Study. *Psychosomatic Medicine*, *77*(9), 1058–1066. doi:10.1097/PSY.0000000000000238 PMID:26428445

Stuart-Edwards, A. (2023). Good begets good? Reciprocal relationships between mindfulness, approach coping, and subjective vitality. *Personality and Individual Differences*, *202*, 111970. doi:10.1016/j.paid.2022.111970

Tang, Y. Y. (2017). *The Neuroscience of Mindfulness Meditation: How the Body and Mind Work Together to Change Our Behavior*. Springer Nature. doi:10.1007/978-3-319-46322-3

Tang, Y. Y., Hölzel, B. K., & Posner, M. I. (2016). Traits and states in mindfulness meditation. *Nature Reviews. Neuroscience*, *17*(1), 59. doi:10.1038/nrn.2015.7 PMID:26631928

Tang, Y. Y., Tang, R., & Gross, J. J. (2019). Promoting Psychological Well-Being through an Evidence-Based Mindfulness Training Program. *Frontiers in Human Neuroscience*, *13*(1), 1–5. doi:10.3389/fnhum.2019.00237 PMID:31354454

Teh, C. K., Ngo, C. W., Binti Zulkifli, R. A., Vellasamy, R., & Suresh, K. (2015). Depression, anxiety and stress among undergraduate students: A cross-sectional study. [CrossRef]. *Open Journal of Epidemiology*, *5*(4), 260–268. doi:10.4236/ojepi.2015.54030

Thanoi, W., Vongsirimas, N., Sitthimongkol, Y., & Klainin-Yobas, P. (2023). Examining Predictors of Psychological Well-Being among University Students: A Descriptive Comparative Study across Thailand and Singapore. *International Journal of Environmental Research and Public Health*, *20*(3), 1875. doi:10.3390/ijerph20031875 PMID:36767238

Tommasi, M., Grassi, P., Balsamo, M., Picconi, L., Furnham, A., & Saggino, A. (2018). Correlations between personality, affective and filial self-efficacy beliefs, and psychological well-being in a sample of Italian adolescents. *Psychological Reports*, *121*(1), 59–78. doi:10.1177/0033294117720698 PMID:28750584

Udhayakumar, P., & Illango, P. (2018). Psychological Wellbeing among College Students. *Journal of Social Work Education and Practice*, *3*(2), 79–89.

Vongsirimas, N., Thanoi, W., & Klainin-Yobas, P. (2017). Evaluating Psychometric Properties of the Connor-Davidson Resilience Scale (10-Item CD-RISC) among University Students in Thailand. *Journal of Nursing Science*, *35*, 25–35.

Wang, X. Q., Ren, T. R., & Wang, J. C. (2017). The Construction of University Aid-receiving Students Gratitude Education Model from the Perspective of Positive Psychology. *Educ. Teach. Forum, 3*, 94–103.

White, L. B. (2004). *The Psychological well-being and academic achievement of children raised by single parents* [Master dissertation, University of Wisconsin Stout]. http://www.uwstout.edu/lib /thesis/2004

World Health Organization. (2021). *Mental Health.* WHO. https://www.who.int/healthtopics/mental-health/#tab=tab

Yurayat, P., & Seechaliao, T. (2021). Effectiveness of Online Positive Psychology Intervention on Psychological Well-Being among Undergraduate Students. *J. Educ. Learn. 10*, 143–155. doi: . v10n4p143. doi:10.5539/jel

Zadow, C., Houghton, S., Hunter, S. C., Rosenberg, M., & Wood, L. (2017). Associations between Positive Mental Well-Being and Depressive Symptoms in Australian Adolescents. [CrossRef]. *Educ. Dev. Psychol*, *34*, 95–105.

# Chapter 14
# Innovative Ways to Boost Well-Being Among Students in Higher Education

**Sindu Padmanabhan**
https://orcid.org/0000-0001-8267-1112
*Bharathiar University, India*

## ABSTRACT

*More than 700,000 people die by suicide each year, according to WHO 2022. One fatality out of every 100 is suicide around the world. The fourth most common cause of death for people between the ages of 15 and 29 is suicide. The importance of mental health awareness in higher education institutions has grown in recent years. For students' general well-being and academic progress, it is essential to identify and treat mental health conditions. Academic performance, retention, and graduation rates can all be improved on campuses that put a strong emphasis on the welfare of their students. Higher motivation, more self-assurance, and higher levels of engagement and accomplishment are common among university students who feel more at home and like they belong. Additionally, they exhibit greater critical thinking skills, improved cultural awareness, higher levels of volunteerism, and a higher likelihood of being compassionate citizens.*

## INTRODUCTION

Well-being is an essential component of student success and satisfaction in higher education. This abstract outline innovative approaches to enhance the well-being of students in higher education institutions. As educational landscapes evolve and face new challenges, institutions must adapt and implement novel strategies to support the physical, mental, and emotional health of their student populations.

This paper explores several groundbreaking methods to promote well-being among students. First, it discusses the importance of fostering a sense of belonging through inclusive and diverse campus environments. Inclusivity efforts, such as affinity groups, peer mentoring, and targeted support for underrepresented student populations, play a crucial role in creating a supportive campus community. Second,

DOI: 10.4018/979-8-3693-2833-0.ch014

the paper highlights the integration of technology and digital platforms in providing mental health and well-being resources. Mobile applications, online counseling services, and virtual support groups offer accessible and convenient ways for students to seek help and information regarding their well-being. Third, the paper examines the role of physical health and its impact on overall well-being. Innovative approaches include wellness programs, fitness and nutrition resources, and the creation of sustainable environments on campus. These initiatives aim to empower students to lead healthier lifestyles. Fourth, the abstract delves into strategies that focus on fostering resilience and stress management among students. Initiatives like mindfulness and meditation programs, stress reduction workshops, and life skills courses empower students to cope with academic and personal challenges effectively. Furthermore, these abstract addresses the importance of personalized support, where higher education institutions offer tailored well-being plans for students. These plans consider individual needs and circumstances, offering a holistic approach to student wellness.

## GROUNDBREAKING METHODS TO PROMOTE WELL-BEING AMONG STUDENTS

Promoting well-being among students in higher education requires a multifaceted approach that incorporates innovative methods. Creating a diverse and inclusive campus culture is vital. This can involve the establishment of affinity groups, cultural centers, and initiatives that celebrate diversity. Encouraging open dialogue and understanding among students from different backgrounds fosters a sense of belonging and support. Leverage technology to offer mental health and well-being resources. Mobile applications, online counseling services, and virtual support groups provide students with convenient and accessible platforms to seek help, and information, and connect with peers facing similar challenges.

Promote physical well-being through wellness programs, fitness facilities, and nutrition resources. Consider initiatives like healthy dining options, fitness challenges, and green spaces on campus to encourage students to lead healthier lifestyles. Offer programs that focus on building resilience and teaching stress management techniques. Mindfulness and meditation programs, stress reduction workshops, and life skills courses can empower students to cope with academic and personal stress effectively (Denovan et al.,2017)

Provide individualized support and well-being plans for students. These plans consider students' unique needs, circumstances, and challenges. Personalized support can encompass academic advising, career counseling, and mental health services tailored to each student's requirements. Conduct mental health awareness campaigns and destigmatization efforts. Encourage open conversations about mental health, share personal stories, and provide resources for seeking help. Break down the barriers that prevent students from seeking assistance when needed (Flora Xuhua et al., 2018)

Establish peer mentorship programs that connect upperclassmen with underclassmen. Peer mentors can provide guidance, emotional support, and assistance with academic and social integration, fostering a sense of community and well-being. Incorporate a holistic well-being curriculum into the academic experience. Introduce courses that address mental and emotional health, stress management, and healthy living to equip students with the knowledge and skills to navigate life's challenges (Worobetz et al.,2020)

Encourage students to engage in creative outlets like art, music, and writing. These forms of self-expression can serve as therapeutic tools and outlets for stress relief, contributing to overall well-being. Implement sustainability and eco-friendly initiatives on campus. Green spaces, community gardens, and eco-conscious practices not only promote environmental well-being but also offer students a peaceful and rejuvenating environment for relaxation and reflection (de Vibe et al 2018)

Innovative methods to promote student well-being require a comprehensive and tailored approach that addresses the diverse needs and challenges faced by students in higher education. Combining these strategies can create a supportive and nurturing environment that enhances the overall well-being of students, contributing to their academic success and personal growth (Ríos-Risquez et al., 2018)

## Case Study on Groundbreaking Methods to Promote Well-Being Among Students

- **Title:** Nurturing Student Well-being: A Real-Time Case Study of Groundbreaking Methods
- **Introduction:** This real-time case study delves into the ongoing journey of "WellNest University" as it pioneers innovative methods to promote well-being among its diverse student body. Recognizing the evolving needs of its students, the university has embarked on a mission to transform the campus environment to support holistic well-being.
- **Background:** WellNest University is a medium-sized institution known for its rigorous academic programs. However, the intense academic environment has taken a toll on student well-being, leading to increased stress levels and mental health challenges. The university saw a need to address these issues proactively.

## Groundbreaking Methods Implemented

- **Holistic Well-being Curriculum:** Wellnest University redefined its curriculum to include a mandatory well-being course in the freshman year. This course covers topics like stress management, resilience, emotional intelligence, and personal growth, instilling well-being as an essential life skill.
- **Peer-Enhanced Support System:** The university established a peer mentorship program where upperclassmen undergo training in active listening, empathy, and well-being support. These mentors provide invaluable peer-to-peer support and serve as a bridge to professional services.
- **Virtual Reality Wellness Center:** A cutting-edge virtual reality (VR) wellness center was created. Students can immerse themselves in soothing natural environments or engage in relaxation exercises using VR headsets, offering a unique and immersive approach to stress reduction.
- **Smart Campus and Well-being App:** Wellnest University launched a campus-wide initiative to build a "smart campus." Sensors track air quality, noise levels, and lighting in common areas, adjusting these elements for optimal comfort and well-being. These data are accessible to students via a well-being app that also provides mental health resources and information on upcoming well-being events.
- **Sustainable Living Initiatives:** The university has placed a strong emphasis on sustainability, with initiatives like community gardens and green spaces. Students are encouraged to participate in eco-friendly practices, fostering a sense of connection with the environment and well-being.
- **Mental Health First Aid Training:** A comprehensive mental health first aid training program was launched for students, faculty, and staff. This training enables the campus community to identify and support individuals facing mental health challenges.

## OUTCOMES (ONGOING)

- **Increased Awareness:** The well-being curriculum and training have heightened awareness and conversations around well-being and mental health throughout the university.
- **Enhanced Peer Support:** The peer mentorship program has fostered a culture of empathy and support among students, creating a strong sense of belonging and emotional well-being.
- **Stress Reduction:** The VR wellness center and smart campus initiatives have contributed to a noticeable reduction in reported stress levels among students.
- **Sustainability and Connection:** The sustainability initiatives have not only contributed to a greener campus but also created opportunities for students to connect with nature, further promoting their well-being.

## CHALLENGES (ONGOING)

- **Resource Allocation:** Implementing groundbreaking methods requires substantial investment, and the university continues to seek funding to support these initiatives.
- **Evaluation and Adaptation:** Regular assessment and adaptation are crucial to ensure these methods remain effective and aligned with student needs.
- **Conclusion:** Well Nest University's ongoing efforts to promote well-being through innovative methods represent a holistic approach to education. The case study showcases the potential for higher education institutions to transform their campus environments and support the well-being of their students. While challenges persist, the results suggest a positive impact on the well-being, sense of community, and academic performance of the student body. This case study serves as a real-time model for other institutions seeking to nurture holistic well-being among their students.

## INTEGRATION OF TECHNOLOGY AND DIGITAL PLATFORMS IN PROVIDING MENTAL HEALTH AND WELL-BEING RESOURCES

The integration of technology and digital platforms in providing mental health and well-being resources has the potential to make support more accessible and effective for students in higher education. Develop and promote mobile applications specifically designed for mental health and well-being. These apps can offer features like mood tracking, relaxation exercises, cognitive-behavioral therapy tools, and access to resources, making it easier for students to manage their mental health on the go (Rupert, P. A et al.,2019)

Offer online counseling and therapy services through secure and confidential platforms. This allows students to connect with mental health professionals for one-on-one sessions, reducing the barriers of in-person appointments, stigma, and scheduling conflicts. Create virtual support groups or forums where students can connect with peers who may be facing similar challenges. These platforms enable students to share their experiences, provide mutual support, and access a community of understanding individuals. Implement telehealth services for mental health assessments and consultations. This approach can help students receive timely assessments and care, even if they are unable to visit the campus health center in person (Stawarz et al., 2019)

Develop AI-powered chatbots that offer 24/7 support and information on mental health issues. These chatbots can engage in text-based conversations with students, providing immediate assistance and referrals to appropriate resources. Create a comprehensive online repository of well-being resources, including articles, videos, self-help guides, and assessment tools. These resources can be accessible through the institution's website and cater to various aspects of well-being (Lattie et al.,2019)

Incorporate e-learning modules or courses that focus on mental health and well-being. These modules can be integrated into the curriculum, offering students the opportunity to build skills for managing stress, developing resilience, and promoting self-care. Develop gamified apps or platforms that encourage students to engage in activities that promote well-being. Gamification can make well-being initiatives more engaging and enjoyable, helping students stay motivated and committed to self-improvement (Bucci, S et al, 2019)

Use social media platforms to disseminate information about mental health and well-being, promote awareness campaigns, and share success stories. Social media can also be a medium for students to connect with campus support services. Utilize data analytics to track and monitor the well-being of students. By analyzing data from apps, online services, and surveys, institutions can identify trends and areas where additional support is needed (McGorry et al., 2022)

Implement anonymous reporting tools that allow students to report concerns about their well-being or the well-being of their peers. These tools can help institutions identify and respond to potential issues early. Encourage the use of wearable devices that monitor physical and emotional well-being indicators, such as heart rate, sleep patterns, and stress levels. Institutions can provide incentives for students to adopt these technologies and offer guidance on interpreting the data.

The integration of technology and digital platforms offers opportunities to reach students where they are and provide support in a manner that is convenient, stigma-reducing, and tailored to individual needs. However, it's essential to ensure the privacy and security of student data and to complement digital resources with human support when necessary (Walker, R et al., 2021).

## Case Study on Integration of Technology and Digital Platforms in Providing Mental Health and Well-Being Resources

- **Title:** Bridging the Gap: Real-Time Case Study of Integrating Technology for Student Mental Health and Well-being
- **Introduction:** This real-time case study highlights the ongoing efforts at "Tech Savvy University" to integrate technology and digital platforms into the provision of mental health and well-being resources. Recognizing the increasing demand for mental health support among its student population, Tec Savvy University has embarked on a journey to leverage technology to provide innovative solutions.
- **Background:** Tech Savvy University is a large urban institution with a diverse student body, including many international and commuter students. The university's counseling services were overwhelmed by demand, and students often faced long wait times for in-person appointments. To address this challenge and enhance overall student well-being, the university initiated a series of tech-driven interventions.

## INTEGRATING TECHNOLOGY

- **Mental Health Mobile App:** The university developed and launched a mental health mobile app, "MindWell," which offers features such as mood tracking, guided meditation, self-help resources, and crisis helplines. The app aims to provide students with immediate access to mental health tools and information.
- **Teletherapy Services:** Tech Savvy University established a teletherapy platform for students. This service enables students to schedule virtual appointments with licensed counselors, therapists, and psychologists. The platform ensures students receive timely support, especially during peak demand periods.
- **Online Support Groups:** To foster a sense of community and emotional support, the university introduced online support groups through video conferencing platforms. These groups address a variety of topics, from stress management to mental health awareness, and provide students with a safe space to share their experiences.
- **Artificial Intelligence Chatbot:** The university integrated an AI-powered chatbot, "WellBot," on its website. WellBot offers 24/7 support, answers common mental health questions, provides immediate intervention for crises, and guides students to appropriate resources.
- **Data Analytics and Student Feedback:** Tech Savvy University collects and analyzes data on app usage, teletherapy appointments, and chatbot interactions to identify trends and areas that require additional support. Additionally, they regularly seek feedback from students through surveys and focus groups to improve the effectiveness of their tech-driven initiatives.

## OUTCOMES (ONGOING)

- **Increased Accessibility:** The mental health mobile app and teletherapy services have significantly improved the accessibility of mental health support, reduced wait times and offering options for students who may not be comfortable with in-person counseling.
- **Enhanced Privacy:** The technology-driven solutions provide a level of privacy and anonymity that some students prefer when seeking mental health support, thereby reducing stigma.
- **Customized Support:** Data analytics and feedback mechanisms have allowed the university to tailor resources and support based on the specific needs and preferences of the student body.
- **24/7 Availability:** The AI chatbot ensures that students have access to mental health information and resources at any time, including during non-business hours.

## CHALLENGES (ONGOING)

- **Digital Equity:** Ensuring that all students have equal access to technology and are comfortable using it can be a challenge, especially for those with limited digital literacy or resources.
- **Data Privacy and Security:** Protecting students' sensitive mental health data is a top priority, and the university has implemented strict security measures.
- **Conclusion:** Tech Savvy University's ongoing efforts to integrate technology and digital platforms into the provision of mental health and well-being resources demonstrate the potential for

innovation in higher education. While challenges remain, the results indicate a positive impact on student well-being, accessibility, and privacy. This case study serves as a dynamic example of how technology can be harnessed to meet the evolving needs of students in an ever-changing higher education landscape.

## ROLE OF PHYSICAL HEALTH AND ITS IMPACT ON OVERALL WELL-BEING

The role of physical health is paramount in its impact on overall well-being, especially for students in higher education. Physical health is intricately connected to mental, emotional, and social well-being, and addressing it can significantly enhance the overall quality of life and academic success of students.

Physical health directly influences energy levels. Regular exercise and a balanced diet promote physical vitality, reducing fatigue and enhancing students' ability to concentrate, stay alert, and engage in academic activities effectively. Physical activity, such as exercise and yoga, stimulates the release of endorphins, which act as natural mood lifters. Regular physical activity helps reduce stress, anxiety, and depression, contributing to improved mental and emotional well-being (Herbert et al.,2020)

Good physical health is linked to improved cognitive function. Exercise increases blood flow to the brain, enhances memory, and supports better problem-solving and critical-thinking skills, which are essential for academic success. A healthy lifestyle promotes better sleep patterns, which are crucial for overall well-being. Adequate sleep enhances memory consolidation, mood regulation, and stress management, all of which are vital for students in higher education.

A strong immune system is essential for well-being, as it helps the body fight off illness and infection. Students who maintain their physical health are less likely to be disrupted by illness, allowing them to stay on track with their academic goals. Physical health can also impact social well-being. Engaging in physical activities, such as team sports or group fitness classes, can promote social connections and foster a sense of belonging and community among students Knifsend, C. A. (2020).

Maintaining physical health can boost self-esteem and self-confidence. When students feel good about their physical well-being, they tend to have a more positive self-image, which can positively influence their overall mental and emotional health. Establishing healthy habits during the college years can lead to a lifelong commitment to well-being. Students who prioritize their physical health are more likely to continue these habits post-graduation, reaping the long-term benefits (Liao, C., et al.,2023)

Engaging in physical health practices, including exercise and a balanced diet, can help reduce the risk of chronic diseases such as diabetes, heart disease, and obesity. This not only enhances well-being during the college years but also supports a healthier future. Physical health contributes to resilience. Physically healthy students are better equipped to handle stress and adversity, bounce back from setbacks, and persist in their academic pursuits (Casimiro-Andújar et al.,2023)

Good physical health is an essential component of an overall high quality of life. It enables students to enjoy their college experience, pursue extracurricular activities, and maintain a healthy work-life balance. Incorporating physical health practices, such as regular exercise, a balanced diet, adequate sleep, and stress management, into a student's daily routine is essential for fostering overall well-being. Educational institutions can play a crucial role by providing resources, fitness facilities, and wellness programs that promote physical health and encourage students to prioritize it as an integral part of their academic journey.

## Case Study on the Role of Physical Health and Its Impact on Overall Well-Being

- **Title:** A Holistic Approach to Student Well-being: A Real-Time Case Study on the Role of Physical Health
- **Introduction:** This real-time case study explores the ongoing initiatives at "Active University" to emphasize the pivotal role of physical health in the overall well-being of its student population. Acknowledging the interconnectedness of physical and mental health, the university has committed to a multifaceted approach to support students in achieving their optimal well-being.
- **Background:** Active University is a mid-sized institution with a robust academic environment and a diverse student body. The university recognized that the physical health of students plays a crucial role in their overall well-being. Many students struggled with academic stress, lack of exercise, and poor dietary choices, which adversely affected their physical health and emotional well-being.

## STRATEGIES IMPLEMENTED

- **Wellness Centers:** Active University established wellness centers across campus, providing access to fitness facilities, nutrition counseling, and relaxation spaces. These centers encourage students to prioritize physical health as a key component of their overall well-being.
- **Healthy Dining Options:** The university revamped its dining services, offering healthier food options, nutritional information, and a focus on locally sourced, sustainable ingredients. This initiative promotes good dietary habits and the well-being of students.
- **Outdoor Activity Spaces:** Active University invested in outdoor activity spaces such as sports fields, walking trails, and community gardens. These spaces are not only for physical exercise but also serve as areas for students to relax, connect with nature, and enhance their mental well-being.
- **Fitness Challenges:** The university introduced friendly fitness challenges and competitions to encourage students to adopt active lifestyles. These events, often tied to rewards and recognition, have motivated students to prioritize their physical health.
- **Mental Health Integration:** Recognizing the strong connection between physical and mental health, the university integrated mental health services with physical health programs. Counseling services, stress management resources, and mental health workshops are offered at wellness centers.
- **Stress Reduction Workshops:** Active University conducts workshops on stress reduction and relaxation techniques. Students learn to manage stress through yoga, meditation, and mindfulness, ultimately improving their emotional and physical well-being.

## OUTCOMES (ONGOING)

- **Increased Physical Activity:** The introduction of outdoor activity spaces and fitness challenges has led to a noticeable increase in physical activity among students, contributing to improved physical health.

- **Healthy Eating Choices:** The availability of healthy dining options and nutritional information has encouraged students to make more nutritious food choices, leading to better dietary habits and overall well-being.
- **Stress Reduction:** The integration of stress reduction workshops and mental health support at wellness centers has contributed to lower stress levels among students and improved emotional well-being.
- **Community Building:** The outdoor activity spaces have fostered a sense of community and connection among students, contributing to their social well-being.

## CHALLENGES (ONGOING)

- **Changing Habits:** Encouraging students to adopt and maintain healthier lifestyles can be a challenge, requiring ongoing education and support.
- **Resource Allocation:** Developing and maintaining wellness centers and outdoor spaces can be resource-intensive, necessitating careful budgeting and fundraising efforts.
- **Conclusion:** Active University's ongoing commitment to prioritizing physical health as an integral part of student well-being exemplifies a holistic approach to higher education. This real-time case study highlights the potential for academic institutions to significantly impact the well-being of their students by promoting physical health. Despite challenges, the university's efforts are producing positive outcomes in terms of physical, emotional, and social well-being, serving as a model for other institutions seeking to prioritize student well-being.

## STRATEGIES THAT FOCUS ON FOSTERING RESILIENCE AND STRESS MANAGEMENT AMONG STUDENTS

Fostering resilience and stress management among students in higher education is essential for their well-being and academic success. Introduce mindfulness and meditation programs on campus to help students develop awareness and stress management skills. These practices can improve emotional regulation and enhance resilience. Organize stress reduction workshops that teach practical techniques for managing stress, including deep breathing, progressive muscle relaxation, and time management strategies (Quinn, J. E. et al., 2019).

Offer counseling services with a focus on stress management and resilience-building. Trained counselors can work with students to develop coping strategies and provide a safe space for discussing stressors. Incorporate resilience training courses into the curriculum. These courses can teach students how to bounce back from adversity, develop problem-solving skills, and build emotional strength. Create peer support groups where students can share their experiences, challenges, and coping strategies. These groups offer a sense of belonging and provide opportunities for students to learn from their peers (Li, Z.-S et al.,2020)

Promote healthy living through wellness initiatives that include exercise, nutrition, and sleep. Physical well-being can enhance resilience and stress management capabilities. Provide workshops or courses on time management and organizational skills. These skills can help students manage their academic workloads more effectively and reduce stress related to deadlines. Offer academic support services, such as tutoring and study skills workshops. These services can help students feel more confident in their academic abilities, reducing academic-related stress (Lopez et al.,2018)

Encourage self-care through workshops that teach students the importance of setting boundaries, managing their schedules, and prioritizing their mental and emotional health. Develop crisis intervention plans to support students facing acute stress or emergencies. These plans should outline clear steps for identifying, supporting, and referring students in crisis. Establish peer mentorship programs that pair experienced students with newcomers. Mentors can guide managing stress, setting goals, and navigating the challenges of higher education (Jennifer First et al.,2018)

Create an online repository of stress management resources, including articles, videos, and self-help tools. This ensures that students have access to information and guidance at any time. Offer workshops focused on building resilience as a professional skill. These workshops can prepare students for future career challenges and help them adapt to changes in the job market. Promote a healthy work-life balance by emphasizing the importance of taking breaks, having hobbies, and maintaining social connections outside of academic commitments (Chew et al.,2022)

Conduct awareness campaigns to reduce the stigma associated with seeking help for stress and mental health issues. Encourage open dialogue and make students aware of available resources.

Create feedback mechanisms for students to express concerns and suggestions related to stress management and resilience-building initiatives. This ensures that programs remain responsive to students' evolving needs. By implementing these strategies, higher education institutions can empower students to develop the skills and support systems needed to manage stress effectively, enhance their resilience, and thrive in their academic pursuits.

## Case Study on Strategies That Focus on Fostering Resilience and Stress Management Among Students

- **Title:** Nurturing Resilience: A Real-Time Case Study on Strategies for Student Stress Management
- **Introduction:** This real-time case study examines the ongoing initiatives at "Resilience University" aimed at fostering resilience and stress management skills among its diverse student population. Recognizing the increasing prevalence of stress-related issues, the university has adopted a multifaceted approach to empower students with the tools they need to thrive in the face of adversity.
- **Background:** Resilience University is a mid-sized institution known for its rigorous academic programs and diverse student body. The university observed that students were increasingly struggling with stress, anxiety, and academic pressures, affecting their overall well-being and academic performance.

## STRATEGIES IMPLEMENTED

- **Resilience and Coping Skills Courses:** The university introduced resilience and coping skills courses as part of the core curriculum. These courses focus on building resilience, emotional intelligence, and stress management techniques. Students are required to take these courses in their first and second years.

- **Mindfulness and Meditation Spaces:** Resilience established designated mindfulness and meditation spaces across campus. These spaces provide a tranquil environment for students to practice stress reduction techniques and promote emotional well-being.
- **Peer-Led Support Groups:** The university-initiated peer-led support groups where students can connect with peers facing similar challenges. These groups provide a safe space for sharing experiences and learning from one another's strategies for managing stress.
- **Mental Health First Aid Training:** Students, faculty, and staff are offered mental health first aid training. This program equips individuals with the skills to identify signs of distress, offer initial support, and provide referrals to appropriate resources.
- **Resilience Mobile App:** Resilience developed a mobile app that offers a range of resilience-building resources, including guided meditation, stress management exercises, and tips for enhancing emotional well-being. The app is accessible to students and staff.
- **Stress Reduction Workshops:** The university conducts regular stress reduction workshops that provide practical tools for managing stress, time management, and improving work-life balance.

## OUTCOMES (ONGOING)

Resilience and coping skills courses have resulted in students reporting increased emotional resilience and adaptability in the face of challenges. The availability of mindfulness spaces, stress reduction workshops, and the mobile app have led to a noticeable reduction in reported stress levels among students. Peer-led support groups have fostered a strong sense of community and support among students, contributing to their social well-being. Mental health first aid training has facilitated early intervention and support for students facing mental health challenges, potentially reducing the severity of issues.

## CHALLENGES (ONGOING)

Implementing these initiatives requires the allocation of resources, including faculty training, space utilization, and technology development. Maintaining ongoing support for these initiatives and ensuring they remain effective is an ongoing challenge that requires consistent evaluation and adaptation. Resilience University's real-time case study demonstrates the potential for academic institutions to prioritize the well-being of their students through targeted strategies focused on fostering resilience and stress management. Despite challenges, the university's efforts are resulting in positive outcomes in terms of student resilience, stress reduction, and community building, serving as an inspiring model for other institutions seeking to enhance the well-being of their students.

In conclusion, the well-being of students in higher education is a multifaceted challenge that requires innovative and diverse strategies. By promoting inclusivity, utilizing technology, enhancing physical health, building resilience, and providing personalized support, institutions can boost the overall well-being of their students, ultimately contributing to their academic success and personal growth.

## REFERENCES

Ang, W. H. D., Chew, H. S. J., Dong, J., Yi, H., Mahendren, R., & Lau, Y. (2022). Digital training for building resilience: Systematic review, meta-analysis, and meta-regression. *Stress and Health*, *38*(5), 848–869. doi:10.1002mi.3154 PMID:35460533

Bucci, S., Schwannauer, M., & Berry, N. (2019). The digital revolution and its impact on mental health care. *Psychology and Psychotherapy: Theory, Research and Practice*, *92*(2), 277–297. doi:10.1111/papt.12222 PMID:30924316

Casimiro-Andújar, A. J., Checa, J. C., Lirola, M.-J., & Artés-Rodríguez, E. (2023). Promoting physical activity and health in the workplace: A qualitative study among university workers, Spain. *International Journal of Environmental Research and Public Health*, *20*(3), 2350. doi:10.3390/ijerph20032350 PMID:36767715

de Vibe, M., Solhaug, I., Rosenvinge, J. H., Tyssen, R., Hanley, A., & Garland, E. (2018). Six-year positive effects of a mindfulness-based intervention on mindfulness, coping and well-being in medical and psychology students; Results from a randomized controlled trial. *PLoS One*, *13*(4), e0196053. doi:10.1371/journal.pone.0196053 PMID:29689081

Denovan, A., & Macaskill, A. (2017). Stress and subjective well-being among first year UK undergraduate students. *Journal of Happiness Studies*, *18*(2), 505–525. doi:10.100710902-016-9736-y

First, J., First, N. L., & Brian Houston, J. (2018). Resilience and Coping Intervention (RCI): A Group Intervention to Foster College Student Resilience. *Social Work with Groups*, *41*(3), 198–210. doi:10.1080/01609513.2016.1272032

He, F. X., Turnbull, B., Kirshbaum, M. N., Phillips, B., & Klainin-Yobas, P. (2018). Assessing stress, protective factors and psychological well-being among undergraduate nursing students. *Nurse Education Today*, *68*, 4–12. doi:10.1016/j.nedt.2018.05.013 PMID:29870871

Herbert, C., Meixner, F., Wiebking, C., & Gilg, V. (2020). Regular physical activity, short-term exercise, mental health, and well-being among university students: The results of an online and a laboratory study. *Frontiers in Psychology*, *11*, 509. doi:10.3389/fpsyg.2020.00509 PMID:32528333

Holt, E. W., Lombard, Q. K., Best, N., Smiley-Smith, S., & Quinn, J. E. (2019). Active and passive use of green space, health, and well-being amongst university students. *International Journal of Environmental Research and Public Health*, *16*(3), 424. doi:10.3390/ijerph16030424 PMID:30717193

Knifsend, C. A. (2020). Intensity of activity involvement and psychosocial well-being among students. *Active Learning in Higher Education*, *21*(2), 116–127. doi:10.1177/1469787418760324

Lattie, E. G., Adkins, E. C., Winquist, N., Stiles-Shields, C., Wafford, Q. E., & Graham, A. K. (2019). Digital mental health interventions for depression, anxiety, and enhancement of psychological well-being among college students: Systematic review. *Journal of Medical Internet Research*, *21*(7), e12869. doi:10.2196/12869 PMID:31333198

Li, Z.-S., & Hasson, F. (2020). Resilience, stress, and psychological well-being in nursing students: A systematic review. *Nurse Education Today*, *90*(104440), 104440. doi:10.1016/j.nedt.2020.104440 PMID:32353643

Liao, C., Nong, L., Wu, Y.-F., Wu, Y.-T., & Ye, J.-H. (2023). The relationships between university students' physical activity needs, involvement, flow experience and sustainable well-being in the post-pandemic era. *Sustainability (Basel), 15*(11), 8719. doi:10.3390u15118719

Lopez, V., Yobas, P., Chow, Y. L., & Shorey, S. (2018). Does building resilience in undergraduate nursing students happen through clinical placements? A qualitative study. *Nurse Education Today, 67*, 1–5. doi:10.1016/j.nedt.2018.04.020 PMID:29704800

McGorry, P. D., Mei, C., Chanen, A., Hodges, C., Alvarez-Jimenez, M., & Killackey, E. (2022). Designing and scaling up integrated youth mental health care. *World Psychiatry; Official Journal of the World Psychiatric Association (WPA), 21*(1), 61–76. doi:10.1002/wps.20938 PMID:35015367

Ríos-Risquez, M. I., García-Izquierdo, M., Sabuco-Tebar, E., Carrillo-Garcia, C., & Solano-Ruiz, C. (2018). Connections between academic burnout, resilience, and psychological well-being in nursing students: A longitudinal study. *Journal of Advanced Nursing, 74*(12), 2777–2784. doi:10.1111/jan.13794 PMID:29992596

Rupert, P. A., & Dorociak, K. E. (2019). Self-care, stress, and well-being among practicing psychologists. *Professional Psychology, Research and Practice, 50*(5), 343–350. doi:10.1037/pro0000251

Stawarz, K., Preist, C., & Coyle, D. (2019). Use of smartphone apps, social media, and Web-based resources to support mental health and well-being: Online survey. *JMIR Mental Health, 6*(7), e12546. doi:10.2196/12546 PMID:31301126

Walker, R., Usher, K., Jackson, D., Reid, C., Hopkins, K., Shepherd, C., Smallwood, R., & Marriott, R. (2021). Connection to... Addressing digital inequities in supporting the well-being of young Indigenous Australians in the wake of COVID-19. *International Journal of Environmental Research and Public Health, 18*(4), 2141. doi:10.3390/ijerph18042141 PMID:33671737

Worobetz, A., Retief, P. J., Loughran, S., Walsh, J., Casey, M., Hayes, P., Bengoechea, E. G., O'Regan, A., Woods, C., Kelly, D., Connor, R. O., Grath, D. M., & Glynn, L. G. (2020). A feasibility study of an exercise intervention to educate and promote health and well-being among medical students: The 'MED-WELL' programme. *BMC Medical Education, 20*(1), 183. doi:10.118612909-020-02097-2 PMID:32493427

# Chapter 15
# Emotional Wellbeing of Students in Higher Education Institutions

**Oluwakemi Bolanle Ajayi**
*University of the Witwatersrand, South Africa*

## ABSTRACT

*The emotional well-being of students at higher education institutions was examined in this chapter. The study used a conceptual review as its framework, and data from published results presented in this chapter showed that most students in higher education institutions faced emotional challenges as a result of their new environment, financial challenges, academic-related stress, anxiety, and depression. Furthermore, many students in higher education are still adjusting to their new experiences and finding their fit in order to achieve in their academic pursuits. It is recommended that higher education institutions adopt innovative techniques to increase students' emotional wellbeing, such as boosting student awareness, building and designing a culture of wellbeing, and providing digital mental services.*

## INTRODUCTION

Emotional well-being is characterised as a sense of calm and freedom from tension (Jordan, 2021). Emotional well-being measures how well people control their thoughts, feelings, and actions in order to function in their daily lives. People's emotional well-being has been found to influence their mental health (Jordan, 2021). Positive emotional well-being is essential for achieving balanced mental health and general well-being. According to research, people with positive emotional health are better able to cope with everyday challenges and problems, resulting in more stable mental health and general well-being (Lister, Seale & Douce, 2021). Research has shown that emotional distress increases vulnerability to physical sickness by altering the immunological response, resulting in poor health conditions. As a result, a convincing intervention aimed at improving an individual's emotional well-being is likely to have a good impact on their overall health (Walker, 2022; Lister et al, 2021).

DOI: 10.4018/979-8-3693-2833-0.ch015

Emotional wellbeing is the ability of a person to accept and control their emotions as well as deal with obstacles in life. How well someone is able to function on a daily basis or how they are able to handle change or uncertainty can both be influenced by their emotional health. A person's mental and physical health may suffer as a result of emotional difficulties (Douwes et al., 2023). Many college students are struggling with well-being difficulties such as psychological and emotional distress, anxiety and depressive symptoms, and a higher risk of burnout (Wang, 2020). Centres for Disease Control and Prevention (CDC) defines wellbeing as the presence of positive emotions and moods (contentment or happiness), the absence of negative emotions (depression or anxiety), satisfaction with life, fulfilment, and positive functioning (Izutsu et al., 2020; CDC, 2018). Academic achievement is fundamentally reliant on student welfare. According to the CDC and other top public health organisations, wellbeing has both individual and aggregate effects on a range of outcomes of interest to students in higher education. These effects can be both negative and positive. A vast body of research has demonstrated that mental health issues have a major impact on academic achievement and graduation rates in higher education, which goes beyond simply having happy students (Cage et al., 2020). Well-being is crucial for degree completion, just as it is for students' success in their day-to-day lives. However, based on the state of affairs as they are today, far too many students in higher education institution lack the emotional stability necessary for them to excel in the academic setting and realise their full potential (Cage et al., 2020).

Although managing stress is a normal part of life, stress can have a negative impact on some students' physical, emotional, and mental health (Lister, 2021). The dropout rates for students who have a diagnosable mental health issue range from 43 percent to as high as 86 percent (Teixeira et al., 2021). Given that most mental diseases initially manifest in youth and early adulthood, this risk is especially important for institutions of higher education (Teixeira et al., 2021). Children and teenagers may experience mental health concerns. According to a review of related literature, girls are more likely than boys to experience mental health issues as they get older (Cage et al., 2020). As a result, a lot of graduate and undergraduate students arrive on campus suffering from an undetected mental illness that manifests itself throughout their time in school. Attention is being paid to the health of students in higher education institution. In full-time higher education, students' ages typically range from 17 to 24. According to Truschel (2020), this is also the important age for the start of psychological and emotional issues. Truschel (2020) asserts that student well-being is receiving more attention in higher education since it affects academic performance and drop-out rates. Due to the detrimental effects on the emotional health of students in higher education, the COVID-19 epidemic and its effects, such as social exclusion, lockdowns, and online education, have increased this emphasis (Manap et al., 2019).

Some of the challenges that relate to the emotional wellbeing of students in higher institutions are presented below.

## CHALLENGES RELATING TO THE EMOTIONAL WELLBEING OF STUDENTS IN HIGHER EDUCATION INSTITUTIONS

Young adulthood is defined as an identity-forming period in which individuals go through emotional, behavioural, sexual, economic, academic, and social transformations, as well as different conflicts. Students are more likely than the overall population to suffer from mental health disorders. Statistically, more than half of American public university students suffer from depression and anxiety (Cage et al, 2020). Similarly, a survey of undergraduate students at Coventry University in the United Kingdom in

2006 (Lattie et al, 2022) discovered that many students had suffered from mental health illnesses such as anxiety and depression. Maser et al. (Lattie et al, 2022) found that the prevalence of mental health disorders such as anxiety and depression is higher in medical school than in the general non student community of the same age, lending credence to these findings. These studies have revealed that the prevalence of emotional health disorder among students has remained higher than in the general population over the last two decades.

According to research from developing nations, "12 to 46 percent of students at university experience mental health problems" (Auerbach et al., 2018; Holt et al, 2016). During the pandemic, students in Brazil suffered high levels of stress, anxiety, and depression (Bezerra et al., 2021). Another South African study discovered that the prevalence of depression and anxiety symptoms among university students increased dramatically during the pandemic (Naidoo et al., 2021). During the pandemic, financial stress was also a serious concern for students in the global south and southern Africa. Financial stress was found to be a significant predictor of poor mental health outcomes among students in a study conducted in Nigeria (Ojediran & Emeke, 2021). Furthermore, mental health treatments are usually constricted or unavailable in the global south and southern Africa, and the epidemic has exacerbated this problem. According to a study conducted in Ghana, students have limited access to mental health services, and those who do have access to services are dissatisfied with the quality of care (Tagoe et al., 2020). The epidemic has interrupted academic timetables and moved learning to online platforms, affecting students' academic performance significantly. According to a study conducted in Uganda, students reported worse academic performance during the pandemic, which was linked to higher stress and anxiety (Kabagenyi et al., 2020).

The COVID-19 epidemic in South Africa may have worsened existing imbalances and increased learning losses for vulnerable children (Eloff, 2021). According to the findings of a large student mental health survey involving 26 publicly funded universities in South Africa and 29 000 students - which was initiated by Universities South Africa (USAf) in 2022 - 20% of students in higher education institutions in South Africa require mental health support, and more than 70% of those students do not receive it (Walker, 2022). According to an ISB survey, many overseas students studying in the United Kingdom during the epidemic were disillusioned and unsatisfied with their experience, with some questioning the value of their degree (Morgan, 2021). According to a study undertaken by researchers at the University of Johannesburg, many students were disillusioned with online learning during the pandemic, with some believing that their education had been jeopardised and that they were not getting good value for money (Phatudi, Mphahlele, & Mashele, 2021). The purpose of this study was to investigate and comprehend students' experiences of wellness in the education faculty of a large urban university in South Africa during the Covid-19 pandemic.

For students in higher education, well-being issues are frequently complicated; concerns include:

## Family Issues

There are numerous elements influencing students' mental health, but the particular function of family as one of the most crucial growing environments cannot be overlooked. Counsellors will frequently encounter psychological problems among students, greedy talk to students, and the process of psychological inquiry discovered that after entering the university students showed a significant portion of the psychological problem as a teenager problem left or accumulation, in the process of student growth, family factors to students' emotional, physical, and mental development has a huge impact (Lister et al, 2021). In China, a youngster spends about two-thirds of his or her life in the family, from birth to college.

Family economic situations, family structure, parent's education level, and so on have a non-negligible impact on students' mental health, particularly a parent-child relationship, including family upbringing style, which has a significant impact on students' mental health (Lister et al, 2021).

The influence of the husband-wife connection, including the relationship between husband and wife, getting along with the family, will have an impact on the child's mental health. For example, if the couple's relationship is not good, they frequently quarrel, and the fight creates an unsafe environment for the child, the child lacks care, lacks a sense of security, may be irritable, pessimistic, loathing, and even depressed, there may be a certain tendency to violence and behaviour, and heterosexual relationship and marital life cognition may also produce deviation (Hawkins, 2019). The relationship between father and son, as well as mother and daughter, will have an effect on students' mental health. The mutual respect, equality, and harmony relationship will make the youngsters feel more cared for and valued. A child's mind is healthy when he feels protected, loved, and respected, his needs are addressed, and his self-awareness and view of the outer world are good. As a result, parents should focus on developing a harmonious, personal family emotional environment, establishing a healthy parent-child relationship, and promoting the child's mental health growth (Evans et al, 2018).

The parent-child interaction is critical for the establishment of stable attachment between the parent and the child beginning at birth (Maunder & LaMothe, 2020). Attachment theory seeks to define a variety of brain systems and behavioural processes that contribute to an infant's bonding or attachment to his or her parents during childhood. This attachment promotes the infant's social and emotional development (Hawkins, 2019). Abdullahi et al (2020) revealed a statistically significant relationship between stable attachment and "later good functioning" of the child. A benefit of building a healthy attachment to parents is that it provides a solid foundation from which the child may face emotional and life's challenges (Abdullahi et al, 2020). That is why a "strong, mutual emotional attachment" (Bruffaerts et al, 2018) promotes a young person's growth and leads to the internalisation of adaptive conduct. In contrast, there is a strong link between early insecure attachment and later emotional and behavioural problems (Maunder & LaMothe, 2020). Similarly, attachment theory suggests that disruption of the attachment bond (between primary carer and child) may result in "uncontrolled forms" (Bullivant, 2021) of fear, anger, distorted emotional communication, and psychopathology in the young person. As a result, where a secure attachment did not develop and adults are unable to establish secure relationships that can mitigate the impact of stress, children grow up with insecure attachment as a risk factor for their emotional wellbeing due to serious stress, which may cause harm later in life (Bullivant, 2021).

Furthermore, strained parent-child relationships during childhood and adolescence have been associated to the beginning of mental health problems such as major depression, anxiety disorders, and schizophrenia (Bullivant, 2021; Eloff, 2021) propose that trauma can alter the brain, making young people experiencing extreme forms of stress more prone to metal health issues such as behavioural, emotional, and social difficulties, mood disorders, PTSD, and personality disorders (Farrell, 2021). Patterson et al (2021) discovered that ineffective parenting contributes to poor emotional and psychological adjustment; thus, it is reasonable to argue that a negative relationship between the parent and child, particularly one that causes significant stress for the young person, may be the "single strongest" (Paton, 2021 p27) determinant of high-risk outcomes for the developing young person. The next section discusses the financial challenges and wellbeing.

## Financial Challenges and Wellbeing

Financial stress can have an impact on a person's capacity to operate well in both their personal and professional lives. Individuals who are under financial stress may struggle to concentrate, make decisions, and solve problems. They may also have a low sense of self-worth and self-esteem. In recent decades, the increased engagement of young people in higher education has focused attention on student emotional well-being, as well as concerns about the impact of financial hardship (Simkins, 2016).

A number of studies have found a link between student debt and mental health problems in students, but other investigations have found no link (Seligman, 2018). Given the significant literature on the association between debt and mental health in the general population, such links may be expected. A 2013 systematic study (Seligman, 2018) discovered that higher levels of debt were linked to depression, suicide, drug and alcohol addiction, and psychotic disorders. Loneliness is exacerbated by societal influences. Given the available information, it is impossible to infer with certainty if financial stress is connected with students' mental health, or which domain of financial stress is most important, the quantity of debt, previous financial issues, or debt anxiety (Eloff, 2021). Furthermore, it is unclear whether the correlations are bidirectional or resistant to adjustment for potential confounders such as socioeconomic background and prior mental health disorders. As a result, the current study attempted to quickly describe the existing literature in this field, with a focus on students in higher education institutions (Farrell, 2021).

Young adulthood is frequently linked to an increased risk of mental health disorders (Soldevila-Domenech et al, 2021). It is also a big life shift that is usually accompanied by an increase in financial responsibility. An assessment of existing literature on debt and mental health in college students suggests that there should be a greater emphasis on the study of college students' financial and psychological well-being. Sapiro (2020) discovered a correlation between college students' poor financial situations and their low mental and physical health. Patterson et al (2021) discovered that financial pressures were connected with higher levels of anxiety and depression among college students in the United Kingdom. Academic achievement has also been connected to financial hardship. Another study of British university student discovered a link between poor mental health and financial pressures such as trouble paying bills on time (Nielsen, 2021). Furthermore, students who pondered leaving their academic programmes before completing them due to financial constraints reported poorer emotional and psychological wellbeing.

In South Africa, 2015 may go down in history with 1976 as a year when students displayed their power to change the direction of education history. The #FeesMustFall campaign compelled the government to consider the myriad difficulties confronting South Africa's higher education industry. Decades of rapidly growing access, along with declining government subsidies, have presented a variety of problems to higher education institutions. Higher education institutions must strive to satisfy enrolment targets while also providing high-quality education (Simkins, 2016). Students who have been accepted into one of South Africa's higher education institutions encounter a plethora of problems that may have an impact on their lives and subjective perceptions of their wellbeing. This is particularly true for first generation college students. They have no prior familial experience with higher education and so no reservoir of information from which to draw to adapt to their new lifestyles (Barry et al, 2017). As a result, intense emotions such as displacement, worry, and guilt can exist alongside the more often accepted emotional responses of hopeful anticipation, enjoyment, and higher self-esteem in the daily lives of first-generation students (Spies, 2022).

The high rates of depression and even suicide among South Africa's student population present prima facie evidence that our understanding of the elements influencing students' subjective wellbeing needs to be re-evaluated and deepened. More research, according Holt et al, (2016), is needed to investigate the psychological characteristics related with these events, particularly within the cultural and socioeconomic context of South Africa. This paper seeks to respond to this challenge by examining the levels and trends in SWB of successive batches of first-year economics students at a comprehensive university in Gauteng's heartland between 2014 and 2017. Students in comprehensive universities come from a variety of educational backgrounds, each with their own set of features and situations (Wiens et al, 2017).

## Stress, Anxiety and Depression

Stress is defined as a specific interaction between a person and his or her environment that the person perceives as exhausting or exceeding his or her resources and harming his or her well-being (Mahon, 2021). The idea of stress has received a lot of attention in regard to student emotional well-being, and reports of high levels of felt stress among these groups are common (Farrell, 2021). Every student faces the challenges of course work, a new environment and new people, and for those living away from home for the first time, learning to cope financially, emotionally, and socially on their own. Furthermore, other potential sources of stress for healthcare students include the emotions involved in dealing with patients and the development of applied clinical skills (Farrell, 2021). Stress has been linked to increased levels of depression (Farrell, 2021), drug and alcohol use, anxiety and attrition in healthcare students.

The cost of training healthcare professionals is a big investment, and attrition has a significant financial impact in addition to being terrible for the student concerned. Consequently, it becomes critical to identify students who may find their course more stressful than their colleagues in order to target them early for guidance and support. Various psychological and psychiatric research undertaken in a variety of industrialised and developing nations over the past decades have revealed that the prevalence of stress, anxiety, and depression (Wang, 2020) is higher among university students than in the general population. Stress anxiety and depression, as a multi-factorial illness, is widely known to generate personal, health, societal, and occupational concerns (Teixeira et al, 2021), all of which can directly influence and be influenced by quality of life. According to self-reported tests and surveys, the level of stress is inversely connected to life quality and well-being (Wang, 2020).

Untreated poor mental health can cause distress among students and, as a result, have a negative impact on their quality of life and academic performance, including, but not limited to, lower academic integrity, alcohol and substance abuse, reduced empathetic behaviour, relationship instability, lack of self-confidence, and suicidal thoughts (Teixeira et al, 2021). Mental health issues affect students and young people as well. Students encounter numerous academic challenges, such as the load of tests and assignments, a lack of sleep, and anxieties about future job, societal expectations, and higher education. According to research, students have a high prevalence of depression, anxiety, and stress symptoms. A research of secondary school girls in the Kingdom of Saudi Arabia (KSA) found that 73% had signs of at least one of the three investigated disorders (depression, anxiety, and stress), and 50% had symptoms of at least two. According to the study, the prevalence of depression was 42%, anxiety was 66%, and stress was 53% among participating students. Students' despair, anxiety, and stress levels were likewise positively and strongly connected. Another research of Turkish university student revealed similar percentages of depression, anxiety, and stress (27%, 47%, and 27%, respectively), while anxiety and stress scores were greater among female students than male students. According to the study, first- and second-year students exhibited higher levels of sadness, anxiety, and stress than other students. Students who were content with their academic achievement, on the other hand, showed lower levels of sadness, anxiety, and stress than those who were not (Morgan & Simmons, 2021).

Anxiety, according to World Health Organisation (2021), is a dynamic emotional state characterised by tension, unease, concern, and other uneasy feelings caused by a person's impending or potential threat. Unnecessary anxiety reduces students' motivation in studying and impedes their academic achievement (Paton, 2021), but reasonable anxiety promotes learning effectiveness and engagement by improving the brain's reaction time and attentiveness (Paton, 2021). Anxiety and fear are obvious on a personal and institutional level. Since the global reaction to the COVID-19 outbreak (isolation through lockdown) prioritised physical health over mental health, the impact on people's mental health has been ignored. Evidence of the consequences on emotional health appears to imply that anxiety has surpassed work-related stress as the students in higher education institution primary concern (WHO, 2021). Students' skill and expertise in providing instruction in the current context (online) is a crucial element leading to their heightened anxiety levels.

It is normal to feel depressed from time to time, but if that poor mood persists day after day, it could indicate depression. Major depression is defined as a period of melancholy or apathy accompanied by other symptoms that lasts at least two weeks and is severe enough to interfere with daily activities. Depression does not indicate a lack of strength or a nasty disposition. A melancholy mood and/or loss of interest in life are the basic signs of depression. Activities that were once enjoyable have lost their allure (Ojediran & Emeka, 2021). Students in challenging situation may also experience feelings of guilt or worthlessness, as well as a loss of hope and recurring thoughts of death or suicide.

In the University of Pennsylvania study published by Bullivant (2021), 61 percent of survey respondents classified anxiety as a significant student mental condition. Anxiety disorder symptoms are commonly misdiagnosed as ordinary stress or dismissed as the result of someone being unduly anxious. Panic attacks may be misdiagnosed as a medical condition, such as a tension headache or heart attack, depending on how your body reacts to high levels of particular chemicals (Bullivant, 2021). Because each person's symptoms manifest differently, what indicates the presence of anxiety in one person may not be the same in another (Hamza et al, 2021). As a result, the reasons of anxiety vary from individual to person; yet, several causes are widespread among university students. Anxiety is typically caused by stress, life experiences, genetics, and brain chemicals (Hamza et al, 2021). As a result, suitable steps of uttermost zeal are required to ensure that the condition is removed from the learners' lives.

Despite all attempts to raise awareness and address mental health issues among university students, there is still an upsurge in depression and suicide among students (Kunjiapu & Kunasegaran, 2021), demonstrating that the measures in place are ineffective. In addition to an increase in the prevalence of mental health concerns, a comparison of students and non-college-attending peers revealed an increase in the severity of psychiatric diseases for which students receive treatment (Truschel, 2020). Suicide rates among adolescents, for example, have risen dramatically in recent decades (Truschel, 2020). Suicide as a result of neglected mental health is, in fact, the second leading cause of death among American college students (Truschel, 2020), highlighting the significance of identifying and addressing risk factors linked with stress, anxiety and depression.

## Academic Pressure

Academic pressure is a typical phenomenon among students, either as a result of the transition from high school to university or as a result of the increasing difficulty level of courses and assignments as necessary in university. Academic pressure refers to the sense of having too many stresses and demands, stressing about tests and academic work, and being unable to manage because the calendar is simply too hectic for students to handle (Kidd, 2021). Adolescence is a perilous phase in which young people struggle with self-organization and role insecurity. Academic assessments, interpersonal relationships, relationship troubles, life changes, and career exploration are the main sources of stress for them. Such stress is often associated with emotional issues (Hughes & Spanner, 2019). Students have distinct expectations, goals, and values that they desire to fulfil while studying in educational institutions, which is only achievable if the students' expectations, goals, and values are merged with those of the institutions. However, if it does not match, students may be subjected to academic pressure (Hughes & Spanner, 2019).

Academic pressure may be the single most important stressor affecting students' emotional well-being at higher education institutions. Some student groups may be more stressed than others, and the coronavirus (COVID-19) pandemic may aggravate the stress response even further (Kabagenyi et al, 2020). Academic stress, combined with bad interpersonal interactions with friends and family, is a critical element in adolescents' emotional well-being. Stressful occurrences typically occur when students perceive a situation to be hazardous or difficult and lack the necessary coping abilities to deal with it (WHO, 2021). These are occasions in which the individual believes it is critical to respond but an adequate solution is not readily available.

Students' stress is multifaceted and can be ascribed to a range of contributing variables. A rising body of evidence demonstrates that academic-related stress is a significant factor in higher education (Kidd, 2021). For example, 87% of college students polled across the United States identified education as their top source of stress. University students face new academic challenges such as a heavy academic course load, significant studying, time management, classroom competition, financial concerns, familial obligations, and adjusting to a new environment (Soldevila-Domenech et al, 2021). Academic stress can impair motivation, impede academic progress, and increase dropout rates among students. Academic stress is perceived differently by different categories of higher education students (Tagoe et al, 2020). Female university students, for example, report higher levels of stress than their male colleagues. Male and female students respond to pressures in various ways (Wiens et al, 2021). Furthermore, non-binary students report more stressors and mental health difficulties than their cisgender peers (Wiens et al, 2021). Students' academic year of study has also been demonstrated to influence academic stress levels.

However, the influence of perceived academic stress on mental wellbeing is complex and is dependent on both internal and external personal resources, such as coping and social support (Morgan & Hoffman, 2018). The level of perceived academic stress is determined by underlying variables or stressors. Isolation can deplete personal resources, worsening the link between perceived academic stress and mental well-being. Academic stress had a greater influence on mental wellbeing among international students, owing to a lack of assistance coping and social interactions (Levula Wilson & Harré, 2016). Personality influences the relationship between perceived academic stress and mental well-being. Self-critical perfectionism was found to have a substantial positive relationship with depression and stress symptoms (Bernstein et al, 2023), whereas students who are open to new experiences and surroundings were found to have much less academic stress and were better able to adjust to new workload (Bernstein et al, 2023). Finally, using the appropriate coping style is critical in dealing with academic stress since it prevents the development of its (potentially) negative repercussions (Barbayannis et al, 2022). Students' ability to cope with stressors is connected to the number of mental health problems they face (Barbayannis et al, 2022; Montagni et al, 2020). Approach coping, also known as problem-focused coping, appears to attenuate the relationship between perceived academic stress and mental well-being (Kurki et al, 2021).

The most impactful stressor, academic pressure, had a direct influence on emotional wellness that was not explained by perceived stress. Approach coping and emotional stability reduce the negative influence of perceived stress on emotional well-being (Rochin Demong et al, 2023). To safeguard mental health of students, it is critical to reduce perceived stress and build students' resilience. To lessen students' perceived stress, academic pressure must be reduced. Furthermore, assisting students in developing emotional well-being competencies by teaching approach-related coping methods and resilience abilities (Rochin Demong et al, 2023).

## CHALLENGES THAT RESULT FROM NEW ENVIRONMENT

Stress is defined as an individual's response to external expectations and pressures that might be perceived as dangerous or overwhelming (Spies, 2022). The degree to which various situations are perceived to be stressful is referred to as perceived stress (Maunder & LaMothe, 2022). There is a danger of lower mental wellness when one lacks personal resources to lessen perceived stress (lack of coping). Perceived stress has a significant impact on students' emotional well-being. There is evidence that university students' reported stress level has increased in recent years (Maunder & LaMothe, 2022).

A good environment that is sustained supports student social, mental, and emotional growth, as well as behavioural and learning outcomes, while also ensuring physical and social safety (Abdullahi et al, 2020; Anglim et al, 2020). Positive environment has been linked to improved academic achievement and performance, adaptive psychosocial adjustment, school satisfaction, sense of belonging, academic value and self-concept, motivation to learn, decreased behavioural problems, and overall positive health and wellbeing (Utami et al, 2021; Wang, 2020). Adjustment to a new environment can also lead to student burnout, lower student retention, and increase student stress, all of which can have an impact on students' emotional well-being (Rochin Demong et al, 2023, Widdicks, 2020).

Individual connectedness or a sense of belonging describes the quality of social relationships within the academic environment: the extent to which students feel like they belong in their new environment and are cared for by the school (Amaya et al, 2019; Montagni et al, 2020), and is associated with higher academic achievement, good attendance, social relationships, and increased mental and emotional well-being of students (Barbayannis et al, 2020; Barry et al, 2017). A smoother secondary school transition and fewer classroom, peer, and emotional problems influence higher levels of school connectedness in students (Maunder & LaMothe, 2020), whereas social isolation, feeling unsafe at school, and poor classroom management are threats to school connectedness (Eloff, 2021).

Individual-level school environment assessments of feeling safe at university, linked to the new environment, and peer support after transitioning to university. While most students enjoy the move to higher education, for some, the change in school context is marked by social, intellectual, and structural problems, and it can be the beginning of school separation and academic disengagement (Patterson et al, 2021). According to (Jordan, 2021), while feeling safe at school, connected at school, and peer support were all important predictors of mental and emotional well-being, peer support was the most significant protective factor during the transition phase from secondary school to higher education (Paton, 2021).

Peer interactions at school have been proven to be the most important contributors to students' well-being (Soldevila-Domenech et al, 2021), as social and emotional issues during the transition phase can lead to dissatisfaction and anxiety, resulting in negative or disruptive behaviours (Cohen & Smerdon, 2009). Social issues during the transition period can include increasing feelings of isolation when friendship groups change and teenagers make new friendships and lose acquaintances during a time when peer interactions are highly valued (Phatudi-Mphahlele & Mashele, 2021).

The challenges mentioned above are some of the factors that influence students' emotional well-being. However, problems can be mitigated when higher education institutions develop intervention programmes that promote emotional wellbeing among students, as detailed below.

## INVENTIVE APPROACHES TO IMPROVING STUDENTS' EMOTIONAL WELLBEING

Leaders agree that in order for students to achieve academically, they should promote health and develop campus environments that emphasise wellbeing as a value. Similarly, efforts are being made to reduce stigmas associated with mental health concerns. Campuses that prioritise student well-being can improve academic performance, retention, and graduation rates. University students who have a stronger sense of belonging and wellbeing tend to be more motivated, have more self-confidence, and achieve more (Douwes et al, 2023). They also demonstrate higher levels of cultural understanding, critical thinking, and community involvement, and are more likely to be compassionate citizens.

Here are a few ways of how emotional wellness programmes can help institutions advance.

### Raising Awareness and Tackling Stigma

Leadership may minimise obstacles to mental health support facilities while also destigmatizing the need for mental health care. In this case, integrated peer-to-peer programming and student-led outreach initiatives can start talks about better understanding and supporting student needs. These can also help students empathise with one another, appreciate sharing similar experiences, and promote awareness about mental health supports that are available (Izutsu et al, 2015).

The success of any anti-stigma intervention is strongly dependent on the intervention's content and manner, as well as the selection of an acceptable measure and technique to assess its impact. It is unrealistic to expect that raising knowledge of mental health will result in changes in attitudes and behaviour. Other educational courses have typically had little effect on modifying behaviour. Adolescent risk behaviour has not altered considerably as a result of efforts to teach teenagers about safe sexual practises to prevent HIV/AIDS infection. Similarly, anti-tobacco campaigns aimed at educating youth about the dangers of smoking have frequently failed to curb smoking (Bernstein, Haiman, & Mayer, 2023). Lessons must be drawn from such experiences in order to determine strategies that are most likely to have the greatest impact. To effectively evaluate stigma-reduction initiatives, a deeper understanding of the diverse manifestations of stigma is required first. Then, strategies for maximising the impact of such treatments can be created and tested. Promotion of such research and its subsequent dissemination would provide a scientific contribution both locally and globally, allow for stronger evidence-based policy, and influence future anti-stigma campaign design (Bernstein, Haiman, & Mayer, 2023).

## Creating and Building a Culture of Wellbeing

To solve the student mental health issue, institutions should recruit more counsellors. Upstream remedies, such as training initiatives focused on resiliency, stress management, and other behavioural difficulties, are recommended by organisations such as SADAG in South Africa. These may aid in the prevention of future issues. Wake Forest University's and Ohio State University's student wellness centres have developed models that ensure student well-being on numerous levels, including emotional, physical, social, intellectual, and financial dimensions (Douwes et al, 2023).

Wellness programmes have traditionally been oriented at the student population throughout the history of academic institutional wellness programming. Executive leadership, professors, and staff are becoming more aware of the barriers to student performance, such as sleeplessness, anxiety, stress, depression, bad eating habits, lack of activity, and general poor coping mechanisms. Despite the fact that many academic institutions have initiated wellness programmes for students and/or employees, only a few have developed complete, systematic, and integrated approaches to health and wellbeing (Wiens et al, 2017). Academic institutions have a unique potential and obligation to deliver transformative education, to engage student voices, to produce new knowledge and understanding, to lead by example, and to advocate to decision-makers for the benefit of society (Amaya, Donegan, Conner, Edwards & Gipson, 2019). Higher education institutions are uniquely positioned in the emerging knowledge society to develop, distribute, and use information and research discoveries to improve the health of citizens and communities today and in the future. The sheer number of individuals who live, work, and visit academic institutions can lead to a higher collective influence when work is done cooperatively in transdisciplinary and cross-sector ways. Higher education institutions can model and evaluate ways for the larger community and society by incorporating health promotion ideals and concepts into their purpose, vision, and strategic objectives (Amaya et al, 2019).

## Digital Mental Health Services

Technology solutions, such as smartphone apps, make advisors more accessible, and as a result, students are more likely to reach out and seek help. Technology can also assist with tracking data and analytics, and data solutions can enable equity and foster belonging in order to properly measure the success of mental health programmes on campuses (Izutsu et al, 2015).

Digital mental health services are an essential component of health literacy, and they contribute to public health measures to prevent and promote mental illness. Understanding how to attain and maintain excellent mental health, understanding mental diseases and their treatment, reducing stigma, and increasing help-seeking behaviour are the four components of this (Kurki et al, 2021). Digital mental health services promote mental health awareness and positive attitudes towards the resources available for mental health difficulties, lowering the barrier to seeking help and utilising appropriate treatment (Kurki et al, 2021). Poor mental health literacy, on the other hand, may result in greater stigma, a lack of information of how to detect mental problems, and barriers to getting treatment, such as confidentiality and confidence in potential sources of aid. These circumstances have been linked to decreased well-being, quality of life, and performance (Montagni et al, 2020).

When technology, such as the internet, mobile phones, computers, or other electronic devices, is used in the delivery of a psychological intervention aimed at improving mental health outcomes, it is termed digital. Digital therapies for various severity mental health problems have quickly emerged as an innovation that promises greater access, acceptance, scalability, and cost-effectiveness when compared to traditional face-to-face services alone (Bernstein et al, 2023). Students' concerns about stigma, time restrictions, and unfamiliarity with health-care systems may be alleviated by digital interventions for university students (Lister et al, 2021). Furthermore, due to high rates of smartphone access and experience with mixed modes of study, most university students are extremely open to digital modes of health assistance (Eloff, 2021). Other worldwide causes, such as the COVID-19 pandemic, have hastened the adoption of digital interventions as solutions for addressing restrictions associated with traditional health care settings for young people (Barbayannis et al, 2022).

Previous research has demonstrated that digital mental health services programmes for teenagers in high schools can improve mental health knowledge and skills (Eloff, 2021). A thorough evaluation, however, found that university-based mental health teaching programmes did not change students' attitudes towards getting help or stigma. Moving from a home context to independent living is a significant transition stage in the life of a young adult, especially when combined with the academic responsibilities of university study (Kurki et al, 2021). Mental health literacy interventions, for example, can raise mental health awareness and minimise the stigma associated with mental health disorders when implemented in university settings. This fosters happiness. In the United Kingdom, medical students were given access to an evidence-based Mental Health First Aid e-learning course that focused on general mental health awareness and recognising mental health problems and mental disorders (Lister et al, 2021). This yielded positive outcomes in terms of increased student emotional well-being. The workshop also enhanced participants' attitudes towards assisting others suffering from mental illnesses. Kurki et al. (2021) compared the outcomes of first-year postsecondary students who participated in the Canadian Transitions intervention to those of a control group who did not two months after the programme finished in 2021. Students in the intervention group had better mental health awareness, less stigma, more positive attitudes towards seeking help, more help-seeking behaviour, and less stress. Furthermore, after the programme, the participants felt more prepared for their academic courses (Kurki et al, 2021).

## Personalization and Belonging

According to surveys, students see online communities as critical to their mental health and adaptability needs throughout the pandemic. Almost 30% said online networks provide them a sense of belonging to their institution, while 25% said they help them feel better. Students observe that receiving personalised communication demonstrates that their institutions are invested in their achievement (Thuraiselvam & Thang, 2015).

Personalised learning, the broad concept of adapting learning to an individual student's requirements, talents, and interests, has been around for a while, but it has grown in popularity in recent years, aided by technological and digital content advancements (Rochin Demong et al, 2023). Although there is no universal definition of personalised learning, there is some overlap amongst approaches. In addition to personalising education to individuals, there is an emphasis on student-teacher collaboration to establish a shared understanding of how to satisfy student educational goals and requirements (Rochin Demong et al, 2023). Students are active participants in their education, unlike traditional educational techniques that use uniform curricula, and are involved in every step of the process, from creating goals to tracking progress and selecting how competency will be demonstrated (Abdullahi et al, 2020). Instructors are essential to the process since they are in charge of education, design, and maintenance of the learning environment, as well as assisting students in taking greater ownership of their learning (Utami et al, 2021). There is minimal but growing evidence that personalised learning is successful. According to research, most schools that used personalised learning in their study saw statistically significant increases in student academic performance and achievement, with growth that was higher than comparison groups of similar students. In comparison to their peers, the lowest-performing students made tremendous improvements (Anglim et al, 2020).

Emotional well-being refers to an individual's total level of health and contentment in their lives. It is significantly influenced by the individual's physical, psychological, and social variables (Rochin Demong et al, 2023). Understanding the factors of emotional well-being is critical for developing personalised methods to improve students' lives. Personality traits are psychological features that can influence an individual's social well-being (Anglim et al., 2020). It is critical to identify and comprehend students' personality features in order to build personalised tactics to promote their social well-being (Tuzovic & Kabadayi, 2021).

## Conduct Ongoing Surveys and Assessments

Mental health support personnel and instructors should be given access to tools for conducting online well-being assessments. Simple questionnaires distributed to students can assist the school evaluate student stress levels while learning what works, what doesn't, and what the next steps should be (Douwes et al, 2023).

Some institutions provide mental and emotional health assessments as part of orientation to help students understand critical signals related to overall well-being and to have a baseline understanding of their current well-being (Abdullahi et al, 2020). While these assessments are not diagnostic, may overestimate prevalence rates, and cannot replace a licenced professional's examination, they can offer students with a knowledge of what warning indicators of distress look like in themselves and others. Screening sessions can also give students with information on campus health and wellness services, as well as connect them to other resources that can help them improve their emotional well-being (Widdicks, 2020).

Almost every higher education institute offers some form of mental health and substance abuse counselling and treatment, often through a counselling and psychological services centre (Maunder & LaMothe, 2020). This institutionalised function may encourage college and university officials to believe that simply expanding their counselling services will enough to address the mental health and well-being issues that today's students face (McKinney et al, 2016). It is the obligation of the institutions to perform frequent and continuous surveys and assessments in order to meet the issues posed by the rising frequency of mental health problems among students in higher education. This would entail allocating greater resources to build capacity for promoting wellbeing and helping students who require assistance with a mental health issue (Baik et al, 2019).

# CONCLUSION

Predisposing variables for mental health and social well-being are a source of worry in the community, particularly among undergraduates. The prevalence of mental problems is higher among college and university students, generating concerns about determining some of the underlying causes of the phenomena. Family concerns, financial difficulties, stress, anxiety, and depression are all risk factors. Academic accomplishment places pressure on pupils and elicits a variety of emotional responses.

Students' feelings and failure to satisfy their expectations place them in mental states that may last for some time. In the university, a change in surroundings and a desire to adjust to a new way of life results in a change in lifestyle. Interaction and other socioeconomic aspects are also important for a student's mental health, which can lead to illnesses if they are disregarded. As a result, the education community would be prudent to implement new approaches to improve students' emotional well-being, such as raising student awareness, creating and establishing a culture of wellbeing, and delivering digital mental services. This action will contribute to the development of a mentally healthy society among students in higher education institutions in the future.

## REFERENCES

Abdullahi, A. M., Orji, R., Rabiu, A. M., Kawu, A. A. (2020). Personality and Subjective Well-Being: Towards Personalized Persuasive Interventions for Health and Well-Being. *Online Journal Public Health Information, 12*(1). . doi:10.5210/ojphi.v12i1.10335

Amaya, M., Donegan, T., Conner, D., Edwards, J., & Gipson, C. (2019). Creating a Culture of Wellness: A Call to Action for Higher Education, Igniting Change in Academic Institutions. *Building Healthy Academic Communities Journal, 3*(2), 27–40. doi:10.18061/bhac.v3i2.7117

Anglim, J., Horwood, S., Smillie, L. D., Marrero, R. J., & Wood, J. K. (2020). Predicting psychological and subjective well-being from personality: *A meta-analysis. Psychological Bulletin, 146*(4), 279–323. doi:10.1037/bul0000226 PMID:31944795

Auerbach, R. P., Alonso, J., Axinn, W. G., Cuijpers, P., Ebert, D. D., Green, J. G., & Zaslavsky, A. M. (2018). Mental disorders among college students in the World Health Organization World Mental Health Surveys. *Psychological Medicine, 48*(4), 554–567. doi:10.1017/S0033291717001665 PMID:28805169

Baik, C., Larcombe, W., & Brooker, A. (2019). How universities can enhance student mental wellbeing: The student perspective. *Higher Education Research & Development, 38*(4), 674–687. doi:10.1080/07294360.2019.1576596

Barbayannis, G., Bandari, M., Zheng, X., Baquerizo, H., Pecor, K. W., & Ming, X. (2022). Academic Stress and Mental Well-Being in College Students: Correlations, Affected Groups, and COVID-19. *Frontiers in Psychology, 13*(5), 886344. doi:10.3389/fpsyg.2022.886344 PMID:35677139

Barry, M. M., Clarke, A. M., & Dowling, K. (2017). Promoting social and emotional well-being in schools. *Health Education, 117*(5), 434–451. doi:10.1108/HE-11-2016-0057

Bernstein, C. A., Haiman, C., & Mayer, L. E. (2023). Raising Awareness and Ensuring Access to Mental Health Resources. *Caring for Caregivers to Be: A Comprehensive Approach to Developing Well-Being Programs for the Health Care Learner*, 196.

Bezerra, I. M. P., da Silva, R. A. B., da Silva, E. R. A., & Dantas, L. C. A. (2021). Anxiety, depression and stress in the context of the COVID-19 pandemic: A cross-sectional study with undergraduate students from Brazil. *Ciencia & Saude Coletiva, 26*(suppl 2), 3433–3442. doi:10.1590/1413-81232021268.2.21112020

Bruffaerts, R., Mortier, P., Kiekens, G., Auerbach, R. P., Cuijpers, P., Demyttenaere, K., Green, J. G., Nock, M. K., & Kessler, R. C. (2018). Mental health problems in college freshmen: Prevalence and academic functioning. *Journal of Affective Disorders, 225*, 97–103. doi:10.1016/j.jad.2017.07.044 PMID:28802728

Bullivant, N. (2021). *Student wellbeing and motivation during the pandemic: A UK survey*. Higher Education Policy Institute (HEPI) and Youth Sight. https://www.hepi.ac.uk/2021/01/28/ student-wellbeing-and-motivation-during-the-pandemic-a-uk-survey

Cage, E., Stock, M., Sharpington, A., Pitman, E., & Batchelor, R. (2020). Barriers to accessing support for mental health issues at university. *Studies in Higher Education, 45*(8), 1637–1649. doi:10.1080/03075079.2018.1544237

Douwes, R., Metselaar, J., Pijnenborg, G. H. M., & Boonstra, N. (2023). Well-being of students in higher education: The importance of a student perspective. *Cogent Education, 1*(8), 1–17. doi:10.1080/2331186X.2023.2190697

Eloff, I. (2021). College students' well-being during the COVID-19 pandemic: An exploratory study. *Journal of Psychology in Africa, 31*(3), 254–260. doi:10.1080/14330237.2021.1939055

Evans, D., Borriello, G. A., & Field, A. P. (2018). A review of the academic and psychological impact of the transition to secondary education. *Frontiers in Psychology, 9*, 1482. doi:10.3389/fpsyg.2018.01482 PMID:30210385

Farrell, E. (2021). *Darkness, Wellness and World Views: The University's Role in Shaping Students' Experiences of Mental Health and Distress. In the Promise of the University*. Springer. doi:10.1007/978-981-16-5277-6_11

Hamza, C. A., Ewing, L., Heath, N. L., & Goldstein, A. L. (2021). When social isolation is nothing new: A longitudinal study on psychological distress during COVID-19 among university students with and without pre-existing mental health concerns. *Canadian Psychology, 62*(1), 20–30. doi:10.1037/cap0000255

Hawkins, Y. (2019). Mental wellbeing: let's find new ways to support students. *Office for Students*. https://www.officeforstudents.org.uk/news-blog-and-events/blog/mental-wellbeing-let-s-find-new-ways-to-support-students/

Holt, R. J., Graham, J. M., Whitaker, K. J., Hagan, C. C., Ooi, C., Wilkinson, P. O., & Suckling, J. (2016). Functional MRI of emotional memory in adolescent depression. *Developmental Cognitive Neuroscience, 19*, 31–41. doi:10.1016/j.dcn.2015.12.013 PMID:26802367

Hughes, G., & Spanner, L. (2019). *The university mental health charter*. Student Minds.

Izutsu, T., Tsutsumi, A., Minas, H., Thornicroft, G., Patel, V., & Ito, A. (2015). Mental health and well-being in the Sustainable Development Goals. *The Lancet. Psychiatry, 2*(12), 1052–1054. doi:10.1016/S2215-0366(15)00457-5 PMID:26613844

Jordan, L. (2021). *Disillusioned, Disenchanted, Disembodied? Towards a Collective Imagination of the University. In the Promise of the University*. Springer. doi:10.1007/978-981-16-5277-6_14

Kabagenyi, A., Baiden, F., Schmied, V., & Javanparast, S. (2020). The impact of the COVID-19 pandemic on academic performance and wellbeing of university students: Implications for policy and practice. *International Journal of Educational Development, 85*, 102388. doi:10.1016/j.ijedudev.2020.102388

Kidd, I. J. (2021). *Character, Corruption, and 'Cultures of Speed' in Higher Education. In the Promise of the University*. Springer. doi:10.1007/978-981-16-5277-6_2

Kunjiapu, S., & Kunasegaran, M. (2021). Psychological Wellbeing Among Undergraduates of Higher Learning Institutions in Malaysia. *Psychology and Education, 58*(2), 9179–9187.

Kurki, M., Gilbert, S., Mishina, K., Lempinen, L., Luntamo, T., Hinkka-Yli-Salomäki, S., & Sourander, A. (2021). Digital mental health literacy-program for the first-year medical students' wellbeing: A one group quasi-experimental study. *BMC Medical Education, 21*, 1–11.

Lattie, E. G., Cohen, K. A., Hersch, E., Williams, K. D. A., Kruzan, K. P., & MacIver, C. (2022). *Uptake and effectiveness of a self-guided mobile app platform for college student mental health.* Internet Intervention. doi:10.1016/j.invent.2021.100493

Levula, A., Wilson, A., & Harré, M. (2016). The association between social network factors and mental health at different life stages. *Quality of Life Research: An International Journal of Quality of Life Aspects of Treatment, Care and Rehabilitation, 25*(7), 1725–1733. doi:10.100711136-015-1200-7 PMID:26669317

Lister, K., Seale, J., & Douce, C. (2021). Mental health in distance learning: A taxonomy of barriers and enablers to student mental wellbeing. *Open Learning*. doi:10.1080/02680513.2021.1899907

Mahon, Á. (2021). *The Promise of the University: Reclaiming Humanity, Humility, and Hope* (Vol. 10). Springer Nature. doi:10.1007/978-981-16-5277-6_1

Manap, R., Hamid, A. S., & Ghani, A. M. (2019). Depression, Anxiety and Stress Among Undergraduate Students. *Journal of Social Sciences and Humanities, 16*(2), 1–7.

Maunder, R. E., & LaMothe, J. (2020). Using mobile phones to capture emotions and experiences in situation: A study of feasibility and user experience. *Journal of Mixed Methods Research, 14*(4), 416–435.

Mayaba, N. N., Ralarala, M. K., & Angu, P. (2018). Student voice: Perspectives on language and critical pedagogy in South African higher education. *Educational Research for Social Change, 7*(1), 1–12. doi:10.17159/2221-4070/2018/v7i1a1

McKinney, C., Morse, M., & Pastuszak, J. (2016). Effective and Ineffective Parenting: Associations with Psychological Adjustment in Emerging Adults. *Journal of Family Issues, 37*(9), 1203–1225. doi:10.1177/0192513X14537480

Montagni, I., Tzourio, C., Cousin, T., Sagara, J. A., Bada-Alonzi, J., & Horgan, A. (2020). Mental health-related digital use by university students: A systematic review. *Telemedicine Journal and e-Health, 26*(2), 131–146. doi:10.1089/tmj.2018.0316 PMID:30888256

Morgan, B., & Simmons, L. (2021). A 'PERMA' response to the pandemic: an online positive education programme to promote wellbeing in university students. In *Frontiers in Education, 6*. Frontiers Media South Africa. doi:10.3389/feduc.2021.642632

Morgan, D., & Hoffman, K. (2018). Focus groups. In *U. Flick The sage handbook of qualitative data collection* (pp. 250–263). SAGE Publications Ltd. doi:10.4135/9781526416070.n16

Morgan, J. (2021). International student perceptions of the UK higher education experience during the pandemic. *International Student Barometer*. https://services.isb.world/reports/2021/ISB_UK_HEI_COVID_19_Whitepaper_2021.pdf

Naidoo, P., Theron, L., & Esterhuizen, T. M. (2021). Mental health outcomes during the COVID-19 pandemic among South African university students. *South African Journal of Psychology. Suid-Afrikaanse Tydskrif vir Sielkunde, 51*(2), 204–216. doi:10.1177/00812463211017913

Nielsen, I., Newman, A., Smyth, R., Hirst, G., & Heilemann, B. (2017). The influence of instructor support, family support and psychological capital on the well-being of postgraduate students: A moderated mediation model. *Studies in Higher Education, 42*(11), 2099–2115. doi:10.1080/03075079.2015.1135116

Ojediran, T. D., & Emeka, E. A. (2021). Prevalence and predictors of poor mental health outcomes among Nigerian university students during the COVID-19 pandemic. *Frontiers in Psychiatry, 12*, 652028. doi:10.3389/fpsyt.2021.652028

Paton, G. (2021). Students' mental health and motivation hit by pandemic; UK survey finds. *Times Higher Education*. https://bit.ly/41ZZZQk

Patterson, Z.R., Gabrys, R.L., Prowse, R.K., Abizaid, A.B., Hellemans, K.G. & McQuaid, R. J. (2021). The influence of COVID-19 on stress, substance use, and mental health among postsecondary students. Emerging Adulthood, 9(5), pp.516-530. https://doi.org/10.1177/21676968211014080 doi:10.1177/21676968211014080

Phatudi-Mphahlele, B., & Mashele, M. (2021). South African students' experience of online learning during the Covid-19 pandemic: A case of a higher education institution. *International Journal of Educational Technology in Higher Education, 18*(1), 1–19. doi:10.118641239-021-00278-2

Rochin Demong, N. A., Shahrom, M., Abdul Rahim, R., Omar, E. N., & Yahya, M. (2023). Personalized recommendation classification model of students' social well-being based on personality trait determinants using machine learning algorithms. *Journal of Information and Communication Technology, 22*(4), 545–585. doi:10.32890/jict2023.22.4.2

Sapiro, B., & Ward, A. (2020). Marginalized youth, mental health, and connection with others: A review of the literature. *Child & Adolescent Social Work Journal, 37*(4), 343–357. doi:10.100710560-019-00628-5

Seligman, M. (2018). PERMA and the building blocks of well-being. *The Journal of Positive Psychology, 13*(4), 333–335. doi:10.1080/17439760.2018.1437466

Simkins, C. (2016). Funding. South African higher education reviewed: two decades of democracy. In: Kagisano, (10), 39-115.

Soldevila-Domenech, N., Forero, C. G., Alayo, I., Capella, J., Colom, J., Malmusi, D., Mompart, A., Mortier, P., Puértolas, B., Sánchez, N., Schiaffino, A., Vilagut, G., & Alonso, J. (2021). Mental well-being of the general population: Direct and indirect effects of socioeconomic, relational and health factors. *Quality of Life Research: An International Journal of Quality of Life Aspects of Treatment, Care and Rehabilitation*, *30*(8), 2171–2185. doi:10.100711136-021-02813-5 PMID:33847868

Spies, J. (2022). *Exploring Teacher Experiences of Subjective Well-Being During a Pandemic.* [Master's thesis, University of Pretoria]. https://hdl.handle.net/2263/82445

Tagoe, M., Quarshie, E. N. B., Ahiaku, A. E., & Ansong, E. (2020). Utilization of mental health services among university students in Ghana. *Journal of College Student Psychotherapy*, *34*(2), 109–124. doi: 10.1080/87568225.2019.1674669

Teixeira, R. J., Brandão, T., & Dores, A. R. (2021). Academic stress, coping, emotion regulation, affect and psychosomatic symptoms in higher education. *Current Psychology (New Brunswick, N.J.)*, 1–10. doi:10.100712144-020-01304-z

Thuraiselvam, S., & Thang, R. B. (2015). Factors That Affect Students' Mental Health: A Study at Taylor's University School of Hospitality. *Tourism and Culinary Arts Final Year Students*. Springer, Singapore. 10.1007/978-981-287-399-6_10

Truschel, J. (2020). *Depression Definition and DSM-5 Diagnostic Criteria: What is Depression?* PsyCom. https://www.psycom.net/depression-definition-dsm-5-diagnostic-criteria/

Utami, N. A., Maharani, W., & Atastina, I. (2021). Personality classification of Facebook users according to Big Five personality using SVM (Support Vector Machine) Method. *Procedia Computer Science*, *179*, 177–184. doi:10.1016/j.procs.2020.12.023

Walker, J. G. (2022). *Towards improving the mental health of students at South African universities.* Universities South Africa. https://www.usaf.ac.za/towards-improvingthe-mental-health-of-students-at-south-african-universities/

Wang, Y. (2020). College students' trait gratitude and subjective well-being mediated by basic psychological needs. *Social Behavior and Personality*, *48*(4), 1–10. doi:10.2224bp.8904

Widdicks, K. (2020). When the good turns ugly: Speculating next steps for digital well-being tools. *Proceedings of the 11th Nordic Conference on Human-Computer Interaction: Shaping Experiences*, Shaping Society, Tallinn, Estonia. 10.1145/3419249.3420117

Wiens, K., Williams, J. V., Lavorato, D. H., Duffy, A., Pringsheim, T. M., Sajobi, T. T., & Patten, S. B. (2017). Is the prevalence of major depression increasing in the Canadian adolescent population? Assessing trends from 2000 to 2014. *Journal of Affective Disorders*, *210*, 22–26. doi:10.1016/j.jad.2016.11.018 PMID:28012349

World Health Organization. (2021). *Mental health and COVID-19.* WHO. https://www.who.int/teams/mental-health-and-substance-use/covid-19

# Chapter 16
# The Benefits of Self-Talk and Imagination for Your Mental Health and Happiness Adolescence in Higher Education

**Vijendra Nath Pathak**
https://orcid.org/0000-0002-4298-9211
*Lovely Professional University, India*

**Prattusha Chatterjee**
*Lovely Professional University, India*

## ABSTRACT

*In the contemporary, fast-paced world, adolescents are confronted with unparalleled challenges and pressures to excel. The core objective of this chapter is to furnish readers, particularly mental health professionals and adults, with pragmatic methodologies to aid adolescents in navigating the challenges that beset their lives. In conclusion, this chapter serves as a valuable reservoir of knowledge for those who are concerned about the well-being of adolescents in today's fiercely competitive and demanding milieu. It furnishes a comprehensive comprehension of self-talk and its various manifestations, elucidating their profound influence on an individual's thoughts, emotions, and actions. Ultimately, the chapter advocates for a proactive approach to adolescent well-being, underscoring the primacy of prevention over remediation.*

## INTRODUCTION

Imagine that you have a younger brother or sister, as I am guessing many of you might have. What kind of company would you want for your sibling? The answer will be obviously good company. A very well

DOI: 10.4018/979-8-3693-2833-0.ch016

known proverb comes to mind 'A man is known by the company that he keeps'. But why? Lets start this chapter with an example, imagine that your younger sibling has just started college. There are a lot of difficult situations that your sibling will face like all the others who join college, for example: managing the college work with assignments, studies, exams, taking care of one self, managing time, fulfilling expectation and even clashes with peers, breaking of romantic relationships, etc. Now imagine the individual is going through these different situations with a company of friends who are constantly saying things 'there is no need to study', 'nothing comes out of hard work, we just need to be smart to copy', 'studying wont give a future, lets just start to do some random work, earning easy money is important', etc. What can be the possible effects of listening to these statements continuously for the major part of the day? The effect will differ from person to person. However, we cannot deny that such an exposure has a high possibility of effecting an individual in an unhealthy manner. Some may be effected more then others but that is a topic for another discussion. Some might accept these statements as true and get influenced i.e. they may start behaving in ways that are aligned with these statements from that particular company of friends. These kinds of peer influences have been commonly seen in colleges. Decent kids getting into so called negative or bad company and their grades start falling, they may start getting into trouble. The good news is that this doesn't happen with every one. Many students may end up being part of this bad or negative company but they end up realizing that 'this is not what I want for myself' and make the choice of parting ways with those peers, but for that to happen the student will have to tell themselves what they really want for themselves and their lives.

Now let's imagine some positive company for this person in the above example i.e. the group of friends that the person has is constantly talking about their goals and aims in life, how there are so many opportunities available now a days with education, doing good with studies will lead to a good job and a better life style, always aiming to be more involved in projects, discussing things that are taught in class and also helping to learn it better. In this scenario how will the person in question be effected? The chances are that the person might feel more motivated to work towards ones own future.

Both scenarios seem very obvious and natural – that when we are constantly listening to negative or unhealthy content or when we are constantly in a negative company it will have some negative effect on us until we choose to leave. While if we are constantly listening to some thing positive or we are with positive company, a positive impact can be seen. When some one talks to us negatively about ourselves or the world, how does that feel? We know that some parts of it may be true but it still doesn't feel very great. You must have come across certain people who are crying and complaining all the time, who talk in a very discouraging manner sometimes even insulting, taunting or criticizing. Does it feel nice to be around these people? When we don't like what the other person is saying or when we realize that the company we are in, is not good we may choose to walk away from them, spend less time with them or we may even start to avoid them.

Now pause for a couple of minutes and ask yourself self, 'how do I talk to myself?' Some individuals may even say I don't talk to myself at all. But upon closer examination it can be observed that there is some thing going on in our mind almost all the time. When we start observing we realize that there is constant conversation going on in our minds. For example - When you are standing in front of your wardrop choosing cloths for the day there is a dialogue or a conversation in your mind about what you want to wear and why, why you don't like certain cloths but you may like the others or that you don't have anything nice to wear you need to buy something new. For some one who is looking at you while you stand in front of your wardrop it might feel like you are doing nothing just standing. However, there is great deal of deliberation going on in your mind. Some thing like – 'who are the people I may meet today? What should I wear? Will this look good? No I don't think this color suits me. This is not in trend at all. I want Tom to look at me. And I also want to look better then Tina. What will the others wear today? Should I check with my friend if this is okay?'. If it's a bad day the conversation in the head would be more like – 'I don't look good in anything, it doesn't matter what I wear. I am just ugly and fat. Tom will never look at me there are better looking people in the class. I don't even want to go close to Tina why would she want me as her friend?'

The more you observe, the more you will start to notice these conversations are happening in your mind about everything and almost always, for example – when you are waiting for a bus, when you are standing in the que for a ticket, when you are in the class and the teacher is teaching, when you are with your friends but you are verbally not saying anything, when you are upset or when you are sad or happy or angry or irritated. There is something going on all most all the time. We cannot leave ourselves and go somewhere else, we cannot avoid ourselves like we can avoid others. If we can learn how to talk to ourselves in a healthy manner then we can guide our own behavior, we can manage crisis situations better and keep ourselves on the path that we desire for ourselves.

Adolescence is a time of great change and development. Adolescents are transitioning from childhood to adulthood, and they are faced with a wide range of new challenges and responsibilities. They face humongous amounts of competition, there is pressure from families, educational institutes to do well as well as self created pressure. They are on the path to develop their own identity, master skills that are required in the world today and also have a personal social life that comes with its own challenges. They are looking at creating a unique identity of their own but also to fit in with others at the same time. There is a persistent exposure to social media and other kinds of media creating more competition and continuous comparisons. With these challenges popping up adolescents experiencing mental health concerns are on the rise. Emotional issues, body image issues, depression, anxiety, relationship concerns, peer pressure and various kinds of addictions can be seen more commonly among today's adolescents. During this time, it is important for adolescents to develop a strong sense of self-esteem and confidence. One way to do this is through developing a self-talk that is either positive or neutral in nature. However, before diving deeper into what is positive self talk and how to use it, the understanding of what is self talk, how it is developed, what are the various kinds of self talk and the current research done in the area are important areas to be explored.

This chapter will help us understand, explore and look at various ways of incorporating this fairly new concept of self talk into our lives. The aim of this chapter is for adolescents to be able to help themselves through their own self talks and for adults to be able to help them develop proper ways of talking to themselves. For example – from 'I am failure, I cannot do anything right' to 'I am learning new ways of doing things, let me understand new skills that I can learn to do this task'.

## Self–Talk

The idea of self-talk is not new, glimpses can be found in all the religions across the world where importance is given to having positive thoughts. There is no clear distinction between positive thoughts and positive self talk, for now we are going to consider them similar in nature because both are internal cognitive processes. The ancient teachings by Buddha, according to whom human beings are a result of the thoughts they have, which is an internal dialogue that has the potential to shape the individual. Importance of self-talk can also be seen in the Tibetan religious discipline known as 'Bon', they would practice positive thinking as a part of their life because they believed that thoughts can have the ability to be transformed into energies and hence positive thinking can lead to positive emotions followed by positive action (Hardy, 2004). The following ideas about self-talk had developed after a critical review of self-talk literature (Hardy, 2006) where the discrepancies in self-talk definitions are discussed in detail giving the guidelines for a working definition of self-talk. which can be divided into 5 parts:

"(a) verbalizations or statements addressed to the self; (b) multidimensional in nature; (c) having interpretive elements association with the content of statements employed; (d) is somewhat dynamic; and (e) serving at least two functions; instructional and motivational". The American Psychological Association defines self-talk as - "an internal dialogue in which an individual utters phrases or sentences to himself or herself". Self-talk is also referred to as intra-personal communication (Oles et al., 2020) and can be seen in almost all individual who are able to use language either vocally or in a speech (Heavy et al., 2008). Moreover, the importance of these internal dialogues and the role they play in an individual's life is worth exploring because of the important cognitive and regulatory functions served by the phenomenon of self-talk (Day et al., 2015; Hardy, 2006).

More simply put self-talk is the internal dialogue that we have with ourselves. It is the way that we talk to ourselves about ourselves, our thoughts, our feelings, and our experiences. While there are many different definitions of self-talk, an old definition of self talk is the one of the most commonly used that is, "the internal dialogue that people have with themselves" (Meichenbaum, 1977). There is no denying in the contribution that the environment has in developing the personality of a child. The child learns tremendously by imitation or through observing how others around are behaving. Learning self talk is no exception. The child learns to talk to themselves and others in ways that others talk to the child. Early experiences and influences, such parents, teachers, peers, immediate environment including neighborhood and media have the potential to shape our beliefs and attitudes about our self and the world, these in return affect how we interpret and react to events. When we repeatedly think and behave in certain ways they create habits i.e. patterns of thinking and behaving which has the capacity to become automatic and are hard to change, until one becomes aware of them and how these patterns are affecting our daily lives. By becoming more aware of what we are thinking we become aware of what we are telling ourselves. For example – a students who didn't do well in the exams or a student who might have failed a particular test, he/she can choose to think/tell themselves that, "I am failure. I can never do things right. What is the point of this any ways." Or can choose to think/tell themselves that, "let me understand my mistakes better. Let me think where I went wrong. I want to do better in the next test." It is important to understand how the first set of statements ("I am failure. I can never do things right. What is the point of this any ways.") will make an individual feel. Will this thought/self talk motivate the student to improve and prepare for the next test? Now let's focus on the second set of statements ("let me understand my mistakes better. Let me think where I went wrong. I want to do better in the next test."). This second thought/self talk has the capacity to motivate the student and also guide his/her behavior because a part of the statement is giving instructions ("let me understand my mistakes better"). This is called as instructional self talk.

## Types of Self–Talk

Now that we fairly understand what is self talk lets look at the various types of self talk that are most applicable to us.

## Positive and Negative Self-Talk

The most used broad segregation is negative and positive self-talk. Weinberg, (1984) had defined positive self-talk as a technique that allows the individual to maintain their focus on the task at hand while ignoring the past failures and maintaining the focus on the desired future. Neck et al., (1992) introduced the idea of self-leadership describing it as the individual's ability to become "self-directional and self-motivated to perform". According to them these abilities could be developed through self-talk and mental imagery. If the individual resorts to positive self-talk then the they will be experiencing positive mental imagery corresponding to that self-talk while the use of negative self-talk will lead to negative mental imagery. Self-talk can create a level of alertness and conscientiousness for the individual allowing a better organizational ability to integrate ideas while the corresponding mental imagery allows the person to visualize that outcome favorably in order to build confidences towards a particular performance. This strategy is most commonly explored and used in sports psychology. Thus it has been observed again and again that positive self-talk brings positive outcomes and negative self-talks brings negative outcomes (Raalte, 1995; Dagrou et al., 1992). With positive and negative self talk as its types, it has been discovered that negative self-talk has been associated in the maintenance of anxiety (Yaratan et al., 2010) and can predict peer loneliness, especially specially threatening self-talk (Ford, 2015) while positive self-talk with an autonomy-supportive style has the potential of positively influencing individuals' enjoyment and perseverance along with psychological need satisfaction playing the role of an intervention (Muynck et al. 2017). The literature indicates that self-talk can play an important role and can be applied in various other areas of life eg: positive self-talk is considered as one of the important psychological skills, the improvement of which can help improve performance of emergency medical service providers under stress (Lauria et al., 2017). In women it has also been observed that negative self- talk in combination with negative imagery declines self-confidence significantly (Khodarahmi R et al, 2015). In simple terms negative self talk is when we say mean things to ourselves and positive self – talk is when we say good things to our selves.

## Motivational and Instructional Self-Talk

Two other types of self talks i.e. motivational and instructional self-talk have also been proven to be very useful (Hatzigeorgiadis, 2006). Motivational self talk is when the individual is self motivating him/herself through the use of their inner dialogue. Instructional self talk is when an individual is giving themselves instructions through the use of inner dialogue. For example – motivational self talk: 'I can do it, I will keep trying'; instructional self talk: 'I have an assignment to complete. Today evening I am going to spend an hour understanding the things that I don't understand about this assignment.' OR 'I have 2 hours before parents come home. I need to clean up my room before that.' OR 'this group of students are always missing class and getting into trouble. May be I should stay away from them.' Or 'this movie won't run away anywhere, it will be there on Netflix for a while so I can watch it after I finish at least a part of this assignment or may be the whole assignment.' Motivational self-talk having a greater impact on the effort that an individual is exerting, in comparison to instructional self-talk. However, their observed effects on attention, effort, confidence, anxiety control, and automaticity can be the same for both instructional and/or motivational self-talk (Hatzigeorgiadis, 2006). Brinthaupt (2009) has studied self-talk extensively giving the Self talk scale (Brinthaupt, 2009). He segregates self talk on the basis of the functions that the self talk is serving or performing which according to his theory are – self criticism self talk, self reinforcement self talk, social assessment self talk and self managing self talk.

- **Social-Assessment self-talk:** Involves the instances of going through something said to another person in ones mind again and again or at least frequently and imagining the reaction of others to what has been said.
- **Self-Reinforcement self-talk:** Includes the self-talk emerging from the feeling of pride but not vanity i.e. when the individual feels that he/she has done something good or when something good has happened. It is encouragement provided to the self by the self.
- **Self-Criticism self-talk:** Involves the self-talk that comes from the feeling of being discouraged about oneself and/or criticizing the self for something said or done, it can be easily considered the opposite of self reinforcement self talk.
- **Self-Management self-talk:** Involves giving oneself instructions, more like instructional self talk. It implies giving directions about what needs to be done or said in a given situation or scenario or in general. The Social-Assessment and Self-Criticism seem to represent more of the negative aspects of self-talk, whereas the Self Reinforcement and Self-Management appears to represent more of the positive aspects of self-talk. Too much of social assessment or self critical self talk can hamper ones confidence and can create negative emotional states. These kinds of self talk can be found more in intensity and frequency among individuals going through depression and anxiety. More and more use of self reinforcing self talk and self management self talk has been seen in sports psychology while training athletes and even in Olympic trainings as they have been found to increase confidence, manage ones own goals and stay focused.

## Field Observation of the Different Types of Self-Talk

It was being observed by the author that individuals who are experiencing intense negative emotion exhibit negative self talk. It may become difficult in these intense negative emotional states to understand or transition into a positive self-talk. Resorting to positive self talk from that point of negativity may seem even impossible while the individual is in the state of heavy emotional distress. It is very important to remember, for the positive self talk to have any beneficial effect on the individual he/she should be able to have some amount of belief in that positive statement, if the person is not able to believe in the positive statement that he/she is telling the self then achieving the beneficial effects those positive self talks is not possible. Being able to believe in the positive self talk while in the midst of a very negative circumstance can be a difficult feat to achieve. This is a very common experience and also one reason why many people might feel that saying something positive to oneself doesn't work. Mainly because many would choose to mindlessly repeat positive affirmations without being able to believe in them or at least relate to them. This transition from negative to positive can seem like a huge impossible step. This process can be made smoother by introducing neutral self talk. Or rather neutral self talk can be used as a bridge to reach positive self talk from negative self – talk.

For example – "I cannot do it", becomes a clear negative statement in the context of learning a new skill required to cope with a difficult situation. On the other hand "I can do it", becomes a clear positive statement. However, when the client says "I can do it" but they are not able to believe in it as there is no proof for the same then this positive statement gets confronted by other self critical self talk statements, for e.g.: "how will I do this? I have failed till now? I have never been able to do this?". Hence, they either remain in that negative state or the self critical statements can even intensify the negative state making them feel worse and creating a belief that this doesn't work. In this scenario neutral self talk have the possibility to reduce anxiety as they are neither positive nor negative, making them more believable, directing the self towards goal formation and taking steps in that direction. For e.g.: "I cannot do it yet. This doesn't mean that I would never be able to do it in the future. What can I do to learn in different ways".

*Table 1. Self-talk*

| Negative self talk | Neutral self talk | Positive self-talk |
|---|---|---|
| I cannot do it. | I cannot do it yet but everything can be learned. | I can do it. |

Another segregation that was found to help was dividing positive self talk into:

1. **Unrealistic positive self-talk:** Statements that are positive but don't seem achievable.
2. **Realistic positive self-talk:** Statements that are positive and seem achievable.

*Table 2. Self-talk*

| Unrealistic positive self talk | Realistic positive self talk |
|---|---|
| I am completely healthy and healed, everything is going to be All right. | I am willing to be healthy, I am taking steps in that direction, cooperating with my treatment. There is a high possibility that I am going to return to better health. |

The understanding of what is self talk and its types are very helpful but without the knowledge of its functions and the impact that it causes our understanding is incomplete.

## Self-Talk: A Way for Self-Regulation of One's Own Behaviour

A plethora of research indicate that self talk is a very important activity. Self-talk plays a vital role in assisting the construction of self (Jemmer, 2010; Qualter et al., 2015). Self-talk when looked at psychologically can be referred to as an internal way to develop self- awareness, understanding, motivation or direction (Brithaupt et al., 2012) which is consistent with the observations of Mischel et al., 1996. He noted that self-talk can have an impact on the process of inhibition of impulses, guiding one's courses of actions, and monitoring one's goal progress through instructional self talk. Similarly self-talk can reflect "meta monitoring" (Carver et al., 1998) which is an indication of one's behaviors and the progress that is being made toward one's goals. They also emphasized on how self-talk can influence emotional reactions and responses to difficult situations or behavioral deficits.

A number of old researches have linked self-talk to the cognitive development of the self and the ability to elicit the practice of self-awareness (Piaget, 1959; Bandura, 1977; Tudge et al, 1993; Leong et al., 2006). The concept of self-awareness which is found very frequently while one acquaints himself in the area of psychological therapies or mental health can be referred to as the ability to manufacture and/or adopt our internal and external perceptions of reality. Self awareness and self regulation can go hand in hand. This idea of self-awareness is also typically negotiated by the use of self-talk (Morrin, 1995; Hardy et al., 2001; Haughton and Neck 2002). Studies on the process of self-regulation indicates that self-talk can be an important component of this process of self awarness. (Berk, 1992; Morin, 1993; Vygotsky, 1987). Benjamin (1994) gave the structural analysis of social behavior which incorporated and emphasized the patterns of state-specific self-talk, for example: the kind of self talk that a person resorts to while failing or succeeding in a particular endeavor.

It has also been observed that self- talk can help an individual in persuading themselves to avoid negative thinking and negative imagery (Gibson, Et al., 2007). Even though this observation has been made with respect to athletes, understanding it's applicability with other population especially among the adolescents of today can help enhance the development of therapeutic approaches targeted for them.

Self-talk and mental imagery are considered cognitive activities (Khodarahmi et al, 2015) and the nature of cognitive activities can influence behavior (Martin et al, 1989). Through this it is safe to infer that the nature of self-talk can influence behavior.

## Self-Talk and Psychological States

Positive self-talk overall has been seen to enhance performance in sports and also for various psychological states like confidence (Vargas, Tonsing et al., 2004). Another psychological state that can be seen to be influenced by self talk is self esteem. What implications can this influence have? Low self-esteem has been connected to negative self- talk (Brinthaupt et al., 2012). In a study by Ford, 2015 it has been observed that positive and negative self-talk can predict self-esteem in adolescence, for example, positive self-talk leading to high self-esteem, however personal failure self-talk significantly predicts low self-esteem. According to the American Psychological Association Self esteem is the degree to which the qualities and characteristics contained in one's self-concept are perceived to be positive. There are two models that speak about the relation between self-esteem and depression - the vulnerability model (Beck, 1967) and the Scar model (Shahar et al., 2003). According to the Vulnerability model low self-esteem makes an individual vulnerable towards depression and according to the Scar Model low self-esteem is the consequence of depression because depression can have a greater impact on the self-concept of an individual in the form of an invisible scar. However, both these models are found to not be mutually exclusive but to be operating at the same time in parallel to each other (Orth et al., 2008). However, there is more support for the vulnerability model as compared to the scar model (Sowislo et al., 2013). The vulnerability effect can be seen across gender; age; affective, emotional, and cognitive as well as somatic symptoms of depression. Further a longitudinal study of Mexican youth diagnosed with depression supports the vulnerability model saying that low self-esteem is a prospective risk factor for depression steaming from self worth (Orth et al., 2014; Orth, et al., 2018). While establishing the Self Talk Scale and its psychometric properties it was found that 3 subscales of the self talk scale were correlated with self-esteem. Self-esteem was found to be negatively associated with Social Assessment self talk and Self-Criticism self talk. Moreover, it was found to be positively associated with Self Reinforcement self talk while Self-Management self talk and self-esteem were unrelated (Brinthaupt et al,

2009). Thus we can see how self talk can influence self esteem and self esteem can influence depression. Traits like mindfulness and self compassion are also found to have a moderate positive correlations, where as a significant negative correlation is seen between negative self-talk and the trait of mindfulness (Grzybowski et al., 2022). This is a possible indication that the different types of self talks can have an impact on the different psychological states that are experienced by people.

## Self-Talk and Coping

Teaching self-talk techniques and positive empathy have found to be considerably helpful for reducing deficient attitude, hopelessness and suicidal thoughts in women with breast cancer (Babakhanloo A et al., 2017). Even though it seems like a different population with different problems and we can observe problems of similar nature (varying in their intensities) being faced by our adolescents. While it might seem obvious that positive self talk have the potential to help in the development of healthier copping strategies, the use of it is still very rare. Another study done during covid – 19 points out a significant positive relationship between self-talk and problem-centered coping style. A significant negative relationship between self-talk and emotional coping style, death anxiety, and obsessive-compulsive disorder was also observed while self-talk was also found to predict problem-centered style, emotional-coping style, death anxiety, and obsessive-compulsive disorder among 354 adults living in Ardabil, Iran, (Damirchi et al., 2020). If we can help you adolescents develop a healthier style of talking to themselves while they are young we are indirectly helping them to become healthier adults.

## Self-Talk and Psychotherapy

The focus on self- talk can also be found in psychological therapies like CBT (Beck, 1993). CBT became a much-preferred means of treating clinically pathological symptomologies, because it was trying to replace negative thinking with positive ones. Zastrow, 1988 suggest that any positive changes in therapies can be accredited to modifications in their use of self-talk. The observation that the ratio of positive and negative self talk can have an impact on the state of mind in association with different types of pathologies (Schwartz et al., 1989) can help in understanding the implications of self talk in the field of psychotherapy. This can also be seen in the work of narrative psychologist. They along with other psychotherapy researchers frequently infused self talk in their models because of the evidence (e.g., Bruner, 1990; Dennett, 1992) which suggested the "self" is a product of self-narration or self-talk. Narrative psychologist also found self talk to have another important role, it has been found that self-narratives can assist in the assimilation of difficult experiences (Honos-Webb et al., 1998). Studies with athletes have shown that self-talk can be used to enhance motivation and bring improvement in performance through acquisition of skills, creating self-confidence, self-efficacy and helps in the modification of ineffective habits (Magnusson et al., 2013). The work of a therapist while treating a psychological dysfunction, lies on the same lines of acquiring new skills that can help the individual cope better with the situation along with increasing self-confidence and self-efficacy while modifying inappropriate behaviors. We can also see the focus on self talk for new therapies like Transactional Analysis while focusing on the narratives that individuals develop and also in Neuro Linguistic Programing.

We now understand that thoughts and feelings are influenced by our mood, stress level, and expectations, all of which can be given a direction through the use of self talk. Our habits are patterns, which are formed by repeatedly being involved in, or using certain types of thoughts and behaviors making these patterns automatic. Once automatic they can be hard to change as they are slowly becoming a part of our personality the more we use them. If we just look at the over all segregation of Self-talk, it can majorly be either positive or negative. Positive self-talk is characterized by encouraging, supportive, and optimistic messages that one chooses to give to one self while negative self-talk, on the other hand, is characterized by critical, judgmental, and pessimistic messages that are communicated to the self. However, we can create a middle path of neutral self talk. Neutral self talk keeps in mind the reality, avoids unrealistically positive self talk without action. It also can help in the reduction of negative self talk, which leads to negative emotional experience along with negative copping behaviors. Nothing can ever beat taking an action step towards a goal. It does not matter how tiny the step is. Having a healthy internal dialogue or self talk is a tool that can move us towards taking that physical action step towards achieving that goal.

## Action Steps for Changing Self-Talk

1. **Observe your self-talk when you are experiencing a negative emotion:** Teaching adolescents to be more aware of the nature of their thoughts can be very helpful. It can also help them prepare for the times and situations when they commonly experience a surge of negative thoughts beforehand. Awareness is the first step towards helping oneself change. When they are aware they can catch themselves engaging in negative self-talk and challenge those thoughts to replace them with more positive or neutral ones. With practice we can make this new more helpful form of copping a habit. One way of developing this new habit is to simply pay attention to the way that we talk to ourselves.
2. **Journaling:** Journaling is an ancient way of venting out, having a space to freely open up without being judged. It also a process that helps in becoming more aware of one self i.e. of ones own actions, thoughts, behaviors and their impact on our and the lives of others around us. Answering reflection questions while journaling can unravel our thoughts. Questions like what do I think about (a person, place, situation)? What were my thoughts when I (felt an intense negative emotional reaction towards something, place, person or situation like anger, jealousy, depressed, etc)? What was I telling myself when I reacted (to something, place, person or situation in a manner that I regret)? Does this way of thinking or talking to myself helpful? What existing negative patterns can I see in my life? What do I tell myself about these patterns? What new and different ways of thinking can help in removing these patterns from my life? The internet is flooded with different forms of journals that already have formats in them to venture in this area of self-help work. Huge number of journaling probe questions are also available. However, these questions need to be answered without judging the self. There is also the possibility of emotional content coming on the surface through journaling which needs to be processed in a healthy fashion. Some adolescents may be able to do these kinds of self-help activities on their own but not every one might will be in a position to be able to go through this process on their own. It can be more beneficial to do these activities under the guidance of a Counsellor or talk to an adult when the adolescent feels emotional overwhelmed.
3. **Other thought record technique:** Like journaling there are different kinds of worksheets that can help in reaching more awareness of the nature of the thoughts that we experience. These worksheets aim at recording our thoughts, emotions, actions and their consequences providing more clarity about our own selves. Below is an example of one such form of thought record technique through the use of worksheets. After going through a triggering or emotional provocative situation the adolescent can use these worksheets to reflect. Step 1 is recording/describing the event. Step 2 is looking back at

the kind of thoughts or self talk that was present during the event. Step 3 is becoming more aware of the emotion that was experienced in the same event. Step 4 is to understand the way the self reacted through actions during the event. The sequence of this process helps in understanding that a change in the thought or self talk that was triggered by the event and was followed up by related emotions and consequences. If we can change our talk to the self differently in that moment then there is a high possibility of arriving at a different emotional state leading to different actions and different consequences. If you look at the example below, one would realize the emotional and behavioral consequence of the thought that 'This always happens to me, I am a failure and I am not good enough' is so different from the possible consequence of the thought that 'I am a human being. I have both strengths and weaknesses. The future can hold a different and even a better outcome, if I learn from my mistakes and work differently this time'. Creating this alternate self talk statements can help in creating more healthier ways of looking at difficult situations.

4. **Creating positive and neutral statements/scipts for the self:** Identifying the negative self talk through journaling, using worksheets or by observing how we think and feel is important. However, replacing these negative self statements and challenging them with new ones is the next more important step. These new statements, scripts or narratives as some choose to call them can be created by the help of a counsellor/psychologist. One can do it by them selves as well. Listening to the positive affirmations or reading about them can help in creating new inner dialogues for ourselves. But it is important to understanding that not everyone will be able to feel and believe in the same statements. So, the statements that has worked for one person might not always work for another person. It is important to be able to believe in what we are telling ourselves. Repeating the statement that 'I am good enough' throughout the day might not work if I am not able to believe in it. Neutral statements can be less anxiety provoking and hence more believable. For example - 'its okay to make a mistake, I am only a human being, let me learn from this to avoid unnecessary problems in the future'.
5. **Practice replacing of the negative thoughts/self talk with the new more positive or neutral but healthier thoughts/self talk:** We are talking to ourselves almost all the time. This gives us a good opportunity to look at what we are saying and replacing it with the new statement. Talking to ourselves the way we talk to our best friend in times of crises to console them and make them feel better can be of advantage and thus can be adopted for our own selves as well. These new ways of conversing with the self can be achieved with practice like every other thing in life. The more we practice talking to our selves positively or in a neutral fashion the more automatic and natural it becomes. This practice aids in the latter use of these techniques. We can choose to motivate ourselves, give our selves good instructions to follow goals, encourage and reinforce ourselves in the direction that we want to venture in. When we start this practice it is better if we are in an emotionally peaceful mental space. When an individual is already stressed or upset or is going through an intense emotional state introducing these new positive or neutral statements may be very difficult. However, if the individual has practiced these ways of talking to the self before then it can be comparatively easier for the person to use these techniques when experiencing an emotionally negative state.
6. **Creating new, healthy and positive exposures for the self:** It is important to take charge when it might feel its very easy to give up and succumb to the negative thoughts and the negative dialogue that is either going on in the mind through out the day or in certain situations in an intense manner. Without a different form of exposure which is positive in nature the mind might continue to be

on the negative thinking direction. It a choice that we can help the adolescents make by exposing them to positive and healthy media content. The world we leave in is amazingly filled with people who are striving hard to create a good path for themselves in spite of the negative situations that they might find them selves in. Offering these stories to the adolescents can help them see that they always have a choice to turn themselves around by making different choices. There are well known people as well as ordinary individuals who have been through tremendous hardships, personal, emotional, physical, social or situational in nature. They have fallen and got back up on their feet again. For example – fighting with abuse in the family, social injustice, physical problems/ disabilities, chronic illness likes cancer, mental health issues, etc. We have books, movies, other videos and audios available all over the internet. Movies like Homeless to Havard, The King's Speech, Wonder just to name a few. Similarly there are inspirational books as well. Since we can observe that watching something nice and interesting can capture the interest in today's adolescent, schools can occasionally screen these movies in the class. Similarly more inspirational material can be discussed in class along with their study material. Students can be given projects to meet local people who have faced hardships in their life and come out it stronger and as a better person. How these individuals have copped with the situation should be discussed more often then the discussion of the problems alone. Some times only discussing the problems of the day can become very gloomy and feelings of despair take a greater grip on the person leading to the self talk of, 'nothing can be done about my state or the state that the society is in'. This thought creates only more despair and helplessness ultimately resulting into more anger, negative coping and also inaction at times. Calling known inspirational people to share their story in schools and colleges or other places where adolescents frequent more also increase their exposure to stories of hope, courage, love. What these individuals went through and the ways through which they copped would help in making an adolescent feel that they are not alone. 'There are others who are going through similar things and even others who have gone through it and survived through the difficult time', this thought or this form of self talk leads to hope and motivation to do something about the stressful situation. 'If some one similar to me can go through so much and still survive while creating a good life for themselves, then why cant I?' this is a statement that we would want them to think about. Similarly listening to songs that can motivate and pep us up for future is a good idea while we are feeling down. Positive, healthy, encouraging and motivational media content can help in the creation of a healthier internal dialogue because what we see and hear more frequently shapes the way we think, talk to others and ourselves.

7. **Increasing the availability of counselling services and other guidance programs:** The current position that our adolescents are in can be very emotional taxing, overwhelming and confusing. The pressure and the competition is surmounting. The exposure that they have in todays world can be baffling creating a fog in their minds over what is right or wrong. So many adolescents are going through depression, having suicidal thoughts and giving into unhealthy peer influences. Self worth issues, body image issues, and similar problems confront them on a regular biases. Some times they are able to handle things on their own but that might not be the plight of all. Under these circumstances having a judgement free space to talk about what they are going through can be helpful. A counsellor or a psychologist can play the role of a guide helping them develop a different and a more healthy perspective, healthy copping coping strategies and a positive way of talking to one self.

*Table 3. Self-talk and experience vs. alternatives*

| Event | My Thought or self talk | My Emotional experience | My Behavioral reaction & the consequence I faced | Alternate thought/ counter self talk |
|---|---|---|---|---|
| Failing in a test or an exam | This always happens to me, I am a failure and I am not good enough | Anger on the self, Disappointment, lack of motivation and sadness | Did not study for the next test which caused more problems latter. | I am a human being. I have both strengths and weaknesses. The future can hold a different and even a better outcome, if I learn from my mistakes and work differently this tim |

There is no denying that the type of self-talk that we engage in can have a significant impact on our wellbeing. Positive self-talk when used mindfully can boost our self-esteem, increase our confidence, and improve our mood. It can also help us to cope with stress, persevere through challenges, and achieve our goals. Negative self-talk if not kept under check can damage our self-esteem, lower our confidence, and lead to anxiety, depression, and other mental health problems. For adolescents, positive self-talk can be especially important. During adolescence, young people are often faced with a lot of new and challenging experiences. They may be starting high school, going through puberty, or dealing with peer pressure. In these challenging times, positive self-talk can provide them with the support and encouragement they need to succeed from within themselves.

## CONCLUSION

this chapter serves as a valuable reservoir of knowledge for those who are concerned about the well-being of adolescents in today's fiercely competitive and demanding milieu. It furnishes a comprehensive comprehension of self-talk and its various manifestations, elucidating their profound influence on an individual's thoughts, emotions, and actions. By disseminating the knowledge and techniques expounded in this chapter, adults and mental health professionals can assume a pivotal role in furnishing adolescents with the competencies requisite for thriving in an ever-evolving and demanding environment. Ultimately, the chapter advocates for a proactive approach to adolescent well-being, underscoring the primacy of prevention over remediation.

## REFERENCES

Alderson-Day, B., & Fernyhough, C. (2015). Inner Speech: Development, Cognitive Functions, Phenomenology, and Neurobiology. *Psychological Bulletin*, *141*(5), 931–965. doi:10.1037/bul0000021 PMID:26011789

Babakhanloo, A., Jalilvand, M., & Shoghi, B. (2017). Effectiveness of self-talk technique and positive empathy on deficient attittudes, hopelessness, and suicidal thoughts in women with breast cancer. *International Journal Of Medical Toxicology And Forensic Medicine*, *7*(1), 1–10. doi:10.22037/ijmtfm.v7i1(Winter).13178

Bandura, A. (1977). Self-efficacy: Toward a unifying theory of behavioral change. *Psychological Review*, *84*(2), 191–215. doi:10.1037/0033-295X.84.2.191 PMID:847061

Beck, A. T. (1993). Cognitive therapy: Past, present, and future. *Journal of Consulting and Clinical Psychology*, *61*(2), 194–198. doi:10.1037/0022-006X.61.2.194 PMID:8473571

Berk, L. E. (1992). Children's private speech: An overview of theory and the status of research. In R. M. Diaz & L. E. Berk (Eds.), *Private speech: From social interaction to self-regulation* (pp. 17–53). Lawrence Erlbaum Associates, Inc.

Brinthaupt,T.M., Benson,S.A., & Moore, Z.D. (2015). *Assessing the accuracy of self reported self-talk.* Frontiers. doi:10.3389/fpsyg.2015.00570

Brinthaupt, T. M., & Dove, C. T. (2012). Differences in self-talk frequency as a function of age, only-child, and imaginary childhood companion status. *Journal of Research in Personality*, *46*(3), 326–333. doi:10.1016/j.jrp.2012.03.003

Brinthaupt, T. M., Hein, M. B., & Kramer, T. E. (2009). The self-talk scale: Development, Factor Analysis, and Validation. *Journal of Personality Assessment*, *91*(1), 82–92. doi:10.1080/00223890802484498 PMID:19085287

Bruner, J. (1990). *Acts of meaning*. Harvard University Press.

Carver, C. S., & Scheier, M. F. (1998). *On the self-regulation of behavior.* Cambridge University Press., doi:10.1017/CBO9781139174794

Dagrou, E., Gauvin, L., & Halliwell, W. (1992). The effects of positive, negative and neutral self-talk on motor performance. *Canadian Journal of Sport Sciences*, *17*(2), 145–147. PMID:1324109

Dennett, D. (1992)... *The Self as a Center of Narrative Gravity*, *46*. doi:10.5209/revASEM.2013.v46.42862

Gibson, A. S. C. (2007). The role of self-talk in the awareness of physiological state and physical performance. *Sports Medicene*, *37*(12), 1–10.

Greer, J. A., Jacobs, J. M., El-Jawahri, A., Nipp, R. D., Gallagher, E. R., Pirl, W. F., Park, E. R., Muzikansky, A., Jacobsen, J. C., Jackson, V. A., & Temel, J. S. (2018). Role of Patient Coping Strategies in Understanding the Effects of Early Palliative Care on Quality of Life and Mood. *Journal of Clinical Oncology*, *36*(1), 53–60. doi:10.1200/JCO.2017.73.7221 PMID:29140772

Grzybowski, J., & Brinthaupt, T. M. (2022). Trait Mindfulness, Self-Compassion, and Self-Talk: A Correlational Analysis of Young Adults. *Behavioral Sciences (Basel, Switzerland)*, *12*(9), 300. doi:10.3390/bs12090300 PMID:36135104

Hardy, J. (2006). Speaking clearly: A critical review of the self-talk literature. *Psychology of Sport and Exercise*, *7*(1), 81–97. doi:10.1016/j.psychsport.2005.04.002

Hardy, J., Gammage, K., & Hall, C. (2001). A descriptive study of athlete self-talk. *The Sport Psychologist*, *15*(3), 306–318. doi:10.1123/tsp.15.3.306

Hardy, J., Hall, C. R., & Hardy, L. (2004). A Note on Athletes' Use of Self-Talk. *Journal of Applied Sport Psychology*, *16*(3), 251–257. doi:10.1080/10413200490498357

Hatzigeorgiadis, A. (2006). Instructional and motivational self-talk: An investigation on perceived self-talk functions. *Hellenic Journal of Psychology*, *3*(2), 164–175. https://www.researchgate.net/publication/284903463_instructional_and_motivational_self-talk_An_investigation_on_perceived_self-talk_funvtion

Heavey, C. L., & Hurlburt, R. T. (2007). The phenomena of inner experience. *Consciousness and Cognition*. doi:10.1016/j.concog.2007.12.006 PMID:18258456

Iddon, J. L., & Grant, L. (2013). Behavioural and cognitive treatment interventions in depression:An analysis of the evidence base. *Open Journal of Depression*, *2*(2), 1–10. doi:10.4236/ojd.2013.22003

Jemmer, P. (2010). Self-talk: The spells of Psycho-chaotic Sorcery. *European Journal of Clinical Hypnosis*, *9*(1), 51–58.

Lauria, M. J., Gallo, I. A., Rush, S., Brooks, J., Spiegel, R., & Weingart, S. D. (2017). Psychological Skills to Improve Emergency Care Providers' Performance Under Stress. *Annals of Emergency Medicine*, *70*(6), 884–890. doi:10.1016/j.annemergmed.2017.03.018 PMID:28460863

Leong, D., & Bodrova, E. (2006). Developing self-regulation: The vygotskian view. *Academic Exchange Quarterly*, *10*(4), 1–10.

Li,C.T., Cao,J., & Li,T.M.H.(2016). *Eustress or distress: an empirical study of perceived stress in everyday college life*, 1209-1217. ACM. doi:10.1145/2968219.2968309

Magnusson, J. E., & van Roon, C. A. (2013). Determining the Effectiveness of Personalized Versus Prescribed Self-Talk on Athletic Performance for Elite and Novice Athletes. *American Journal of Applied Psychology*, *1*(1), 1–6. doi:10.12691/ajap-1-1-1

Martin, J., Martin, W., & Slemon, A. G. (1989). Cognitive-mediational models of action-act sequences in counseling. *Journal of Counseling Psychology*, *36*(1), 8–16. doi:10.1037/0022-0167.36.1.8

Mehnert, A., Berg, P., Henrich, G., & Herschbach, P. (2009). Fear of cancer progression and cancer-related intrusive cognitions in breast cancer survivors. *Journal Of The Psychological. Psycho-Oncology*, *18*(12), 1273–1280. doi:10.1002/pon.1481 PMID:19267364

Mischel, W., Cantor, N., & Feldman, S. (1996). Principles of self-regulation: The nature of willpower and self-control. In E. T. Higgins & A. W. Kruglanski (Eds.), *Social Psychology: Handbook of basic principles* (pp. 329–360). Guilford.

Morin, A. (1993). Self-talk and self-awareness:On the nature of the relation. *Journal of Mind and Behavior*, *14*(3), 223–234. https://philpapers.org/rec/MORSAS

Morin, A. (1995). Preliminary data on a relation between self-talk and complexity of the self-concept. *Psychological Reports*, *76*(1), 1–10. doi:10.2466/pr0.1995.76.1.267 PMID:7770579

Muynck, G., Vansteenkiste, M., Delrue, J., & Aelterman, N. (2017). The effects of feedback valence and style on need satisfaction, self-talk, and perseverance among tennis players: An experimental study. *Journal of Sport & Exercise Psychology*, *39*(1), 1–38. doi:10.1123/jsep.2015-0326 PMID:28253062

Neck, C. P., & Manz, C. C. (1992). Thought self-leadership: The influence of self-talk and mental imagery on performance. *Journal of Organizational Behavior*, *13*(7), 681–699. doi:10.1002/job.4030130705

Orth, U., & Robins, R. (2018). Development of self-esteem across the lifespan. *Handbook of personality development,* 328-344. Research Gate. https://www.researchgate.net/publication/329512803_Development_of_SelfEsteem_Across_the_Lifespan

Orth, U., Robins, R. W., & Roberts, B. W. (2008). Low self-esteem prospectively predicts depression in adolescence and young adulthood. *Journal of Personality and Social Psychology*, *95*(3), 695–708. doi:10.1037/0022-3514.95.3.695 PMID:18729703

Orth, U., Robins, R. W., Widaman, K. F., & Conger, R. D. (2014). Is low self-esteem a risk factor for depression? Findings from a longitudinal study of Mexican-origin youth. *Developmental Psychology*, *50*(2), 622–633. doi:10.1037/a0033817 PMID:23895172

Sadri Damirchi, E., Mojarrad, A., Pireinaladin, S., & Grjibovski, A. M. (2020). The Role of Self-Talk in Predicting Death Anxiety, Obsessive-Compulsive Disorder, and CopingStrategies in the Face of Coronavirus Disease (COVID-19). *Iranian Journal of Psychiatry*, *15*(3), 182–188. doi:10.18502/ijps.v15i3.3810 PMID:33193766

Shahar, G., & Davidson, L. (2003). Depressive symptoms erode self-esteem in severe mental illnesss:A three-wave, cross-lagged study. *Journal Of Consulting and Clinical*, *71*(5), 21-31. doi:10.1037/0022-006X.71.5.890

Sowislo, J. F., & Orth, U. (2013). Does low self-esteem predict depression and anxiety? A meta-analysis of longitudinal studies. *Psychological Bulletin*, *139*(1), 213–240. doi:10.1037/a0028931 PMID:22730921

Stiles, W. B., Honos-Webb, L., & Surko, M. (1998). Responsiveness in psychotherapy. *Clinical Psychology : a Publication of the Division of Clinical Psychology of the American Psychological Association*, *5*(4), 439–458. doi:10.1111/j.1468-2850.1998.tb00166.x

Tomai, M., & Lauriola, M. (2019). Biopsychosocial correlates of adjustment to cancer during chemotherapy: The key role of health-related quality of life. *TheScientificWorldJournal*, *2019*(5), 1–12. doi:10.1155/2019/9750940 PMID:30983914

Vargas-Tonsing, T. M., Myers, N. D., & Feltz, D. L. (2004). Coaches' and Athletes' Perceptions of Efficacy-Enhancing Techniques. *The Sport Psychologist*, *18*(4), 397–414. doi:10.1123/tsp.18.4.397

Visser, M. M., Aben, L., Heijenbrok-Kal, M. H., Busschbach, J. J., & Ribbers, G. M. (2014). The relative effect of coping strategy and depression on health-related quality of life in patients in the chronic phase after stroke. *Journal of Rehabilitation Medicine*, *4*(6), 514–519. doi:10.2340/16501977-1803 PMID:24687167

Weinberg, R. S., Smith, J., Jackson, A., & Gould, D. (1984). Effect of association, dissociation and positive self-talk strategies on endurance performance. *Canadian Journal of Applied Sport Sciences*, *9*(1), 25–32. https://psycnet.apa.org/record/1985-00646-001 PMID:6705126

Yaratan, H., & Yucesoylu, R. (2010). Self-esteem,self-concept,self-talk and significant others statements in fifth grade students: Differences according to gender and school type. *Procedia: Social and Behavioral Sciences*, *2*(2), 3506–3518. doi:10.1016/j.sbspro.2010.03.543

Zastrow, C. (1988). What really causes psychotherapy change? *Journal of Independent Social Work*, *2*(3), 5–16. doi:10.1300/J283v02n03_02

# Chapter 17
# Flourishing on Campus:
## Promoting Mental Health and Coping Skills in Higher Education Institutions

**S. C. Vetrivel**
https://orcid.org/0000-0003-3050-8211
*Kongu Engineering College, India*

**T. Mohanasundaram**
https://orcid.org/0000-0003-4511-7539
*Ramaiah Institute of Technology, India*

## ABSTRACT

*Mental health concerns among college students have become a growing issue in higher education institutions worldwide. The transition to college life often comes with various stressors, such as academic pressure, social adjustments, and financial challenges, which can negatively impact students' well-being. To address this issue, higher education institutions are increasingly focusing on promoting mental health and coping skills to foster student flourishing. This abstract explores the importance of implementing initiatives and programs that support mental health and coping skills on college campuses. Firstly, it is essential to understand the concept of flourishing, which encompasses positive emotions, engagement, meaning, positive relationships, and accomplishment. Promoting flourishing on campus involves creating an environment that not only addresses mental health issues but also nurtures students' overall well-being.*

## 1. INTRODUCTION

### 1.1 Background and Significance of Mental Health in Higher Education Institutions

Over the past few decades, there has been a growing recognition of the profound impact that mental health issues can have on students, faculty, and staff within these institutions. The transition to college or university life can be a period of heightened stress, academic pressure, and social adjustment, making

DOI: 10.4018/979-8-3693-2833-0.ch017

individuals vulnerable to mental health challenges such as anxiety, depression, and substance abuse. Additionally, the COVID-19 pandemic has exacerbated these concerns, with many students facing increased isolation and disrupted learning environments. The deteriorating mental well-being of students in tertiary and higher education has become a growing focal point in public health and policy discussions (Association of Colleges, 2017; Hughes & Spanner, 2019; Sivertsen et al., 2019). The consequences of untreated mental health issues in higher education can be severe, including impaired academic performance, increased dropout rates, and a negative impact on overall well-being.

Recognizing the significance of this issue, higher education institutions have been taking proactive steps to address mental health concerns. They are implementing comprehensive mental health programs, offering counseling services, and creating more inclusive and supportive campus environments. This not only improves the well-being of students but also fosters a conducive learning environment. Furthermore, research in this area has also grown, shedding light on the prevalence of mental health challenges, the unique stressors faced by individuals in higher education, and effective intervention strategies. As a result, the importance of mental health in higher education has transcended beyond a campus issue; it has become a societal concern, with implications for workforce productivity and the overall health of future generations. Preventing poor mental health and supporting positive mental wellbeing needs to be based on an evidence informed understanding what factors influence the mental health of students.(Campbell et al., 2022).The background and significance of mental health in higher education institutions underscore the need for continued attention, resources, and research to ensure the well-being and success of individuals pursuing higher education.

## 2. UNDERSTANDING MENTAL HEALTH IN HIGHER EDUCATION

### 2.1 Prevalence and Impact of Mental Health Issues Among College Students

The prevalence and impact of mental health issues among college students have become a growing concern in recent years. A substantial body of research indicates that mental health problems are widespread in higher education settings. According to studies, approximately one in three college students experiences significant symptoms of anxiety or depression, making these conditions some of the most common mental health challenges on campuses. The factors contributing to this prevalence are multifaceted and include academic pressures, social isolation, financial stress, and the transition to adulthood.

The impact of these mental health issues is profound and far-reaching. They can hinder a student's ability to succeed academically, affecting their grades and overall performance. Moreover, untreated mental health conditions can lead to a range of negative outcomes, including increased dropout rates, substance abuse, and even suicidal ideation. College students facing mental health challenges may also struggle with forming and maintaining relationships, both socially and romantically. The stigma surrounding mental health can further exacerbate the problem, as students may be hesitant to seek help due to fear of judgment. To address this crisis, many colleges and universities are expanding their mental health services and raising awareness about the importance of emotional well-being, recognizing that the mental health of their students is not only essential for their academic success but also for their overall quality of life.

## 2.2 Factors Contributing to Mental Health Challenges in Higher Education

Mental health challenges are prevalent among students in higher education, and several factors contribute to these issues. It's essential for higher education institutions to prioritize the mental health and well-being of their students by providing support services, raising awareness, and creating a supportive campus environment. Depression and anxiety were both prevalent and widespread in students; all colleges reported students experiencing depression and 99% reported students experiencing severe anxiety (Bayram & Bilgel, 2008; Pereira et al., 2019). Students should be encouraged to seek help when needed and practice self-care to manage their mental health effectively.

It's important to recognize that these factors can vary from person to person, but some common contributors include:

- **Academic Pressure:** The high expectations, rigorous coursework, and competitive environment in higher education can lead to academic stress, anxiety, and depression. Students often feel pressured to excel academically, which can negatively impact their mental health.
- **Financial Stress:** Many students face financial difficulties, including tuition costs, living expenses, and student loan debt. Financial stress can contribute to anxiety and depression, as students worry about their ability to afford their education and meet their basic needs.
- **Social Isolation:** Transitioning to college or university can be challenging, and some students may struggle to make new friends or maintain existing social connections. Feelings of isolation and loneliness can have a significant impact on mental health.
- **Homesickness:** Moving away from home for the first time can trigger homesickness, which can lead to feelings of sadness and loneliness. This emotional strain can contribute to mental health challenges.
- **Pressure to Succeed:** There is often pressure to succeed not only academically but also in extracurricular activities and career planning. This constant pressure to excel can lead to burnout and mental health problems.
- **Sleep Deprivation:** Irregular schedules, late-night studying, and social activities can disrupt students' sleep patterns. Sleep deprivation can exacerbate mental health issues, including anxiety and depression.
- **Substance Abuse:** Some students turn to alcohol or drugs as a way to cope with stress and mental health challenges. Substance abuse can worsen mental health problems and lead to addiction.
- **Lack of Access to Mental Health Services:** Inadequate access to mental health resources, including counseling services and therapy, can make it difficult for students to seek help when needed.
- **Discrimination and Stigma:** Discrimination based on factors such as race, gender, sexual orientation, or disability can contribute to mental health challenges. Stigma around seeking help for mental health issues can also prevent some students from seeking support.
- **Balancing Multiple Responsibilities:** Many students juggle multiple responsibilities, such as work, family obligations, and care giving, in addition to their studies. This can lead to increased stress and decreased time for self-care.
- **Uncertainty About the Future:** The uncertainty about post-graduation plans, including employment prospects and student loan repayment, can cause anxiety and stress among students.
- **Pre-existing Mental Health Conditions:** Some students enter higher education with pre-existing mental health conditions, which can be exacerbated by the stressors of academic life.

## 2.3 Stigma and Barriers to Seeking Help

Stigma surrounding mental health remains a formidable barrier to individuals seeking help for their psychological well-being. This pervasive societal stigma often leads to discrimination, misunderstanding, and prejudice against those facing mental health challenges. People may fear being labeled as "crazy" or "weak" if they admit to struggling with their mental health, which can result in a reluctance to disclose their issues or seek professional assistance. This reluctance perpetuates a culture of silence, making it difficult for individuals to access the support they desperately need. Moreover, cultural, religious, or familial beliefs can exacerbate the stigma, discouraging people from acknowledging their mental health concerns or seeking help. As a result, many suffer in silence, potentially leading to the exacerbation of their conditions. Combatting stigma requires a concerted effort from society, including education, awareness campaigns, and fostering an environment of acceptance and empathy, to break down these barriers and encourage individuals to prioritize their mental health without fear of judgment.

## 2.4 Importance of Addressing Mental Health on Campus

Addressing mental health on campus is of paramount importance for several reasons. Firstly, a student's mental well-being significantly influences their academic performance and overall college experience. When students are struggling with mental health issues, their ability to concentrate, learn, and engage in campus activities can be severely compromised, leading to lower grades and decreased satisfaction with their education. Secondly, the college years are a time of significant personal growth and development, and untreated mental health problems can hinder this process, potentially impacting a student's future success and happiness. Moreover, fostering a supportive and inclusive campus environment that prioritizes mental health sends a powerful message to students that their well-being matters, reducing stigma and encouraging individuals to seek help when needed. Additionally, addressing mental health on campus can contribute to a safer community by identifying and assisting students who may be at risk of harming themselves or others. Ultimately, creating a campus culture that promotes mental health not only benefits individual students but also strengthens the overall academic community, leading to healthier, more successful, and happier graduates.

# 3. PROMOTING MENTAL HEALTH AWARENESS AND EDUCATION

## 3.1 The Role of Awareness Campaigns in Reducing Stigma

Awareness campaigns play a crucial role in reducing the stigma surrounding mental health by raising public consciousness, challenging stereotypes, and fostering empathy and understanding. These campaigns typically utilize various media channels, including television, social media, and community events, to disseminate information about mental health issues, their prevalence, and the importance of seeking help. By providing accurate and relatable information, they help debunk myths and misconceptions, such as the idea that mental health problems are a sign of personal weakness or that they affect only a small minority. Moreover, awareness campaigns often feature personal stories and testimonials from individuals who have experienced mental health challenges, which humanizes the issue and encourages open conversations.

These campaigns encourage people to talk openly about mental health, which is a crucial step in reducing stigma. When individuals feel comfortable discussing their own struggles or supporting loved ones, it helps normalize the topic. Furthermore, by emphasizing the prevalence of mental health issues, awareness campaigns show that these problems can affect anyone, regardless of age, gender, or background, fostering a sense of collective responsibility and compassion. In addition to public awareness, these campaigns often promote available resources and avenues for seeking help, reducing barriers to access. They may also highlight the importance of early intervention and the positive outcomes that can result from treatment and support. By addressing stigma through education and empathy, awareness campaigns contribute significantly to creating a more inclusive and supportive society for individuals dealing with mental health challenges.

## 3.2 Strategies for Promoting Mental Health Education on Campus

Promoting mental health education on a college campus is crucial for the well-being of students and the overall campus community. Promoting mental health education is an ongoing process, and it requires a commitment from the entire campus community. By implementing these strategies, we can create a campus environment that prioritizes mental well-being and provides the necessary resources for students to thrive.

Following are some strategies to help effectively promote mental health education on campus:

1. **Create a Mental Health Awareness Campaign:** Develop a comprehensive awareness campaign that includes posters, flyers, and social media posts to inform students about the importance of mental health education. Use relatable messaging and visuals to capture their attention.
2. **Host Workshops and Training Programs:** Organize workshops and training sessions on topics such as stress management, coping skills, and mental health first aid. Invite qualified mental health professionals to facilitate these sessions and provide students with practical tools and knowledge.
3. **Incorporate Mental Health Into Orientation Programs:** Integrate mental health education into orientation programs for new students. This sets the tone for the importance of mental well-being from the start of their college journey.
4. **Offer Supportive Services:** Ensure that counseling and mental health services are easily accessible on campus. Promote these services through various channels and emphasize their confidentiality.
5. **Peer Support Programs:** Establish peer support programs where trained student volunteers can provide a listening ear and guidance to their peers. These programs can help reduce stigma and encourage open conversations about mental health.
6. **Collaborate with Student Organizations:** Partner with student organizations to co-host events and activities related to mental health. Student-led initiatives can be highly effective in reaching their peers.
7. **Utilize Online Resources:** Create a dedicated website or portal with resources, self-help tools, and information related to mental health. Ensure that this resource is user-friendly and regularly updated.
8. **Faculty and Staff Training:** Provide training to faculty and staff on recognizing signs of mental distress in students and how to offer support or referrals. They play a critical role in identifying students in need.

9. **Promote a Healthy Campus Environment:** Encourage healthy lifestyle choices by promoting physical activity, good nutrition, and adequate sleep. These factors are closely linked to mental well-being.
10. **Address Stigma and Myths:** Develop campaigns that challenge stigmas and misconceptions surrounding mental health. Encourage open dialogue and create safe spaces for discussing mental health issues.
11. **Student Surveys and Feedback:** Conduct surveys to gauge students' mental health needs and gather feedback on existing mental health programs. Use this information to tailor the efforts effectively.
12. **Collaborate with Local Mental Health Organizations:** Partner with local mental health organizations to provide resources and support for students. This can include referrals to off-campus services and joint events.
13. **Promote Self-Care Practices:** Educate students about self-care practices such as mindfulness, meditation, and relaxation techniques. Encourage them to prioritize self-care as part of their daily routine.
14. **Evaluate and Adapt Programs:** Continuously assess the effectiveness of mental health education programs and make necessary adjustments based on feedback and outcomes.
15. **Promote a Culture of Compassion and Inclusivity:** Foster an inclusive and compassionate campus culture that emphasizes empathy, support, and understanding among students, faculty, and staff.

## 3.4 Incorporating Mental Health Into Academic Curriculum

Incorporating mental health into the academic curriculum is a crucial step towards addressing the growing mental health crisis among students. By integrating mental health education into the curriculum, educational institutions can foster a more holistic and supportive learning environment. This initiative involves teaching students about the importance of emotional well-being, stress management, self-care, and resilience alongside traditional subjects. It includes creating space for open discussions about mental health, reducing the stigma surrounding it, and providing resources for seeking help when needed. By doing so, students can develop a better understanding of their own mental health and that of their peers, helping to create a more empathetic and inclusive academic community. Furthermore, this approach equips students with essential life skills, enhancing their ability to cope with the challenges they may face during their educational journey and beyond. Ultimately, integrating mental health into the academic curriculum not only benefits students individually but also contributes to a healthier and more productive society as a whole.

## 3.5 Peer-Led Initiatives and Student Organizations Promoting Mental Health

Peer-led initiatives and student organizations play a vital role in promoting mental health on college campuses and in the broader community. These initiatives are characterized by the involvement of students who are passionate about mental health advocacy and support. They create safe spaces where individuals can openly discuss their mental health concerns, reducing the stigma surrounding these issues. Peer-led support groups, often led by trained student facilitators, provide a platform for sharing experiences and coping strategies. Additionally, these initiatives organize awareness campaigns, workshops, and events to educate students about mental health, stress management, and self-care. Such organizations empower students to take charge of their mental well-being and foster a sense of belonging and solidarity. By offering a peer-to-peer approach, they enhance accessibility to mental health resources and create a supportive environment that contributes to the overall well-being of students, addressing a critical need in today's educational institutions.

## 4. CREATING SUPPORTIVE CAMPUS ENVIRONMENTS

### 4.1 Developing a Comprehensive Mental Health Policy

Developing a comprehensive mental health policy is a multifaceted endeavor that requires careful planning and execution. Such a policy should encompass a wide range of strategies to address the unique challenges faced by students, faculty, and staff within these academic settings. According to a cohort study conducted in the UK, there is an observed rise in psychological distress when students enter university (Bewick et al., 2010). Additionally, recent findings indicate a growing incidence of mental health issues among university students, such as self-harm and suicide (Hughes & Spanner, 2019; Sivertsen et al., 2019). This alarming trend has led to an increased demand for mental health support services for students, with reports from some universities indicating a doubling in the number of students seeking assistance (Thorley, 2017). Firstly, it should prioritize destigmatizing mental health issues by fostering a culture of openness and understanding, where seeking help is encouraged and normalized. To achieve this, awareness campaigns and educational programs can be implemented to increase mental health literacy. Furthermore, the policy should allocate resources to establish accessible and affordable mental health services on campus, such as counseling centers staffed with trained professionals. These centers should offer a variety of support options, including individual therapy, group counseling, and crisis intervention. Additionally, the policy should emphasize preventative measures, such as stress management workshops, mindfulness programs, and resilience-building activities, to equip students and staff with coping skills and emotional resilience.

Inclusivity is another vital aspect of the policy, ensuring that the mental health needs of diverse populations, including marginalized groups, are recognized and addressed appropriately. Collaborations with community mental health organizations can extend the reach of these services beyond campus boundaries. Furthermore, data collection and evaluation mechanisms should be integrated to continuously assess the effectiveness of the policy, enabling adjustments and improvements over time. A comprehensive mental health policy for higher education institutions should strive to create a supportive environment that fosters the holistic well-being of all stakeholders, facilitating not only academic success but also personal growth and fulfillment. It should be adaptable, evolving in response to changing circumstances and emerging best practices, with a long-term commitment to nurturing mental health as an integral part of the educational experience.

### 4.2 Enhancing Accessibility and Availability of Mental Health Services

In recent years, the recognition of the mental health challenges faced by students has grown significantly, and it has become clear that proactive measures are needed to support their well-being. To achieve this, universities and colleges must invest in a multifaceted approach. Firstly, providing easily accessible on-campus counseling services with flexible hours and well-trained mental health professionals can reduce barriers to seeking help. Telehealth options should also be expanded, allowing students to access services remotely, especially during the COVID-19 pandemic and for those who may have physical or scheduling constraints. Additionally, promoting mental health literacy through educational programs and workshops can empower students with the knowledge and skills necessary to manage stress, anxiety, and other mental health issues. Collaborative efforts between academic departments, counseling centers, and student organizations can further destigmatize mental health discussions and encourage a culture of open communication. There is a clear association between a student's mental health and financial well-being (Benson-Egglenton, 2019), with "increased financial concern being consistently associated with worse health" (Jessop et al., 2005). By prioritizing the mental well-being of their students and implementing these strategies, higher education institutions can create a supportive environment that fosters resilience, coping skills, and ultimately, academic success.

## 4.3 Establishing Counseling Centers and Student Support Programs

Mental health is a critical aspect of overall well-being, and it significantly impacts a student's academic success, personal growth, and future prospects. In higher education institutions, students often face various stressors, including academic pressures, social challenges, and personal issues, which can lead to mental health issues if not addressed effectively. To promote mental health and coping skills among students, it is essential to establish counseling centers and implement student support programs within higher education institutions.

### 4.3.1 Establishing Counseling Centers

1. Comprehensive Counseling Services:
    a. Establish dedicated counseling centers on campus, staffed by qualified mental health professionals, including psychologists, counselors, and social workers.
    b. Offer a wide range of services, including individual therapy, group therapy, crisis intervention, and psychoeducation.
2. Accessibility and Availability:
    a. Ensure easy access to counseling services by providing multiple channels for students to seek help, such as in-person appointments, teletherapy, and crisis hotlines.
    b. Extend counseling center hours to accommodate diverse student schedules, including evenings and weekends.
3. Awareness and Destigmatization:
    a. Launch awareness campaigns to destigmatize seeking help for mental health issues and promote a culture of openness and acceptance.
    b. Encourage faculty and staff to support mental health initiatives and refer students to counseling services when needed.
4. Tailored Support:
    a. Provide specialized support for diverse student populations, including LGBTQ+ students, international students, students with disabilities, and students from underrepresented backgrounds.

### 4.3.2 Implementing Student Support Programs

1. Mental Health Education:
    a. Integrate mental health education into the curriculum, offering courses or workshops that teach coping skills, stress management, and emotional intelligence.
    b. Provide online resources and self-help materials for students to access at their convenience.
2. Peer Support Programs:
    a. Develop peer support programs, where trained students can offer a listening ear and guidance to their peers.
    b. Create a mentorship system to connect incoming students with experienced peers who can assist with the transition to college life.
3. Wellness Initiatives:
    a. Promote holistic wellness through initiatives like yoga and mindfulness classes, fitness programs, and healthy eating campaigns.
    b. Offer relaxation spaces on campus for students to unwind and de-stress.
4. Crisis Response and Prevention:
    a. Establish crisis response teams that can quickly address emergencies and provide immediate support to students in crisis.
    b. Develop prevention strategies, including early identification of at-risk students and proactive outreach.
5. Collaboration and Partnerships:
    a. Collaborate with local mental health organizations and hospitals to ensure seamless referral and access to external resources when needed.
    b. Partner with student organizations to organize mental health awareness events and activities.

## 4.4 Addressing the Needs of Specific Student Populations (e.g., International Students, LGBTQ+ Students)

Addressing the needs of specific student populations, such as international students and LGBTQ+ students, is crucial for promoting mental health and coping skills in higher education institutions. These groups may face unique challenges and stressors that require tailored approaches to ensure their well-being. By addressing the specific needs of international students and LGBTQ+ students through these strategies, higher education institutions can promote mental health and coping skills, ultimately contributing to a more inclusive and supportive learning environment for all students. One study (O'Neill et al., 2018) recruited LGBTQ (lesbian, gay, bisexual, transgender, intersex, queer/questioning) students. Some strategies and considerations for addressing their mental health and coping needs given below:

1. Cultural Competence and Sensitivity Training:
    a. Provide cultural competence training for faculty, staff, and mental health professionals to better understand and support international students' diverse backgrounds and experiences.
    b. Conduct LGBTQ+ sensitivity training to create an inclusive and affirming campus environment.

2. Counseling Services:
    a. Offer counseling services specifically tailored to the needs of international students, including counselors who understand the challenges of adjusting to a new culture and educational system.
    b. Employ mental health professionals who are knowledgeable about LGBTQ+ issues and can provide affirming and inclusive counseling.
3. Supportive Communities:
    a. Create safe and welcoming spaces for international students and LGBTQ+ students to connect with peers who share similar experiences. Student organizations and support groups can help foster a sense of belonging.
    b. Encourage the formation of student-led diversity and inclusion clubs or organizations that promote mental health awareness and coping strategies.
4. Mental Health Education:
    a. Offer workshops and seminars that address the unique mental health challenges faced by international students and LGBTQ+ students.
    b. Include mental health and coping skills in orientation programs for these student populations.
5. Access to Resources:
    a. Ensure that international students and LGBTQ+ students are aware of available mental health resources and support services, including counseling centers, crisis hotlines, and online resources.
    b. Make information on health insurance coverage and mental health services easily accessible and understandable for international students.
6. Inclusive Policies and Practices:
    a. Develop and implement inclusive policies that protect the rights and well-being of LGBTQ+ students, such as gender-neutral housing options, restroom facilities, and non-discrimination policies.
    b. Promote inclusivity and diversity in curricula and classroom discussions to create a more welcoming educational environment for all students.
7. Mentoring and Peer Support:
    a. Establish mentoring programs where international students can connect with faculty or senior students who can provide guidance on academic and cultural adjustment.
    b. Encourage peer support initiatives within the LGBTQ+ community to help students build coping skills and share experiences.
8. Data Collection and Assessment:
    a. Collect data on the mental health and well-being of international students and LGBTQ+ students to understand their unique challenges and track progress.
    b. Use assessment results to continually refine support programs and services.
9. Collaboration with Student Services:
    a. Collaborate with various student services, including career counseling, academic advising, and disability support services, to provide holistic support for students' mental health and coping needs.
10. Promote Allyship:
    a. Encourage faculty, staff, and students to act as allies and advocates for international and LGBTQ+ students, creating a more inclusive and supportive campus community.

# 5. BUILDING RESILIENCE AND COPING SKILLS

## 5.1 Understanding Resilience and Its Importance in Higher Education

Recognizing the supreme importance of resilience within today's constantly changing academic environment is crucial in higher education.. Resilience in this context refers to an individual's ability to bounce back from setbacks, adapt to challenges, and maintain a sense of well-being while pursuing their educational goals. In an era marked by rapid technological advancements, shifting societal norms, and unforeseen global crises, resilience is the cornerstone of a successful academic journey. An illustration of this phenomenon is the substantial increase in referrals for young individuals with eating disorders seeking treatment within the NHS. The number of such referrals nearly doubled from 2019 to 2020 (NHS England., 2021). It enables students to navigate academic pressures, manage stress, and persevere through difficulties, ultimately fostering a more positive and effective learning experience. Moreover, resilience equips students with essential life skills that extend beyond the classroom, preparing them for the uncertainties of the future job market and society at large. By fostering resilience in higher education, institutions not only enhance students' capacity to excel academically but also empower them to become adaptable, resourceful, and resilient individuals capable of thriving in an increasingly complex world.

## 5.2 Promoting Stress Management and Self-Care Practices

The demanding nature of higher education can lead to high levels of stress and anxiety, which can negatively impact students' mental and physical health. Given below some strategies to promote stress management and self-care practices in higher education:

- **Incorporate Stress Management Into the Curriculum:** Integrate stress management and self-care topics into the curriculum. Offer courses or workshops on mindfulness, meditation, time management, and coping strategies.
- **Offer Counseling Services:** Provide on-campus counseling services staffed with trained professionals who can offer individual or group therapy sessions to help students manage stress and develop coping skills.
- **Peer Support Programs:** Establish peer support programs or mentoring systems where senior students can guide and support newer students in managing stress and adapting to the demands of higher education.
- **Physical Well-Being Initiatives:** Promote physical health through fitness programs, yoga classes, and access to gym facilities. Physical activity can reduce stress and improve overall well-being.
- **Mental Health Awareness Campaigns:** Run awareness campaigns to reduce the stigma around seeking mental health support. Encourage students to seek help when needed and make them aware of available resources.
- **Time Management Workshops:** Offer workshops on time management and study skills. Teaching students how to effectively manage their time can reduce the pressure they feel from academic responsibilities.
- **Access to Relaxation Spaces:** Create designated relaxation spaces on campus where students can unwind, meditate, or practice mindfulness. These spaces should be quiet and conducive to relaxation.

- **Promote Healthy Eating and Sleep Habits:** Educate students about the importance of nutrition and sleep for stress management. Encourage them to maintain balanced diets and prioritize sleep.
- **Online Resources:** Develop and promote online resources such as articles, videos, and apps that provide tips and techniques for stress management and self-care.
- **Peer Support Groups:** Encourage the formation of peer support groups where students can share their experiences and coping strategies. These groups can provide emotional support and a sense of belonging.
- **Faculty and Staff Involvement:** Involve faculty and staff in promoting stress management and self-care. Encourage them to be understanding of students' challenges and provide flexibility when necessary.
- **Evaluation and Feedback:** Continuously assess the effectiveness of your stress management and self-care initiatives through surveys, focus groups, or other feedback mechanisms. Use this feedback to make improvements.
- **Promote Work-Life Balance:** Emphasize the importance of maintaining a healthy work-life balance. Encourage students to engage in hobbies and activities outside of their academic responsibilities.
- **Crisis Intervention Plans:** Develop clear crisis intervention plans to address severe cases of stress, anxiety, or mental health crises. Ensure that students know how to access emergency support.
- **Collaborate With Student Organizations:** Collaborate with student organizations to organize stress-relief events, wellness fairs, or seminars on self-care practices.

## 5.3 Enhancing Coping Skills Through Workshops and Training Programs

Enhancing coping skills through workshops and training programs for students in higher education is vital in today's fast-paced and demanding academic environment. These initiatives provide students with invaluable tools to navigate the complexities of their academic journey and beyond. Through interactive workshops and targeted training sessions, students learn effective stress management techniques, time management strategies, and emotional resilience. These skills not only empower them to handle the pressures of coursework and exams but also equip them with essential life skills that are transferable to various personal and professional situations. By fostering a supportive and proactive approach to mental health and well-being, universities and colleges are not only investing in the success of their students but also contributing to the development of resilient, adaptable, and confident individuals who can thrive in an ever-changing world.

## 5.4 Integrating Mindfulness and Meditation Practices on Campus

In an increasingly fast-paced and stress-ridden academic environment, these practices offer a powerful toolset for students to cultivate mental clarity, emotional resilience, and overall well-being. By providing accessible resources, such as meditation classes, quiet spaces for reflection, and workshops on mindfulness techniques, universities can empower students to better manage the pressures of academia and navigate the challenges of personal growth. Beyond stress reduction, mindfulness and meditation encourage self-awareness, empathy, and a deeper connection to one's own thoughts and feelings, which can enhance interpersonal relationships and foster a sense of community on campus. Ultimately, integrating these practices not only supports students in their academic journeys but also equips them with lifelong skills to thrive in an ever-evolving world.

# 6. STRENGTHENING SOCIAL CONNECTIONS

## 6.1 Importance of Social Support Networks in Student Well-Being

Social support networks take part in a crucial task in promoting the well-being of students in higher education. This critical period of academic and personal growth can be challenging, often accompanied by stress, anxiety, and feelings of isolation. Having a strong support system, whether it's through friends, family, or university resources, can provide students with a safety net to navigate these difficulties. Social support networks offer emotional support, guidance, and a sense of belonging, which are essential for maintaining mental health and academic success. They provide a platform for students to share their concerns, seek advice, and connect with like-minded individuals, fostering a sense of community that can significantly enhance their overall college experience. Additionally, these networks can act as a buffer against the adverse effects of stress, ultimately contributing to the holistic well-being of students pursuing higher education.

## 6.2 Building Positive Relationships and Fostering Community on Campus

Building positive relationships can enhance the overall college experience, contribute to personal growth, and provide valuable support systems. Given below are some strategies for students to achieve this:

- **Attend Campus Events:** Get involved in on-campus events, such as club meetings, workshops, and social gatherings. These activities are great opportunities to meet people with similar interests.
- **Join Clubs and Organizations:** Join clubs or student organizations that align with your interests or goals. Being part of a group with a common purpose can lead to meaningful friendships.
- **Volunteer:** Participate in community service or volunteer activities. This not only helps you connect with like-minded individuals but also gives you a sense of purpose and fulfillment.
- **Attend Orientation Programs:** Attend orientation events and programs designed to help new students acclimate to campus life. These events are excellent for making initial connections with fellow students.
- **Utilize Social Media:** Join campus-related social media groups or pages to stay informed about events and connect with peers. Many universities have dedicated Facebook groups or online communities for students.
- **Study Groups:** Form or join study groups for your classes. Collaborating with classmates not only helps with academic success but also fosters a sense of camaraderie.
- **Residential Life:** If you live on campus, engage with your dorm or housing community. Attend floor or building meetings, and be open to meeting your neighbors.
- **Participate in Sports and Fitness:** If you're into sports or fitness, consider joining intramural teams or using the campus gym. Physical activity can be a great way to relieve stress and bond with others.

- **Mentorship Programs:** Seek out mentorship programs on campus. These can connect you with experienced students or faculty who can offer guidance and support.
- **Networking:** Attend career fairs, networking events, and workshops related to your field of study. Building professional relationships early can be beneficial for your future career.
- **Open Communication:** Be open and approachable. Smile, introduce yourself, and strike up conversations with classmates, roommates, and instructors.
- **Cultural and Diversity Events:** Explore and attend events celebrating cultural diversity on campus. Embracing different cultures can lead to cross-cultural friendships and a broader perspective.
- **Respect and Inclusivity:** Show respect and inclusivity to all members of the campus community, regardless of their background, beliefs, or identity. A welcoming environment encourages positive relationships.
- **Seek Help When Needed:** If you're struggling with academics or personal challenges, don't hesitate to seek help from counseling services or academic advisors. They can provide guidance and support during difficult times.
- **Organize Your Own Events:** If you have a passion or interest not represented on campus, consider starting your own club or organizing events. This can help you connect with others who share your enthusiasm.

## 6.3 Encouraging Peer Support and Mentorship Programs

Peer support and mentorship programs not only provide a sense of belonging and community but also offer invaluable opportunities for personal and academic growth. By connecting experienced upperclassmen or graduate students with newcomers, institutions can help ease the transition into college life, tackle academic challenges, and navigate the complexities of higher education. only a third of students with mental health problems seek support from counselling services in the UK (Macaskill, 2013). Peer mentors serve as role models, offering guidance on course selection, study strategies, and time management, which can significantly improve students' academic success. Moreover, these initiatives enhance interpersonal skills, promote diversity and inclusion, and create a supportive network that can boost confidence and self-esteem. In sum, fostering peer support and mentorship programs in higher education enriches the overall student experience and contributes to the development of well-rounded, empowered individuals ready to excel both inside and outside the classroom.

## 6.4 Promoting Inclusive and Diverse Social Environments

Promoting inclusive and diverse social environments in higher education is not merely an aspiration; it is very important for fostering a truly enriching and equitable learning experience. Universities and colleges serve as melting pots of diverse backgrounds, cultures, and perspectives. Embracing and celebrating this diversity not only empowers students to become global citizens but also enhances their cognitive and social growth. By actively encouraging inclusivity, educational institutions create spaces where every student, regardless of their race, ethnicity, gender, sexual orientation, or socioeconomic background, feels valued and respected. This inclusive atmosphere fosters open dialogue, encourages critical thinking, and nurtures empathy – all crucial skills for today's interconnected world. Through proactive policies, educational programs, and campus initiatives, higher education institutions can cultivate an environment that not only welcomes diversity but also ensures that it thrives, preparing students to become more compassionate, informed, and adaptable individuals.

## 7. ADDRESSING CRISIS AND EMERGENCIES

### 7.1 Establishing Protocols for Responding to Mental Health Crises

The protocols serve as a crucial framework for colleges and universities to address the diverse and complex mental health needs of their student populations. They typically involve a multi-faceted approach that includes training staff and faculty to recognize signs of distress, providing readily accessible mental health resources, and establishing clear procedures for responding to crises. By promoting a culture of care and understanding, these protocols aim to destigmatize mental health issues and encourage students to seek help when needed. Moreover, they play a pivotal role in fostering a supportive and inclusive educational environment where students can thrive both academically and emotionally.

### 7.2 Training Staff and Faculty in Recognizing and Responding to Emergencies

The training programs equip educators with the knowledge and skills needed to identify potential emergency situations, ranging from natural disasters to medical crises and security threats. By fostering a culture of preparedness, educational institutions empower their staff and faculty to act swiftly and effectively in critical situations, reducing the potential for harm and enhancing the overall security of the campus community. Moreover, such training not only saves lives but also provides a sense of reassurance to students, who can focus on their academic pursuits knowing that their educators are well-prepared to respond to emergencies, thereby creating a conducive and secure learning environment. In today's dynamic world, where unexpected challenges can arise, ongoing training in emergency response is an essential element in the holistic education and care of students in higher education.

### 7.3 Suicide Prevention and Intervention Strategies

Suicide prevention and intervention strategies are of dominant significance in higher education settings, where students often face academic pressures, personal challenges, and a transitional period of increased stress and uncertainty. Creating a supportive and proactive environment is crucial to address this issue. One key approach is to establish comprehensive mental health programs that destigmatize seeking help and provide easy access to counseling services. Faculty and staff should be trained to recognize signs of distress in students and know how to refer them to appropriate resources. Promoting a culture of open communication and peer support is equally vital, as it encourages students to reach out to one another when they suspect someone is struggling. Furthermore, educational institutions should disseminate information on mental health resources, crisis helplines, and self-help tools, ensuring that students are aware of available assistance. Ultimately, by fostering a compassionate and informed community, higher education institutions can play a pivotal role in preventing and intervening in cases of suicide, saving lives and promoting the well-being of their students.

### 7.4 Collaborating With Local Mental Health Resources and Emergency Services

By establishing strong partnerships with community mental health organizations and emergency responders, universities can create a safety net that supports students facing mental health crises. This collaboration allows for timely intervention and access to professional mental health services when needed, helping to prevent or address issues such as anxiety, depression, and suicidal thoughts. Additionally, it enables higher education institutions to provide comprehensive training to faculty, staff, and students on recognizing signs of distress and knowing how to connect individuals to the appropriate resources. Ultimately, these collaborative efforts foster a more caring and resilient campus environment, where students can thrive academically and emotionally.

## 8. EVALUATING AND IMPROVING CAMPUS MENTAL HEALTH INITIATIVES

### 8.1 Importance of Ongoing Evaluation and Assessment

The importance of ongoing evaluation and assessment of Campus Mental Health Initiatives in higher education cannot be overstated. Continuous evaluation allows institutions to gauge the effectiveness of their initiatives, identify areas that require improvement, and tailor their support services to the evolving needs of the student body. Regular assessment not only ensures that resources are allocated efficiently but also provides a mechanism for students to actively participate in the process, voicing their concerns and suggestions. Furthermore, it helps in undeceive mental health, fostering a culture of openness and understanding. In an era where the pressures and challenges faced by students are ever-changing, ongoing evaluation and assessment of Campus Mental Health Initiatives are essential to safeguarding the emotional well-being of those pursuing higher education.

### 8.2 Long-Term Sustainability of Mental Health Initiatives

Long-term sustainability of mental health initiatives in higher education is essential for ensuring the well-being of students and the overall success of academic institutions. These initiatives must extend beyond short-term fixes and reactive measures. A sustainable approach involves creating a culture of mental health awareness, destigmatizing seeking help, and integrating mental health support into the fabric of the educational environment. This means consistently providing access to counseling services, promoting stress reduction and coping strategies, and fostering a supportive community where students can openly discuss their mental health challenges. Moreover, collaboration between students, faculty, and administrators is crucial in developing and maintaining programs that evolve with the changing needs of the student body. By prioritizing long-term sustainability, higher education institutions can contribute to the holistic development of their students and create a nurturing environment where mental health is given the attention and care it deserves.

## 9. CONCLUSION

In recent years, there has been a significant shift in the discourse surrounding mental health on college campuses, reflecting both emerging trends and pressing challenges for students in higher education.

One notable trend is the growing acknowledgment of the importance of proactive mental health support. Universities are increasingly prioritizing prevention and early intervention programs, recognizing that addressing mental health issues before they escalate is crucial. Another key trend is the integration of technology, with virtual counseling services and mental health apps becoming more commonplace, making mental health resources more accessible to students. However, alongside these positive changes, numerous challenges persist. The stigma around mental health remains a formidable barrier to seeking help for many students, and the increased stress and isolation stemming from academic pressures and the pandemic have exacerbated these issues. Moreover, institutions must grapple with resource limitations and the need for a more culturally sensitive approach to mental health support. Thus, as we navigate this evolving landscape, it is imperative for colleges and universities to prioritize the mental well-being of their students, foster open conversations, and adapt to meet the changing needs of their diverse student populations. The state of campus mental health is a matter of utmost concern for higher education institutions. As we reflect on the challenges and opportunities discussed in this discourse, it is imperative that universities and colleges across the globe recognize their pivotal role in fostering a nurturing and supportive environment for their students. We must prioritize mental health as an integral component of the educational experience and commit to destigmatizing seeking help for psychological well-being. To achieve this, higher education institutions must invest in comprehensive mental health programs, increase awareness campaigns, and strengthen collaboration with mental health professionals. Moreover, we urge students to actively engage in self-care practices, reach out to their peers in times of need, and advocate for mental health resources on their campuses. It is only through collective action and a shared commitment to prioritizing mental health that we can create campuses that truly foster the holistic growth and success of our students. Let us embark on this journey together, ensuring that every student feels valued, supported, and empowered to thrive in their academic pursuits and beyond.

## REFERENCES


Association of Colleges. (2017). Ao*C Survey on Students with Mental Health Conditions in Further Education*. AOC.

Bayram, N., & Bilgel, N. (2008). The prevalence and socio-demographic correlations of depression, anxiety and stress among a group of university students. *Social Psychiatry and Psychiatric Epidemiology, 43*(8), 667–672. doi:10.100700127-008-0345-x PMID:18398558

Benson-Egglenton, J. (2019). The financial circumstances associated with high and low wellbeing in undergraduate students: A case study of an English Russell Group institution. *Journal of Further and Higher Education, 43*(7), 901–913. doi:10.1080/0309877X.2017.1421621

Bewick, B., Koutsopoulou, G., Miles, J., Slaa, E., & Barkham, M. (2010). Changes in undergraduate students' psychological well-being as they progress through university. *Studies in Higher Education, 35*(6), 633–645. doi:10.1080/03075070903216643

Campbell, F., Blank, L., Cantrell, A., Baxter, S., Blackmore, C., Dixon, J., & Goyder, E. (2022). Factors that influence mental health of university and college students in the UK: A systematic review. *BMC Public Health, 22*(1), 1778. doi:10.118612889-022-13943-x PMID:36123714

Hughes, G., & Spanner, L. (2019). *The university mental health charter*. Student Minds.

Jessop, D. C., Herberts, C., & Solomon, L. (2005). The impact of financial circumstances on student health. *British Journal of Health Psychology*, *10*(3), 421–439. doi:10.1348/135910705X25480 PMID:16238857

Macaskill, A. (2013). The mental health of university students in the United Kingdom. *British Journal of Guidance & Counselling*, *41*(4), 426–441. doi:10.1080/03069885.2012.743110

NHS England. (2021). *Children and Young People with an Eating Disorder Waiting Times*. NHS England. https://www.england.nhs.uk/statistics/statistical-work-areas/cyped-waiting-times/

O'Neill, S., McLafferty, M., Ennis, E., Lapsley, C., Bjourson, T., Armour, C., Murphy, S., Bunting, B., & Murray, E. (2018). Socio-demographic, mental health and childhood adversity risk factors for self-harm and suicidal behaviour in College students in Northern Ireland. *Journal of Affective Disorders*, *239*, 58–65. doi:10.1016/j.jad.2018.06.006 PMID:29990663

Pereira, S., Reay, K., Bottell, J., Walker, L., Dzikiti, C., Platt, C., & Goodrham, C. (2019). *University Student Mental Health Survey 2018: A large scale study into the prevalence of student mental illness within UK universities*. Insight Network.

Sivertsen, B., Hysing, M., Knapstad, M., Harvey, A. G., Reneflot, A., Lønning, K. J., & O'Connor, R. C. (2019). Suicide attempts and non-suicidal self-harm among university students: Prevalence study. *BJPsych Open*, *5*(2), e26. doi:10.1192/bjo.2019.4 PMID:31068238

Thorley, C. (2017). *Not By Degrees: Not by degrees: Improving student mental health in the UK's universities*. IPPR.

# Chapter 18
# Support Services to Enhance Students' Mental Health in Higher Education Institutions in Namibia

**Emilia Ndapandula Mbongo**
https://orcid.org/0000-0001-6560-8664
*University of Namibia, Namibia*

**Mirjam Sheyapo**
*University of Namibia, Namibia*

## ABSTRACT

*This chapter presents an overview of the support services to enhance students' mental health in higher education institutions in Namibia. In light of the myriad difficulties encountered by students on a daily basis, it is imperative to establish frameworks that guarantee the provision of essential assistance to foster academic excellence. An analysis was conducted by reviewing various sources in order to obtain an understanding of the student affairs and support services offered at three leading universities in Namibia. These services encompass a range of areas, such as counselling services, peer support programs, initiatives promoting mental health awareness, mental health screening, accommodation and support services, and crisis intervention services. Institutional support mechanisms in terms of policy and practice and recommendations for future practice are examined.*

## INTRODUCTION

Mental health is crucial for students to succeed not only in their everyday lives, but most importantly, in their academic lives. However, students encounter numerous obstacles that complicate their lives, jeopardise their mental health, and impede their academic success (Abrams, 2022; Hans-Werner, 2015; Lattie et al. 2019; Pedrelli et al. 2015; Stein, 2013). Research evidence suggests that relationship prob-

DOI: 10.4018/979-8-3693-2833-0.ch018

lems, eating disorders, family issues, bereavement, stress, worry, abuse, and sexuality or gender identity crises are just a few of the problems students face daily (Pedrelli et al. 2015; Gupta et al. 2023). Pedrelli et al. (2015) argue that it is possible for mental health issues to develop for the first time as students get to higher education institutions due to academic pressure and other factors. The period of attending university is accompanied by a transitional phase in which the typical student experiences a new stage of personal growth, resulting in heightened obligations and duties. The importance of student mental health and its link to academic success is well documented (Bostani et al., 2014; Shankar & Park, 2016; Wyatt et al., 2017). Therefore, for students to have sound mental health, it is necessary to have support mechanisms in institutions of higher learning for those facing difficulties in place (Browne, 2017; Buizza et al. 2022; Hans-Werner, 2015; Prince, 2015).

In light of the considerable prevalence of mental health difficulties in student populations (Bantjes, et al. 2023; Katz & Davison, 2014; Macaskill, 2013; Oswalt et al., 2020; Porter, 2018), higher education institutions must provide comprehensive support systems that prioritise the promotion of students' psychological well-being. Indeed, many higher education institutions worldwide have been documented as having comprehensive structures in place, aiming aimed at promoting students' mental well-being and facilitate their academic focus (Cage et al., 2020; DiPlacito-DeRango, 2016; Giamos et al., 2017; Hughes & Spanner, 2019; Priestley et al., 2020). However, little is known about the support structures of students' mental health in institutions of higher education in Namibia. Thus, the chapter provides an overview of various student support services available at institutions of higher education in Namibia.

## BACKGROUND

Mental health is a fundamental human right and an integral component of our overall health and well-being. The World Health Organisation [WHO] (2022) defines mental health as a condition of well-being in which every individual realises their potential, can deal with the pressures of everyday life, is productive in their work, and can make a positive contribution to society. Having sound mental health enables individuals to enhance their capacity for social interaction, cognitive functioning, adaptive coping, and overall well-being. For students to be able to navigate life's challenges in addition to those that are a direct consequence of being a student, mental health is even more crucial. Therefore, the prioritisation of student mental health within the context of higher education institutions should be a central focus in conversations pertaining to the overall welfare of students. According to Goodman (2017), mental health is a significant concern among post-secondary education students due to the unique developmental opportunities presented by institutions of higher education environment. This is because institutions of higher learning offer a crucial platform for equipping students with necessary skills to foster long-term mental health and overall well-being.

Mental health is a concern among the general population, and according to WHO (2022) approximately one in eight people in the world has a mental disorder. The prevalence of mental health difficulties among students is rising in response to the fast pace of modern society (Abelson et al., 2022; Hans-Werner, 2015; Johnson & Lester, 2021; Lattie et al., 2019; Storrie et al., 2010). According to Abrams (2022), today's students face a multitude of challenges encompassing academic demands, interpersonal dynamics, acclimation to the campus environment, financial constraints, societal inequities, instances of widespread violence, and multiple forms of loss. In addition to these challenges, post-secondary education entails heightened academic demands and exposure to new social environments. Brown (2016) noted that many students, particularly first-year students, are living away from home for the first time and may lack direct access to their key support networks while confronting a variety of obstacles. The experience of living away from home can be particularly arduous and challenging for students, especially those grappling with mental health issues (Stein, 2013).

In addition to the new environment and the experience of living alone for many, for the typical tertiary education student, this represents a period during which young individuals experience a maturation phase, characterized by a shift in the environment and increased responsibilities. As Pedrelli et al. (2015) put it, in addition to academic stress, many students may have to take on more adult responsibilities without yet having mastered adulthood skills and cognitive maturity. There is evidence that the post-secondary education phase is associated with an increased susceptibility to the development of prevalent mental diseases. For instance, Ballester et al. (2020) conducted a study among university students in Spain, which revealed that almost 42% of the participants had indications of at least one potential mental condition. A national survey on the mental health of university students in South Africa revealed that common mental disorders are highly prevalent in South African university students (Bantjes et al. 2023). Over one-third of the participants in a study conducted by Mhata et al. (2023) on medical students at the University of Namibia displayed indications of depression and exhaustion, while just under one-third displayed symptoms of anxiety. Mhata et al' s study further reported that a considerable majority of participants (77%) reported a cold, negative disposition marked by a gradual disengagement from academic endeavours, an..d 68% reported profound fatigue and emotional exhaustion.

Research evidence indicates that students who encounter mental health difficulties primarily exhibit symptoms of anxiety, depression, eating disorders, and difficulties in regulating self-worth (Hans-Werner, 2015; Lattie et al., 2019; Pedrelli et al., 2015). As a sound and healthy mind is almost always the key to academic success and achievement, these mental health issues could have a significant negative effect on students' academic success. Multiple studies (such as Bostani et al., 2014; Shankar & Park, 2016; Wyatt et al., 2017) have provided evidence of a significant correlation between academic performance and mental well-being.

The demands for mental health services in institutions of higher education have increased (Hans-Werner, 2015). As such, higher education institutions should have sufficient mental health support services for their student populations to cope with their mental health challenges (Buizza et al., 2022). In addition, Bantjes et al.'s (2023) study of undergraduate students from universities in South Africa highlighted an urgent need to develop institution-based interventions to deal with students' mental health problems. Having functional structures to enhance student mental health in place in institutions of higher education would prevent inadequate mental health support services, which have been identified as a problem in some universities. Priestley et al. (2022) highlighted that service accessibility and availability was a critical challenge that compromised university mental health services. In developing countries such as Namibia, the provision of student mental health support within higher education institutions may be inadequate.

In recent years, there has been a notable rise in student enrolment in institutions of higher education in Namibia. According to the National Council for Higher Education (NCHE) reports, there was a notable increase in the student population in institutions between 2015 and 2020. Specifically, the number of student enrolment in institutions of higher education rose from 49,678 in 2015 to 66,656 in 2020, representing a significant growth of 34%. Given the increasing number of students enrolled in higher education institutions, it is imperative that their well-being, particularly their mental well-being, be accorded the utmost importance. In recent years, there has been a notable surge of interest in the area of mental health care in Namibia, particularly within the educational context. This has resulted in a plethora of studies focusing on the provision of guidance and counselling services in schools (Sekibo et al., 2022; Hako & Mbongo, 2018; Mbongo et al., 2016). However, there has been a lack of emphasis on the mental well-being of students in higher education institutions, as well as the support systems available within these institutions. In particular, there is a dearth of research regarding the provision of mental health services within institutions of higher education in Namibia. Thus, this chapter looks at how institutions of higher education in Namibia support students' mental health.

## Types of Institutional Support to Enhance Students' Mental Health

Institutions of higher education provide, or ought to have, support services that are specifically designed to enhance the mental well-being of students. Hartrey et al (2017) define institutional support as the provision of targeted help, encompassing both personal and environmental factors, which facilitates their participation in everyday academic activities and their integration into the academic community. According to Hughes and Spanner (2019), the range of services offered can differ according to the size and nature of the institution. They added that student support services in institutions of higher learning typically encompass a blend of mental health teams, counselling services, disability support teams, wellbeing teams, nursing teams, pastoral care services, residential or accommodation teams, and financial advisory services. In the subsequent discussion, we look at the common student support services offered at institutions of higher education.

*Figure 1. Student support services in institutions of higher education*

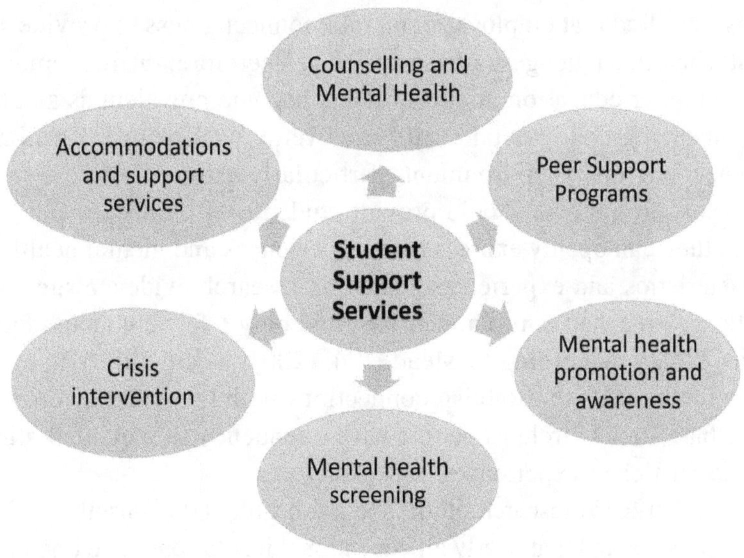


### Counselling and Mental Health

Many educational institutions offer complementary counselling services to students. These services usually are provided by mental health professionals who can provide individual or group therapy. According to Hans-Werner (2015), psychological counselling services are part of an academic tradition and a particular society, so their history, status, and importance to individuals vary. It is believed that counselling services within higher education institutions are very important for the delicate evolutionary phase that students experience (Buizza et al., 2022). Research evidence suggests that there has been an increase in the demand for counselling services in institutions of higher education as students' mental health has been on the rise (Lattie et al., 2019: Prince, 2015). An observation was also made that more students are now seeking out counselling services in numbers unprecedented in the history of counselling (Prince, 2015). This is due to the fact that, as stated by Browne (2017), if students' mental struggles are not effectively addressed, they have the potential to impede students' paths toward productive careers and future mental health and well-being. Furthermore, Prince (2015) asserts that failure to address students' mental health concerns can result in the deterioration of their academic performance and also have an impact on other students within campus living situations and classrooms.

It has been found that counselling and therapy is very beneficial to students experiencing mental health challenges. An instance can be observed in Bentley's (2018) research conducted among university students, which yielded findings suggesting that counselling interventions facilitated greater involvement in academic activities and were perceived as contributing to improved academic performance. Therefore, Bentley's conclusion suggests that counselling services in universities have the potential to expand the understanding of university counselling as a supplementary educational experience in addition to academic instruction.

## Peer Support Programmes

Peer counselling is a method that employs social interconnectedness to provide support to students experiencing mental health challenges (Abrams, 2022). Therefore, the implementation of peer support programmes in higher education institutions has become prevalent as an effective strategy to assist students in enhancing their mental health and overall well-being, as well as facilitating their adjustment to the new university environment, particularly among first-year students (Collings et al., 2014). Peer support programme should provide students with a secure and non-judgmental environment in which they can openly express their experiences and mental health issues with others with similar characteristics and experiences. There is research evidence suggesting that students experiencing challenges reached out to a peer first and only a few contacted faculty staff or other personnel (Abrams, 2022). According to Mead et al. (2001, as cited in Jonh et al., 2018), there is a higher likelihood for students to establish connections with their peers, compared to individuals outside their immediate social circle as people have a tendency to seek affiliation with those who share similar characteristics or experiences.

According to Prince's (2015) research on the mental health and counselling of university students in the United States, it was found that nearly all educational institutions have implemented peer-to-peer counselling or education initiatives in collaboration with their respective campus counselling centres. Peer support counselling has been found to yield benefits not only for individuals receiving peer counselling but also for those who are offering peer support. Crisp et al. (2020) conducted a study examining the expectations and experiences of students who were recruited as facilitators for a peer support programme at a university. The findings of the study revealed that although the facilitators encountered some challenges, they perceived the experience as rewarding.

## Mental Health Promotion and Awareness

Promoting education and fostering awareness about mental health is a key factor in addressing and effectively managing mental health concerns. As such, educational institutions must provide educational programmes and resources to promote mental health awareness and reduce the stigma associated with mental illness. According to Mahmoud et al. (2012), cited in Giamos (2017), a lack of understanding and education regarding mental health and coping strategies and the perception of stigma associated with mental illnesses are significant problems among students in higher education. Hughes and Spanner (2019) assert that the promotion and awareness of mental health could significantly contribute to shifting the discourse away from interventions, and instead focus on the comprehensive influence of universities and the need for proactive support of students and staff in maintaining positive mental well-being. Brewster et al. (2022) maintain the same argument and argue that universities should go beyond merely offering reactive services or individual interventions. Instead, institutions of higher education should advocate for a proactive and comprehensive approach that integrates cultural and structural changes throughout the entire institution (Brewster, 2022). The objective is to promote positive well-being results for the entire university community.

Institutions of higher education can engage in several activities to promote student mental health, one of which is the implementation of mental health campaigns. Prince (2015) reports that many institutions in the United States of America engage in public information campaigns and other extensive prevention initiatives aimed at raising knowledge about mental health resources and reducing the stigma that prevents students from seeking help.

## Mental Health Screening

Higher education institutions should provide mental health screening services to help students identify potential mental health problems. Research evidence suggests that mental health screening is linked to early identification and intervention, hence reducing the likelihood of students being neglected (Goodman-Scott, 2019). Screening instruments may include questionnaires or evaluations that evaluate the mental health status of students and provide recommendations for further assessment or treatment. Prince (2015) states that numerous university counselling centres provide online diagnostic and screening tools for prevalent mental health issues like depression and eating disorders. In addition, these centres also offer access to a variety of psycho-educational videos and written materials. Early mental health screening is of utmost importance, as, for example, research has demonstrated that individuals who exhibit suicidal ideation in the future tend to exhibit higher levels of mental health issues, such as depression and anxiety, at baseline compared to those who do not (Shim & Jeong, 2018; Tran et al. 2020).

## Accommodations and Support Services

Institutions may provide academic accommodations and support services to students with mental health conditions, such as additional time on exams, assistance with note-taking, and other accommodations to support academic success. According to the findings of Brockelman and Scheyett (2015), university students who have mental health issues can effectively navigate crises and achieve stability and academic success when provided with appropriate accommodations and support. They further stated that university personnel must possess an understanding of mental health, including the strategies necessary for students to navigate mental crises, as well as how universities can help students address their mental health challenges.

Academic accommodations commonly provided for students facing mental health challenges encompass a range of strategies. These include granting deadline extensions, allowing additional time for examinations, engaging in discussion with the student to address the issue, permitting absences when necessary, providing separate examination venues, and referring the student to counselling services (Becker et al., 2002; Brokelman & Scheyet, 2015; Martin, 2010 as cited in Hartrey et al., 2017). According to the findings of Steins (2013), accommodations were effective in addressing the many issues associated with psychological difficulties among students. The participants in Stein's study recounted the significance of accommodations and other forms of assistance offered by the university's support service, emphasizing their indispensable role in facilitating their academic successes. They further acknowledged that their academic objectives would remain unattainable in the absence of these supportive measures. This was particularly evident among individuals who self-identified as experiencing anxiety or mood disorders, such as depression or bipolar disorder.

### Crisis Intervention

Certain situations necessitate immediate intervention, particularly when a student poses a threat to themselves or others. It is important that institutions have established high-quality crisis intervention services to aid students in mental health crises (Wang, 2018). Yao and Zhang (2018) argue that the objective is to effectively handle the welfare and safety issues faced by students, while also ensuring that students with pressing mental health concerns receive suitable assistance from experienced healthcare practitioners. These services may include hotlines available around the clock, emergency counselling, and referrals to local mental health resources.

## Tertiary Institutions in Namibia

There are two categories of higher education institutions in Namibia: public institutions and private institutions. The University of Namibia (UNAM), Namibia University of Science and Technology (NUST) and Namibia Open College of Learning (NAMCOL), make up the three public institutions in Namibia. As of 2020, there were 14 private institutions of higher learning and these include the International University of Management (IUM), the Institute of Open Learning (IOL) and Welwitchia Health Training Centre, among others (National Council for Higher Education [NCHE], 2020). More than 70% of students are enrolled in public educational institutions, with 45.3%, 18.4%, and 6.9% enrolled at UNAM, NUST, and NAMCOL, respectively (NCHE, 2020). The remaining students are enrolled at private institutions, with IUM and ILO accounting for 14.9% and 7.2% of the total, respectively (NCHE, 2020). This indicates that UNAM, NUST, and IUM enrol the greatest number of students in Namibia, making them the leading institutions of higher education in terms of enrolment. This chapter focuses on the student support structures at these three prominent universities in Namibia, which collectively account for about 80% of the country's university student population.

In keeping up with global trends in education, the top three universities in Namibia have made efforts to address students' basic needs in accordance with the 1998 World Declaration on Higher Education's call for universities to "place students and their needs at the centre of their concern" (Ludeman et al. 2009). Furthermore, the 2009 World Health Conference on Higher Education urged institutions of higher learning to provide services and programmes outside of the classroom, commonly referred to as student affairs and services (Ludeman et al. 2009). Consequently, these efforts should be designed to enable and empower students to concentrate more intently on their studies and on their personal growth and maturation, both cognitively and emotionally (Ludeman et al. 2023). Accordingly, numerous tertiary institutions worldwide have made significant efforts to establish student affairs and support services within their institutions aimed at promoting students' mental well-being and facilitating their academic focus (Cage et al., 2020; DiPlacito-DeRango, 2016; Giamos et al., 2017; Hughes & Spanner, 2019; Priestley et al., 2020). Luescher-Mamashela et al. (2013) observed a rising inclination towards the professionalization of student affairs in Africa. They highlighted the emergence of academic programmes, specifically dedicated to student affairs in various African universities during the past decade.

## Student Support Services at the University of Namibia (UNAM)

Through the Office of the Directorate of Student Affairs, students at the leading institution of higher learning in Namibia (UNAM) have access to mental health services. The Directorate of Student Affairs consists of two divisions: Student Support Services & Residences and Career Services & Student Experiences. The Career Services and Student Experiences offers individual, and group counselling sessions on wellness, academic, career and psycho-social support to all university students (UNAM, 2023). Five sub-divisions comprise the Career Services and Student Experiences.

*Figure 2. UNAM's student affairs directorate*

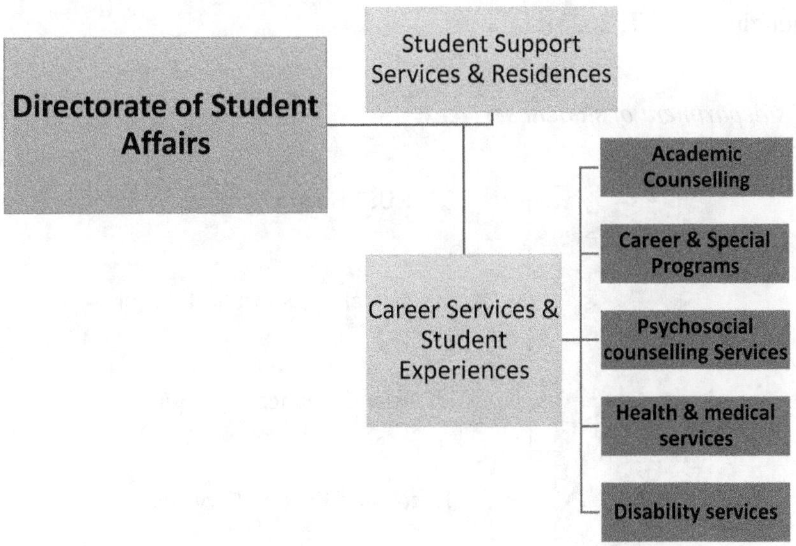


Whereas all divisions under the Directorate of Student Affairs are geared toward the well-being of students at the institution, the university's website indicates that the academic counselling and psychosocial counselling offices are particularly geared toward catering for and supporting students' mental health. The institution employs a Clinical Psychologist and Academic Counsellors who regularly handle student cases related to anxiety disorders, panic attacks, depressive disorders, bipolar mood disorders, substance use and dependency, psychotic disorders as well as academic problems such as motivation and concentration, and any other psychosocial challenges (UNAM, 2023). The Psychosocial Counselling Services Office provides professional support and counselling to students experiencing personal, social and life challenges that make it difficult for students to focus on their studies (UNAM, 2023). In line with various authors and researchers who noted the challenges faced by students, the Psychological Counselling Services Office deals with students experiencing adjustment challenges, homesickness and loneliness, social skills, self-esteem, confidence building, individuation away from home and being away from home, loss and bereavement, trauma and crisis intervention, rape, sexual assault and harassment, HIV/AIDS counselling, sexual identity and orientation, addiction issues and family problems (Abrams, 2022; Hans-Werner, 2015; Lattie et al, 2019; Pedrelli et al. 2015; Stein, 2013; UNAM, 2023). The institution has a multi-disciplinary team of mental health professionals, including social workers, psychologists, nurses and peer counsellors.

## Student Support Services at Namibia University of Science and Technology (NUST)

Namibia's second-largest university caters for students' mental health under its Social Welfare Services section under the Department of Student Services (DSS). The DSS provides institutional leadership for development and delivery of a broad range of student services essential to the achievement of the educational goals of the university (NUST, 2023). As such, the university indicates that student services are designed to contribute to the health, social, academic, career, sports, cultural moral, intellectual, and physical well-being of students. In addition to the core business of the university, which are teaching and research, the university strives to build within each student a sense of personal worth, self-confidence and sense of belonging (NUST, 2023).

*Figure 3. NUST's department of student services*

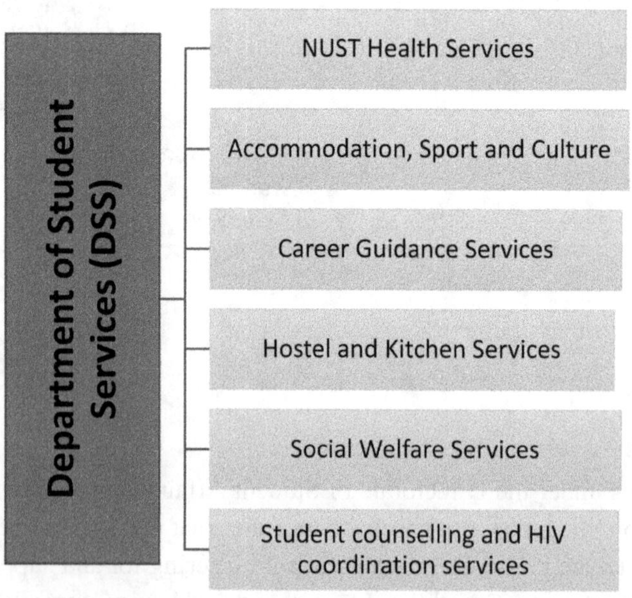

The DSS comprises six divisions/sections, namely: NUST health services, accommodation, sport and culture, career guidance services, hostel and kitchen services, as well as student counselling and HIV coordination services. Mental health falls under the social welfare services, with the section focusing on social problems and promoting good mental health for students (NUST, 2023). The section is proactive in supporting students' mental health in that they provide social welfare development workshops focusing on relationships, dating, rape and sexual harassment, stress management and self-esteem. They go a step further and provide social welfare programmes like orientation programmes for new students, violence against women and children and alcohol and substance abuse (NUST, 2023). An Early Alert Programme (EAP) was established at this institution to identify and help the at-risk and under-prepared students. Although the programme is hosted under the DSS, each faculty member has a representative to facilitate identifying at-risk students and referrals for timely interventions (Mwewa & McNally, 2018). The institution has a multi-disciplinary team of health professionals, including social workers, nurses, student counsellors and relevant departments that deal with academic, financial and social student issues.

## Student Support Services at the International University of Management (IUM)

At the third largest university in Namibia (IUM), student mental health support falls under the Office of the Dean of Students (ODS). The ODS Office '*serves as a point of information and a response unit for students*' (IUM, 2023). The ODS office further coordinates clinics for blood donations, voluntary HIV/AIDS testing and family planning, in collaboration with the Faculty of Health Sciences, the IUM clinic and the Student Counsellor. In contrast with the two public institutions discussed above, Namibia's largest private institution of higher education seems to be limited in its endeavours to address student mental health.

As demonstrated above, tertiary institutions in Namibia are devoting considerable resources and effort to support student well-being. The three leading higher education institutions have indeed made commendable initiatives in establishing frameworks aimed at promoting student mental well-being. All three institutions provide student counselling services, with UNAM and NUST specifying that they offer both academic and psychosocial counselling. UNAM has included peer counsellors as a component of their multidisciplinary mental health professions, whereas NUST and IUM are silent on this aspect. On mental promotion and awareness, NUST was very progressive in having a programme (Early Alert Programme) to identify and help at-risk and under-prepared students. The promotion and awareness of mental health is vital as it could contribute to shifting the discourse away from interventions, and instead focus on the comprehensive influence of universities and the need for proactive support of students and staff in maintaining positive mental well-being (Hughes & Spanner, 2019). Mental health screening appears to be absent from each of the three reviewed institutions. Crisis intervention is another aspect of student mental health support and institutions must establish high-quality crisis intervention services to aid students in mental health crises. These services may include hotlines available around the clock, emergency counselling, and referrals to local mental health resources. The three institutions have explicitly stated their crisis intervention services. Overall, the three universities have made considerable efforts to have student mental health support systems in place.

However, the effectiveness of student support within the established frameworks at these institutions to improve student mental health is yet to be fully determined. In a recent study conducted in Namibia, Sheyapo et al. (2023) discovered a deficiency in the provision of counselling services for marginalised students in institutions of higher education. The absence of efficacy in mental health support services within tertiary institutions in Namibia, as identified by Sheyapo et al. (2023), is not an isolated incident. This observation aligns with the findings of other researchers, including Dhillon et al. (2008), Bobga (2016), and Joan et al. (2021), who have also reported comparable outcomes. Among the obstacles and barriers to the success of students' mental health support are student resistance to referrals, a lack of awareness about available services, a lack of self-help-seeking behaviour among students, a lack of resources and shortages of qualified mental health professionals (Cage et al. 2020).

## Recommendations for Improved Mental Health Support in Institutions of Higher Learning in Namibia

The afore-mentioned section highlights the efforts made by the top three tertiary institutions in Namibia to prioritize the well-being of their students through the establishment of various structures aimed at promoting mental health. The authors observed the lack of qualified mental health professionals, particularly clinical psychologists and psychological counsellors at the three institutions. We recommended that universities employ qualified mental health professionals to adequately care for students presenting mental health challenges such as depression, anxiety and eating disorders as conditions that many students suffer from (Hans-Werner, 2015; Lattie et al. 2019; Mhata, 2015; Pedrelli et al. 2017).

The peer support component of institutional support structures to improve student mental health appears to be deficient, according to the reviews conducted. Only UNAM mentioned peer counsellors as part of their establishment. NUST and IUM did not explicitly mention peer support programmes as part of their structures for promoting the mental health of students. The paper therefore recommends that these institutions implement peer support programmes, as such programmes have been found to be advantageous for both receiving and providing students (Abrams, 2022; Collings, 2014; Crisp, 2020).

Research evidence suggests that mental health screening is linked to early identification and intervention, hence reducing the likelihood of students being neglected (Goodman-Scott, 2019). Mental health screening services aim to ensure the timely and proactive identification for at-risk students, which encourages self-help-seeking behaviour (Grotan, Sund, & Bjerkeset, 2019). The absence of this particular aspect of mental health support is evident within the three higher education institutions under consideration. Consequently, it is recommended that these institutions incorporate mental health screening as an integral component of their institutional mental health support services.

Furthermore, among the three reviewed post-secondary institutions, only NUST seems to have a strong programme for mental health education and awareness. UNAM and IUM need to strengthen their mental awareness and education programmes. We recommend that institutions raise more awareness about mental health and the services they offer to improve mental health. In addition, higher education institutions should provide clear guidelines to students and staff on accessing the available support services.

Insufficient attention has been given to the topic in existing scholarly works, indicating the need for more investigation into the mental health challenges faced by students in Namibian institutions of higher education (Bartholomew, 2016). The chapter, additionally, proposes the assessment and evaluation of existing mental health programmes and services, with a focus on determining their efficacy in addressing the mental health needs of students.

## CONCLUSION

This chapter presented an overview of student support services that are specifically designed to improve mental health within the three leading higher education institutions in Namibia. Consistent with prevailing global trends in higher education, Namibia's three prominent institutions of higher learning have made significant efforts to build support systems aimed at improving the mental well-being of their students. As is the case with UNAM and NUST, these institutions have departments comprising several subsections, whose purpose is to tend to and promote the general well-being and mental health of students. UNAM and NUST student affairs offices comprise a multi-disciplinary team of mental health professionals, including social workers, psychologists, nurses, peer counsellors and relevant departments that deal with academic, financial and social student issues. IUM's student affairs office has a Student Counsellor at each of their campuses. The absence of psychologists at NUST and IUM may be attributed to the scarcity of psychologists in the country. Peer support programmes, mental health screening, and mental health education and awareness were found to be deficient in the institutional support services intended to improve mental health at these three institutions. On paper, the student support structures for improving mental health in higher education institutions appear good. However, the effectiveness of student support within the established frameworks at these institutions for the purpose of improving student mental health needs to be determined. Further research is needed to understand the experiences of students accessing and making use of the student support services, aimed at enhancing student mental health at tertiary institutions in Namibia.

## REFERENCES

Abelson, S., Lipson, S. K., & Eisenberg, D. (2023). Mental health in college populations: A multidisciplinary review of what works, evidence gaps, and paths forward. In L. W. Perna (Ed.), *Higher education: Handbook of Theory and Research* (Vol. 37). Springer. doi:10.1007/978-3-030-76660-3_6

Abrams, Z. (2022). Student mental health is in crisis: Campuses are rethinking their approach. American Psychological Association.

Bahari, S. & Amla, S. (n.d.). Clients' Perception of Counseling Variables in Relation to Counselling Outcomes. *Malaysian Online Journal of Counselling*, 1–14.

Ballester, L., Alayo, I., Vilagut, G., Almenara, J., Cebrià, A. I., Echeburúa, E., Gabilondo, A., Gili, M., Lagares, C., Piqueras, J. A., Roca, M., Soto-Sanz, V., Blasco, M. J., Castellví, P., Mortier, P., Bruffaerts, R., Auerbach, R. P., Nock, M. K., Kessler, R. C., & Jordi, A. (2020). Mental disorders in Spanish university students: Prevalence, age-of-onset, severe role impairment and mental health treatment. *Journal of Affective Disorders*, *273*, 604–613. doi:10.1016/j.jad.2020.04.050 PMID:32560960

Bantjes, J., Kessler, M., Lochner, C., Breet, E., Bawa, B., Roos, J., Davids, C., Muturiki, M., Kessler, R. C., & Stein, D. J. (2023). The mental health of university students in South Africa: Results of the national student survey. *Journal of Affective Disorders*, *321*, 217–226. doi:10.1016/j.jad.2022.10.044 PMID:36349649

Bartholomew, T. T. (2016). Mental Health in Namibia: Connecting Discourses on Psychological Distress, Western Treatments and Traditional Healing. *Psychology and Developing Societies*, *28*(1), 101–125. doi:10.1177/0971333615622909

Bentley, A. (2018). 'I was just like, Wow!': Students' perceptions of how counselling benefitted their academic experience. *Counselling & Psychotherapy Research*, *18*(2), 215–219. doi:10.1002/capr.12149

Bobga, T. J. (2016). An Appraisal of Effective Provision of Guidance and Counseling Services in Cameroon State Universities; Trends and Challenges. International Journal of Humanities, Social. *Sciences and Education*, *3*(9), 75–90. doi:10.20431/2349-0381.0309010

Bostani, M., Nadri, A., & Nasab, A. R. (2014). A study of the relation between mental health and academic performance of students of the Islamic Azad University Ahvaz Branch. *Procedia: Social and Behavioral Sciences*, *116*, 163–165. doi:10.1016/j.sbspro.2014.01.186

Brewster, L., Jones, E., Priestley, M., Wilbraham, S. J., Spanner, L., & Hughes, G. (2022). 'Look after the staff and they would look after the students' cultures of wellbeing and mental health in the university setting. *Journal of Further and Higher Education*, *46*(4), 548–560. doi:10.1080/0309877X.2021.1986473

Brockelman, K. F., & Scheyett, A. M. (2015). Faculty perceptions of accommodations, strategies, and psychiatric advance directives for university students with mental illnesses. *Psychiatric Rehabilitation Journal*, *38*(4), 342–348. doi:10.1037/prj0000143 PMID:26053532

Brown, P. (2016). *The Invisible Problem?: Improving students' mental health*. Higher Education Policy Institute.

Browne, V., Munro, J., & Cass, J. (2017). The Mental Health of Australian University Students. *JANZSSA. Journal of the Australian and New Zealand Student Services Association*, *50*(2), 51–62. doi:10.30688/janzssa.2017.16

Buizza, C., Cela, H., Costa, A., & Ghilardi, A. (2022). Coping strategies and mental health in a sample of students accessing a university counselling service. *Counselling & Psychotherapy Research*, *22*(3), 658–666. doi:10.1002/capr.12519

Cage, E., Stock, M., Sharpington, A., Pitman, E., & Batchelor, R. (2020). Barriers to accessing support for mental health issues at university. *Studies in Higher Education*, *45*(8), 1637–1649. doi:10.1080/03075079.2018.1544237

Collings, R., Swanson, V., & Watkins, R. (2014). The impact of peer mentoring on levels of student wellbeing, integration and retention: A controlled comparative evaluation of residential students in UK higher education. *Higher Education*, *68*(6), 927–942. doi:10.100710734-014-9752-y

Crisp, D. A., Rickwood, D., Martin, B., & Byrom, N. (2020). Implementing a peer support program for improving university student wellbeing: The experience of program facilitators. *Australian Journal of Education*, *64*(2), 113–126. doi:10.1177/0004944120910498

Dhillon, J. K., McGowan, M., & Wang, H. (2008). How effective are institutional and departmental systems of student support? Insights from an Investigation into the Support Available to Students at one English University. *Research in Post-Compulsory Education*, *13*(3), 281–293. doi:10.1080/13596740802346472

DiPlacito-DeRango, M. L. (2016). Acknowledge the Barriers to Better the Practices: Support for Student Mental Health in Higher Education. *The Canadian Journal for the Scholarship of Teaching and Learning*, *7*(2). https://ir.lib.uwo.ca/cjsotl_rcacea/vol7/iss2/2. doi:10.5206/cjsotl-rcacea.2016.2.2

Giamos, D., Lee, A., Suleiman, A., Stuart, H. & Chen, S.-P. (2017). Understanding Campus Culture and Student Coping Strategies for Mental Health Issues in Five Canadian Colleges and Universities. *Canadian Journal of Higher Education / Revue canadienne d'enseignement supérieur, 47*(3), 136–151. doi:10.7202/1043242ar

Goodman, L. (2017). Mental Health on University Campuses and the Needs of Students They Seek to Serve. *Building Healthy Academic Communities Journal*, *1*(2), 31–44. doi:10.18061/bhac.v1i2.6056

Goodman-Scott, E., Donohue, P., & Betters-Bubon, J. (2019). The case for universal mental health screening in schools. *Counseling Today*, *62*(3), 40–45. https://digitalcommons.odu.edu/chs_pubs

Grotan, K., Sund, E. R., & Bjerkeset, O. (2019). Mental health, academic self-efficacy and study progress among college students - The SHoT study, Norway. *Frontiers in Psychology*, *10*(JAN), 1–11. doi:10.3389/fpsyg.2019.00045 PMID:30733694

Gupta, K., Parimal, B. S., & Narang, N. (2023). Academic stress among first-year undergraduate college students: role of emotional intelligence in coping with academic stress. In P. Aloka & K. Mukuna (Eds.), *Handbook of Research on Coping Mechanisms for First-Year Students Transitioning to Higher Education* (pp. 191–210). IGI Global. doi:10.4018/978-1-6684-6961-3.ch004

Hako, A. N., & Mbongo, E. N. (2018). Beneficiaries' satisfaction with the School Counselling Services in Namibia: A case study of a selected region. *Namibia CPD Journal for Educators*, *4*(1), 20–35.

Hans-Werner, R. (2015). Students' mental health and psychological counselling in Europe. *Mental Health & Prevention*, *3*(1–2), 34–40. doi:10.1016/j.mhp.2015.04.006

Hartrey, L., Denieffe, S., & Wells, J. S. G. (2017). A systematic review of barriers and supports to the participation of students with mental health difficulties in higher education. *Mental Health & Prevention*, *6*, 26–43. doi:10.1016/j.mhp.2017.03.002

Hughes, G., & Spanner, L. (2019). *The University Mental Health Charter*. Student Minds.

Joan, C., Finson, B., & Wilson, K. (2021). Challenges that Students Face at The University that May Require Counselling. *International Journal of Academic Research in Business & Social Sciences*, *11*(9), 18–34. doi:10.6007/IJARBSS/v11-i9/10968

John N.M., Page O., Martin S.C. &Whittaker P. (2018). Impact of peer support on student mental wellbeing: a systematic review. *MedEdPublish, 7*, 170 (https://doi.org/ doi:10.15694/mep.2018.0000170.1

Johnson, A. P., & Lester, R. J. (2021). Mental health in academia: Hacks for cultivating and sustaining wellbeing. *American Journal of Human Biology*, *34*(S1), e23664. doi:10.1002/ajhb.23664 PMID:34357661

Katz, D. S., & Davison, K. (2014). Community College Student Mental Health: A Comparative Analysis. *Community College Review*, *42*(4), 307–326. doi:10.1177/0091552114535466

Lattie, E. G., Adkins, E. C., Winquist, N., Stiles-Shields, C., Wafford, Q. E., & Graham, A. K. (2019). Digital mental health interventions for depression, anxiety, and enhancement of psychological well-being among college students: Systematic review. *Journal of Medical Internet Research, 21*(7), e12869. doi:10.2196/12869 PMID:31333198

Ludeman, R. B., Osfield, K. J., Hidalgo, E. I., Oste, D., & Wang, H. S. (Eds.). (2009). *Student Affairs and Services in Higher Education: Global Foundations, Issues and Best Practices*. UNESCO.

Luescher-Mamashela, T., Moja, T., & Schreiber, B. (2013). Towards a professionalisation of student affairs in Africa. *Journal of Student Affairs in Africa, 1*(1&2). doi:10.14426/jsaa.v1i1-2.181q1

Macaskill, A. (2013). The mental health of university students in the United Kingdom. *British Journal of Guidance & Counselling, 41*(4), 426–441. doi:10.1080/03069885.2012.743110

Mbongo, E.N., Möwes, A.D. & Chata, C.C. (2016). Factors impacting the implementation of guidance and counselling in secondary schools in the Ohangwena Region of Namibia. *International Journal for innovation, education and research, 4*(5).

McNally, A., & Susan, M. (2018). *Early Alert Programme Presentation Orientation*. NUST.

Mhata, N. T., Ntlantsana, V., Tomita, A. M., Mwambene, K., & Saloojee, S. (2023). Prevalence of depression, anxiety and burnout in medical students at the University of Namibia. *The South African Journal of Psychiatry : SAJP : the Journal of the Society of Psychiatrists of South Africa, 31*(29). doi:10.4102ajpsychiatry.v29i0.2044 PMID:37292521

Musika, F., & Bukaliya, R. (2015). The Effectiveness of Counseling on Students' Learning Motivation in Open and Distance Education. *International Journal of Research in Humanities and Social Studies, 2*(7), 85.

Namibia Council of Higher Education (NCHE). (2020). *2019 Namibia higher education statistical yearbook*. Ministry of Higher Education, Technology and Innovation.

Namibia Council of Higher Education (NCHE). (2021). *2020 Namibia higher education statistical yearbook*. Ministry of Higher Education, Technology and Innovation.

Namibia University of Science and Technology. (2023). *NUST social welfare services*. NUST. https://www.nust.na/dss/social-welfare

Oswalt, S. B., Lederer, A. M., Chestnut-Steich, K., Day, C., Halbritter, A., & Ortiz, D. (2020). Trends in college students' mental health diagnoses and utilization of services, 2009–2015. *Journal of American College Health, 68*(1), 41–51. doi:10.1080/07448481.2018.1515748 PMID:30355071

Pedrelli, P., Nyer, M., Yeung, A., Zulauf, C., & Wilens, T. (2015). College students: Mental health problems and treatment considerations. *Academic Psychiatry, 39*(5), 503–511. doi:10.100740596-014-0205-9 PMID:25142250

Porter, S. (2018). *A descriptive study of post-secondary student mental health crises*.

Priestley, M., Broglia, E., Hughes, G., & Spanner, L. (2022). Student Perspectives on improving mental health support services at University. *Counselling & Psychotherapy Research, 22*(1), 197–206. doi:10.1002/capr.12391

Prince, J. P. (2015). University student counseling and mental health in the United States: Trends and challenges. *Mental Health & Prevention, 3*(1-2), 5–10. doi:10.1016/j.mhp.2015.03.001

Sekibo, I., Tinibu, J., & Balogun, M. (2022). School Counselling Programme and Students' Academic Development. *Journal Educational Verkenning, 3*(1), 1–9. https://hdpublication.com/index.php/jev/article/view/140

Shankar, N. L., & Park, C. L. (2016). Effects of stress on students' physical and mental health and academic success. *International Journal of School & Educational Psychology, 4*(1), 5–9. doi:10.1080/21683603.2016.1130532

Sheyapo, M., Haihambo, C. K., & Mbongo, E. N. (2023). The roles of institutions in addressing the needs of students from marginalised backgrounds in higher education in Namibia. Edulearn23 Proceedings.

Shim, G., & Jeong, B. (2018). Predicting suicidal ideation in college students with mental health screening questionnaires. *Psychiatry Investigation, 15*(11), 1037–1045. doi:10.30773/pi.2018.08.21.3 PMID:30380820

Stein, K. F. (2013). DSS and Accommodations in Higher Education: Perceptions of Students with Psychological Disabilities. *Journal of Postsecondary Education and Disability, 26*(2), 145–161.

Storrie, K., Ahern, K., & Tuckett, A. (2010). A systematic review: Students with mental health problems—A growing problem. *International Journal of Nursing Practice, 16*(1), 1–6. doi:10.1111/j.1440-172X.2009.01813.x PMID:20158541

Tran, A., Tran, L., Geghre, N., Darmon, D., Rampal, M., Brandone, D., Gozzo, J.-M., Haas, H., Rebouillat-Savy, K., Caci, H., & Avillach, P. (2017). Health assessment of French university students and risk factors associated with mental health disorders. *PLoS One, 12*(11), e0188187. doi:10.1371/journal.pone.0188187 PMID:29176864

University of International Management (IUM). (2023). *Administrative departments*. IUM. https://ium.edu.na/

University of Namibia (UNAM). (2023). *Directorate of student affairs*. UNAM. https://www.unam.edu.na/student-affairs

Wang, X. (2018). Research on college students' mental health and crisis intervention. *International Workshop on Advances in Social Sciences (IWASS 2018)*. SAMHSA.

World Conference on Higher Education (WCHE). (1998). Higher Education in the Twenty-first Century: Vision and Action. *World Declaration on Higher Education for the Twenty-first Century; Framework for Priority Action for Change and Development in Higher Education.* UNESCO.

Wyatt, T. J., Oswalt, S. B., & Ochoa, Y. (2017). Mental Health and Academic Performance of First-Year College Students. *International Journal of Higher Education, 6*(3), 178–187. doi:10.5430/ijhe.v6n3p178

Yao, F., & Zhang, A. (2021). Integration of education management and mental health in psychological crisis intervention in colleges and universities. *ASP Transactions on Psychology and Education, 1*(1), 31–38.

# Chapter 19
# Institutional Support Available to Enhance the Mental Health of Students in Higher Education Institutions

**Janet Auma Odhiambo**
*Jaramogi Oginga Odinga University of Science and Technology, Kenya*

**Enos Barasa Mukadi**
*Laikipia University, Kenya*

## ABSTRACT

*Mental health is important in every individual's life right from childhood through to adulthood. A state of good mental health accounts for an individual's ability to cope with life stressors and attain quality life. Students at the institutions of higher learning are exposed to a range of psychological variables ranging from financial constraints, family problems, and sicknesses, to social relations, which adversely affect their mental well-being. A majority of students are not able to deal with the risk factors or challenges that may affect their mental health. Some feel overwhelmed and experience various adjustment problems, which may eventually lead to mental illness. The services that are provided at school need to take care of all the areas that can be productive and counterproductive to the learning environment. There is a need for human resources who are experts in shaping the student's behavior and overall adjustment at school.*

## INTRODUCTION

Mental health is defined as a state of well-being in which each person realizes his or her own potential and can cope with the normal stresses of life, develop her or himself productively and fruitfully, and be able to contribute to him or herself and the community (Haile, et al., 2017). However, the admission and attendance of students at the university could affect their emotional state, since this formative period is considered critical and very stressful as they leave their homes, have to adapt

DOI: 10.4018/979-8-3693-2833-0.ch019

to a new social environment, must face greater academic pressure as previously described and have more access to the consumption of alcoholic beverages and psychoactive substances. Mental health issues affect 10-20% of individuals globally and the onset age of such individuals is at 14 years of age. Unattended mental health escalates to treatment gap which may be as a result of care seeking attitude. Hurdles of mitigating mental conditions in the institutions of higher learning include limited treatment options and the implied costs of treating mental illness. Mental health support services help students who are vulnerable and are at risk in developing coping mechanisms. A great deal of information is required for mitigation purposes in terms of utilization of mental health services for the improvement of mental wellbeing of students. Blanco et al., (2008) indicated that mental health problems are very common among college students. This may be since attending college corresponds to a challenging time for many traditional and non-traditional undergraduate students. Traditional college students start college after completing high school, are typically younger, depend on parents for financial support, and do not work or work part-time. Thus, in addition to stress related to academic load, these students may have to face the task of taking on more adult-like responsibilities without having yet mastered the skills and cognitive maturity of adulthood. Thus, this group of students may have to cope with meeting work and family demands in addition to academic requirements. In these contexts, many college students may experience the persistence, exacerbation, or first onset of mental health and substance use problems while possibly receiving no or inadequate treatment. With the increasing recognition of child mental health issues and the use of more psychotropic medications, the number of young adults with mental health problems entering college has significantly increased. For example, in a survey of 274 institutions, 88% of counseling center directors reported an increase in "severe" psychological problems over the previous 5 years including learning disabilities, self-injury incidents, eating disorders, substance use, and sexual assaults (Gallagher, Gill & Sysko, 2000). Nonmedical use of prescription medications often co-occurs with heavy alcohol use a worrisome occurrence given that alcohol taken in combination with analgesic opioids may further inhibit activity in the central nervous system, increasing the risk of oversedation, respiratory depression, and death. Regrettably, college students do not appear to view prescription drug abuse as problematic. Practitioners should communicate with college students about the ethical, medical, psychological, addictive, and legal issues of prescription drug abuse. College students should be advised to take their medications as prescribed and not give or sell their medications to others. Safe storage of controlled substances such as benzodiazepines or stimulants is important (Arria & DuPont, 2010). The extent to which the increase in poor mental health is also being seen amongst non-students of a similar age is not well understood and warrants further study. However, the increase in poor mental health specifically within students in higher education highlights a need to understand what the risk factors are and what might be done within these settings to ensure young people are learning and developing and transitioning into adulthood in environments that promote mental wellbeing. Commencing higher education represents a key transition point in a young person's life. It is a stage often accompanied by significant change combined with high expectations of high expectations from students of what university life will be like, and also high expectations from themselves and others around their own academic performance. Relevant factors include moving away from home, learning to live independently, developing new social networks, adjusting to new ways of learning, and now also dealing with the additional greater financial burdens that students now face (Campbell, et al., 2022).

## BACKGROUND

When students get to institutions of higher learning, they are reported to have significantly higher level of emotional stress Klein (2010). While quite a good number of students can deal with the challenges and adjust to high school life successfully, some feel overwhelmed and experience various adjustment problems (Bernier, Larose & Whipple, 2005). In addition, Aloka, Opondo and Ooko (2023) argues that transition to higher education from secondary school can be a complex and challenging task for the first-year students. The higher education environment and secondary school contexts are quite different in terms of the teaching, learning and expectations for the first-year students. The first year of study is a critical period for students as it is a transitional step from secondary school (high school) to more adult life. The beginning years in higher education institutions is a crucial period for mitigating risks of attrition as this is the time when students develop a sense of belonging, and academic and personal connections. Furthermore, Aloka, Opondo and Ooko (2023) reiterate that first-year attrition presents adverse consequences for first-year students and their institutions. When students withdraw from college during their initial year, they often do not return and face low socio-economic outcomes due to not acquiring credentials or skill sets that lead to a career path. It is also reported that individuals often move away from home for the first time during this period and are cut off from family and friends who have provided significant social support in their lives. Mental health and mental health-related issues have been a matter of concern for quite a long time earning little regard and interest from the respective healthcare facilities and systems. Governments have put inadequate measures to ensure that citizens' mental challenges are handled rightfully to achieve high levels of mentally healthy people. The perpetuated issue has also developed in various sectors of society. The current situation in a learning institution is worth raising eyebrows, and therefore it deserves serious attention. Most of the undergraduate students and yet to graduate college students depict high levels of mental illness among the students, thus, depicting discomfort of the students and the level of neglect the health sector is faced with. The majority of today's people who are suffering from mental issues in society constitute college and university students (Larson et al., 2022).

The significance of psychological wellbeing among students in the institutions of higher learning has been recorded by recent research revealing that student with poor mental health experience poor academic achievement, lower rate of completion, less social contact with their fellow students and less enthusiasm in studies (Regehr, Glancy & Pitts, 2013). Despite the challenges faced by students, studies show that the students are reluctant to seek help which could be attributed to perceived stigma and lack of knowledge about available support services at the institutions (Gulliver, Griffiths & Chistensen, 2010). Some of the students also believe in their own wisdom of going about the challenges they encounter and underestimate the consequences of their mental ill health on their success in life (Givens & Tjia 2002). In one study students perceived as having mental health issues were more likely to report impaired academic achievements than those with stable mental health (Keyes, Eisenber, Perry, Dube, Kroenke & Dhingra,2012). Aloka (2022) study reported that barriers to work wellness among staff in higher education institutions include but are not limited to aspects such as personal barriers, environmental barriers, organizational barriers, and legal barriers. In another research, Aloka, Ooko, Ooko and Onyango, (2023) also indicates that students do not perform in class at similar levels and that there are individual differences among them, even when family background and school and teacher quality are controlled for. This implies that individual differences play an important role in determining whether children thrive or fail in school.

One of the most important goals of education has become to help students acquire self-regulation skills that to improve learning during school years. Self-regulation looks at the triadic interaction between the person, their behavior, and the environment.

According to Gruttadaro and Crudo (2010), a survey carried out among 765 high school students diagnosed with mental health shows that stigma was identified as the number one reason for them not to seek mental services while at campus. As a result of such challenges, there is need of robust available support systems at the institutions that should be explored for early intervention purposes. Provision of mental health services in the institutions of higher learning is critical for effective intervention strategies among students with psychological challenges. According to Baker & Sinyk (1984), the process of getting used to being in an institution of higher learning is described mainly by identifying four types of adjustments which include social adjustment, academic adjustments and goal commitment or institutional attachment. However, Gee & Chwalisz (2007), identifies risk factors for adjustment to College life to be attributed to low income, academic performance and relationships or interpersonal problems. Bonhert, Aikins & Edidin (2007), on the other hand reiterate that three main risk factors affect students, relationship with friends, participation in social activities and leisure time management. Aloka (2022) indicate that students' attitudes towards online learning are generally positive, but in developing countries, the attitudes are generally negative in the beginning phases. The study recommends that teachers of English as foreign language should create more space in schools for activities that develop students' creative thinking skills.

Students mental wellbeing are mostly affected during late adolescence and early childhood. These periods in life is their transitional period marked by major psychological changes (Arnette,2000). Blanco et al 2008 similarly reports that indeed many mental health disorders including depression, anxiety and substance abuse disorders begin during this period. A growing body of evidence suggests that academic related stress plays a significant role among college students (Misra & Mc Keen, 2000). Students are exposed to academic stressors such as extensive academic course load, time management, financial concerns, family pressures, and adapting to new environment (Misra & Castillo, 2004). The American Psychological Association reports 45% of students seeking help in college because of stress and the main cause being anxiety and depression. While all students can be vulnerable to stress, some groups of students may experience more stress than others and some may be able to cope better than others. Stress among students can be overwhelming and can affect the student's mental well-being. Psychological well-being is key to positive mental health and this comprises robust stress management strategies, happiness, proper psychological functioning and general life satisfaction. The state of mental health has been shown to be predictive of both negative and positive quality of life. Poor mental wellbeing has been shown to affect academic performance of students in general (Freire et al.2016). Academic stress can lead to reduction of motivation, low academic achievement and less completion rate (Pasho et al. 2020). Aloka (2022) study indicate that the opportunities for online learning include personal enabler factors; use of metacognitive and compensation strategies; increased interactive and motivating sessions; increased amount of leisure time; teachers' technological and pedagogical knowledge; use of collaboration, networking, and communication initiatives; availability and use of modern technologies; and flexibility of learning. The challenges reported include digital divide as a hindrance to students, insufficient online resources and platforms for online teaching, poor adaptation among students, inadequate information technology skills and resilience among teachers, behavioral and individual personality challenges, lack of social interaction among students, increased anxiety and depression among students, loss of interests and motivation to learn, and finally, inadequate parental supervision.

At early stages in life, children have a lot of faith and trust in their parents. However, as they grow into teenage, they tend to withdraw from their previous attachments to parents and freedom of expression. The free communication may be transferred to friends or they just keep to themselves. At this age, the children's frustrations are manifested in other ways such as irritability, mood swings, headaches, withdrawal from friends and family, change in sleeping habits, decreased concentrations, negative attitudes, substance abuse and signs of depression which can easily escalate to mental disorder. Students may not be free to talk about their fears and worries simply because they want to please their parents by giving the impression that all is well with them and by sharing, their parents and friends may see them as weak and unable to handle school demands. The bottling up of challenging issues impacts negatively on their mental well-being. It is for this reason that support services should be made available at the institutions of higher learning to support vulnerable students who are at risk.

## ELEMENTS OF MENTAL WELL- BEING

### Emotional Intelligence

Emotional Intelligence is one's ability to recognize and understand their own emotions and the emotions pf those around them and the ability to use this awareness to manage one's own behavior and relationship with others (Bradberry, Travis & Greaves (2009). Emotional intelligence is an aspect of human intelligence that involves emotional awareness and how to use the emotions appropriately in decision making and the ability to cope with life's psychological trauma and mental disorders. It is the ability to monitor an individual's own and others feelings and regulate the emotions in order to promote emotional and intellectual growth. Emotional intelligence is key for living a successful life, it helps in maintaining healthy relationships with others as the human world is all about relationships. For one to have a state of mental wellbeing, there is need to have an understanding and management of one's own emotions and that of others through effective self-awareness and self-control as this would be of great benefit to a state of good mental health (Goleman & Daniel,2006).

Emotional intelligence services are those services that can be applied to train students to become more conscious of their feelings alongside other people's feelings and the influence emotions have on people's decisions, behavior and performance. It is important that students develop a stronger understanding of their own emotions and that of others as well as how those emotions relate to the world around them. Emotional intelligence plays a positive role in helping students deal with stress, development of relationships, and handling transitional changes that they would face in life. Research show that when students are in an environment where they and their peers have developed emotional intelligence, they see higher levels of engagement, have better classroom leadership and organization, experience less bullying, manage test anxiety better and have higher academic achievement (Checa & Fernandez-Berrocal, 2019) all these attributes results to stronger interpersonal relationships and a state of mental wellbeing. The main goal of being trained in emotional intelligence is to shape student's response to challenges. Students who go through emotional intelligence training get skills that enables them navigate their way around obstacles successfully. It enables them to weigh situations and come up with better mitigation strategies. It is therefore important to infuse emotional intelligence training in the institutions of higher learning as this would enable them use their emotions effectively in an adaptive manner. It would as well assist students to draw meaningful links between emotional intelligence, mental health and overall well-being.

According to Zysberg (2018), the relevance of emotional intelligence as a personal resource associated with health outcomes, wellbeing, task performance and cognitive performance. There are researchers who have argued that emotional intelligence has two components that comprise of the emic and etic perspectives that facilitate human interaction. The emic helps an individual to understand and regulate their own emotions whereas the etic aids in relating with emotions in situations such as empathizing and responding to other people's emotions (Ng & Earley,2006). Emotional intelligence is considered as one of the major contributing factors to academic performance. This comes about as a result of attitude, emotional skills, resilience, personal traits, self-regulation and motivation (Gutman & Schoong,2013).

## Self-Awareness

This is the conscious knowledge of one's own feelings and behavior which involves self-concept, thoughts, feelings and emotions. Self-awareness gives an individual the ability and power to influence achievements in life. It is how one perceives self and he perceptions are mostly derived from individuals' experiences, their expectations of themselves in future and the belief in their capabilities. It enables an individual to become a better decision maker and gives more confidence. Self-awareness enables an individual to understand things from multiple perspectives which is free from assumptions and biases. It is easier for individuals to build self-esteem only when they are able to understand themselves better.

Self-awareness enables students to navigate their relationships with confidence giving them the ability to make sound decisions. It enables students to encourage themselves by adopting optimistic feelings as they pursue their goals in life. It helps individuals not to focus on challenges of life but to appreciate their potentials even as they struggle with life's challenging issues. In most cases, self-awareness enables individuals to identify the skills gap they experience in life and give students the opportunity to exploit their strengths and cope with their weaknesses. Students with healthy self-concept are more likely to cope with challenges in life and are capable of achieving set goals successfully. It is important that the vulnerable students who are at risk of low self-concept are trained to make effort to change how they perceive themselves. This may be easier for some vulnerable students and might be much harder for others. However, with help the change can be possible. Proper training of students within the institutions can enable the learners to keep their minds from pessimistic thoughts such as hatred, anger, fear and greed as all these may escalate to mental disorders.

## Thoughts

Thoughts are formulated ideas and beliefs about individuals and the world around them within their mind. Peoples thoughts are tied to their emotions. It is heathy when moderate amount of mental stress is stimulated as it can lead into productive thinking. However, when too much stress is stimulated then ones thinking ability can be negatively affected. Thoughts may become confused, jumbled and be diverted to worries. Once one is preoccupied with worries then it becomes difficult to make sound decisions and find solutions to problems. For students to be aware of their emotions they need to understand their thinking processes first. It is important for students to take note of what they think and say about themselves and how they perceive the situations they find themselves in. Students need to be trained on how to reflect on their negative thoughts and find ways of influencing them to be positive. The key to mental well-being is to think positively. This can only be done through learning effective techniques to think positively.

### Feelings

Students need to be trained on the identification of feelings associated with their experiences. They need to identify their feelings and keep track of any patterns that may impact negatively to their mental well-being and find a way of avoiding them.

### Body

Thoughts sometimes get accompanied with physical responses. Students need to be trained on how to respond physically to their feelings. They need to understand if their feelings show physically in their facial expressions, voice, heart beat or any other form of body language and the ways to restrain these physical knee jerk reactions.

### Emotions

Individuals with higher levels of emotional intelligence have the ability to recognize and accept their varying emotional states. Students knowledge of their emotional state may enable them to enhance their personal relationships. With proper support services at the institutions of higher learning, the students may effectively manage and control emotional outbursts and maintain healthier mental well-being.

## STRESSORS AMONG STUDENTS

Even though research show that moderate stress is healthy and can act as motivator for students to work hard and excel in their academic achievement, too much stress on the other hand can have negative impact on their mental well-being. Research show that 70% of students report anxiety and depression while at school. Chronic stress can result to decreased motivation, poor academic achievement and students dropping out of school. It is therefore important that educators are able to recognize what triggers stressors and the mitigation measures necessary.

Overscheduling has been reported as one of the major causes of stress to students. Feelings of having too much to do but not enough time to do them may lead to numerous stress related symptoms such as headaches, exhaustion, irritability, insufficient sleep, stomach ulcers and several health issues that results to chronic stress and unstable mental health. Squeezing many activities into students' schedules results into poor organization habits. Students who are not well organized are prone to suffer more stress as a result of missing important deadlines. When students lack balance in scheduling their time, they end up being overworked and stressed. It is therefore a requirement that students should have expert time management skills.

Another form of stressor among students is parental pressure. Even though it is normal for parents to want their children to have good performance in academics, there are certain times when this does more harm than good to the students. Research show that 66% of students report parental pressure as a source of prominent stress (Arnett, 2000). Putting pressure on students by parental high expectations can make the students to improve on their academic performance but too much pressure to consistently meet these expectations may result to negative consequences on their overall mental well-being and their academic performance.

## TRAININGS FOR MENTAL WELL-BEING AT SCHOOL

Exercising is an effective way of reducing stress levels as it produces hormones that relieve pain and stress in the body system. Physical body activity has the ability to counteract the negative effects of stress such as fatigue and contractions. Avoidance of procrastination is away of trying to complete tasks before the set deadlines. This can control and limit stressful situations that students might be exposed to. Students need to be trained on how to give priorities when surrounded with deadlines. It is better to create a time table for revision sessions or make a to do list of all tasks to be done in a day with their deadlines. Research show that effective time management is a powerful mediator of stress and has been positively correlated with better academic performance by students (Zysberg, 2012).

Development of proper sleep routine. Research has established that sleep and mood go hand in hand. Students who regularly report better sleep quality have been found to have better academic performance. Students need to train themselves to set regular bed time that can enable them have quality sleep. Sticking to a sleep schedule has been found to have one of the greatest positive impacts on academic performance. Communication has been equally identified to be therapeutic when one is stressed. It is important to talk to someone whenever one feels stressed. Talking to teachers, parents or friends can be a big relief whenever students feel overwhelmed. Talking would also help in developing social network or support team instead of suffering in silence. This can aid in developing proper mental and physical well being which is more important than achievement of excellent grades. Having this support system within the institutions of higher learning can help improve student's ability to cope and act as a stress buffer which eventually improves individual's performance and resilience.

## CONCLUSION

It is important that all the institutions of higher learning have support systems in place for mental well-being of students. Creation of awareness on Institutional available support system on matters of mental well being among students is critical and will equip them with essential information that will help them to navigate the emotional stressors and challenges associated with college life. This would aid them to realize their abilities and live meaningful and purposeful life as they form positive relationships and make positive contribution to the society. Most of the learning institutions have tight schedules and continuous sequences of study, which affects the students' performance and their mental well-being. Challenges and the predisposing factors that affect the students are bound to result from their school environment or their history; therefore, the growth environment and interaction play a significant role in determining one's health. Some of the predisposing factors are avoidable, while others are accustomed and tied to the students. Therefore, it is prudent to come up with measures to ensure control and regulation of the inherent situation of the undergraduate students who make up the future and continuity of our current society.

## REFERENCES

Aloka, P. J. (2022). Barriers to Work Wellness among Academic Staff in Higher Education Institutions. In C. Alexander & A. Tureen (Eds.), *Leadership Wellness and Mental Health Concerns in Higher Education* (pp. 22–42). IGI Global. doi:10.4018/978-1-7998-7693-9.ch002

Aloka, P. J., Ooko, M., Ooko, P. A., & Onyango, P. (2023). Self-Regulated Learning and Student Success, Retention, and Engagement in Online Courses. In J. Keengwe (Ed.), *Handbook of Research on Innovative Frameworks and Inclusive Models for Online Learning* (pp. 238–255). IGI Global. doi:10.4018/978-1-6684-9072-3.ch012

Aloka, P. J., Opondo, C. M., & Ooko, M. (2023). Expectations, Culture, and Adaptation to Higher Education Institutions by First-Year Students. In P. Aloka & K. Mukuna (Eds.), *Handbook of Research on Coping Mechanisms for First-Year Students Transitioning to Higher Education* (pp. 1–20). IGI Global. doi:10.4018/978-1-6684-6961-3.ch001

Aloka, P. J. O. (2022). Students' Self-Directed Learning Techniques and Attitudes toward Online English Language Learning. In W. El-Henawy & M. del Mar Suárez (Eds.), *English as a Foreign Language in a New-Found Post-Pandemic World* (pp. 51–66). IGI Global. doi:10.4018/978-1-6684-4205-0.ch003

Aloka, P. J. O. (2022). Social Impact of Digital English Language Learning Environments. In W. El-Henawy & M. del Mar Suárez (Eds.), *English as a Foreign Language in a New-Found Post-Pandemic World* (pp. 207–225). IGI Global. doi:10.4018/978-1-6684-4205-0.ch010

American Psychological Association. (2020). *Stress in America: A national Mental Health Crisis*. American Psychological Association.

Arnett, J. J. (2000). Emerging adulthood: A theory of development from the late teens through the twenties. *The American Psychologist*, *55*(5), 469–480. doi:10.1037/0003-066X.55.5.469 PMID:10842426

Arria, A. M., & DuPont, R. L. (2010). Nonmedical prescription stimulant use among college students: Why we need to do something and what we need to do. *Journal of Addictive Diseases*, *29*(4), 417–426. doi:10.1080/10550887.2010.509273 PMID:20924877

Baker, P. W., & Siryk, B. (1984). Measuring adjustment to college. *Journal of Counseling Psychology*, *2*, 45–56.

Bernier, A., Carlson, S. M., & Whipple, N. (2010). Future Directions in Childhood Adversity & Youth Psychology. *Journal of Clinical Child and Adolescent Psychology*, *45*(3), 361–382. doi:10.1080/15374416.2015.1110823

Blanco, C., Okuda, M., Wright, C., Hasin, D. S., Grant, B. F., & Liu, S. M. (2008). Mental Health of College Students and their non-college peers: Results from the National Epidemiologyic study on Alcohol and Related Conditions. *Archives of General Psychiatry*, *65*(12), 1429–1437. doi:10.1001/archpsyc.65.12.1429 PMID:19047530

Bradberry, T., & Greaves, J. (2009). *Emotional Intelligence*.

Cage, E., Stock, M., Sharpington, A., Pitman, E., & Batchelor, R. (2020). Barriers to accessing Support for mental health issues at University. *Studies in Higher Education, 45*(1), 1–13. doi:10.1080/03075079.2018.1544237

Campbell, F., Blank, L., Cantrell, A., Baxter, S., Blackmore, C., Dixon, J., & Goyder, E. (2022). Factors that influence mental health of university and college students in the UK: A systematic review. *BMC Public Health, 22*(1), 1778. doi:10.118612889-022-13943-x PMID:36123714

Checa, P., & Fernández-Berrocal, P. (2019). Cognitive Control & Emotional Intelligence: Effect of the Emotional Content of Task. *Frontiers in Psychology, 10*, 195. doi:10.3389/fpsyg.2019.00195 PMID:30792680

Freire, C., Ferradas, M., Rgueiro, B., Rodriguez, S., Valle, A., & Nunez, J. C. (2020). *Coping Strategies and Self -efficacy in University Students: A person centered approach.* Nova Publishers.

Freire, C., Ferradas, M. D., Valle, A., Nunez, J. C., & Vallejo, G. (2016). Profiles of Psychological well-being & Coping Strategies among University Students. *Frontiers in Psychology, 23*, 67–76. doi:10.3389/fpsyg.2016.01554 PMID:27790168

Gallagher, R., Gill, A. M., & Sysko, H. B. (2000). *National survey of counseling directors, 2000.* International Association of Counseling Centers, Inc.

Givens, J. L., & Tjia, J. (2002). Depressed medical students use of mental health services and barriers to use. *Academic Medicine, 2*, 34–46. PMID:12228091

Greer, T. M., & Chwalisz, K. (2007). Minority-related Stressors and Coping Processes among African American College Students. *Journal of College Student Development, 2*(4), 32–46. doi:10.1353/csd.2007.0037

Guilliver, A., Griffiths, K. M., & Christensen, H. (2010). Perceived barriers and facilitators to mental health-help seeking in young people. *Systematic Reviews, 1*, 32–45.

Gutman, L. M., & Schoon, I. (2013). *The Impact of Non-Cognitive Skills on Outcomes for Young People.* Education Endowment Foundation. Leading Education and Social Research.

Haile, Y., Alemu, S., & Habtewold, T. (2017). Common mental disorder and its association with academic performance among Debre Berhan University students, Ethiopia. *International Journal of Mental Health Systems, 11*(1), 34–45. doi:10.118613033-017-0142-6 PMID:28473869

Keyes, C. L. M., Eisenberg, D., Perry, G. S., Dube, S. R., Kroenke, K., & Dhingra, S. S. (2012). The Relationship of level of positive mental health with current mental disorders in predicting suicidal behavior and academic impairment in college students. *Journal of American College Health, 2*(2), 34–46. doi:10.1080/07448481.2011.608393 PMID:22316409

Klein, J. T. (2010). A taxonomy of Interdisciplinary. The oxford handbook of Interdisciplinary. In R. Frodeman, J. T. Klein, & C. Mitcham (Eds.), *The Oxford Handbook of Interdisciplinarity* (pp. 15–30). Oxford University Press.

Larson, L. R., Mullenbach, L. E., Browning, M. H., Rigolon, A., Thomsen, J., Metcalf, E. C., Reigner, N. P., Sharaievska, I., McAnirlin, O., D'Antonio, A., Cloutier, S., Helbich, M., & Labib, S. M. (2022). Greenspace and park use associated with less emotional distress among college students in the united states during the COVID-19 pandemic. *Environmental Research, 2022*(204), 112367. doi:10.1016/j.envres.2021.112367 PMID:34774510

Misra, R., & Castillo, L. G. (2004). Academic Stress among College Students: Comparison of American &b International Students. *International Journal of Stress Management, 3*(2), 1–10. doi:10.1037/1072-5245.11.2.132

Misra, R., McKean, M., West, S., & Russo, T. (2000). Academic Stress of College Students: Comparison of student and faculty perceptions. *College Student Journal, 34*(2), 236–245.

Ng, K. Y., & Earley, P. C. (2006). Cultural intelligence as predictor of individuals adaptive performance. *International Area Studies Review, 17*(4), 394–413. doi:10.1177/2233865914550727

Pascob, M. C., Hetrick, S. E., & Parker, A. G. (2020). The Impact of stress on students in Secondary School and higher education. *International Journal of Adolescence Psychology, 3*, 46–56.

Rgehr, C., Glancy, D., & Pitts, A. (2013). Interventions to reduce stress in University Students. A review and Meta-analysis. *Journal of Affective Disorders, 1*(1), 1–10. doi:10.1016/j.jad.2012.11.026 PMID:23246209

Zysberg, L. (2012). *Emotional antecedents of psychological loneliness. In book: Loneliness: Psychosocial Risk Factors, Prevalence and Impacts on Physical and Emotional Health. Publisher*. Nova Science Publishers.

# Chapter 20
# Institutional Support Available to Enhance the Mental Health of Students at the University of Namibia

**Daniel Opotamutale Ashipala**
https://orcid.org/0000-0002-8913-056X
*University of Namibia, Namibia*

**Fransisco Chindongo Ntjamba**
*University of Namibia, Namibia*

## ABSTRACT

*This chapter critically examines the institutional support systems aimed at supporting the mental health of students within the University of Namibia. The shift from childhood to adulthood brings with it special difficulties, leaving students open to a range of stresses that can negatively impact their mental health. This research examines common mental health problems among students, such as stress and anxiety, with a particular focus at the University of Namibia. The study highlights the necessity of an all-encompassing strategy that considers social, emotional, and intellectual aspects in order to create an environment where students can flourish both academically and mentally. This chapter adds to the continuing conversation on mental health in higher education by advocating for additional improvements and identifying successful initiatives. This chapter adds to the continuing conversation on mental health in higher education by advocating for additional improvements and identifying successful initiatives.*

## INTRODUCTION

The mental health of university students is a topic of increasing concern, both globally and within the context of the University of Namibia (Pillay, 2022). Mental health emphasises the need to face life difficulties without the student collapsing under pressure. Campbell et al. (2022) explain that mental health

DOI: 10.4018/979-8-3693-2833-0.ch020

challenges among university students is a rising concern. Furthermore, a study by Mutinta (2022) found that mental distress is more prevalent in student communities than in the general population. This is supported by Agrawal and Sharma (2022), who state that many mental disorders present among young people within the age range of 18 to 24 years, corresponding to the average enrolment in higher education institutions, an observation which is worrying. Mental health encompasses an extricable relationship between three factors: social, emotional and psychological wellbeing (Agrawal & Sharma, 2022). In addition, harmony between the three leads to mental wellbeing, signifying a process where the individual can think, feel, and react in varying conditions based on their decisions. When one or more of the three experiences distress, negative consequences will disturb the student 's mental wellbeing (Neupert, 2022). It is critical for higher education institutions to consider students' mental health by providing supportive environment that will ensure harmony between their social, emotional and psychological wellbeing. A supportive environment for students is one which provides relevant services and supportive policies for students in higher institutions of learning can helps them to successfully overcome their psychological challenges that may be encountered during their academic life. Alternative sources of support could help students to cope with psychological challenges and study skill adversities, which are some of the challenges experienced in higher education (Barrable et al., 2018). The term "student support" describes a broad range of services, tools and programmes that educational institutions offer to help students with many elements of their overall, academic and personal development (Huijser et al., 2022). These services are intended to improve students' success and overall wellbeing throughout their academic careers. Academic support, mental health and counselling services, financial aid, career counselling, and access to resources are just a few of the many aspects of student support that contribute to students' development, wellbeing and success in both academic and extracurricular contexts (Cenko & Canollari-Baze, 2018). The purpose of student support is to provide a welcoming, inclusive learning environment that promotes students' holistic development and assists them in overcoming obstacles they may face while pursuing their education (Simpson, 2018). The available institutional support services include counselling sessions, financial aid programs, and specialized resources designed to assist students in overcoming mental health challenges. This background underscores the vital need for continued institutional support, emphasizing the significance of targeted interventions, awareness campaigns, and the availability of resources to enhance the mental health and well-being of students at UNAM.

The psychological challenges faced by students during the COVID-19 pandemic, such as isolation, a sense of threat and transiting to e-learning, exposed certain strengths and weaknesses in the mental health support system at universities (lisiecka et al., 2023). A good understanding of factors that contribute to mental health distress among university students is crucial for higher education institutions. Positive diversity of mental health support for students at higher education institutions can help them to deal with stressors and future challenges without crumbling under pressure (Pandya & Lodha, 2022). In order to assist students' mental health, teachers are extremely important (Udah & Francis, 2022). They must be aware of the particular difficulties that students experience and offer chances for socialisation and emotional assistance. However, faculty members frequently lack the requisite expertise to recognise and successfully handle mental health issues (Ford & Parker, 2016). Institutions must therefore offer training courses that give teachers the knowledge and skills they need to support students' mental health. Institutions should also develop a learning atmosphere that supports students' overall wellbeing (Yao, 2023). This entails establishing a feeling of community, offering tools for mental health support, and putting into practice regulations that give students' mental health top priority. The University of Namibia (UNAM) can improve its efforts to promote the mental health of its students and foster an environment that is favourable for their general wellbeing by taking these actions. Additionally, it is crucial to establish a learning atmosphere that supports students' wellbeing (Capozza et al., 2021). This includes building what is described as "bonding social capital" – emotional bonds between students and between students and lectures. By including opportunities for engagement and emotional support in their courses, lecturers can help to facilitate these connections (Committee on Mental Health et al., 2021). For many students, the transition from high school to college can be difficult and frequently results in mental health problems (Xu et al., 2023). University students are vulnerable because of things like scholastic pressure, social adjustment and the demands of young adulthood. These issues have been made worse by the COVID-19 pandemic, and the move to online learning has added new stressors (Yang et al., 2022).

At its foundation, student support includes a vast array of programmes and tools intended to promote students' overall wellbeing, going beyond academic goals and addressing their emotional, social and psychological needs. This all-encompassing approach to student support is not just a goal at UNAM; it is a real commitment embedded in the very fabric of the school (Henry et al., 2020). In recent years, there has been a tremendous increase in the understanding of how important student mental health is to both their academic performance and general wellbeing. There is a definite link between mental health and academic achievement, according to study by Bas, (2021). In order to fulfil their commitment to providing students with a comprehensive education, universities all around the world, including UNAM, have been urged to prioritise student mental health. The ground-breaking study by Lipson et al. (2017) emphasises the following significant points: Reduced academic involvement among students who are dealing with mental health issues frequently results in lower marks and higher dropout rates. Depression, anxiety and stress are just a few of the different ways that mental health problems can present themselves (Ulla & Lena, 2023). These can all have a negative impact on a student's ability to do well in the classroom. For academic institutions to foster a culture of wellbeing and eliminate the stigma associated with mental health disorders, proactive mental health support and awareness are crucial (Mihai, 2021).

## Institutional Policy on Student Support Framework Services

This theoretical framework outlines student support services, aligning with Hyseni et al. (2023) principles, which emphasise the provision of readily accessible services in accordance with institutional policies. Hyseni et al. (2023) study found that higher education students typically have access to support for their mental health without the restrictions that persons in the larger community frequently suffer. This is because on-campus health and counselling facilities are readily available. It has been demonstrated that the higher education environment has a greater impact on health-related behaviours than health literacy alone. Hyseni et al. (2023), reported that higher education institutional policy offers a variety of support services to students in fields as varied as counselling, emotional wellbeing, safeguarding and special educational needs.

It is important to clarify the notion of student support before examining specific UNAM programmes and systems. Beyond the classroom, student assistance includes academic counselling, emotional well-being, safeguarding, special educational needs (SEN support), career advice, mental health resources, financial help, and a sense of community within the university (Dos Santos, 2022). Broglia et al. (2021) acknowledged that students are more than just passive users of knowledge, but rather distinct persons going through a life-changing stage, which allows for a deeper comprehension of their various demands and difficulties. The framework's (Hyseni et al. 2023) central concept is "Student Support". This represents the main hub of the resources and services an institution offers to help students with various

*Figure 1. Institutional policy on student support framework services*
*(Hyseni et al. 2023)*

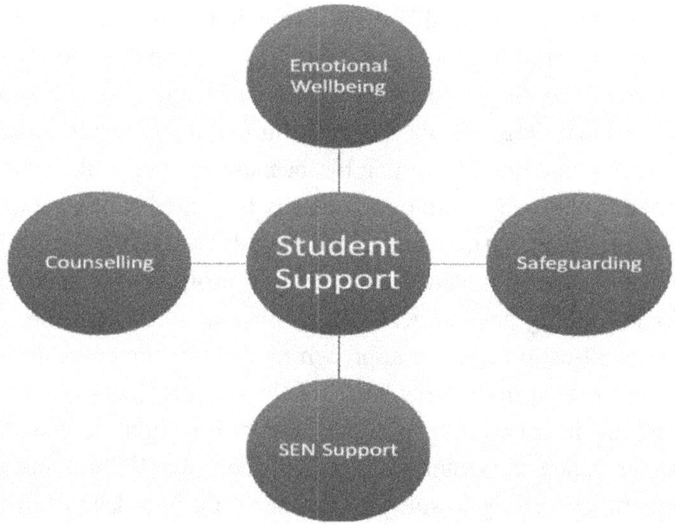


elements of their academic journey and personal development. In addition, Zungu (2022) reported that student support services such as academic advice, counselling, career coaching and assistance with a variety of issues that students could run into while enrolled at the school are just a few of the services that fall under the umbrella of "student support". Such support seeks to produce an atmosphere in which students can flourish academically, emotionally and socially.

## Types of Institutional Support to Enhance Students' Mental Health

### Counselling

A crucial component of student support is counselling services. This concentrates on treating the emotional and psychological wellbeing of the students (Courtney et al. 2019). To assist students in overcoming a range of issues, including stress, anxiety, depression, marital problems and personal challenges, qualified counsellors and mental health specialists provide both individual and group counselling sessions (Rosli et al. 2023). Counselling strives to give students a private, secure setting in which they can examine their feelings, learn coping mechanisms and enhance their mental health (Kılıç et al. 2023). Through these counselling interventions, students are empowered to confront their challenges head-on, fostering resilience and enhancing their mental health. The approach is holistic, considering not only the immediate issues at hand but also focusing on long-term emotional well-being. By providing a supportive environment and professional guidance, counselling services contribute significantly to creating a nurturing atmosphere within higher education institutions. Research conducted by Clements et al. (2023) underscores the importance of such services, emphasizing the positive impact they have on students' overall mental health and well-being. Ultimately, these counselling initiatives play a pivotal role in equipping students with the tools and emotional strength necessary to navigate the complexities of academic life and beyond.

## Safeguarding

Safeguarding measures serve as a fundamental pillar in ensuring the holistic well-being of students within educational environments. The paramount objective of these procedures is to uphold the rights, security, and welfare of students, fostering an atmosphere where they can thrive academically and personally (Porter et al. 2020). In the educational setting, safeguarding encompasses a multifaceted approach, meticulously designed to shield students from various forms of harm, abuse, harassment, and prejudice. Central to these initiatives is the creation of a safe and inclusive campus environment where every student feels valued, supported, and protected. Safeguarding policies and procedures are comprehensive, incorporating a range of preventative, reporting, and intervention measures (Courtney et al. 2019). Preventative measures are proactively implemented to create awareness, educate students and staff, and establish a culture of respect and understanding. These initiatives not only deter potential issues but also contribute to building a positive and respectful campus culture (Kılıç et al. 2023). To safeguard the rights, security and welfare of students, safeguarding procedures are implemented. In the educational setting, this includes making sure that students are safe from harm, abuse, harassment and prejudice. To build a welcoming and secure campus in which all students feel supported and protected, safeguarding policies and procedures frequently include preventative, reporting and intervention measures (Coleman, 2022).

## Emotional Wellbeing

Emotional wellbeing, a crucial facet of student support, underscores the paramount importance of nurturing students' mental and emotional wellness throughout their academic journey (Chase et al. 2020). This multifaceted element delves into a spectrum of initiatives, encompassing diverse programs and tools meticulously designed to enhance emotional stamina, reduce stress, and promote overall wellbeing among students (Mergler et al.2020). Educational institutions, cognizant of the profound impact that emotional health has on academic performance and personal growth, have pioneered efforts to address this vital aspect comprehensively. These institutions recognize that students who are emotionally balanced are better equipped to navigate the challenges of higher education effectively. Consequently, they have instituted a myriad of services and programs aimed at improving students' mental and emotional wellbeing (Chase et al. 2020). This element focuses on the significance of fostering students' mental and emotional wellness. This includes programmes and tools that promote emotional stamina, stress reduction and general wellbeing. Educational institutions understand that students' emotional health has a big impact on their academic performance and personal growth. As a result, they offer services and programmes to improve students' mental and emotional wellbeing (Joyce-Beaulieu & Zaboski, 2020).

## Special Educational Needs (SEN)

Special Educational Needs (SEN) exemplify an institution's unwavering commitment to catering to the diverse requirements of students facing disabilities or learning challenges (Earle & Curry, 2017). Within the educational landscape, SEN initiatives stand as a testament to the institution's dedication to inclusivity and equity. These programs are meticulously designed to ensure that students with SEN not only have equal access to educational opportunities but also receive specialized support, accommodations, and resources tailored to their specific needs (Ashcroft et al. 2021). Central to this approach is the recognition that every student, regardless of their challenges, deserves an equitable learning environment.

Specialized support services encompass a wide array of interventions, ranging from assistive technologies and adaptive learning materials to individualized teaching methods and personalized tutoring sessions. These measures are essential in addressing the unique learning styles and pace of students with SEN, fostering an environment where they can flourish academically and personally (Ashcroft et al. 2021). The institution's dedication to meeting the varied needs of students with disabilities or other learning challenges is highlighted by SEN. In order to guarantee that students with SEN have equal access to educational opportunities, specialised support, accommodation and resources should be provided. This element demonstrates how inclusive the organisation is and how committed it is to giving every student an equitable learning environment (Earle & Curry, 2017).

## REVIEW OF RELATED LITERATURE

This review of relevant literature attempts to document a detailed coverage of the current research and scholarly work on the mental health issues faced by college students. The work of Marquez (2019) has shown that mental health problems are becoming more common among college students. Among the most prevalent mental health issues identified are mood and anxiety disorders. It is significant to observe that the diagnostic cut off has increased rather than decreased, indicating a genuine rise in the prevalence of mental disease among young individuals (Nwoke at al., 2020). The pressures of emerging adulthood, social adjustment and academic pressure all add to university students' vulnerability. Additionally, because of systems like racism, sexism and economic marginalisation, marginalised students may experience additional stressors, which can increase their exposure and vulnerability to stressful life events (Committee on Mental Health et al., 2021). It is widely accepted that educators play a crucial role in promoting students' mental health. It is easier for instructors to recognise and treat mental health disorders since they are frequently in contact with students and can see changes in their behaviour over time. However, faculty staff frequently lack the requisite training to effectively support students' mental health. This emphasises the requirement for educational institutions to offer training courses that give lecturers the expertise and abilities to identify and address mental health issues (Canady, 2020). Goodwin (2016) reported that universities could improve their ability to recognise students who are at risk and make the right referrals to support services by spending money on faculty training. Supporting student wellbeing in the classroom is essential for promoting mental health. The development of "bonding social capital", often known as emotional relationships between students and teachers, has been proven advantageous. By including opportunities for engagement and emotional support in their courses, instructors can help to facilitate these connections. Institutions should also allocate funds for mental health support and put in place regulations that give priority to students' mental health in order to foster a welcoming and inclusive campus climate (Marthoenis, 2018). According to Dangore and Bhivgade (2023), there is no one demographic that is more susceptible to mental health issues than university students. It is important to understand that mental health problems can affect students from all backgrounds, even though some marginalised groups may experience additional stressors and discrimination that worsen their mental health issues. Mardhiyah (2021) stated that instructors should adopt a proactive strategy to support the wellbeing of all students rather than making assumptions about which students are most likely to experience mental health challenges. In summary, addressing the mental health issues university students experience calls for a thorough and proactive strategy.

UNAM, as the model institution of higher learning in Namibia: UNAM has made admirable progress in building a solid system of support services for its students (Manalo, 2018). These services are created to satisfy and address a wide range of requirements and difficulties that students experience during their academic careers. Important components of this assistance network include:

- **Academic guidance:** UNAM provides academic counselling services to assist students in understanding their course requirements, selecting majors and effectively planning their academic careers.
- **Mental health and counselling services:** UNAM has established counselling services aimed at offering emotional support and assistance to students in recognition of the significant impact that mental health has on academic achievement and general wellbeing.
- **Financial aid and scholarships:** UNAM is dedicated to making sure that financial limitations do not obstruct academic advancement. Access to education is a fundamental right. To those who qualify, financial help and scholarships are offered.
- **Student organizations and leadership:** The University promotes active involvement in student organisations to help students develop their leadership abilities and sense of belonging.
- **Health and wellness programmes:** UNAM place a high priority on students' physical and emotional wellbeing and provides health services, wellness initiatives, and fitness centres to support this goal.

## GOVERNANCE IN HIGHER EDUCATION INSTITUTIONS

Effective governance frameworks within higher education institutions have a big impact on how supportive services are provided (Bouri & Maalouf, 2017). The key to understanding how institutional assistance is handled is to comprehend these systems. An actual illustration of how a well-organised framework can improve the entire student experience is seen in the governance structure of the UNAM. This structure is crucial in determining the policies, choices and support services that have an immediate impact on students' lives. This framework is intended to promote the values of openness, responsibility and diversity, ensuring that governance is consistent with the institution's overarching goal of fostering students' wellbeing.

## GOVERNANCE STRUCTURE OF THE DIRECTORATE OF STUDENT AFFAIRS AT THE UNIVERSITY OF NAMIBIA

The Director of Student Affairs is a body established to assist students throughout their academic lifecycle with the UNAM and also providing referrals for counselling and community services. All university students have a right to the various professional services offered at the university.

Figure 2 presents the structure of the Directorate of Student Affairs (DSA) governance at the UNAM, which supports students to cope well academically and overcome stress, anxiety, depression, suicidal thoughts and any other issues that prevent students from thriving. This figure presents the hierarchical structure of Student Affairs at UNAM beginning with the Director at the top to the faculty representatives

*Figure 2. Structure of the Student Affairs (DSA) governance at the UNAM*

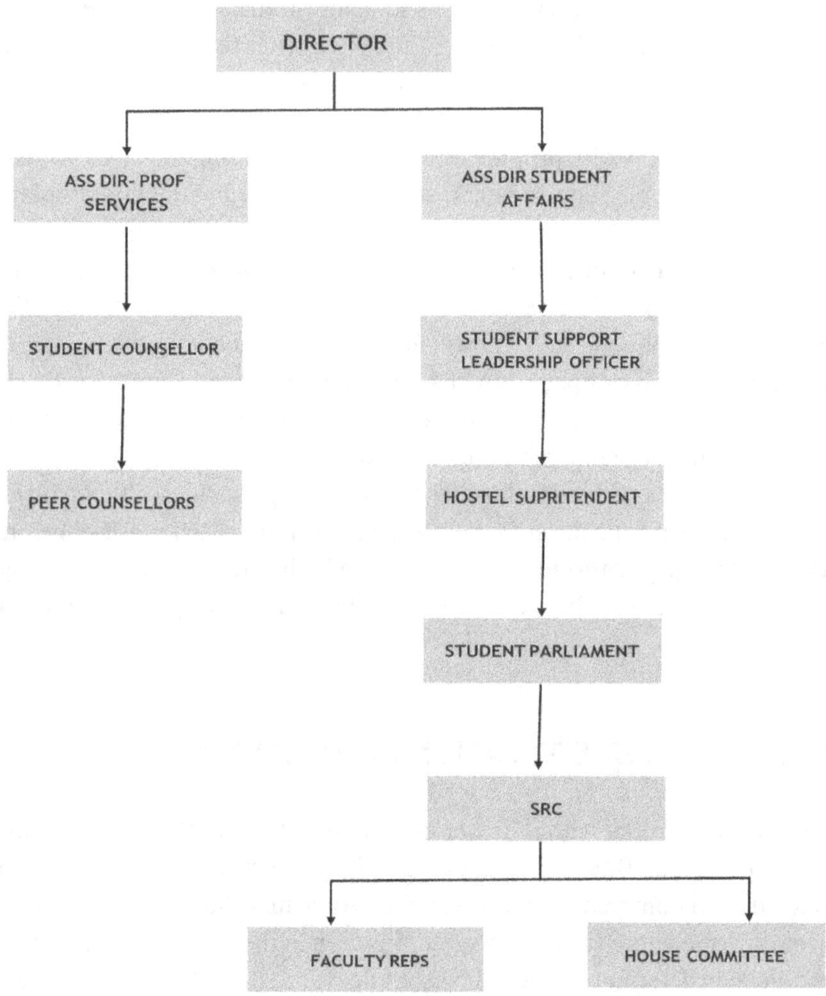


and house committees below, as this reveals the channel which is readily available to enhance student support at UNAM.

## Director

At UNAM, the director of DSA oversees and manages all aspects of the institution's student affairs. The success of the students is their main priority, and they provide strategic direction and oversee all facets of student support services. The Director collaborates with other DSA employees to provide a strong support system.

## Assistant Director: Professional Services (Ass. Dir-Prof Services)

This position probably entails giving expert direction and leadership in a variety of student affairs areas. This may include academic support services, career counselling and student administrative support at

UNAM. The Associate Director ensures that these services are efficiently coordinated and in line with the objectives of the organisation.

## Student Counsellor

In order to meet the emotional and psychological requirements of students, UNAM's student counsellors are extremely important, providing counselling services to assist students in overcoming their own obstacles, stress and mental health problems. Maintaining students' emotional health requires this support.

## Peer Counsellors

In order to give peer-to-peer support, peer counsellors collaborate with the student counsellor. They foster a welcoming environment where students feel free to express their worries. Peer counsellors can lessen the stigma attached to obtaining mental health care, which will make it simpler for students to ask for help.

## Assistant Director (ASS DIR) Student Affairs

At UNAM, this position is responsible for a wide range of student issues. It involves duties connected to co-curricular activities, campus life and student engagement. The associate director ensures that students can participate in a welcoming and active campus community.

## Student Support Leadership Officer

At UNAM, this post promotes coordination and communication among various student support services. They make sure that services are coordinated and offer students a comprehensive support system. The effective integration of support activities is facilitated by this function.

## Hostel Superintendent

Students living in dorms or other campus housing are under the supervision and care of the hostel superintendent. They guarantee that students live in a welcoming, affordable and secure environment. This assistance is crucial for students who live on campus.

## Student Parliament

The Student Parliament at UNAM speaks for all students. It has several branches, including:

- **Student Representative Council (SRC):** The SRC represents students' interests and makes sure that the university administration is aware of and responsive to their issues.
- **Faculty representatives:** These representatives customise their support and advocacy to the particular needs and problems within their individual academic faculties.
- **House committees:** In hostel settings, house committees promote a sense of community. They plan events and programmes that encourage harmony and wellbeing among dormitory inmates.

Every element of the DSA organisation at UNAM contributes significantly to improving student support. Together, they build a vast network of resources and services that cater to the intellectual, social and emotional requirements of students. This multifaceted strategy helps create a supportive and encouraging learning environment, ultimately assisting students in achieving academic success.

The participation of student leaders in the creation and implementation of assistance programmes is a distinctive feature of student support at UNAM. In order to make sure that student issues are recognised and properly addressed, student leaders frequently serve as a point of contact between the student population and the university administration (Hughes, 2021). They are essential in determining the student experience and pushing for better support services. Understanding UNAM's governance structure is essential in order to comprehend the context in which student support services function. The governance of UNAM is distinguished by a dedication to openness, responsibility and diversity. A comprehensive set of policies and procedures that outline the university's operations, particularly those pertaining to student affairs and support services, serve as its compass (Rheeder, 2021). The DSA is essential to the delivery of student support services at UNAM, acting as the hub of student life and managing numerous facets of student welfare, such as housing, counselling and involvement (Massey, 2019). Understanding the DSA's governing structure is essential to understanding the ways in which student support is provided. This backdrop prepares the scene for a thorough investigation of the governance and support systems for students at UNAM. DSA has a very specific mission: to give students unwavering assistance during their time at the university. This mandate covers a broad range of services that are crucial for creating a supportive and encouraging atmosphere (Massey, 2019). One of the goals of the DSA is making sure that students have access to a variety of services to meet their academic, social and emotional needs (Shikulo & Lekhetho, 2020).

The DSA takes on tasks like the following within the context of student welfare:

- **Accommodation Services:** UNAM is aware of the value of providing students with secure and affordable housing. The DSA oversees housing facilities, working to provide welcoming surroundings where students can live and prosper.
- **Counselling and psychological support:** Counsellors at UNAM are trained mental health specialists that are licensed and qualified. They are qualified to offer students both individual and group counselling since they have degrees in psychology, counselling or similar subjects. These therapists are adept at handling a variety of challenges such as stress, anxiety, depression, marital problems and academic stress. UNAM employs psychologists in addition to counsellors. Because they frequently hold doctoral degrees in psychology, psychologists can offer specialised psychological evaluations and interventions to students who have more complicated mental health requirements. To guarantee all-encompassing care, they collaborate closely with counsellors.
- **Student engagement and activities:** The DSA plans a variety of events, clubs and activities to enhance the student experience while encouraging holistic growth and a feeling of community.
- **Health services:** The DSA makes sure that healthcare facilities and services are available to meet medical needs because students' wellbeing also includes their physical health. A vital part of the student assistance system is the UNAM Clinic, sometimes referred to as the UNAM Health

Services. The clinic offers a variety of services to take care of students' medical requirements, promoting their general wellbeing and ensuring they have access to healthcare while they are pursuing their education. Here are some further details about UNAM Clinic:

- **Medical Services:** The UNAM Clinic provides a range of medical services, including general medical consultations for ailments and health issues that are widespread. The clinic offers medical evaluations, diagnoses and treatment to students for a variety of health conditions.
- **Nursing care:** To provide crucial healthcare services, registered nurses and nursing personnel are on hand. They can offer first aid for minor wounds, deliver immunisations and educate students about health.
- **Health promotion and education:** To spread awareness of preventative health measures, the clinic frequently runs health promotion initiatives and educational programmes. Workshops, seminars and awareness campaigns on subjects including diet, sexual health and disease prevention are a few examples of these programmes.
- **Immunisations:** The UNAM Clinic provides immunisation services to make sure that students are up to day on the immunisations necessary for their health and compliance with public health requirements.
- **Counselling and health guidance:** The clinic personnel may offer fundamental health assistance and guidance, although this is not a substitute for psychological counselling services. They can make suggestions on how to have a healthy lifestyle, deal with stress and make wise health decisions.
- **Referrals:** The clinic may refer students to other healthcare organisations or facilities for additional assessment and treatment in circumstances when specialised medical attention is required.

## REFERRAL PROCEDURES AT THE UNIVERSITY OF NAMIBIA

The referral process described here is a methodical and considerate strategy created to cater to the various demands of students in a university setting. It provides an essential foundation for recognising, evaluating and supporting students who may be dealing with academic, emotional or personal difficulties that go beyond the purview of standard university services.

### Counselling Service Guidelines on Referral Introduction

For some students being at university can prove to be a very challenging and stressful experience. The range of supportive services provided throughout the university are significant in assisting students to cope effectively and successfully in achieving academic success and maintaining personal wellbeing. However, there are times when more specialist intervention is required in order to address specific issues that may arise. It is at these times that a referral to the counselling services may be appropriate. The following guidelines on signs and symptoms that present may be helpful in making that assessment.

## Signs and Symptoms

1. When you become concerned around academic issues such as:
    a. inconsistent work
    b. procrastination
    c. poor attendance or performance
    d. repeated requests for extensions or special consideration
2. When you are conscious of marked behavioural changes in a student such as:
    a. changes in mood or behaviour
    b. tearfulness or intense emotional expression
    c. obvious lack of emotion
    d. high levels of irritability or violent outburst
    e. notable changes in grooming or personal hygiene
    f. dramatic weight gains or loss
    g. signs of excessive alcohol or drug use
    h. falling asleep in class
3. When you become aware of marked changes in interpersonal interactions such as:
    a. increased dependency on your support or that of others
    b. social withdrawal or isolation
    c. complaints from peers regarding the student's behaviour
    d. unexpected changes in personal relationships
4. When you become concerned for the student's safety due to:
    a. expressed feelings of persecution
    b. expressed feelings of hopelessness
    c. references to suicide or self-destructive behaviour
5. When you become conscious of your own boundaries in relation to a student's demands or issues. This may include:
    a. when dealing with the student is taking too much of your time
    b. when you feel the student is becoming too dependent on your support
    c. when you feel you are covering the same ground over and over again with the student
    d. when you are unsure of what to do or how to respond
    e. when you feel out of your depth
    f. when the situation is depleting you of your own emotional resources
    g. when your suggestions are constantly rejected
    h. when no change is evident

## Responding to a Student

When a student presents with a particular concern that you feel might best be dealt with by another service or professional it is important to note the following guidelines:

- Talk to the student in private.
- Reassure and affirm the student for choosing to confide in you.
- Express your concerns and observations openly and in a straightforward way directly to the student.

- Explain clearly to the student what you can provide in terms of your time and the type of support you can offer.
- Inquire how the student is attempting to handle the problem.
- If a student is very upset, ask if there anyone you can contact.
- If and when a referral to counselling is appropriate or necessary, express this recommendation clearly to the student. You can validate your suggestion by indicating the specific behaviours or concerns that the student has presented with. In addition, you may wish to point out that the issues presented go beyond the boundaries or competency of your professional role.
- The decision to enter counselling is always a personal choice on the part of the student. However, providing information on the service can often help to dispel some of the myths and misconceptions that prevail about counselling. If unsure about any details, please contact the service and check these in the presence of the student.
- Encourage students to make appointments themselves. This ensures a degree of personal responsibility and motivation on their part. There are times, however, when it is important to assist a student in making the appointment. Allowing the student to phone from your office is helpful.
- In the event of a student agreeing to attend for counselling it is important that you clarify any follow up offered by you or your department. This reassures the student of your interest and can provide a comprehensive management of the situation.
- There are times when a student may refuse to attend for counselling. This decision must be respected, as the student may need more time to consider this as an option. In the event of such a refusal, it is important that you do not become a substitute for the professional help they may need. It may be helpful to document your interactions with the student for future reference.

## Making a Referral

On making a referral to the counselling services it is helpful to:

- Discuss the referral with the student.
- Reassure the student that self-referral to the counselling services is welcomed and encouraged.
- Provide accurate information on how to access the service. The counselling services information leaflet and business card are useful for this purpose. Copies are available on request from the counselling services.
- Reassure the student that the counselling service is a confidential, professional service for assessment purposes and not a commitment to therapy.

In the event of an emergency or a crisis, it is important to state this on contacting the counselling services. In such instances, it is important that you provide an escort for the student to the counselling services.

## Confidentiality

Counselling is a professional service, which abides by a strict code of ethics and confidentiality as outlined in the policy. Confidentiality is a central and integral part of the counselling process and is assured to each client who avails themselves of the service. The service offers safety and privacy to those who choose to discuss personal and private concerns. Information given during the counselling session is held in strict confidence. No information, written or verbal, will be disclosed to a third party without the client's written permission. The issue of confidentiality is always discussed with clients during the first session. This provides an opportunity to clarify any concerns that may arise. Counselling services files are not attached to any academic record held within the university.

## Limits to Confidentiality

In exceptional circumstances, counsellors may need to break confidentiality if they believe there is a real intent of serious harm or danger to either their client or another individual. Such circumstances may pertain to issues relating to sexual abuse, rape, self-harm, suicidal ideation or criminal activities.

## Consultations

If in any doubt about how to respond or proceed, students should feel free to consult with a member of the counselling team. This can be done over the phone or by appointment. Seeking clarification is important in effectively managing and addressing the many student issues that present. Such consultations are dealt with in confidence. A group of 50 peer counsellors are also trained to assist students and are supervised by trained staff members.

The referral process for the university's counselling service serves as a crucial part of an all-encompassing system of student support. This process plays a critical role in promoting academic performance and personal wellbeing within the university community by offering a clear and systematic framework for identifying, assessing and reacting to students' individual needs. The referral process displays the institution's dedication to providing for its students' overall needs by methodically identifying signs and symptoms, having confidential, compassionate dialogues, and thoughtfully recommending counselling services as necessary. UNAM Clinic is usually prepared to respond to medical crises on campus, offering immediate care and, if necessary, coordinating with local emergency services.

## Scholarships and Financial Aid

The DSA runs a number of financial aid programmes and scholarships to help students enter higher education despite their financial challenges.

The participation of student leaders in the creation and implementation of assistance programmes is a distinctive feature of student support at UNAM. In order to make sure that student issues are recognised and properly addressed, student leaders frequently serve as a point of contact between the student population and the university administration (Ray & Radimer, 2019). They are essential in determining the student experience and pushing for better support services. Understanding UNAM's governance structure is essential in order to comprehend the context in which student support services function. The governance of UNAM is distinguished by a dedication to openness, responsibility and diversity (Warren, 2017). Additionally, establishing a comprehensive and unambiguous code of student behaviour is a key component of creating a supportive academic environment (Venugopal-Wairagade, 2016).

The student code of conduct at UNAM establishes the rights and obligations of students while fostering a climate of decency, honesty and academic performance. It establishes standards for conduct within the university community and acts as a manual for moral and responsible behaviour. Students at

UNAM benefit from a supportive environment that pushes them to become well-rounded individuals with traits like academic excellence, leadership and initiative, diversity and cultural sensitivity. While UNAM is committed to offering wide-ranging support services, it is crucial to recognise that students may face obstacles. These obstacles can include everything from monetary hardships to academic stress, from adjusting to university life to juggling academic and personal obligations (Jitaru et al., 2022). It is crucial to comprehend the particular difficulties that UNAM students experience in order to customise support services to meet their needs and make sure that every student has the chance to succeed academically and personally. In conclusion, this section has offered an overview of the multifaceted idea of student support, the different support services offered at UNAM, the function of student leadership, the governance structure of UNAM, the duties of the DSA, the student code of conduct, the qualities UNAM students can be expected to possess and the difficulties they might face.

## RECOMMENDATIONS AND SOLUTIONS

UNAM should increase funding for its mental health services. More counsellors and mental health specialists should be recruited to shorten appointment waiting times and give students individualised help. It is crucial to provide a friendly and stigma-free environment for people seeking mental health care. UNAM could establish an online portal where students can conveniently schedule appointments, get information on available resources and access self-help resources for mental health, academic support and career guidance. UNAM could also help to improve awareness of mental health concerns, lessen stigma and give students' coping mechanisms and resilience skills, incorporate mental health education into the curriculum or provide workshops and seminars. UNAM has to set up a method for gathering student opinions on the efficacy of support services. Regular evaluations and surveys can assist in locating areas that require improvement and provide guidance for the development of assistance programmes.

## STRENGTHS, LIMITATIONS, AND FUTURE DIRECTIONS FOR RESEARCH

This chapter focuses on University of Namibia (UNAM) as a case study. This is because UNAM is seen as a model for other universities globally to learn from globally on how they can design a structure that is more responsive to student mental health needs. This chapter is however limited because it exclusively focusing on UNAM as case study consequently limiting the applicability of this discussion to many different universities worldwide. Longitudinal research could be conducted on mental health trends to monitor changes in UNAM students' mental health over time. Such a study could shed light on how a student's mental health requirements change over the course of their academic career and pinpoint key moments when support is most required. To find best practices in student mental health support, comparative studies could be done with other institutions in the area or throughout the world. In addition, the possible advantages of including trained peer educators in initiatives to promote mental health could be investigated, the best ways for peer educators to spread knowledge, lessen stigma and promote help-seeking behaviour could be examined, and the way UNAM students improve their resilience and coping mechanisms analysed. The goal of institutional support is to ensure students have the proper support for the right problem at the right time, so they can successfully progress in their academic journey.

Thus, the findings in the current study have the potential to have implications for policymakers, service planners, and strategic planning of institutional resources and budgets.

## CONCLUSION

In summary, addressing the mental health issues university students experience calls for a thorough and proactive strategy. The literature review emphasises how crucial it is to address students' mental stress, reduce stigma, offer extensive support services, incorporate mental health into course design, and prioritise self-care and wellbeing. Universities should provide faculty training to give lecturers the information and abilities they need to promote students' mental health. Universities should use this chapter to establish a favorable climate that promotes student wellbeing and supports their mental health needs by putting these suggestions and solutions into practice.

## REFERENCES

Agrawal, S., & Sharma, N. (2022). *Barriers and role of higher educational institutes in students' mental wellbeing: A critical analysis.* Atlantis Highlights in Social Sciences, Education and Humanities. doi:10.2991/ahsseh.k.220105.021

Ashcroft, K., Bigger, S., & Coates, D. (2021). Students with special educational needs. *Researching into Equal Opportunities In Colleges and Universities*, (pp. 84-103). Taylor & Francis. doi:10.4324/9781315041711-5

Barrable, A., Papadatou-Pastou, M., & Tzotzoli, P. (2018). Supporting mental health, wellbeing and study skills in higher education: An online intervention system. *International Journal of Mental Health Systems, 12*(1), 54. doi:10.118613033-018-0233-z PMID:30323858

Bas, G. (2021). *Relation between student mental health and academic achievement revisited: A meta-analysis.* Health and Academic Achievement - New Findings., doi:10.5772/intechopen.95766

Bouri, E., & Maalouf, M. (2017). The impact of governance in higher education institutions on scientific research in the Arab World. *Higher Education Governance in the Arab World*, 65–82. doi:10.1007/978-3-319-52060-5_4

Broglia, E., Millings, A., & Barkham, M. (2021). Student mental health profiles and barriers to help seeking: When and why students seek help for a mental health concern. *Counselling & Psychotherapy Research, 21*(4), 816–826. doi:10.1002/capr.12462

Campbell, F., Blank, L., Cantrell, A., Baxter, S., Blackmore, C., Dixon, J., & Goyder, E. (2022). Factors that influence mental health of university and college students in the UK: A systematic review. *BMC Public Health, 22*(1), 1778. doi:10.118612889-022-13943-x PMID:36123714

Canady, V. A. (2020). College students with MH issues find support by staff lacking. *Mental Health Weekly, 30*(43), 5–5. doi:10.1002/mhw.32578

Capozza, F., Moghani, V., & Acampora, M. (2021). *Mental health literacy and demand for mental health support among University students.* AEA Randomized Controlled Trials. doi:10.1257/rct.8406-2.1

Cenko, E., & Canollari-Baze, A. (2018). The role of academic support services in ensuring student success and wellbeing: A case study in the Albanian higher education context. *EDULEARN Proceedings*. INTED. 10.21125/edulearn.2018.2430

Chahine, S. A., & Damaj, I. (2020). Review of governance policies and practices in lebanese higher-education institutions. *Higher Education in the Arab World*, (pp. 265–277). Springer. doi:10.1007/978-3-030-58153-4_10

Chase, E., & Allsopp, J. (2020). Emotional and mental wellbeing. *Youth Migration and the Politics of Wellbeing*, (pp. 153-172). Cambridge Press. doi:10.1332/policypress/9781529209020.003.0009

Clements, S., & Paramova, P. (2023). Institutional and psychological predictors of university students' mental health help-seeking intentions. *British Journal of Guidance & Counselling*, 1–13. doi:10.1080/03069885.2023.2176823

Coleman, M. E. (2022). Mental health in the college classroom: Best practices for instructors. *Teaching Sociology*, *50*(2), 168–182. doi:10.1177/0092055X221080433

Dangore, A. R., & Bhivgade, S. (2023). Common mental health problems for students. *Journal of Mental Health Issues and Behavior*, (33), 1–4. doi:10.55529/jmhib.33.1.4

Dos Santos, L. M. (2022). The stress, mental health issues, and mental wellbeing of COVID-19 survivors: An interpretative phenomenological analysis study of male University students. *The Journal of Men's Health*, *18*(9), 180. doi:10.31083/j.jomh1809180

Earle, K., & Curry, G. (2017). Meeting special educational needs and disabilities. *Addressing Special Educational Needs and Disability in the Curriculum*, *1–5*, 1–5. doi:10.4324/9781315446721-1

Faragher, R. M. (2023). Individual student characteristics, abilities, personal qualities, and the teacher's role in improving mathematics-learning outcomes. *The Evolution of Research on Teaching Mathematics*, 227–253. doi:10.1007/978-3-031-31193-2_8

Ford, T., & Parker, C. (2016). Emotional and behavioural difficulties and mental (ill)health. *Emotional & Behavioural Difficulties*, *21*(1), 1–7. doi:10.1080/13632752.2016.1139300

Goodwin, A. B. (2016). Mental health and students at risk. *New Directions for Student Services*, *2016*(156), 65–75. doi:10.1002s.20192

Guo, F., Liu, J., & Li, L. (2022). Student support and services in Chinese higher education institutions: Practices and impacts. *Student Support Services*, 113–143. doi:10.1007/978-981-16-5852-5_45

Henry, T. L., Jetty, A., Petterson, S., Jaffree, H., Ramsay, A., Heiman, E., & Bazemore, A. (2020). Taking a closer look at mental health treatment differences: Effectiveness of mental health treatment by provider type in racial and ethnic minorities. *Journal of Primary Care & Community Health*, *11*, 2150132720966403. doi:10.1177/2150132720966403 PMID:33089752

Hope, J. (2017). Comprehensive student support efforts lead to impressive outcomes. *Student Affairs Today*, *20*(10), 6–6. doi:10.1002ay.30422

Hughes, G. (2021). The challenge of student mental wellbeing: Reconnecting students services with the academic universe. *Student Support Services*, 1–23. doi:10.1007/978-981-13-3364-4_6-1

Huijser, H., Kek, M. Y., & Padró, F. F. (2022). Introduction: Student support services in an overall ecology for learning. *Student Support Services*, 3–10. doi:10.1007/978-981-16-5852-5_49

Hyseni Duraku, Z., Davis, H., & Hamiti, E. (2023). Mental health, study skills, social support, and barriers to seeking psychological help among university students: A call for mental health support in higher education. *Frontiers in Public Health*, *11*, 1220614. doi:10.3389/fpubh.2023.1220614 PMID:37920583

Jitaru, O., Axinte, R., & Vatavu, C. (2022). The role of personal development in students adapting to the academic life. *Scientific Research and Education in the Airforce*. doi:10.19062/2247-3173.2021.22.10

Joyce-Beaulieu, D., & Zaboski, B. (2020). Raising the emotional wellbeing of students with anxiety and depression. *Fostering the Emotional Wellbeing of our Youth*, (pp. 435–458). Oxford press. doi:10.1093/med-psych/9780190918873.003.0022

Kalagher, S. S., & Curran, R. D. (2023). Crafting and revising your student conduct code. *Student Conduct Practice*, (pp. 36–57). Taylor & Francis. doi:10.4324/9781003447177-4

Kılıç, C., & Karahan, F. Ş. (2023). Mental health problems among graduate students in Turkey: A cross-sectional study. *International Journal for the Advancement of Counseling*, *45*(4), 634–650. doi:10.100710447-023-09514-3 PMID:37359032

Lipson, S. K., & Eisenberg, D. (2017). Mental health and academic attitudes and expectations in university populations: Results from the healthy minds study. *Journal of Mental Health (Abingdon, England)*, *27*(3), 205–213. doi:10.1080/09638237.2017.1417567 PMID:29265935

Lisiecka, A., Chimicz, D., & Lewicka-Zelent, A. (2023). Mental health support in higher education during the COVID-19 pandemic: A case study and recommendations for practice. *International Journal of Environmental Research and Public Health*, *20*(6), 4969. doi:10.3390/ijerph20064969 PMID:36981877

Manalo, E. (2018). Teaching and learning support services. *Wellbeing in Higher Education*, (pp. 161-173). Taylor & Francis. doi:10.4324/9781315641539-16

Mardhiyah, S. A. (2021). Mental health literacy and psychological distress as predictors of psychological well-being in Sriwijaya University students. *Mental Health: Global Challenges*, *4*(1), 49–60. doi:10.32437/mhgcj.v4i1.114

Marquez, C. G. (2019). A review on first-generation college students: Challenges they face in college when dealing with mental health issues. *UC Merced Undergraduate Research Journal*, *11*(2). doi:10.5070/M4112043709

Marthoenis,. (2018). Cultural background, social support and mental health of college students. *Proceedings of the Aceh International Nursing Conference*. ScitePress. doi:10.5220/0008396702210227

Massey, K. D. (2019). Student affairs and services in Canadian higher education. *Preparing Students for Life and Work*, (pp. 78–97). Brill. doi:10.1163/9789004393073_005

Mergler, A., & Boman, P. (2020). Promoting good mental health and supporting social and emotional wellbeing. *Developing Positive Classroom Environments*, (pp. 228-244). Taylor & Francis. doi:10.4324/9781003115335-18

Mihai, A. (2021). *Mental health stigma on campus: The promotion of mental wellbeing to Ryerson students.* Toronto Metropolitan University. doi:10.32920/ryerson.14668134.v1

Mutinta, G. (2022). undefined. *BMC Psychology, 10*(1). doi:10.118640359-022-00903-8 PMID:35982493

National Academies of Sciences. (2021). Engineering; and Medicine, Health and Medicine Division, Policy and Global Affairs, Board on Health Sciences Policy, Board on Higher Education and Workforce, & Committee on Mental Health; Substance Use; and Wellbeing in STEM Undergraduate and Graduate Education. Mental health, substance use, and wellbeing in higher education: Supporting the whole student. National Academies Press.

Neupert, S. (2022). *Mental health, stress and student wellbeing*. Wicked Problems, Wolfpack Solutions. doi:10.52750/300976

Nwoke, C. N., Okpalauwaekwe, U., & Bwala, H. (2020). Mental health professional consultations and the prevalence of mood and anxiety disorders among immigrants: Multilevel analysis of the Canadian community health survey. *JMIR Mental Health, 7*(9), e19168. doi:10.2196/19168 PMID:32801115

Pandya, A., & Lodha, P. (2022). Mental health consequences of COVID-19 pandemic among college students and coping approaches adapted by higher education institutions: A scoping review. *SSM. Mental Health, 2*, 100122. doi:10.1016/j.ssmmh.2022.100122 PMID:35665095

Patton, L. D., Renn, K. A., Guido, F. M., & Quaye, S. J. (2016). *Student development in college: Theory, research, and practice*. John Wiley & Sons.

Pillay, J. (2022). University students' mental health: A concern for all. In S. Deb & B. A. Gerrard (Eds.), *Handbook of health and wellbeing* (pp. 277–293). doi:10.1007/978-981-16-8263-6_12

Porter, L. (2020). Safeguarding students: Physical and emotional security. *Student Behaviour*, (pp. 209-224). Taylor & Francis. doi:10.4324/9781003117520-11

Ray, D. C., & Radimer, S. (2019). Preparing student affairs professionals to serve in urban institutions. *Student Affairs in Urban-Serving Institutions*, (pp. 128–150). Taylor & Francis. doi:10.4324/9781351043366-7

Rheeder, C. (2022). Student affairs and services leadership in trying times: Student social behaviour project and psycho-social support interventions at a comprehensive university in South Africa. *Journal of Student Affairs in Africa, 10*(2). doi:10.24085/jsaa.v10i2.4369

Rosli, I. N., & Harun, M. M. (2023). The relationship between mental health, coping strategies and attitudes towards seeking counselling services among University students. *International Journal of Academic Research in Business & Social Sciences, 13*(7). doi:10.6007/IJARBSS/v13-i7/17443

Shikulo, L., & Lekhetho, M. (2020). undefined. *Cogent Social Sciences, 6*(1). doi:10.1080/23311886.2020.1737401

Simpson, O. (2018). Student support face to face. I O. Simpson, O. (Ed.), Supporting students in online, open and distance learning (pp. 78–87). Taylor & Francis. doi:10.4324/9780203417003-7

Udah, H., & Francis, A. (2022). COVID-19 and mental health and wellbeing of higher education international students. In H. Udah & A. Francis (Eds.), *Mental health and higher education in Australia* (pp. 303–320). Routledge. doi:10.1007/978-981-16-8040-3_18

Ulla, D., & Lena, R. (2023). Sustainable development work aimed at promoting mental health among municipal adult students with mental health problems. *Insights on the Depression and Anxiety, 7*(1), 016–017. doi:10.29328/journal.ida.1001037

Venugopal-Wairagade, G. (2016). Creating a supportive learning environment for better student engagement. *2016 International Conference on Learning and Teaching in Computing and Engineering (LaTICE)*. IEEE. 10.1109/LaTiCE.2016.26

Warren, J. M. (2017). *School consultation for student success.* Springer. doi:10.1891/9780826177780

Xu, J., & Lee, S. G. (2023). Problems with complex college admissions policies and overloaded after-school private education on middle- and high-school students' mental health in South Korea. *Journal of Global Health Reports, 7.* doi:10.29392/001c.84099

Yang, J., Zhang, Y., Li, P., Zhang, H., & Liu, T. (2022). College students' academic stressors on mental health during the COVID-19 pandemic: A comparison between graduating students and non-graduating students. *International Journal of Mental Health Promotion, 24*(4), 603–618. doi:10.32604/ijmhp.2022.019406

Yao, J. (2023). Starting with the mental health of students. In J. Yao (Ed.), *Psychological communication between teachers and students* (pp. 3–22). Routledge. doi:10.4324/9781003360094-2

Zungu, S. (2022). *Student support services: Opening TVET education in South Africa through the provision of student support.* ScienceOpen.com. doi:10.47622/9781928502425_P07

## ADDITIONAL READING

Boykin, A. W., & Noguera, P. (2011). *Creating the opportunity to learn: Moving from research to practice to close the achievement gap.* ASCD.

Evans, N. J., Forney, D. S., Guido, F. M., Patton, L. D., & Renn, K. A. (2009). *Student development in college: Theory, research, and practice.* John Wiley & Sons.

Quaye, S. J., Harper, S. R., & Pendakur, S. L. (Eds.). (2019). *Student engagement in higher education: Theoretical perspectives and practical approaches for diverse populations.* Routledge. doi:10.4324/9780429400698

Simpson, O. (2013). *Supporting students for success in online and distance education.* Routledge. doi:10.4324/9780203095737

## KEY TERM DEFINITIONS

**Governance Structure:** The framework of leadership roles, duties and decision-making procedures that direct an institution's policies, practices and support services is referred to as the governance structure in the context of higher education institutions (Chahine et al., 2020).

**Student Attributes and Qualities:** These qualities and characteristics cover the traits and abilities required of students, such as critical thinking, drive, resiliency, and effective communication, which support their success in the classroom and personal growth (Faragher, 2023).

**Student Code of Conduct:** The student code of conduct is a set of rules, regulations and ethical guidelines that outline expected behaviour and standards of conduct for students within an academic institution. It serves as a guide for ethical decision-making and conflict resolution (Kalagher et al., 2023).

**Student Support:** The term "student support" refers to a complex approach used in institutions of higher learning. It includes a wide range of services and resources aimed at empowering students, meeting their many needs, and promoting their success both academically and personally (Guo et al., 2022).

# Compilation of References

(2022). RUDN. *Journal of Political Science*, *24*(1), 166–174.

Abbott-chapman, J. (2011). Making the most of the mosaic: Facilitating post-school transitions to higher education of disadvantaged students. *Australian Educational Researcher*, *38*(1), 57–71. doi:10.100713384-010-0001-9

Abdelwahed, N. A. A., Aldoghan, M. A., Moustafa, M. A., & Soomro, B. A. (2022). Factors affecting online learning, stress and anxiety during the COVID-19 pandemic in Saudi Arabia. *International Journal of Human Rights in Healthcare*. doi:10.1108/IJHRH-03-2022-0012

Abdullahi, A. M., Orji, R., Rabiu, A. M., Kawu, A. A. (2020). Personality and Subjective Well-Being: Towards Personalized Persuasive Interventions for Health and Well-Being. *Online Journal Public Health Information*, *12*(1). . doi:10.5210/ojphi.v12i1.10335

Abelson, S., Lipson, S. K., & Eisenberg, D. (2023). Mental health in college populations: A multidisciplinary review of what works, evidence gaps, and paths forward. In L. W. Perna (Ed.), *Higher education: Handbook of Theory and Research* (Vol. 37). Springer. doi:10.1007/978-3-030-76660-3_6

Abrams, Z. (2022). Student mental health is in crisis: Campuses are rethinking their approach. American Psychological Association.

Acosta, J., Chinman, P., Ebener, P., Malone, A., Phillips, A., & Wilks, A. (2019). Understanding the relationship between perceived school climate and bullying: A mediator analysis. *Journal of School Violence*, *18*(2), 200–215. doi:10.1080/15388220.2018.1453820 PMID:30778279

Acutt, J., & Hattingh, S. B. (2016). *Occupational health: Management and practice for health practitioners* (5th ed.). Juta.

Adan, M., Ansari, A., & Yasmeen, B. (2022). The effects of institutional environment on academic performance at higher level of learning: A case of Punjab University Lahore. *Bulletin of Business and Economics*, *11*(1), 104–112.

Adasi, G. S., Amponsah, K. D., Mohammed, S. M., Yeboah, R., & Mintah, P. C. (2020). Gender differences in stressors and coping strategies among teacher education students at University of Ghana. *Journal of Education and Learning*, *9*(2), 123–133. doi:10.5539/jel.v9n2p123

Adewale, A. S., & Abdulsalam, I. (2017). Impact of higher education management and leadership. *Malaysian Online Journal of Educational Management*, *5*(2), 23–34. doi:10.22452/mojem.vol5no2.5

Adqasuraq, G., & Kualaga, O. (2012). Exploring the Role of Teachers in the Lives of Teenage Learners. *Journal of Humanities*, *37*(7), 203–211.

Affum, P. K., Kusi, H., Mensah, D. K. D., & Afful-Broni, A. (2013). "Serving 'Two Masters' in The Ghanaian Educational Context": The Experiences of Working Post Graduate Students, at the Department of Psychology and Education, University of Education, Winneba, Ghana. *African Journal of Inter Disciplinary Studies.*, *6*(2), 13–22.

Agardh, A., Priebe, G., Emmelin, M., & Palmiere, J. (2020). Sexual harassment among employees and students at a large Swedish university: Who are exposed, to what, by whom and where – a cross-sectional prevalence study. *BMC Public Health*, *22*(1), 1–14. PMID:31898494

Agrawal, S., & Sharma, N. (2021). *Barriers and role of higher educational institutes in students' mental well-being: A critical analysis*. Atlantis Press International.

Agrawal, S., & Sharma, N. (2022). *Barriers and role of higher educational institutes in students' mental wellbeing: A critical analysis*. Atlantis Highlights in Social Sciences, Education and Humanities. doi:10.2991/ahsseh.k.220105.021

Ahmed, A. M. (2019). The real core competencies in premed culture. *Academic Medicine*, *94*(5), 611. doi:10.1097/ACM.0000000000002616 PMID:31021862

Aitken, M. E., Mccarthy, M. L., Slomine, B. S., Ding, R., Durbin, D. R., Jaffe, K. M., Paidas, C. N., Dorsch, A. M., Christensen, J. R., & MacKenzie, E. J. (2009). Family Burden after Traumatic Brain Injury in Children. *Pediatrics*, *123*(1), 199–206. doi:10.1542/peds.2008-0607 PMID:19117883

Ajandi, J. (2011). Single Mothers by Choice: Discourses of the Family through Social Justice Alternatives. *International Journal of Child, Youth & Family Studies : IJCYFS*, *3*(4), 410–431. doi:10.18357/ijcyfs23/420117757

Akinci, Z., Yurcu, G., & Ekin, Y. (2018). Relationships between student personality traits, mobbing, and depression within the context of sustainable tourism education: The case of a faculty of tourism. [Al]. *Sustainability (Basel)*, *10*(10), 3418. doi:10.3390u10103418

Akparep, J. (2019). An examination of the causes of students-management conflicts in university for development studies from 1999 to 2009 January. *Open Journal of Leadership*, *8*(2), 75–94. doi:10.4236/ojl.2019.82005

Akram, M., & Rana, S. (2013). Positive schooling and subjective well-being of Pakistani children (A qualitative study). *Pakistan Journal of Social and Clinical Psychology*, *11*(1), 42–51.

Alabri, A. (2022). Fear of missing out (FOMO): The effects of the need to belong, perceived centrality, and fear of social exclusion. *Human Behavior and Emerging Technologies*, *2022*, 1–12. doi:10.1155/2022/4824256

Alderson-Day, B., & Fernyhough, C. (2015). Inner Speech: Development, Cognitive Functions, Phenomenology, and Neurobiology. *Psychological Bulletin*, *141*(5), 931–965. doi:10.1037/bul0000021 PMID:26011789

Alkhawaldeh, A., Al Omari, O., Al Aldawi, S., Al Hashmi, I., Ann Ballad, C., Ibrahim, A., Al Sabei, S., Alsaraireh, A., Al Qadire, M., & ALBashtawy, M. (2023). Stress Factors, Stress Levels, and Coping Mechanisms among University Students. *TheScientificWorldJournal*, *2023*, 2023. doi:10.1155/2023/2026971 PMID:37426577

Allen, T. D., & Eby, L. T. (2003). Relationship effectiveness for mentors: Factors associated with learning and quality. *Journal of Management*, *29*(4), 469–486. doi:10.1016/S0149-2063(03)00021-7

Allott, K., & Lin, A. (2020). Cognitive risk factors for psychosis. *Risk Factors for Psychosis*, 269-287. doi:10.1016/B978-0-12-813201-2.00014-4

Aloka, P. J. O. (2022). Barriers to work wellness among students in higher education institutions. In C. Alexander & A. Tureen (Eds.), *Leadership Wellness and Mental Health Concerns in Higher Education* (pp. 22–42). IGI Global. doi:10.4018/978-1-7998-7693-9.ch002

Aloka, P. J. O. (2022). Social Impact of Digital English Language Learning Environments. In W. El-Henawy & M. del Mar Suárez (Eds.), *English as a Foreign Language in a New-Found Post-Pandemic World* (pp. 207–225). IGI Global. doi:10.4018/978-1-6684-4205-0.ch010

Aloka, P. J. O. (2022). Students' Self-Directed Learning Techniques and Attitudes toward Online English Language Learning. In W. El-Henawy & M. del Mar Suárez (Eds.), *English as a Foreign Language in a New-Found Post-Pandemic World* (pp. 51–66). IGI Global. doi:10.4018/978-1-6684-4205-0.ch003

Aloka, P. J., Ooko, M., Ooko, P. A., & Onyango, P. (2023). Self-Regulated Learning and Student Success, Retention, and Engagement in Online Courses. In J. Keengwe (Ed.), *Handbook of Research on Innovative Frameworks and Inclusive Models for Online Learning* (pp. 238–255). IGI Global. doi:10.4018/978-1-6684-9072-3.ch012

Aloka, P. J., Opondo, C. M., & Ooko, M. (2023). Expectations, Culture, and Adaptation to Higher Education Institutions by First-Year Students. In P. Aloka & K. Mukuna (Eds.), *Handbook of Research on Coping Mechanisms for First-Year Students Transitioning to Higher Education* (pp. 1–20). IGI Global. doi:10.4018/978-1-6684-6961-3.ch001

Alorani, O., & Alradaydeh, M. (2018). Spiritual well-being, perceived social support, and life satisfaction among university students. *International Journal of Adolescence and Youth*, *23*(3), 291–298. doi:10.1080/02673843.2017.1352522

Alsubaie, M. M., Stain, H. J., Webster, L. A., & Wadman, R. (2019). The role of sources of social support on depression and quality of life for university students. *International Journal of Adolescence and Youth*, *24*(4), 484–496. doi:10.1080/02673843.2019.1568887

Altbach, P. G. (2013). Advancing the national and global knowledge economy: The role of research universities in developing countries. *Studies in Higher Education*, *38*(3), 316–330. doi:10.1080/03075079.2013.773222

Amanvermez, Y., Rahmadiana, M., Karyotaki, E., de Wit, L., Ebert, D. D., Kessler, R. C., & Cuijpers, P. (2020). Stress management interventions for college students: A systematic review and meta-analysis. *Clinical Psychology: Science and Practice*. https://psycnet.apa.org/doi/10.1111/cpsp.12342

Amaya, M., Donegan, T.E., Conner, D.R., Edwards, J., & Gipson, C.S. (2019). Creating a Culture of Wellness: A Call to Action for Higher Education, Igniting Change in Academic Institutions. *Building Healthy Academic Communities Journal.*

Amaya, M., Donegan, T., Conner, D., Edwards, J., & Gipson, C. (2019). Creating a Culture of Wellness: A Call to Action for Higher Education, Igniting Change in Academic Institutions. *Building Healthy Academic Communities Journal*, *3*(2), 27–40. doi:10.18061/bhac.v3i2.7117

American College Health Association. (2019). Academic impacts. *American College Health Association.* https://www.acha.org/documents/ncha/NCHAII_SPRING_2019_US_REFERENCE_GROUP_EXECUTIVE_SUMMARY.pdf

American College Health Association. (2019). *American College Health Association-national College Health Assessment II: Canadian consortium executive summary.* ACHA.

American Psychiatric Association. (2013). *Diagnostic and statistical manual of mental disorders* (5th ed.). APA. doi:10.1176/appi.books.9780890425596

American Psychological Association. (2013, January 1). *Stress and sleep.* APA. https://www.apa.org. https://www.apa.org/news/press/releases/stress/2013/sleep

American Psychological Association. (2020). *Stress in America: A national Mental Health Crisis.* American Psychological Association.

American Psychological Association. (2020a). *Coping strategy.* American Psychological Association. https://dictionary.apa.org/coping-strategy

American Psychological Association. (2020b). *Stress*. American Psychological Association. https://dictionary.apa.org/stress

Amholt, T., Dammeyer, J., Carter, R., & Niclasen, J. (2020). *Child indicators research*. Springer.

Amos, P. M., Amoako, B. M., Antwi, T., & Amoah, H. (2021). Motherhood and higher education in Ghana: Experiences of student-nursing mothers. *International Journal of Didactical Studies*, *2*(1), 1–9. doi:10.33902/IJODS.2021167163

Analisah, C. D., & Indartono, S. (2019). Ecological theory: preventing student bullying to promote culture of peace. *Joint Proceedings of the International Conference on Social Science and Character Education (IcoSSCE 2018) and International Conference on Social Studies, Moral, and Character Education (ICSMC 2018)*. Atlantis Press. 10.2991/icossce-icsmc-18.2019.44

Anderson, D. L., & Graham, A. P. (2016). Improving student wellbeing: Having a say at school. *school effectiveness and school improvement, 27*(3), 348-366.

Anderson, M. S. (2017). Barriers to the Utilization of Mental Health Services on College Campuses by African-American Students1. *McNair Scholar Research Journal*, *11*(3), 1–12.

Andretta, J. R., & McKay, M. T. (2020). Self-efficacy and well-being in adolescents: A comparative study using variable and person-centered analyses. *Children and Youth Services Review*, *118*, 105374. doi:10.1016/j.childyouth.2020.105374

Anglim, J., Horwood, S., Smillie, L. D., Marrero, R. J., & Wood, J. K. (2020). Predicting psychological and subjective well-being from personality: *A meta-analysis. Psychological Bulletin*, *146*(4), 279–323. doi:10.1037/bul0000226 PMID:31944795

Ang, W. H. D., Chew, H. S. J., Dong, J., Yi, H., Mahendren, R., & Lau, Y. (2022). Digital training for building resilience: Systematic review, meta-analysis, and meta-regression. *Stress and Health*, *38*(5), 848–869. doi:10.1002mi.3154 PMID:35460533

Anho, J., Kporhobo, J., & Aweto, J. (2023). Students unrest in Nigerian universities: Types, causes and administrative strategies to the challenges. *World Journal of Advanced Research and Reviews*, *18*(03), 376–385. doi:10.30574/wjarr.2023.18.3.1072

Ansah, T., & Tiwaah, W. E. (2007). Perceived Social and Psychological Challenges of Adolescent Mothers in Manso Nkwanta. *Journal of Social Sciences and Education*, *3*(7), 423–431.

Appleton, J. J., Christenson, S. L., & Furlong, M. J. (2008). Student engagement with school: Critical conceptual and methodological issues of the construct. *Psychology in the Schools*, *45*(5), 369–386. doi:10.1002/pits.20303

Aragon, T. J. (2020.) epitools: Epidemiology tools. *R package version 0.5-10.1*. Cran. https://cran.r-project. org/web/packages/epitools/epitools.pdf.

Arday, J. (2022). No one can see me cry: Understanding mental health issues for Black and minority ethnic staff in higher education. *Higher Education*, *83*(1), 79–102. doi:10.100710734-020-00636-w

Arensman, E., Scott, V., De Leo, D., & Pirkis, J. (2020). Suicide and suicide prevention from a global perspective. *Crisis*, *41*(Supplement 1), S3–S7. doi:10.1027/0227-5910/a000664 PMID:32208759

Arnett, J. J. (2000). Emerging adulthood: A theory of development from the late teens through the twenties. *The American Psychologist*, *55*(5), 469–480. doi:10.1037/0003-066X.55.5.469 PMID:10842426

Arnett, J. J. (2007). Emerging adulthood: What is it, and what is it good for? *Child Development Perspectives*, *1*(2), 68–73. doi:10.1111/j.1750-8606.2007.00016.x

Aron, E. N. (1996). *The highly sensitive person: How to thrive when the world overwhelms you.* Perpus. https://perpus.univpancasila.ac.id/index.php?p=show_detail&id=124394

Arria, A. M., & DuPont, R. L. (2010). Nonmedical prescription stimulant use among college students: Why we need to do something and what we need to do. *Journal of Addictive Diseases*, *29*(4), 417–426. doi:10.1080/10550887.2010.509273 PMID:20924877

Arseneault, L., Bowes, L., & Shakoor, S. (2010). Bullying Victimization in Youths and Mental Health Problems: 'Much Ado about Nothing'? *Psychological Medicine*, *40*(5), 717–729. doi:10.1017/S0033291709991383 PMID:19785920

Arshad, M., Shahzadi, E., & Mahmood, A. (2016). Parents Involvement at University Level Education: Students Perception in Under Developing Country. *European Scientific Journal*, *12*(22), 294–304. doi:10.19044/esj.2016.v12n22p294

Arslan, G. (2023). Psychological Well-Being and Mental Health in Youth: Technical Adequacy of the Comprehensive Inventory of Thriving. *Children (Basel, Switzerland)*, *10*(7), 1269. doi:10.3390/children10071269 PMID:37508766

ARTE. (2018). *Demain, l'école (2/2) - Les innovations dans le monde* [Video]. Youtube. https://www.youtube.com/watch?v=9POzTRzuQnw

ARTE. (2021). *Dans la tête des champions* [Video]. ARTE Boutique. https://boutique.arte.tv/detail/dans-la-tete-des-champions

ARTE. (2022, September 17). *Peut-on se fier à soi-même? | 42, la réponse à presque tout.* [Video]. YouTube. https://www.youtube.com/watch?v=jeAfbTKmZng

Aselton, P. (2012). Sources of stress and coping in American college students who have been diagnosed with depression. *Journal of child and adolescent psychiatric nursing: Official publication of the Association of Child and Adolescent Psychiatric Nurses*, *25*(3), 119–123.

Ashcroft, K., Bigger, S., & Coates, D. (2021). Students with special educational needs. *Researching into Equal Opportunities In Colleges and Universities*, (pp. 84-103). Taylor & Francis. doi:10.4324/9781315041711-5

Ashipala, D. O., Albanus, F. S., & Nghole, T. M. (2023). Overview and management of burnout among academics. In A. ul Haque (Ed.), Handbook of research on dissecting and dismantling occupational stress in modern organizations (pp. 200-215). IGI Global. doi:10.4018/978-1-6684-6543-1.ch015

Ashipala, D. O., & Shilunga, A. P. (2023). Overview and Management of Anxiety. In *Acceleration of the Biopsychosocial Model in Public Health* (pp. 194–210). IGI Global.

Ashipala, D. O., & Shilunga, A. P. (2023). Overview and management of anxiety. In S. G. Taukeni (Ed.), *Acceleration of the biopsychosocial model in public health* (pp. 194–210). IGI Global.

Asif, S., Mudassar, A., Shahzad, T. Z., Raouf, M., & Pervaiz, T. (2020). Frequency of depression, anxiety and stress among university students. [CrossRef]. *Pakistan Journal of Medical Sciences*, *36*(5), 971–976. doi:10.12669/pjms.36.5.1873 PMID:32704273

Association of Colleges. (2017). AoC *Survey on Students with Mental Health Conditions in Further Education.* AOC.

Astuti, B., Sugiyatno, S., & Aminah, S. (2017). The development of early childhood sex education materials for early childhood education (ECE) teachers. [Jurnal Pendidikan dan Pemberdayaan Masyarakat]. *JPPM*, *4*(2), 113–120. doi:10.21831/jppm.v4i2.14869

AtterayaM. S. (2020). Acculturation stressors and academic adjustment among Nepalese students in South Korean higher education institutions. doi:10.1101/2020.12.07.414441

Auerbach, R. P., Alonso, J., Axinn, W. G., Cuijpers, P., Ebert, D. D., Green, J. G., Hwang, I., Kessler, R. C., Liu, H., Mortier, P., Nock, M. K., Pinder-Amaker, S., Sampson, N. A., Aguilar-Gaxiola, S., Al-Hamzawi, A., Andrade, L. H., Benjet, C., Caldas-de-Almeida, J. M., Demyttenaere, K, & Bruffaerts, R. (2016). Mental disorders among college students in the World Health Organization world mental health surveys. *Psychological Medicine*, *46*(14), 2955–2970. doi:10.1017/S0033291716001665 PMID:27484622

Auerbach, R. P., Alonso, J., Axinn, W. G., Cuijpers, P., Ebert, D. D., Green, J. G., & Zaslavsky, A. M. (2018). Mental disorders among college students in the World Health Organization World Mental Health Surveys. *Psychological Medicine*, *48*(4), 554–567. oi:10.1017/S0033291717001665 PMID:28805169

Auerbach, R. P., Mortier, P., Bruffaerts, R., Alonso, J., Benjet, C., Cuijpers, P., Demyttenaere, K., Ebert, D. D., Green, J. G., Hasking, P., Murray, E., Nock, M. K., Pinder-Amaker, S., Sampson, N. A., Stein, D. J., Vilagut, G., Zaslavsky, A. M., & Kessler, R. C. (2018). WHO World Mental Health Surveys International College Student Project: Prevalence and distribution of mental disorders. *Journal of Abnormal Psychology*, *127*(7), 623–638. doi:10.1037/abn0000362 PMID:30211576

Awodiji, O. (2023). Students' unrest in higher education: A perspective from The 4IR in book: A compendium of response to student unrest in African Universities. (pp.185-318): Axiom Academic Publishers (PTY) Ltd.

Ayo, V. (2019). *Effects of sexual harassment on the academic performance of female students at Makerere University*. [Unpublished Bachelor's Degree Dissertation, Makerere University, Uganda].

Azañedo, C. M., Artola, T., Sastre, S., & Alvarado, J. M. (2021). Character strengths predict subjective well-being, psychological well-being, and psychopathological symptoms, over and above functional social support. *Frontiers in Psychology*, *12*, 661278. Advance online publication. doi:10.3389/fpsyg.2021.661278 PMID:34621205

Babakhanloo, A., Jalilvand, M., & Shoghi, B. (2017). Effectiveness of self-talk technique and positive empathy on deficient attittudes, hopelessness, and suicidal thoughts in women with breast cancer. *International Journal Of Medical Toxicology And Forensic Medicine*, *7*(1), 1–10. doi:10.22037/ijmtfm.v7i1(Winter).13178

Babicka-Wirkus, A., Wirkus, L., Stasiak, K., & Kozłowski, P. (2021). University students' strategies of coping with stress during the coronavirus pandemic: Data from Poland. *PLoS One*, *16*(7), e0255041. doi:10.1371/journal.pone.0255041 PMID:34310649

Backhaus, I., Varela, A. R., Khoo, S., Siefken, K., Crozier, A., Begotaraj, E., Fischer, F., Wiehn, J., Lanning, B., Lin, P., Jan, S., Zaranza Monteiro, L., Al-Shamli, A., La Torre, G., & Kawachi, I. (2020). Associations between social capital and depressive symptoms among college students in 12 countries: Results of a cross-national study. *Frontiers in Psychology*, *11*, 644. doi:10.3389/fpsyg.2020.00644 PMID:32411038

Backović, D. V., Maksimovic, M. Z., Davidovic, D., Živojinović, J., & Stevanović, D. (2013). Stress and mental health among medical students. *Srpski Arhiv za Celokupno Lekarstvo*, *141*(11-12), 11–12, 780–784. doi:10.2298/SARH1312780B

Bahari, S. & Amla, S. (n.d.). Clients' Perception of Counseling Variables in Relation to Counselling Outcomes. *Malaysian Online Journal of Counselling*, 1–14.

Baig, T., Ganesan, G. S., Ibrahim, H., Yousuf, W., & Mahfoud, Z. R. (2021). The association of parental involvement with adolescents' well-being in Oman: Evidence from the 2015 Global School Health Survey. *BMC Psychology*, *9*(1), 1–9. doi:10.118640359-021-00677-5 PMID:34749828

Baik, C., Larcombe, W., & Brooker, A. (2019). How universities can enhance student mental wellbeing: The student perspective. *Higher Education Research & Development*, *38*(4), 674–687. doi:10.1080/07294360.2019.1576596

Baker, C. (2018). *Mental Health Statistics for England: Prevalence, Services and Funding*. House of Commons Library. http://researchbriefings.files.parliament.uk/documents/SN06988/SN06988.pd

Baker, P. W., & Siryk, B. (1984). Measuring adjustment to college. *Journal of Counseling Psychology*, *2*, 45–56.

Bakır-Ayğar, B., & Kaya, A. (2017). Ortaokul öğrencilerinin okul aidiyet duygusu ile okul temelli yalnızlıkarasındaki ilişkide okul ikliminin aracılık rolü. *E-Uluslararası Eğitim Araştırmaları Dergisi*, *8*(1), 14–27.

Ballester, L., Alayo, I., Vilagut, G., Almenara, J., Cebrià, A. I., Echeburúa, E., Gabilondo, A., Gili, M., Lagares, C., Piqueras, J. A., Roca, M., Soto-Sanz, V., Blasco, M. J., Castellví, P., Mortier, P., Bruffaerts, R., Auerbach, R. P., Nock, M. K., Kessler, R. C., & Jordi, A. (2020). Mental disorders in Spanish university students: Prevalence, age-of-onset, severe role impairment and mental health treatment. *Journal of Affective Disorders*, *273*, 604–613. doi:10.1016/j.jad.2020.04.050 PMID:32560960

Banda, B.C., & Malinga, W. (2021). Coronavirus (COVID-19) and women in higher education in a South African University: Academic and social implications. *African Journal of Gender, Society and Development*, *10*(1), 7–34. doi:10.31920/2634-3622/2021/v10n1a1

Bandura, A. (1977). Self-efficacy: Toward a unifying theory of behavioral change. *Psychological Review*, *84*(2), 191–215. doi:10.1037/0033-295X.84.2.191 PMID:847061

Banko, J., Navraga, H., & Obansa, L. K. (2012). Exploring the Academic Stress of Adolescent Mothers. *Education and Counselling*, *7*, 351–360.

Bantjes, J., Kessler, M., Lochner, C., Breet, E., Bawa, B., Roos, J., Davids, C., Muturiki, M., Kessler, R. C., & Stein, D. J. (2023). The mental health of university students in South Africa: Results of the national student survey. *Journal of Affective Disorders*, *321*, 217–226. doi:10.1016/j.jad.2022.10.044 PMID:36349649

Bantjes, J., Saal, W., Christine Lochner, C., Roos, J., Auerbach, R. P., Mortier, P., Bruffaerts, R., & Ronald, C. (2020). Inequality and mental healthcare utilisation among first-year university students in South Africa. *International Journal of Mental Health Systems*, *14*(1), 5. doi:10.118613033-020-0339-y PMID:31998406

Banyard, V., Demers, J., Cohn, E., Edwards, K. M., Moynihan, M. M., Walsh, W. A., & Ward, S. K. (2020). Academic correlates of unwanted sexual contact, intercourse, stalking, and intimate partner violence: An understudied but Important Consequence for College Students. *Journal of Interpersonal Violence*, *35*(21-22), 4375–4392. doi:10.1177/0886260517715022 PMID:29294800

Barbayannis, G., Bandari, M., Zheng, X., Baquerizo, H., Pecor, K. W., & Ming, X. (2022). Academic Stress and Mental Well-Being in College Students: Correlations, Affected Groups, and COVID-19. *Frontiers in Psychology*, *13*, 886344. doi:10.3389/fpsyg.2022.886344 PMID:35677139

Barden, N., & Caleb, R. (2019). *Student mental health and wellbeing in higher education: A Practical Guide*.Sage eds.

Barkham, M., Broglia, E., Dufour, G., Fudge, M., Knowles, L., Percy, A., Turner, A., & Williams, C. (2019). Towards an evidence base for student wellbeing and mental health. *Counselling & Psychotherapy Research*, *19*(4), 351–357. doi:10.1002/capr.12227

Barkway, P. M. (2006). Creating supportive environments for mental health promotion in the workplace. *Contemporary Nurse*, *21*(1), 131–141. doi:10.5172/conu.2006.21.1.131 PMID:16594890

Barnard, L. K., & Curry, J. F. (2011). Self-compassion: Conceptualizations, correlates, & interventions. *Review of General Psychology*, *15*(4), 289–303. doi:10.1037/a0025754

Barnett, M. (2004). A qualitative analysis of family support and interaction among Black college students at an ivy league university. *The Journal of Negro Education, 73*(1), 53–68. doi:10.2307/3211259

Barnett, P., Arundell, L., Saunders, R., Matthews, H., & Pilling, S. (2021). The efficacy of psychological interventions for the prevention and treatment of mental health disorders in university students: A systematic review and meta-analysis. *Journal of Affective Disorders, 280*, 381–406. doi:10.1016/j.jad.2020.10.060 PMID:33227669

Barnett-Page, E., & Thomas, J. (2009). Methods for the synthesis of qualitative research: A critical review. *BMC Medical Research Methodology, 9*(1), 1–11. doi:10.1186/1471-2288-9-59 PMID:19671152

Barrable, A., Papadatou-Pastou, M., & Tzotzoli, P. (2018). Supporting mental health, wellbeing and study skills in Higher Education: An online intervention system. *International Journal of Mental Health Systems, 12*(1), 54. doi:10.118613033-018-0233-z PMID:30323858

Barr, D. A., Gonzalez, M. E., & Wanat, S. F. (2008). The leaky pipeline: Factors associated with early decline in interest in premedical studies among underrepresented minority undergraduate students. *Academic Medicine, 83*(5), 503–511. doi:10.1097/ACM.0b013e31816bda16 PMID:18448909

Barry, M. M., Clarke, A. M., & Dowling, K. (2017). Promoting social and emotional well-being in schools. *Health Education, 117*(5), 434–451. doi:10.1108/HE-11-2016-0057

Bartholomew, T. T. (2016). Mental Health in Namibia. *Psychology and Developing Societies, 28*(1), 101–125. Advance online publication. doi:10.1177/0971333615622909

Bartley, M., Head, J., & Stansfeld, S. (2007). Is attachment style a source of resilience against health inequalities at work? *Social Science & Medicine, 64*(4), 765–775. doi:10.1016/j.socscimed.2006.09.033 PMID:17129652

Bas, G. (2021). *Relation between student mental health and academic achievement revisited: A meta-analysis.* Health and Academic Achievement - New Findings., doi:10.5772/intechopen.95766

Basta, M., Micheli, K., Koutra, K., Fountoulaki, M., Dafermos, V., Drakaki, M., & Vgontzas, A. N. (2022). Depression and anxiety symptoms in adolescents and young adults in Greece: Prevalence and associated factors. *Journal of Affective Disorders Reports, 8*, 100334. Advance online publication. doi:10.1016/j.jadr.2022.100334

Battashi, N., Al Omari, O., Sawalha, M., Al Maktoumi, S., Alsuleitini, A., & Al Qadire, M. (2021). The relationship between smartphone use, insomnia, stress, and anxiety among university students: A cross-sectional study. *Clinical Nursing Research, 30*(6), 734–740. doi:10.1177/1054773820983161 PMID:33375850

Bayram, N., & Bilgel, N. (2008). The prevalence and socio-demographic correlations of depression, anxiety and stress among a group of university students. *Social Psychiatry and Psychiatric Epidemiology, 43*(8), 667–672. doi:10.100700127-008-0345-x PMID:18398558

Beck, A. T. (1993). Cognitive therapy: Past, present, and future. *Journal of Consulting and Clinical Psychology, 61*(2), 194–198. doi:10.1037/0022-006X.61.2.194 PMID:8473571

Beck, L., & Wright, A. (2019). iGen: What you should know about post-millennial students. *College and University, 94*(1), 21–26.

Bedu-Addo, P. K. A. (2000). *Guidance and Counselling Unmasked* (3rd ed.). Type Company Ltd.

Benoit, V., & Gabola, P. (2021). Effects of Positive Psychology Interventions on the Well-Being of Young Children: A Systematic Literature Review. *International Journal of Environmental Research and Public Health, 18*(22), 12065. doi:10.3390/ijerph182212065 PMID:34831827

Benson-Egglenton, J. (2019). The financial circumstances associated with high and low wellbeing in undergraduate students: A case study of an English Russell Group institution. *Journal of Further and Higher Education, 43*(7), 901–913. doi:10.1080/0309877X.2017.1421621

Bentley, A. (2018). 'I was just like, Wow!': Students' perceptions of how counselling benefitted their academic experience. *Counselling & Psychotherapy Research, 18*(2), 215–219. doi:10.1002/capr.12149

Berke, D. S., Leone, R. M., Hyatt, C. S., Zeichner, A., & Parrott, D. J. (2021). Correlates of men's bystander intervention to prevent sexual and relationship violence: The role of masculine discrepancy stress. *Journal of Interpersonal Violence, 36*(21-22), 9877–9903. doi:10.1177/0886260519880999 PMID:31608781

Berk, L. E. (1992). Children's private speech: An overview of theory and the status of research. In R. M. Diaz & L. E. Berk (Eds.), *Private speech: From social interaction to self-regulation* (pp. 17–53). Lawrence Erlbaum Associates, Inc.

Bernal-Morales, B., Rodríguez-Landa, J. F., & Pulido-Criollo, F. (2015). *Impact of anxiety and depression symptoms on scholar performance in high school and university students, a fresh look at anxiety disorders*. London, UK: IntechOpen. doi:10.5772/60711

Bernier, A., Carlson, S. M., & Whipple, N. (2010). Future Directions in Childhood Adversity & Youth Psychology. *Journal of Clinical Child and Adolescent Psychology, 45*(3), 361–382. doi:10.1080/15374416.2015.1110823

Bernstein, C. A., Haiman, C., & Mayer, L. E. (2023). Raising Awareness and Ensuring Access to Mental Health Resources. *Caring for Caregivers to Be: A Comprehensive Approach to Developing Well-Being Programs for the Health Care Learner*, 196.

Bewick, B., Koutsopoulou, G., Miles, J., Slaa, E., & Barkham, M. (2010). Changes in Undergraduate Students' Psychological Well-being as They Progress through University. *Studies in Higher Education, 35*(6), 633–645. doi:10.1080/03075070903216643

Beyens, I., Pouwels, J. L., van Driel, I. I., Keijsers, L., & Valkenburg, P. M. (2020). The effect of social media on well-being differs from adolescent to adolescent. *Scientific Reports, 10*(1), 10763. doi:10.103841598-020-67727-7 PMID:32612108

Beyer, K., Kaltenbach, A., Szabo, A., Bogar, S., Nieto, F. J., & Malecki, K. (2014). Exposure to Neighborhood Green Space and Mental Health: Evidence from the Survey of the Health of Wisconsin. *International Journal of Environmental Research and Public Health, 11*(3), 3453–3472. doi:10.3390/ijerph110303453 PMID:24662966

Bezabeh, T. S. (2016). *Exploring institutional policies and female students' coping strategies on sexual harassment: A case study of Adi Haki Campus.* [Unpublished Master's thesis, Mekelle University, Ethiopia].

Bezerra, I. M. P., da Silva, R. A. B., da Silva, E. R. A., & Dantas, L. C. A. (2021). Anxiety, depression and stress in the context of the COVID-19 pandemic: A cross-sectional study with undergraduate students from Brazil. *Ciencia & Saude Coletiva, 26*(suppl 2), 3433–3442. oi:10.1590/1413-81232021268.2.21112020

Bhargava, D., & Trivedi, H. (2018). A study of causes of stress and stress management among youth. *IRA-International Journal of Management & Social Sciences, 11*(03), 108–117. doi:10.21013/jmss.v11.n3.p1

Bhatia, D., Roerig, M., Marani, H., King, M., Morales-Vstressedazquez, M., & Allin, S. (2020). Supporting Mental Health and Wellbeing Among Students in Higher Education. Toronto: North American Observatory on Health Systems and Policies. *Rapid Review*, (24).

BhatiaD.RoerigM.MaraniH.KingM.Morales-VazquezM.AllinS. (2020). *Rapid.*

Bhugra, D., Till, A., & Sartorius, N. (2013). What is mental health? *The International Journal of Social Psychiatry, 1*(1), 3–4. doi:10.1177/0020764012463315 PMID:23349505

Biggs, A., Brough, P., & Drummond, S. (2017). Lazarus and Folkman's psychological stress and coping theory. In C. Cooper & J. C. Quick (Eds.), *The handbook of stress and health: A guide to research and practice* (pp. 349–364). Wiley. doi:10.1002/9781118993811.ch21

Bijaraniya, B. (2022). Student's unrest In Higher Education: Nature, cause and effect. *International Journal of Advanced Research in Commerce, Management &. Social Science*, *5*(3), 176–180.

Bireda, A. D., & Pillay, J. (2018). Perceived parent–child communication and well-being among Ethiopian Adolescents. *International Journal of Adolescence and Youth*, *23*(1), 109–117. doi:10.1080/02673843.2017.1299016

Birhanu Ayalew, M. (2022). *Socialization experiences among undergraduate students in higher learning institutions (HLI)*. Higher Education - New Approaches to Accreditation, Digitalization, and Globalization in the Age of Covid. doi:10.5772/intechopen.99007

Birya, G. D. (2020). *The role of communication in crisis management in institutions of higher learning in Kenya: A case of Daystar University student unrest.* [Doctoral dissertation, Daystar University, Kenya].

Bitew, T., & Birhan, W. (2021). The potential effect of depression on academic outcomes of students in higher educational institutions of northwest Ethiopia: A cross-sectional study. *Educational Research Review*, *16*(1), 9–15. doi:10.5897/ERR2020.4055

Błachnio, A., Przepiórka, A., & Rudnicka, P. (2013). Psychological determinants of using Facebook: A research review. *International Journal of Human-Computer Interaction*, *29*(11), 775–787. doi:10.1080/10447318.2013.780868

Black-Hughes, C., & Stacy, P. (2013). Early childhood attachment and its impact on later life resilience: A comparison of resilient and no resilient female siblings. *Journal of Evidence-Based Social Work*, *10*(5), 410–420. doi:10.1080/15433714.2012.759456 PMID:24066631

Blair, B. L., & Perry, N. B. (2019). Parental sensitivity and friendship development: The mediating role of cooperation. *Social Development*, *28*(1), 106–119. doi:10.1111ode.12332

Blanco, C., Okuda, M., Wright, C., Hasin, D. S., Grant, B. F., & Liu, S. M. (2008). Mental Health of College Students and their non-college peers: Results from the National Epidemiologyic study on Alcohol and Related Conditions. *Archives of General Psychiatry*, *65*(12), 1429–1437. doi:10.1001/archpsyc.65.12.1429 PMID:19047530

Bluth, K., & Blanton, P. W. (2014). Mindfulness and self-compassion: Exploring pathways to adolescent emotional well-being. *Journal of Child and Family Studies*, *23*(7), 1298–1309. doi:10.100710826-013-9830-2 PMID:25328369

Bobga, T. J. (2016). An Appraisal of Effective Provision of Guidance and Counseling Services in Cameroon State Universities; Trends and Challenges. International Journal of Humanities, Social. *Sciences and Education*, *3*(9), 75–90. doi:10.20431/2349-0381.0309010

Boehm, J. K., Vie, L. L., & Kubzansky, L. D. (2012). The promise of well-being interventions for improving health risk behaviours. *Current Cardiovascular Risk Reports*, *6*(6), 511–519. doi:10.100712170-012-0273-x

Bøe, T., Serlachius, A. S., Sivertsen, B., Petrie, K. J., & Hysing, M. (2018). Cumulative Effects of Negative Life Events and Family Stress on Children's Mental Health: The Bergen Child Study. *Social Psychiatry and Psychiatric Epidemiology*, *53*(1), 1–9. doi:10.100700127-017-1451-4 PMID:29090324

Bologna, C. (2019). The scary ways an all-nighter messes with your body and brain. *HuffPost.* https://www.huffpost.com/entry/what-happens-when-you-pull-an-allnighter_l_5dd5b559e4b010f3f1d21d30

Bonanno, G. A. (2004). Loss, trauma, and human resilience: Have we underestimated the Human capacity to thrive after extremely aversive events? *The American Psychologist*, *59*(1), 20–28. doi:10.1037/0003-066X.59.1.20 PMID:14736317

Bondarchuk, O., Balakhtar, V., Pinchuk, N., Pustovalov, I., & Pavlenok, K. (2023). Adaptation of coping strategies to reduce the impact of stress and Lonelines on the psychological well-being of adults. *Journal of Law and Sustainable Development*, *11*(10), e1852. doi:10.55908dgs.v11i10.1852

Bondestam, F., & Lundqvist, M. (2020). Sexual harassment in higher education – A systematic review. *Eur J High Educ*, *10*(4), 397–419. doi:10.1080/21568235.2020.1729833

Borenstein, J. (2020, August). *Stigma, prejudice and discrimination against people with mental illness.* American Psychiatric Association. https://www.psychiatry.org/patients-families/stigma-and-discrimination

Borges, L. O., Motta, G. M. V., Garcia-Primo, G. M., Barros, S. C., & Heleno, C. T. (2023). Working Conditions and Mental Health in a Brazilian University. *International Journal of Environmental Research and Public Health*, *20*(2), 1536. doi:10.3390/ijerph20021536 PMID:36674290

Bosch, B. (2013). Balancing the Dual Role of Post Graduate Student and Mother. Edith Cowan University: Brown, V., & Nichols, T. R. (2013). Pregnant and Parenting Students on Campus: Policy and Program Implications for a Growing Population. *Educational Policy*, *27*(3), 499–530. doi:10.1177/0895904812453995

Bostani, M., Nadri, A., & Nasab, A. R. (2014). A Study of the Relation between Mental health and Academic Performance of Students of the Islamic Azad University Ahvaz Branch. *Procedia: Social and Behavioral Sciences*, *116*, 163–165. doi:10.1016/j.sbspro.2014.01.186

Boston consulting group/ IPSOS. (2021, December 3). *Les paradoxes et illusions perdues de la méritocratie en France.* IPSOS. https://www.ipsos.com/. https://www.ipsos.com/sites/default/files/ct/news/documents/2021-12/IpsosxBCG%20-%20Enquete%20meritocratie.pdf

Boulton, C. A., Hughes, E., Kent, C., Smith, J. R., & Williams, H. T. (2019). Student engagement and wellbeing over time at a higher education institution. *PLoS One*, *14*(11), e0225770. doi:10.1371/journal.pone.0225770 PMID:31774878

Bourdon, J. L., Moore, A. A., Long, E. C., Kendler, K. S., & Dick, D. M. (2020). The relationship between on-campus service utilization and common mental health concerns in undergraduate college students. *Psychological Services*, *17*(1), 118–126. doi:10.1037er0000296 PMID:30299149

Bouri, E., & Maalouf, M. (2017). The impact of governance in higher education institutions on scientific research in the Arab World. *Higher Education Governance in the Arab World*, 65–82. doi:10.1007/978-3-319-52060-5_4

Bouvet, E., Cosmini, D., Palaktsoglou, M., & Vanzo, L. (2017). 'Doing good' in Italian through student community engagement: The benefits of language placements. *Australian Review of Applied Linguistics*, *40*(2), 159–175. doi:10.1075/aral.40.2.05bou

Bowers, E. P., Li, Y., Kiely, M. K., Brittian, A., Lerner, J. V., & Lerner, R. M. (2010). The five Cs model of positive youth development: A longitudinal analysis of confirmatory factor structure and measurement invariance. *Journal of Youth and Adolescence*, *39*(7), 720–735. doi:10.100710964-010-9530-9 PMID:20397040

Bradberry, T., & Greaves, J. (2009). *Emotional Intelligence.*

Bram, B. (2022, November). *Involution: the generation turning inward and away from Xi's Chinese dream.* Asia Society. https://asiasociety.org/policy-institute/involution-generation-turning-inward-and-away-xis-chinese-dream

Brar, I.K., Ryu, J., Shaikh, K., Altman, A., & Ng, J.Y. (2012). University Campus Peer Support Centres: Benefits for Student Emotional and Mental Well-Being. *The Meducator*, 1.

Brenneisen Mayer, F., Souza Santos, I., Silveira, P. S. P., Itaqui Lopes, M. H., de Souza, A. R. N. D., Campos, E. P., de Abreu, B. A. L., Hoffman, I. II, Magalhães, C. R., Lima, M. C. P., Almeida, R., Spinardi, M., & Tempski, P. (2016). Factors associated to depression and anxiety in medical students: A multicenter study. *BMC Medical Education*, *16*(1), 282. doi:10.118612909-016-0791-1 PMID:27784316

Brewer, M., van Kessel, G., Sanderson, B., Naumann, F., Lane, M., Reubenson, A., & Carter, A. (2019). Resilience in higher education students: *A scoping review. Higher Education Research & Development*, *38*(6), 1105–1120. doi:10.1080/07294360.2019.1626810

Brewster, L., Jones, E., Priestley, M., Wilbraham, S. J., Spanner, L., & Hughes, G. (2022). 'Look after the staff and they would look after the students' cultures of wellbeing and mental health in the university setting. *Journal of Further and Higher Education*, *46*(4), 548–560. doi:10.1080/0309877X.2021.1986473

Briggs, A. R. J., Clark, J., & Hall, I. (2012). Building Bridges: Understanding Student Transition to University. *Quality in Higher Education*, *18*(1), 3–21. doi:10.1080/13538322.2011.614468

Brinckerhoff, L. C. (1996). Making the Transition to Higher Education. *Journal of Learning Disabilities*, *29*(2), 118–136. doi:10.1177/002221949602900202 PMID:8820197

Brinthaupt,T.M., Benson,S.A., & Moore, Z.D. (2015). *Assessing the accuracy of self reported self-talk.* Frontiers. doi:10.3389/fpsyg.2015.00570

Brinthaupt, T. M., & Dove, C. T. (2012). Differences in self-talk frequency as a function of age, only-child, and imaginary childhood companion status. *Journal of Research in Personality*, *46*(3), 326–333. doi:10.1016/j.jrp.2012.03.003

Brinthaupt, T. M., Hein, M. B., & Kramer, T. E. (2009). The self-talk scale: Development, Factor Analysis, and Validation. *Journal of Personality Assessment*, *91*(1), 82–92. doi:10.1080/00223890802484498 PMID:19085287

Brockelman, K. F., & Scheyett, A. M. (2015). Faculty perceptions of accommodations, strategies, and psychiatric advance directives for university students with mental illnesses. *Psychiatric Rehabilitation Journal*, *38*(4), 342–348. doi:10.1037/prj0000143 PMID:26053532

Broglia, E., Millings, A., & Barkham, M. (2021). Student mental health profiles and barriers to help-seeking: When and why students seek help for a mental health concern. *Counselling and Psychotherapy Research, 21*(4), 816-826.

Broglia, E., Millings, A., & Barkham, M. (2021). Student mental health profiles and barriers to help seeking: When and why students seek help for a mental health concern. *Counselling & Psychotherapy Research*, *21*(4), 816–826. doi:10.1002/capr.12462

Brokaw, K., Tishler, W., Manceor, S., Hamilton, K., Gaulden, A. D., Parr, E., & Wamsley, E. J. (2016). Resting state EEG correlates with memory consolidation. *Neurobiology of Learning and Memory*, *130*, 17–25. doi:10.1016/j.nlm.2016.01.008 PMID:26802698

Bronfenbrenner, U. (1976). The experimental ecology of education. *Educational Researcher*, *5*(9), 5–15. doi:10.2307/1174755

Bronfenbrenner, U. (1979). *The ecology of human development: Experiments by nature and design*. Harvard University Press. https://www.hup.harvard.edu/catalog.php?isbn=9780674224575

Brooks, A. W., Schroeder, J., Risen, J. L., Gino, F., Galinsky, A. D., Norton, M. I., & Schweitzer, M. E. (2016). Don't stop believing: Rituals improve performance by decreasing anxiety. *Organizational Behavior and Human Decision Processes*, *137*, 71–85. doi:10.1016/j.obhdp.2016.07.004

Broonk, L., Gijselaers, H. J. M., Ritzen, H., & Brand-Gruwel, S. (2018). A review of the relationship between parental involvement indicators and academic achievement. *Educational Research Review*, *24*, 10–30. doi:10.1016/j.edurev.2018.02.001

Brougham, R. R., Zail, C. M., Mendoza, C. M., & Miller, J. R. (2009). Stress, sex differences, and coping strategies among college students. *Current Psychology (New Brunswick, N.J.)*, *28*(2), 85–97. doi:10.100712144-009-9047-0

Browne, V., Munro, J., & Cass, J. (2017). The Mental Health of Australian University Students. *JANZSSA. Journal of the Australian and New Zealand Student Services Association*, *50*(2), 51–62. doi:10.30688/janzssa.2017.16

Brown, K. W., Goodman, R. J., & Inzlicht, M. (2013). Dispositional *mindfulness and the attenuation of neural responses to emotional stimuli. Social Cognitive and Affective Neuroscience*, *8*(1), 93–99. doi:10.1093can/nss004 PMID:22253259

Brown, P. (2016). *The Invisible Problem?: Improving students' mental health.* Higher Education Policy Institute.

Brown, T., Bourke-Taylor, H., Isbel, S., Gustafsson, L., McKinstry, C., Logan, A., & Etherington, J. (2019). Establishing similarities and differences among the self-reported academic integrity of Australian occupational therapy undergraduate and graduate-entry Master's students. *The Open Journal of Occupational Therapy*, *7*(3), 1–16. doi:10.15453/2168-6408.1558

Bruffaerts, R., Mortier, P., Kiekens, G., Auerbach, R. P., Cuijpers, P., Demyttenaere, K., Green, J. G., Nock, M. K., & Kessler, R. C. (2018). Mental health problems in college freshmen: Prevalence and academic functioning. *Journal of Affective Disorders*, *225*(1), 97–103. doi:10.1016/j.jad.2017.07.044 PMID:28802728

Bruner, J. (1990). *Acts of meaning*. Harvard University Press.

Bryan, C. J. (2021). *Rethinking Suicide: Why Prevention Fails, and How We Can Do Better*. Oxford University Press. https://www.amazon.com/Rethinking-Suicide-Prevention-Fails-Better/dp/0190050632 doi:10.1093/med-psych/9780190050634.001.0001

Bucci, S., Schwannauer, M., & Berry, N. (2019). The digital revolution and its impact on mental health care. *Psychology and Psychotherapy: Theory, Research and Practice*, *92*(2), 277–297. doi:10.1111/papt.12222 PMID:30924316

Buizza, C., Cela, H., Costa, A., & Ghilardi, A. (2022). Coping strategies and mental health in a sample of students accessing a university counselling service. *Counselling & Psychotherapy Research*, *22*(3), 658–666. doi:10.1002/capr.12519

Buku, D. K., Namale, M. K., & Oppong, R. (2018). Psychosocial Challenges of Adolescent Student Mothers in Senior High Schools: Guidance and Counselling Implications. *International Journal of Basic Education Research & Policy*, *1*(2), 10.

Bullivant, N. (2021). *Student wellbeing and motivation during the pandemic: A UK survey.* Higher Education Policy Institute (HEPI) and Youth Sight. https://www.hepi.ac.uk/2021/01/28/ student-wellbeing-and-motivation-during-the-pandemic-a-uk-survey

Buni, I. (2020). Managing students' unrest in Universities: Unmasking the threat and success implication through Ubuntu. *Multicultural Education*, *6*(2), 27–38.

Busby, D. R., Zheng, K., Eisenberg, D., Albucher, R. C., Favorite, T., Coryell, W., & King, C. A. (2019). Black college students at elevated risk for suicide: Barriers to mental health service utilization. *Journal of American College Health*, 1–7. PMID:31662044

Busch, B. (2017, August 17). Practice makes perfect: why mock exams are great for students' brains. *The Guardian*. https://www.theguardian.com/teacher-network/2015/dec/03/practice-makes-perfect-why-mock-exams-students-brains

Busygina, A., Rudenko, I., Arkhipova, I., Firsova, T., & Murtazina, D. & Shichiyakh. (2019). Study of the features of family education in the process of social adaptation of a child. *Revista de Ciencias Sociales y Humanidades*, *4*(13), 346–352.

Butler, F. C., & Martin, J. A. (2020). Research in Occupational Stress and Well Being: Vol. 123-146. Struggling to survive: Non-family member employees, the family, and stress in family firm startups. Emerald. doi:10.1108/S1479-355520200000018006

Cage, E., Jones, E., Ryan, G., Hughes, G., & Spanner, L. (2021). Student mental health and transitions into, through and out of university: Student and staff perspectives. *Journal of Further and Higher Education*, *45*(8), 1076–1089. doi:10.1080/0309877X.2021.1875203

Cage, E., Stock, M., Sharpington, A., Pitman, E., & Batchelor, E. (2020). Barriers to accessing support for mental health issues at university. *Studies in Higher Education*, *45*(8), 1637–1649. doi:10.1080/03075079.2018.1544237

Cai, D., Zhu, M., Lin, M., Zhang, X. C., & Margraf, J. (2017). The bidirectional relationship between positive mental health and social rhythm in college students: A three-year longitudinal study. *Frontiers in Psychology*, *8*, 1119. doi:10.3389/fpsyg.2017.01119 PMID:28713318

Camacho, E. (2016). Minority student perceptions of mental health. *Journal of Undergraduate Research (Gainesville, Fla.)*, *14*, 35–54. http://openprairie.sdstate. edu/jur/vol14/iss1/6

Campbell, F., Blank, L., Cantrell, A., Baxter, S., Blackmore, C., Dixon, J., & Goyder, E. (2022). Factors that influence mental health of university and college students in the UK: A systematic review. *BMC Public Health*, *22*(1), 1–22. doi:10.118612889-022-13943-x PMID:36123714

Campbell, M., Katikireddi, S. V., Sowden, A., & Thomson, H. (2019). Lack of transparency in reporting narrative synthesis of quantitative data: A methodological assessment of systematic reviews. *Journal of Clinical Epidemiology*, *105*, 1–9. doi:10.1016/j.jclinepi.2018.08.019 PMID:30196129

Canady, V. A. (2020). College students with MH issues find support by staff lacking. *Mental Health Weekly*, *30*(43), 5–5. doi:10.1002/mhw.32578

Cao, W., Fang, Z., Hou, G., Han, M., Xu, X., Dong, J., & Zheng, J. (2020). The psychological impact of the COVID-19 epidemic on college students in China. *Psychiatry Research*, *287*, 112934. doi:10.1016/j.psychres.2020.112934 PMID:32229390

Capozza, F., Moghani, V., & Acampora, M. (2021). *Mental health literacy and demand for mental health support among University students*. AEA Randomized Controlled Trials. doi:10.1257/rct.8406-2.1

Caprara, G. V., Alessandri, G., Barbaranelli, C., & Vecchione, M. (2013). The longitudinal relations between self-esteem and affective self-regulatory efficacy. *Journal of Research in Personality*, *47*(6), 859–870. doi:10.1016/j.jrp.2013.08.011

Carrico, B. A. (2016). *The effects of students' perceptions of campus safety and security on student enrollment.* [Unpublished PhD dissertation Marshall University, USA].

Caruana, V., Clegg, S., & Ploner, J. (2011). *Promoting students' 'resilient thinking' in diverse higher education learning environments.* HE Academy Subject Centre for Sociology, Anthropology and Politics.

Carver, C. S., & Scheier, M. F. (1998). *On the self-regulation of behavior.* Cambridge University Press., doi:10.1017/CBO9781139174794

Casagrande, M., Favieri, F., Tambelli, R., & Forte, G. (2020). The enemy who sealed the world: Effects quarantine due to the COVID-19 on sleep quality, anxiety, and psychological distress in the Italian population. *Sleep Medicine*, *75*, 12–20. doi:10.1016/j.sleep.2020.05.011 PMID:32853913

Casey, S. M., Varela, A., Marriott, J. P., Coleman, C. M., & Harlow, B. L. (2022). The influence of diagnosed mental health conditions and symptoms of depression and/or anxiety on suicide ideation, plan, and attempt among college students: Findings from the healthy minds study, 2018-2019. *Journal of Affective Disorders*, *298*, 464–471. doi:10.1016/j.jad.2021.11.006 PMID:34774646

Casimiro-Andújar, A. J., Checa, J. C., Lirola, M.-J., & Artés-Rodríguez, E. (2023). Promoting physical activity and health in the workplace: A qualitative study among university workers, Spain. *International Journal of Environmental Research and Public Health*, *20*(3), 2350. doi:10.3390/ijerph20032350 PMID:36767715

Catalano, R. F., Berglund, M. L., Ryan, J. A., Lonczak, H. S., & Hawkins, J. D. (2004). Positive youth development in the United States: Research findings on evaluations of positive youth development programs. *The Annals of the American Academy of Political and Social Science*, *591*(1), 98–124. doi:10.1177/0002716203260102

Causer, H., Bradley, E., Muse, K., & Smith, J. (2021). Bearing Witness: A grounded theory of the experiences of staff at two United Kingdom Higher Education Institutions following a student death by suicide. *PLoS One*, *16*(5), e0251369. doi:10.1371/journal.pone.0251369 PMID:33979333

Cenko, E., & Canollari-Baze, A. (2018). The role of academic support services in ensuring student success and wellbeing: A case study in the Albanian higher education context. *EDULEARN Proceedings*. INTED. 10.21125/edulearn.2018.2430

Central Board of Secondary Education. (2018). *Mainstreaming health and physical education*. CBSE. http://cbseacademic.nic.in/web_material/Circulars/2018/Health%20and%20Physical%20Education%20(HPE)%20IX-XII.pdf

Central Board of Secondary Education. (n.d.). *About CBSE*. CBSE. https://www.cbse.gov.in/newsite/aboutCbse.html

Chahine, S. A., & Damaj, I. (2020). Review of governance policies and practices in lebanese higher-education institutions. *Higher Education in the Arab World*, (pp. 265–277). Springer. doi:10.1007/978-3-030-58153-4_10

Chand, S. P., & Arif, H. (2022). *Depression*. StatPearls Publishing. https://www.ncbi.nlm.nih.gov/books/NBK430847/

Chang, K. H., Lu, F. J., Chyi, T., Hsu, Y. W., Chan, S. W., & Wang, E. T. (2017). Examining the stress-burnout relationship: The mediating role of negative thoughts. *PeerJ*, *5*, e4181. doi:10.7717/peerj.4181 PMID:29302397

Chang, T. F., Ley, B. L., Ramburn, T. T., Srinivasan, S., Hariri, S., Purandare, P., & Subramaniam, B. (2022). Online isha upa yoga for student mental health and well-being during COVID-19: A randomized control trial. *Applied Psychology. Health and Well-Being*, *14*(4), 1408–1428. doi:10.1111/aphw.12341 PMID:35064741

Charlton, T., Moulton, C., Sabey, V., & West, R. (2021). A systematic review of the efects of schoolwide intervention programs on student and teacher perceptions of school climate. *Journal of Positive Behavior Interventions*, *23*(3), 185–200. doi:10.1177/1098300720940168

Chase, E., & Allsopp, J. (2020). Emotional and mental wellbeing. *Youth Migration and the Politics of Wellbeing*, (pp. 153-172). Cambridge Press. doi:10.1332/policypress/9781529209020.003.0009

Chávez-Flores, Y. V., Hidalgo-Rasmussen, C. A., & Navarro, S. M. (n.d.). Intrafamily relationships and health-related quality of life in Mexican adolescents who harm themselves without suicidal intent. *Salud y Sociedad*, *9*(2), 130–144.

Chazan, D. (2023, July 13). Mark pupils down for poor French spelling, says education MP. *Times*. https://www.thetimes.co.uk/article/mark-pupils-down-for-poor-french-spelling-says-education-mp-6q86h82ls

Checa, P., & Fernández-Berrocal, P. (2019). Cognitive Control & Emotional Intelligence: Effect of the Emotional Content of Task. *Frontiers in Psychology*, *10*, 195. doi:10.3389/fpsyg.2019.00195 PMID:30792680

Chemutai, B., Onkware, K., & Iteyo, C. (2020). Nature of student unrest in secondary schools in Kericho County Kenya. *International Journal of Social Sciences and Humanities Invention*, *7*(11), 6293–6307. doi:10.18535/ijsshi/v7i011.04

Cheng, Y., Zhang, X. M., Ye, S. Y., Jin, H., & Yang, X. H. (2020). Suicide in Chinese graduate students: A review from 2000 to 2019. *Frontiers in Psychiatry*, *11*, 579745. doi:10.3389/fpsyt.2020.579745 PMID:33424658

Chen, L., Duan, J., & Lu, M. (2019). The Gaokao: A decisive filter for human capital allocation in China. *China Economic Review*, *58*, 101341.

Chen, Y., Zhu, L. J., Fang, Z. M., Wu, N., Du, M. X., Jiang, M. M., Wang, J., Yao, Y., & Zhou, C. C. (2021). The association of suicidal ideation with family characteristics and social support of the first batch of students returning to a college during the COVID-19 epidemic period: A cross sectional study in China. *Frontiers in Psychiatry*, *12*, 653245. doi:10.3389/fpsyt.2021.653245 PMID:34262488

Chen, Z., Xiaoming, L., Yu, L., Shan, Q., Liying, Z., Yuejiao, Z., Zhiyong, S., & And Zhengzhu, T. (2016). Emotional, Physical and Financial Burdens of Stigma against People Living with HIV/AIDS in China. *AIDS Care*, *28*(1), 124–131. PMID:26886415

Chernomas, W. M., & Shapiro, C. (2013). Stress, depression, and anxiety among undergraduate nursing students. *International Journal of Nursing Education Scholarship*, *10*(1), 255–266. doi:10.1515/ijnes-2012-0032 PMID:24200536

Chi, N. C., Demiris, G., Lewis, F. M., Walker, A. J., Langer, S. (2015). Behavioral and Educational Interventions to Support Family Caregivers in End-Of-Life Care: A Systematic Review. *Am J Hosp Palliat Care*, (7).

Chikendu, E. (2022). Student's unrest and academic achievements in Tertiary Institutions In Nigeria. *International Journal of Research Publication and Reviews*, *3*(5), 2452–2457.

Chiluba, B. C. (2019). Strategies for social engagement: The University of Zambia student unrests. *International Journal of Research and Innovation in Social Science*, *3*(7), 267–271.

Chipare, M. A., Mupazvihwo, T., Tapera, R., & January, J. (2021). Mental Health Research in Namibia: A Scoping Review of Literature. *Medical Journal of Zambia*, *48*(2), 119–124. doi:10.55320/mjz.48.2.39

Cho, J., & Yu, H. (2015). Roles of University Support for International Students in the United States: Analysis of a Systematic Model of University Identification, University Support, and Psychological Well-Being. *Journal of Studies in International Education*, *19*(1), 11–27. doi:10.1177/1028315314533606

Choudhary, K. (2018). Student unrest:Causes and cure. *International Journal of Advance Research in Science and Engineering*, *7*(4), 755–762.

Christner, N., Essler, S., Hazzam, A., & Paulus, M. (2021). Children's psychological well-being and problem behaviour during the COVID-19 pandemic: An online study during the lockdown period in Germany. [PMCID.]. *PLoS One*, *16*(6), e0253473. doi:10.1371/journal.pone.0253473 PMID:34161376

Cicognani, E., Pirini, C., Keyes, C., Joshanloo, M., Rostami, R., & Nosratabadi, M. (2008). Social participation, sense of community and social well-being: A study on American, Italian, and Iranian university students. *Social Indicators Research*, *89*(1), 97–112. doi:10.100711205-007-9222-3

Ciobanu, A. M. (2013). The Role of Student Services in the Improving of Student Experience in Higher Education. *Procedia: Social and Behavioral Sciences*, *92*, 169–173. doi:10.1016/j.sbspro.2013.08.654

Clements, S., & Paramova, P. (2023). Institutional and psychological predictors of university students' mental health help-seeking intentions. *British Journal of Guidance & Counselling*, 1–13. doi:10.1080/03069885.2023.2176823

Cleveland Clinic. (2020, September 10). *Stressors: Coping Skills and Strategies*. Cleveland Clinic. https://my.clevelandclinic.org/health/articles/6392-stress-coping-with-lifes-stressors

Clifton, D. O., Anderson, E., & Schreiner, L. A. (2002). *StrengthsQuest*. The Gallup Organization.

Closson, M. C. D. (n.d.). *New Barna's research reveals the extent of America's loss of faith*. FRC. https://www.frc.org/blog/2021/06/new-barna-research-reveals-extent-americas-loss-faith

Colarossi, J. (2022, April 21). *Mental health of college students is getting worse*. The Brink: Pioneering Research from Boston University. https://www.bu.edu/articles/2022/mental-health-of-college-students-is-getting-worse/

Cole, D., Sugioka, H. L., & Yamagata-Lynch, L. C. (1999). Supportive Classroom Environments For Creativity in Higher Education. *The Journal of Creative Behavior*, *33*(4), 277–293. doi:10.1002/j.2162-6057.1999.tb01407.x

Coleman, M. E. (2022). Mental health in the college classroom: Best practices for instructors. *Teaching Sociology*, *50*(2), 168–182. doi:10.1177/0092055X221080433

Coleman, M., & And Thomas, D. (2003). An Economic Model of Locus of Control and the Human Capital Investment Decision. *The Journal of Human Resources*, *38*(3), 701–721. doi:10.2307/1558773

Collier, P. (2017). Why peer mentoring is an effective approach for promoting college student success. *Metropolitan Universities*, *28*(3), 9–19. doi:10.18060/21539

Collings, R., Swanson, V., & Watkins, R. (2014). The impact of peer mentoring on levels of student wellbeing, integration and retention: A controlled comparative evaluation of residential students in UK higher education. *Higher Education*, *68*(6), 927–942. doi:10.100710734-014-9752-y

Community Translational Science Team (CTST). (2016). *Policy Report: Building A Public Health Model for Promoting Emotional Well-Being*. University of California.

Compas, B. E., Vreeland, A., & Henry, L. (2019). Coping models of stress and resilience. The Oxford Handbook of Stress and Mental Health, 584-600. Oxford Press. doi:10.1093/oxfordhb/9780190681777.013.27

Conley, C. S., Shapiro, J. B., Huguenel, B. M., & Kirsch, A. C. (2020). Navigating the College Years: Developmental Trajectories and Gender Differences in Psychological Functioning, Cognitive-Affective Strategies, and Social Well-Being. *Emerging Adulthood*, *8*(2), 103–117. doi:10.1177/2167696818791603

Conley, C. S., Shapiro, J. B., Kirsch, A. C., & Durlak, J. A. (2017). A meta-analysis of indicated mental health prevention programs for at-risk higher education students. *Journal of Counseling Psychology*, *64*(2), 121–140. doi:10.1037/cou0000190 PMID:28277730

Conley, C. S., Travers, L. V., & Bryant, F. B. (2013). Promoting Psychosocial Adjustment and Stress Management in First-Year College Students: The Benefits of Engagement in a Psychosocial Wellness Seminar. *Journal of American College Health*, *61*(2), 75–86. doi:10.1080/07448481.2012.754757 PMID:23409857

Connolly, J., Josephson, W., Schnoll, J., Simkins-Strong, E., Pepler, D., MacPherson, A., Weiser, J., Moran, M., & Jiang, D. (2015). Evaluation of a youth-led program for preventing bullying, sexual harassment, and dating aggression in Middle Schools. *The Journal of Early Adolescence*, *35*(3), 403–434. doi:10.1177/0272431614535090

Conrad, P. (1986). The myth of cut-throats among premedical students: On the role of stereotypes in justifying failure and success. *Journal of Health and Social Behavior*, *27*(2), 150–160. doi:10.2307/2136313 PMID:3734381

Cooper, C. L., Hoel, H., & Faragher, B. (2004). Bullying is Detri-Mental to Health, but not Necessarily Equally Damaging. *British Journal of Guidance & Counselling*, *32*, 367–387. doi:10.1080/03069880410001723594

Cooper, K. M., Gin, L. E., Barnes, M. E., Sara, E., & Brownell, S. E. (2020). Exploratory Study of Students with Depression in Undergraduate Research Experiences. *CBE Life Sciences Education, 19*(2), ar19. doi:10.1187/cbe.19-11-0217 PMID:32412838

Cooper, S., & Nicholas, L. (2013). Counselling and psychotherapy in South Africa: Responding to post-apartheid counselling needs. In R. Moodley, U. P. Gielen, & R. Wu (Eds.), *Handbook of counselling and psychotherapy in an international context* (pp. 61–71). Routledge.

Copeland, M., Fisher, J. C., Moody, J., & Feinberg, M. E. (2018). Different kinds of lonely: Dimensions of isolation and substance use in adolescence. *Journal of Youth and Adolescence, 47*(8), 1755–1770. doi:10.100710964-018-0860-3 PMID:29774451

Copeland, W. E., Bulik, C. M., Zucker, N., Wolke, D., Lereya, S. T., & Costello, E. J. (2015, December). Does Childhood Bullying Predict Eating Disorder Symptoms? A Prospective, Longitudinal Analysis. *International Journal of Eating Disorders, 48*(8), 1141–1149. doi:10.1002/eat.22459 PMID:26337405

Corey, G. (2012). *Theory and practice of counseling and psychotherapy*. Cengage learning.

Corpuz, J. C. G. (2022). Protecting the minority: How do we protect the minority in times of crisis? *Journal of Primary Care & Community Health, 13*, 21501319221108999. doi:10.1177/21501319221108999 PMID:35748429

Corpuz, J. C. G. (2023). Enhancing Well-Being in the University Workplace: The Context of Higher Educational Institution. *Journal of Primary Care & Community Health, 14*, 21501319231181488. doi:10.1177/21501319231181488 PMID:37326366

Corpuz, J. C. G. (2023, April). Workplace mental health in schools. *Workplace Health & Safety, 71*(4), 160–161. doi:10.1177/21650799221147171 PMID:36695164

Corradi, A. (2021). Safety in numbers: Security on campus and the importance of the corporatization of Universities. *Security Journal, 35*(11), 1–21.

Cottini, E., & Lucifora, C. (2013). Mental health and working conditions in Europe. *Industrial & Labor Relations Review, 66*(4), 958–988. doi:10.1177/001979391306600409

Coulter, S., Iosad, A., & Scales, J. (2022, August 23). *Ending the big squeeze on skills: How to Futureproof education in England*. Global Institute. https://www.institute.global/insights/public-services/ending-big-squeeze-skills-how-futureproof-education-england

Cox, E. (2018). *The surprising link between stress and memory* [Video]. TED Talks. https://www.ted.com/talks/elizabeth_cox_the_surprising_link_between_stress_and_memory/transcript.%22%20n.d.%20The%20surprising%20link%20between%20stress%20and%20memory

Crego, A., Carrillo-Diaz, M., Armfield, J. M., & Romero, M. (2016). Stress and academic performance in dental students: The role of coping strategies and examination-related self-efficacy. *Journal of Dental Education, 80*(2), 165–172. doi:10.1002/j.0022-0337.2016.80.2.tb06072.x PMID:26834134

Crisp, D. A., Rickwood, D., Martin, B., & Byrom, N. (2020). Implementing a peer support program for improving university student wellbeing: The experience of program facilitators. *Australian Journal of Education, 64*(2), 113–126. doi:10.1177/0004944120910498

Crowley, B. Z., Cornell, D., & Konold, T. (2021). School climate moderates the association between sexual harassment and student well-being. *School Mental Health, 13*(4), 695–706. doi:10.100712310-021-09449-3

Curtin, S. C., Warner, M., & Hedegaard, H. (2016). Increase in suicide in the United States, 1999–2014. *NCHS Data Brief*, *241*, 1–8. PMID:27111185

Dagrou, E., Gauvin, L., & Halliwell, W. (1992). The effects of positive, negative and neutral self-talk on motor performance. *Canadian Journal of Sport Sciences*, *17*(2), 145–147. PMID:1324109

Dahal, P., Joshi, S. K., & Swahnberg, K. (2022). A Qualitative Study on Gender Inequality and Gender-Based Violence in Nepal. *BMC Public Health*, *22*(1), 2005. doi:10.118612889-022-14389-x PMID:36320057

Dahlum, S., & Wig, T. (2021). Chaos on campus: Universities and Mass Political Protest. *Comparative Political Studies*, *54*(1), 3–32. doi:10.1177/0010414020919902

Dalpati, N., Jena, S., Jain, S., & Sarangi, P. P. (2022). Yoga and meditation, an essential tool to alleviate stress and enhance immunity to emerging infections: A perspective on the effect of COVID-19 pandemic on students. *Brain, Behavior, & Immunity - Health*, *20*, 100420. doi:10.1016/j.bbih.2022.100420 PMID:35072120

Dalton, J. (2022). A review of moral distress in nursing students: Causes and educational methods to address it. *Proceedings of the 2022 AERA Annual Meeting*. Aera. 10.3102/1892355

Dammeyer, J. (2018). *Mental health and psychosocial well-being in deaf and hard-of-Hearing students*. Oxford Scholarship Online. doi:10.1093/oso/9780190880545.003.0021

Dangore, A. R., & Bhivgade, S. (2023). Common mental health problems for students. *Journal of Mental Health Issues and Behavior*, (33), 1–4. doi:10.55529/jmhib.33.1.4

Das, D. (2017). Student indiscipline and student unrest in relation to their socioeconomic background political influence and academic achievement. *International Journal of Humanities and Social Science*, *6*(2), 92–98.

Dasig, J. P. (2020). Challenges of Student-Mothers in the Tertiary Education of University of Perpetual Help System-DALTA. [JWEEP]. *Journal of World Englishes and Educational Practices*, *2*(6), 1–33. doi:10.32996/jweep.2020.2.6.4

Daud, N., Norwani, N. M., & Yusof, R. (2018). Students financial problems in higher education institutions. *International Journal of Academic Research in Business & Social Sciences*, *8*(10). doi:10.6007/IJARBSS/v8-i10/5312

Davies, K., Ekwere, G., & Uyanga, U. (2016). Factors influencing students unrest in institutions of higher learning and its implications on the academic performance of students in University of Uyo, Akwa Ibom State, Nigeria. *Research in Pedagogy*, *6*(1), 26–42. doi:10.17810/2015.21

Davis, R. R., & Olpin, M. (2021). The Effects of Stress Relief Tools and Interventions on Student Well-Being. *ResearchGate*. https://www.researchgate.net/publication/351424377_The_Effects_of_Stress_Relief_Tools_and_Interventions_on_Student_Well-Being

Day-Vines, N., & Terriquez, V. (2008). A strengths-based approach to promoting prosocial behavior among African American and Latino students. *Professional School Counseling*, *12*(2), 170–175. doi:10.5330/PSC.n.2010-12.170

De Caroli, M. E., & Sagone, E. (2014). Generalized self-efficacy and well-being in adolescents with high vs. low scholastic self-efficacy. *Procedia: Social and Behavioral Sciences*, *141*, 867–874. doi:10.1016/j.sbspro.2014.05.152

de Vibe, M., Solhaug, I., Rosenvinge, J. H., Tyssen, R., Hanley, A., & Garland, E. (2018). Six-year positive effects of a mindfulness-based intervention on mindfulness, coping and well-being in medical and psychology students; Results from a randomized controlled trial. *PLoS One*, *13*(4), e0196053. doi:10.1371/journal.pone.0196053 PMID:29689081

De Witte, M., Da Silva Pinho, A., Stams, G. J., Moonen, X., Bos, A. E. R., & Van Hooren, S. (2020). Music therapy for stress reduction: A systematic review and meta-analysis. *Health Psychology Review, 16*(1), 134–159. doi:10.1080/17437199.2020.1846580 PMID:33176590

Delamater, A. M., Guzman, A., & Aparicio, K. (2017). Mental health issues in children and adolescents with chronic illness. *International Journal of Human Rights in Healthcare, 10*(3), 163–173. doi:10.1108/IJHRH-05-2017-0020

Delos Reyes, R. D. G., & Torio, V. A. G. (2021). The relationship of expert teacher–learner rapport and learner autonomy in the CVIF-dynamic learning program. *The Asia-Pacific Education Researcher, 30*(5), 471–481. doi:10.100740299-020-00532-y

Demirtaş, A. S. (2020). Cognitive flexibility and mental well-being in Turkish adolescents: The mediating role of academic, social and emotional self-efficacy. *Anales de psicología/annals of Psychology, 36*(1), 111-121.

Dennett, D. (1992)... *The Self as a Center of Narrative Gravity, 46.* oi:10.5209/revASEM.2013.v46.42862

Denollet, J., & Brutsaert, D. L. (2018). Reducing emotional distress improves prognosis in coronary heart disease: 9-year mortality in a clinical trial of rehabilitation. [PubMed: 11673339]. *Circulation, 104*(17), 23. PMID:11673339

Denovan, A., & Macaskill, A. (2017). Stress and subjective well-being among first year UK undergraduate students. *Journal of Happiness Studies, 18*(2), 505–525. doi:10.100710902-016-9736-y

Denslow, C. (2023, February 12). Pre-med students need our support. The high suicide rates tell as much. *The Daily Orange.* https://dailyorange.com/2023/02/pre-med-students-need-support-high-suicide-rates-tells-as-much/#google_vignette

*Depression.* (2022, October 14). Mayo Clinic. www.mayoclinic.org/diseases-conditions/depression/diagnosis-treatment/drc-20356013

Deshpande, A.G., Johnson, J.R., Casta, A.M., Marien, M.S., & Reiff, M. (2023). The impact of a mindfulness-based stress reduction program on university students' mental health: A mixed-methods evaluation. *Journal of American college health,* 1-11.

Desselle, S. P., Darbishire, P. L., & Clubbs, B. H. (2020). Pharmacy Faculty Burnout: Cause for Concern that Requires Our Support and Use of Best Evidence. *Innovations in Pharmacy, 11*(3), 1–10. doi:10.24926/iip.v11i3.3274 PMID:34007640

Dhabhar, F. S. (2018). The short-term stress response - Mother nature's mechanism for enhancing protection and performance under conditions of threat, challenge, and opportunity. *Frontiers in Neuroendocrinology, 49*, 175–192. doi:10.1016/j.yfrne.2018.03.004 PMID:29596867

Dhanabhakyam, M. & Sarath, M. (2023). Psychological Wellbeing: A Systematic Literature Review. *International Journal of Advanced Research in Science Communication and Technology.* . doi:10.48175/IJARSCT-8345

Dhar, B. K., Ayittey, F. K., & Sarkar, S. M. (2020). Impact of COVID-19 on Psychology among the University Students. [CrossRef]. *Global Challenges (Hoboken, NJ), 4*(11), 2000038. doi:10.1002/gch2.202000038 PMID:33042575

Dhillon, J. K., McGowan, M., & Wang, H. (2008). How effective are institutional and departmental systems of student support? Insights from an Investigation into the Support Available to Students at one English University. *Research in Post-Compulsory Education, 13*(3), 281–293. doi:10.1080/13596740802346472

Díaz, D., Rodríguez-Carvajal, R., Blanco, A., Moreno-Jiménez, B., Gallardo, I., & Valle, C. (2006). The Psychological Well-Being Scales (PWBS)]. [PubMed]. *Psicothema, 18*, 572–577. PMID:17296089

Diener, E., Lucas, R. E., Schimmack, U., & Helliwell, J. (2010). *Well-being for public policy.* Oxford University Press.

Diener, E., Wirtz, D., Tov, W., Kim-Prieto, C., Choi, D. W., Oishi, S., & Biswas-Diener, R. (2010). New well-being measures: Short scales to assess flourishing and positive and negative feelings. *Social Indicators Research, 97*(2), 143–156. doi:10.100711205-009-9493-y

Ding, H., & Rubie-Davies, C. M. (2019). Teacher expectation intervention: Is it effective for all students? *Learning and Individual Differences, 74,* 101751. doi:10.1016/j.lindif.2019.06.005

Dinu, L. M., Dommett, E. J., Baykoca, A., Mehta, K. J., Everett, S., Foster, J. L. H., & Byrom, N. C. (2021). A case study investigating mental wellbeing of university academics during the covid-19 pandemic. *Education Sciences, 11*(11), 702–710. doi:10.3390/educsci11110702

DiPlacito-DeRango, M. L. (2016). Acknowledge the Barriers to Better the Practices: Support for Student Mental Health in Higher Education. *The Canadian Journal for the Scholarship of Teaching and Learning, 7*(2), 2. https://ir.lib.uwo.ca/cjsotl_rcacea/vol7/iss2/2. doi:10.5206/cjsotl-rcacea.2016.2.2

Dong, H., Dai, J., Lipson, S. K., & Curry, L. (2022). Help-seeking for mental health services in Asian American college students: Anexploratory qualitative study. *Journal of American College Health, 70*(8), 2303–2310. doi:10.1080/07448481.2020.1851234 PMID:33289588

Doolan, K. (2021). *Student life during the COVID-19 pandemic lockdown: Europe-wide insights*. European Students' Union.

Dooris, M. (2009). Holistic and sustainable health improvement: The contribution of the settingsbased approach to health promotion. *Perspectives in Public Health, 129*(1), 29–36. doi:10.1177/1757913908098881 PMID:19338133

Dopmeijer, J. M. (2021). *Running on empty. The impact of challenging student life on well-being and academic performance.* [Doctoral dissertation, University of Amsterdam]. Digital Academic Repository.

Dos Santos, L. M. (2022). The stress, mental health issues, and mental wellbeing of COVID-19 survivors: An interpretative phenomenological analysis study of male University students. *The Journal of Men's Health, 18*(9), 180. doi:10.31083/j.jomh1809180

Dou, R., Cian, H., & Espinosa-Suarez, V. (2021). Undergraduate STEM majors on and off the pre-med/health track: A STEM identity perspective. *CBE Life Sciences Education, 20*(2), ar24. doi:10.1187/cbe.20-12-0281 PMID:33856900

Douwes, R., Metselaar, J., Hendrika, G., Pijnenborg, M., & Boonstra, N. (2023). Well-being of students in higher education: The importance of a student perspective. *Cogent Education, 10*(1), 1–17. doi:10.1080/2331186X.2023.2190697

Drazoa, C. (2018). Sexual harassment at African Higher Education Institutions. *Industry and Higher Education, 94*(4), 4–5. doi:10.6017/ihe.2018.0.10553

Dubé, J. P., Smith, M. M., Sherry, S. B., Hewitt, P. L., & Stewart, S. H. (2021). Suicide behaviours during the COVID-19 pandemic: A meta-analysis of 54 studies. *Psychiatry Research, 301,* 113998. doi:10.1016/j.psychres.2021.113998 PMID:34022657

DuBois, C. M., Beach, S. R., Kashdan, T. B., Nyer, M. B., Park, E. R., Celano, C. M., & Huffman, J. C. (2012). Positive psychological attributes and cardiac outcomes: Associations, mechanisms, and interventions. *Psychosomatics, 53*(4), 303–318. doi:10.1016/j.psym.2012.04.004 PMID:22748749

Duerden, M. D., & Witt, P. A. (2010). An ecological systems theory perspective on youth programming. *Journal of Park and Recreation Administration, 28*(2), 108–120.

Duffy, A., Keown-Stoneman, C., Goodday, S., Horrocks, J., Lowe, M., King, N., Pickett, W., McNevin, S. H., Cunningham, S., Rivera, D., Bisdounis, L., Bowie, C. R., Harkness, K., & Saunders, K. E. (2020). Predictors of mental health and academic outcomes in first-year university students: Identifying prevention and early-intervention targets. *BJPsych Open*, *6*(3), e46. doi:10.1192/bjo.2020.24 PMID:32381150

Duffy, A., Saunders, K. E. A., Malhi, G. S., Patten, S., Cipriani, A., McNevin, S. H., MacDonald, E., & Geddes, J. (2019). Mental health care for university students: A way forward? The Lancet. *The Lancet. Psychiatry*, *6*(11), 885–887. doi:10.1016/S2215-0366(19)30275-5 PMID:31324561

Dunlosky, J., Rawson, K. A., Marsh, E. J., Nathan, M. J., & Willingham, D. T. (2013). *Improving students' learning with effective learning techniques: Promising directions from Cognitive and Educational Psychology.* Association for Psychological Science-APS. https://www.psychologicalscience.org/publications/journals/pspi/learning-techniques.html

Durisic, M. & Bunijevac, M. (2017). Parental involvement as a important factor for successful Education. *c e p s Journal, 7*(3), 137-153.

Durkheim, E. (1951). *Suicide: a study in sociology [1897].* The Free Press.

Durso, S. de O., Afonso, L. E., & Beltman, S. (2021). Resilience in higher education: A conceptual model and its empirical analysis. *Education Policy Analysis Archives*, *29*(August - December), 156. doi:10.14507/epaa.29.6054

Eagan, M. K., Stoltenberg, E. B., Zimmerman, H. B., Aragon, M. C., Whang Sayson, H., & Rios-Aguilar, C. (2017). The American freshman: National norms fall. *Higher Education Research Institute.* UCLA. https://www.heri.ucla.edu/monographs/ TheAmericanFreshman2016.pdf

Earle, K., & Curry, G. (2017). Meeting special educational needs and disabilities. *Addressing Special Educational Needs and Disability in the Curriculum, 1–5*, 1–5. doi:10.4324/9781315446721-1

Earnest, D. (2016). Studying: Is it bad for your health to pull an all-nighter? *Texas A&M.* https://www.sciencedaily.com/releases/2016/09/160919162837.htm epidemic.html

Ebert, D. D., Mortier, P., Kaehlke, F., Bruffaerts, R., Baumeister, H., Auerbach, R. P., Alonso, J., Vilagut, G., Martínez, K. U., Lochner, C., Cuijpers, P., Kuechler, A.-M., Green, J., Hasking, P., Lapsley, C., Sampson, N. A., & Kessler, R. C. (2019). WHO World Mental Health-International College Student Initiative collaborators. Barriers of mental health treatment utilization among first-year college students: First cross-national results from the WHO World Mental Health International College Student Initiative. *International Journal of Methods in Psychiatric Research*, *28*(2), e1782. doi:10.1002/mpr.1782 PMID:31069905

Echouffo-Tcheugui, J. B., Conner, S. C., Himali, J. J., Maillard, P., DeCarli, C., Beiser, A. S., Vasan, R. S., & Seshadri, S. (2018). Circulating cortisol and cognitive and structural brain measures. *Neurology*, *91*(21), e1961–e1970. doi:10.1212/WNL.0000000000006549 PMID:30355700

EducationWorld. (2021). *Towards a level playing field in K-12 education.* Education World. https://www.educationworld.in/towards-a-level-playing-field-in-k-12-education/

Eisenbarth, C. A. (2019). Coping with stress: Gender differences among college students. *College Student Journal*, *53*(2), 151–162.

Eisenberg, D., Hunt, J., Speer, M.D., & Nicole, M.S. (2013). Mental Health in American Colleges and Universities: Variation Across Student Subgroups and Across Campuses. *The Journal of Nervous and Mental Disease, 201*(1), 60-67. . doi:10.1097/NMD.0b013e31827ab077

Eisenberg, D., Golberstein, E., & Hunt, J. B. (2009). Mental Health and Academic Success in College. *The B.E. Journal of Economic Analysis & Policy*, *9*(1), 9. doi:10.2202/1935-1682.2191

Ekpoh, U., Edet, O., & Ukpong, N. (2020). Security challenges in Universities: Implications for safe school environment. *Journal of Educational and Social Research*, *10*(6), 112–124. doi:10.36941/jesr-2020-0113

Eleftheriades, R., Fiala, C., & Pasic, M. D. (2020). The challenges and mental health issues of academic trainees. *F1000 Research*, *9*, 104. https://www.ncbi.nlm.nih.gov/pmc/articles/PMC7199285/pdf/f1000research-9-23184.pdf. doi:10.12688/f1000research.21066.1 PMID:32419927

Eloff, I. (2021). College students' well-being during the COVID-19 pandemic: An exploratory study. *Journal of Psychology in Africa*, *31*(3), 254–260. doi:10.1080/14330237.2021.1939055

England, B. J., Brigati, J. R., & Schussler, E. E. (2017). Student anxiety in introductory biology classrooms: Perceptions about active learning and persistence in the major. *PLoS One*, *12*(8), e0182506. doi:10.1371/journal.pone.0182506 PMID:28771564

Enwefa, R., Enwefa, S., & Fagbeyiro, G. (2020). The Epidemic of Mental Health in Higher Education and Its Impact on Students' Academic Success. [IJTIE]. *International Journal of Technology and Inclusive Education*, *1*(9), 1500–1504. doi:10.20533/ijtie.2047.0533.2020.0184

Epstein, J. L. (1995). School/family/community partnerships. *Phi Delta Kappan*, *76*(9), 701.

Erez, A., & Isen, A. M. (2002). The influence of positive affect on the components of expectancy motivation. *The Journal of Applied Psychology*, *87*(6), 1055–1067. doi:10.1037/0021-9010.87.6.1055 PMID:12558213

Eriksson, M., Ghazinour, M., & Hammarstrom, A. (2018). Different uses of Bronfenbrenner's ecological theory in public mental health research: What is their value for guiding public mental health policy and practice? *Social Theory & Health*, *16*(4), 414–433. doi:10.105741285-018-0065-6

Etaneki, A. F., & Okolie, U. C. (2020). students ' unrest : An evaluation of influencing factors and control in tertiary educational institutions in Delta State, Nigeria. *Journal Plus Education*, *25*(1), 192–210.

Evans, M.G. (2000). *Planning for the transition to tertiary study: A literature review*.

Evans, D., Borriello, G. A., & Field, A. P. (2018). A review of the academic and psychological impact of the transition to secondary education. *Frontiers in Psychology*, *9*, 1482. doi:10.3389/fpsyg.2018.01482 PMID:30210385

Eyeberu, A., Getachew, T., Sertsu, A., Sisay, M., Baye, Y., Debella, A., & Alemu, A. (2022). Teenage Pregnancy and Its Predictors in Africa: A Systematic Review and Meta-Analysis. *International Journal of Health Sciences (Qassim)*, *16*(6), 47–60. PMID:36475034

Fadem, B. (2012). *Behavioral science in medicine*. Lippincott Williams & Wilkins.

Faku, T. U., & Kablavoh. (2006). Coping Strategies for Adolescent Mothers Who Return to School after Giving Birth. *The Journal of Psychology and Measurement*, *4*, 361–372.

Falki, S. (2021). Student unrest- Its causes and remedies. *International Journal of Indian Psychology*, *9*(2), 442–469.

Fallesen, P., & Gähler, M. (2020). Family type and parents' time with children: Longitudinal evidence for Denmark. *Acta Sociologica*, *63*(4), 361–380. doi:10.1177/0001699319868522

Family Central. (2021). *Children - so much more than just grades.* Family Central. https://www.family-central.sg/news-articles/children-more-than-grades/

Fang, D. Z., Young, C. B., Golshan, S., Fellows, I., Moutier, C., & Zisook, S. (2010). Depression in premedical undergraduates: A cross-sectional survey. *Primary Care Companion to the Journal of Clinical Psychiatry, 12*(6), e1–e6. doi:10.4088/PCC.10m00958blu PMID:21494338

Fang, D. Z., Young, C. B., Golshan, S., Moutier, C., & Zisook, S. (2012). Burnout in premedical undergraduate students. *Academic Psychiatry, 36*(1), 11–16. doi:10.1176/appi.ap.10080125 PMID:22362430

Faragher, R. M. (2023). Individual student characteristics, abilities, personal qualities, and the teacher's role in improving mathematics-learning outcomes. *The Evolution of Research on Teaching Mathematics*, 227–253. doi:10.1007/978-3-031-31193-2_8

Fares, J., Al Tabosh, H., Saadeddin, Z., El Mouhayyar, C., & Aridi, H. (2016). Stress, burnout and coping strategies in preclinical medical students. *North American Journal of Medical Sciences, 8*(2), 75. doi:10.4103/1947-2714.177299 PMID:27042604

Farrell, E. (2021). *Darkness, Wellness and World Views: The University's Role in Shaping Students' Experiences of Mental Health and Distress. In the Promise of the University*. Springer. doi:10.1007/978-981-16-5277-6_11

Fatima, S., Sharif, S., & Khalid, I. (2018). How does religiosity enhance psychological well-being? Roles of self-efficacy and perceived social support. *Psychology of Religion and Spirituality, 10*(2), 119–127. doi:10.1037/rel0000168

Fedina, L., Holmes, J. L., & Backes, B. L. (2018). Campus sexual assault: A systematic review of prevalence research from 2000 to 2015. *Trauma, Violence & Abuse, 19*(1), 76–93. doi:10.1177/1524838016631129 PMID:26906086

Feller, S. C., Castillo, E. G., Greenberg, J. M., Abascal, P., Van Horn, R., & Wells, K. B. (2018). Emotional well-being and public health: Proposal for a model national initiative. *Public Health Reports (Washington, D.C.), 133*(2), 136–141. doi:10.1177/0033354918754540 PMID:29448872

Fennell, M. (2016). Overcoming low self-esteem: A self-help guide using cognitive behavioural techniques. Hachette UK.

Fernandez, A., Howse, E., Rubio-Valera, M., Thorncraft, K., Noone, J., Luu, X., Veness, B., Leech, M., Llewellyn, G., & Salvador-Carulla, L. (2016). Setting-based interventions to promote mental health at the university: A systematic review. *International Journal of Public Health, 61*(7), 797–807. doi:10.100700038-016-0846-4 PMID:27364779

Fernández-Alonso, R., & Álvarez-Díaz, M. Woitschach, Pamela., Suárez-Álvarez, J., & Cuesta, M. (2017). Parental involvement and academic performance: Less control and more communication. Psicothema, 29(4), 453-461 doi:10.7334/psicothema2017.181

Findlay, L., & Arim, R. (2020). *Canadians Report Lower Self-Perceived Mental Health During The COVID-19 Pandemic*. Statistics Canada. https://www150.statcan.gc.ca/n1/pub/45-28-0001/2020001/article/00003-eng.htm

First, J., First, N. L., & Brian Houston, J. (2018). Resilience and Coping Intervention (RCI): A Group Intervention to Foster College Student Resilience. *Social Work with Groups, 41*(3), 198–210. doi:10.1080/01609513.2016.1272032

Fletcher, J.M., Frank, R.G., Mcguire, T., Meara, E., Stange, K.C., & Vigdor, J.L. (2009). *Mental health and academic success in college.*

Fogelgarn, R., & Burns, E. A. (2020). What constrains passionate teaching? A heuristic exploration. *Issues in Educational Research, 30*(2), 493–511.

Fonseca-Pedrero, E., Paino, M., Sierra-Baigrie, S., Lemos-Giráldez, S., & Muñiz, J. (2012). Psychometric Properties of the "State-Trait Anxiety Questionnaire". *Behav. Psychol. Psicol. Conduct., 20*, 547–561.

Fontinha, R., Easton, S., & Van Laar, D. (2019). Overtime and Quality of Working Life in Academics and Non-academics: The Role of Perceived Work-Life Balance. *International Journal of Stress Management, 26*(2), 173–183. doi:10.1037tr0000067

Fook, C. Y., & Sidhu, G. K. (2015). Investigating Learning Challenges Faced by Students in Higher Education. *Procedia: Social and Behavioral Sciences, 186*, 604–612. doi:10.1016/j.sbspro.2015.04.001

Foong, C. C., Bashir Ghouse, N. L., Lye, A. J., Pallath, V., Hong, H., & Vadivelu, J. (2021). Differences between high- and low-achieving pre-clinical medical students: A qualitative instrumental case study from a theory of action perspective. *Annals of Medicine, 54*(1), 195–210. doi:10.1080/07853890.2021.1967440 PMID:35019800

Ford, T., & Parker, C. (2016). Emotional and behavioural difficulties and mental (ill)health. *Emotional & Behavioural Difficulties, 21*(1), 1–7. doi:10.1080/13632752.2016.1139300

Frajerman, A., Morvan, Y., Krebs, M. O., Gorwood, P., & Chaumette, B. (2019). Burnout in medical students before residency: A systematic review and meta-analysis. *European Psychiatry, 5*, 36–42. doi:10.1016/j.eurpsy.2018.08.006 PMID:30384110

Franke, F., Huffmeier, J., Montano, D., & Reeske, A. (2017). Leadership, followers' mental health and job performance in organizations: A comprehensive meta-analysis from an occupational health perspective. *Journal of Organizational Behavior, 38*(3), 327–350. doi:10.1002/job.2124

Franzen, J., Jermann, F., Ghisletta, P., Rudaz, S., Bondolfi, G., & Tran, N. T. (2021). Psychological Distress and Well-Being among Students of Health Disciplines: The Importance of Academic Satisfaction. *International Journal of Environmental Research and Public Health, 18*(4), 2151. doi:10.3390/ijerph18042151 PMID:33672097

Freire, C., Ferradas, M. D., Valle, A., Nunez, J. C., & Vallejo, G. (2016). Profiles of Psychological well-being & Coping Strategies among University Students. *Frontiers in Psychology, 23*, 67–76. doi:10.3389/fpsyg.2016.01554 PMID:27790168

Freire, C., Ferradás, M., Regueiro, B., Rodríguez, S., Valle, A., & Núñez, J. C. (2020). Coping strategies and self-efficacy in university students: A person-centered approach. *Frontiers in Psychology, 11*, 841. doi:10.3389/fpsyg.2020.00841 PMID:32508707

Freire, C., Ferradas, M., Rgueiro, B., Rodriguez, S., Valle, A., & Nunez, J. C. (2020). *Coping Strategies and Self -efficacy in University Students: A person centered approach.* Nova Publishers.

Frisby, B. N. (2019). The influence of emotional contagion on student perceptions of instructor rapport, emotional support, emotion work, valence, and cognitive learning. *Communication Studies, 70*(4), 492–506. doi:10.1080/10510974.2019.1622584

Frothingham, S. (2023, March 29). *Does caffeine cause anxiety?* Healthline. https://www.healthline.com/health/caffeine-and-anxiety%23caffeine-and-anxiety

Galbicsek, C. (2020). College alcoholism. *Alcohol Rehab Guide.* https://www.alcoholrehabguide.org/resources/college alcoholabuse/#:~:text=Roughly%20 80%20percent%20of%20college, alcohol%20in%20too%20little%20time.

Galderisi, S., Heinz, A., Kastrup, M., Beezhold, J., & Sartorius, N. (2015). Toward a new definition of mental health. *World Psychiatry; Official Journal of the World Psychiatric Association (WPA), 14*(2), 231–233. doi:10.1002/wps.20231 PMID:26043341

Galdi, S., & Guizzo, F. (2021). Media-induced sexual harassment: The routes from sexually objectifying media to sexual harassment. *Sex Roles, 84*(11), 645–669. doi:10.100711199-020-01196-0

Gallagher, R., Gill, A. M., & Sysko, H. B. (2000). *National survey of counseling directors, 2000.* International Association of Counseling Centers, Inc.

Gallagher, R., Gill, A., & Sysko, H. (2000). *National survey of counseling center directors.* International Association of Counseling Services.

Gallagher, S. (2012). Multiple aspects in the sense of agency. *New Ideas in Psychology*, *30*(1), 15–31. doi:10.1016/j.newideapsych.2010.03.003

Gallego, J., Aguilar-Parra, J. M., Cangas, A. J., Langer, Á. I., & Mañas, I. (2014). Effect of a Mindfulness Program on Stress, Anxiety and Depression in University Students. [CrossRef] [PubMed]. *The Spanish Journal of Psychology*, *17*, 17. doi:10.1017jp.2014.102 PMID:26055051

Gall, T. L., Evans, D. R., & Bellerose, S. (2000). Transition to First-Year University: Patterns of Change in Adjustment across Life Domains and Time. *Journal of Social and Clinical Psychology*, *19*(4), 544–567. doi:10.1521/jscp.2000.19.4.544

Gámez-Guadix, M., & Calvete, E. (2016). Assessing the relationship between mindful awareness and problematic Internet use among adolescents. *Mindfulness*, *7*(6), 1281–1288. doi:10.100712671-016-0566-0

Gans, S. E., & Johnson, V. K. (2016). Cortisol response to family interaction as a predictor for adjustment. *Journal of Family Psychology*, *30*(7), 812–821. doi:10.1037/fam0000238 PMID:27559928

Gao, H. (2021). Beijing is worried young Chinese are embracing nihilism. *Foreign Policy*. https://foreignpolicy.com/2021/10/23/china-meritocracy-youth-burned-out/

Gao, W., Ping, S., & Liu, X. (2020). Gender differences in depression, anxiety, and stress among college students: A longitudinal study from China. *Journal of Affective Disorders*, *263*, 292–300. doi:10.1016/j.jad.2019.11.121 PMID:31818792

Garcia, S. L. (2020). *Attending anyway: A qualitative case study of the intersections of family stress, school climate, and school attendance choices within a Northeast Urban High School.* [Unpublished doctoral dissertation, Concordia University, USA].

García, F., & Musitu, G. (2014). *AF5: Autoconcepto Forma 5* [AF5: Form 5 Self-Concept]. TEA Ediciones.

García-Hernández, R. J., Hernández-Sánchez, J. E., & García-Martínez, V. (2020). Sexual harassment in a Higher Education Institution. *Multidisciplinary Journal of Gender Studies*, *9*(3), 210–233. doi:10.17583/generos.2020.5609

García, V. T., Fernández, B. G., & Ruiz-Gallardo, J. R. (2018). Home-based family Involvement and academic achievement: A case study in Primary Education. *Educational Studies*, *44*(3), 361–375. doi:10.1080/03055698.2017.1373636

Gargiulo, I., Garcia, X., Benages-Albert, M., Martinez, J., Pfeffer, K., & Vall-Casas, P. (2020). *Women's safety perception assessment in an urban stream corridor: Developing a safety map based on qualitative GIS. Landscape and urban planning*. Springer.

Garone, S. (2020, August 11). *The health benefits of natural light (and 7 ways to get more of it).* Healthline. https://www.healthline.com/health/natural-light-benefits#benefits

Garriott, P. O., & Nisle, S. (2018). Stress, coping, and perceived academic goal progress in first-generation college students: The role of institutional supports. *Journal of Diversity in Higher Education*, *11*(4), 436–450. doi:10.1037/dhe0000068

Gaspar, T., Gomez-Baya, D., Trindade, J, & Botelho Guedes, F., Cerqueira, A., & Margarida G. de Matos. (2021). Relationship between family functioning, parents' psychosocial factors, and children's well-being. *Journal of Family Issues*, *0*(0), 1–18.

Gebreegziabher, Y., Girma, E., & Tesfaye, M. (2019). Help-seeking behavior of Jimma university students with common mental disorders: A crosssectional study. *PLoS One*, *14*(2), e0212657. doi:10.1371/journal.pone.0212657 PMID:30794639

Gewin, V. (2021). Pandemic burnout is rampant in academia. *Nature*, *591*(7850), 491–493. doi:10.1038/d41586-021-00663-2 PMID:33723408

Giamos, D., Lee, A., Suleiman, A., Stuart, H. & Chen, S.-P. (2017). Understanding Campus Culture and Student Coping Strategies for Mental Health Issues in Five Canadian Colleges and Universities. *Canadian Journal of Higher Education / Revue canadienne d'enseignement supérieur, 47*(3), 136–151. doi:10.7202/1043242ar

Gibson, A. S. C. (2007). The role of self-talk in the awareness of physiological state and physical performance. *Sports Medicene*, *37*(12), 1–10.

Gillham, J., Adams-Deutsch, Z., Werner, J., Reivich, K., Coulter-Heindl, V., Linkins, M., Winder, B., Peterson, C., Park, N., Abenavoli, R., Contero, A., & Seligman, M. E. P. (2011). Character strengths predict subjective well-being during adolescence. *The Journal of Positive Psychology*, *6*(1), 31–44. doi:10.1080/17439760.2010.536773

Giroux, D., & Geiss, E. G. (2019). Evaluating a Student-Led Mental Health Awareness Campaign. *Psi Chi Journal of Psychological Research*, *24*(1), 61–66. doi:10.24839/2325-7342.JN24.1.61

Givens, J. L., & Tjia, J. (2002). Depressed medical students use of mental health services and barriers to use. *Academic Medicine*, *2*, 34–46. PMID:12228091

Glariana, E., & Solar, B. (2015). Status of schools safety and security among elementary schools in the fifthy class municipality. *Asia Pacific Journal of Multidisciplinary Research*, *3*(5), 10–18.

Gloria, C. T., & Steinhardt, M. A. (2016). Relationships among positive emotions, coping, resilience and mental health. *Stress and Health*, *32*(2), 145–156. doi:10.1002mi.2589 PMID:24962138

Godman, H. (2022). Top ways to reduce daily stress. *Harvard Health*. https://www.health.harvard.edu/staying-healthy/top-ways-to-reduce-daily-stress

Goel, D. (2020, May 26). Premed burnout and medical education. *Journal of Young Investigators*. www.jyi.org/blog/2020/5/26/premed-burnout-and-medical-education

Goldman, J. A., & Bell, S. C. B. (2022). Student and faculty coping and impacts on academic success in response to COVID-19. *Journal of Interdisciplinary Studies in Education*, *11*(1), 74–91.

Go, M. (2016). The effects of entrance examination stress on suicide ideation among college entrance examinees - Moderating effect of social support. *Health & Welfare*, *18*, 55. doi:10.23948/kshw.2016.12.18.55

Gong, H., & Jiang, J. (2018). The Psychological Health Promotion and Intervention Strategies of College Teachers from the Perspective of Positive Psychology. *Theor. Pract. Innov. Entrep.*, *10*, 27–33.

Gong, X., Wang, L., Rong, G., Zhang, D., Zhang, A. Y., & Liu, C. (2023). Effects of online mindfulness-based interventions on the mental health of university students: A systematic review and meta-analysis. *Frontiers in Psychology*, *14*, 14. doi:10.3389/fpsyg.2023.1073647 PMID:36844353

Good Therapy. (2018, September 26). Coping Mechanisms. *Good Therapy*. https://www.goodtherapy.org/blog/psychpedia/coping-mechanisms

Goodman, L. (2017). Mental Health on University Campuses and the Needs of Students They Seek to Serve. *Building Healthy Academic Communities Journal*, *1*(2), 31–44. doi:10.18061/bhac.v1i2.6056

Goodman-Scott, E., Donohue, P., & Betters-Bubon, J. (2019). The case for universal mental health screening in schools. *Counseling Today*, *62*(3), 40–45. https://digitalcommons.odu.edu/chs_pubs

Goodwin, A. B. (2016). Mental health and students at risk. *New Directions for Student Services*, *2016*(156), 65–75. doi:10.1002s.20192

Goyal, M., Singh, S., Sibinga, E. M., Gould, N. F., Rowland-Seymour, A., Sharma, R., Berger, Z., Sleicher, D., Maron, D. D., Shihab, H. M., Ranasinghe, P. D., Linn, S., Saha, S., Bass, E. B., & Haythornthwaite, J. A. (2014). Meditation programs for psychological stress and well-being: A systematic review and meta-analysis. *JAMA Internal Medicine*, *174*(3), 357–368. doi:10.1001/jamainternmed.2013.13018 PMID:24395196

Grace, M. K. (2018). Depressive symptoms, burnout, and declining medical career interest among undergraduate pre-medical students. *International Journal of Medical Education*, *9*, 302–308. doi:10.5116/ijme.5be5.8131 PMID:30481160

Grace, M. K. (2020). "They understand what you're going through": Experientially similar others, anticipatory stress, and depressive symptoms. *Society and Mental Health*, *11*(1), 20–37. doi:10.1177/2156869320910773

Gradišek, P. (2021). Character strengths of first-year student teachers and the 5 Cs of the Positive Youth Development framework: A mixed-methods study. In Kozina, A & Wiium, Z (Eds). Positive youth development in contexts (pp. 127). Pedagoški inštitut/Educational Research Institute. doi:10.32320/978-961-270-341-7.127-150

Graham, A., Powell, M. A., & Truscott, J. (2016). Facilitating student well-being: Relationships do matter. *Educational Research*, *58*(4), 366–383. doi:10.1080/00131881.2016.1228841

Grant, J. E., & Chamberlain, S. R. (2020). Family history of substance use disorders: Signifificance for mental health in young adults who gamble. *Journal of Behavioral Addictions*, *9*(2), 289–297. doi:10.1556/2006.2020.00017 PMID:32516117

Gratz, K. L., Mann, A. J. D., & Tull, M. T. (2021). Suicidal ideation among university students during the COVID-19 pandemic: Identifying at-risk subgroups. *Psychiatry Research*, *302*, 114034. doi:10.1016/j.psychres.2021.114034 PMID:34098158

Graves, B. S., Hall, M. E., Dias-Karch, C., Haischer, M. H., & Apter, C. (2021). Gender differences in perceived stress and coping among college students. *PLoS One*, *16*(8), e0255634. doi:10.1371/journal.pone.0255634 PMID:34383790

Grazia, V., & Molinari, L. (2021). School climate multidimensionality and measurement: A systematic literature review. *Research Papers in Education*, *36*(5), 561–587. doi:10.1080/02671522.2019.1697735

Greenleaf, C., Petrie, T. A., & Martin, S. B. (2014). Relationship of weight-based teasing and adolescents' psychological well-being and physical health. *The Journal of School Health*, *84*(1), 49–55. doi:10.1111/josh.12118 PMID:24320152

Green, R. A., Conlon, E. G., & Morrissey, S. A. (2017). Task values and self-efficacy beliefs of undergraduate psychology students. *Australian Journal of Psychology*, *69*(2), 112–120. doi:10.1111/ajpy.12125

Greer, J. A., Jacobs, J. M., El-Jawahri, A., Nipp, R. D., Gallagher, E. R., Pirl, W. F., Park, E. R., Muzikansky, A., Jacobsen, J. C., Jackson, V. A., & Temel, J. S. (2018). Role of Patient Coping Strategies in Understanding the Effects of Early Palliative Care on Quality of Life and Mood. *Journal of Clinical Oncology*, *36*(1), 53–60. doi:10.1200/JCO.2017.73.7221 PMID:29140772

Greer, T. M., & Chwalisz, K. (2007). Minority-related Stressors and Coping Processes among African American College Students. *Journal of College Student Development*, *2*(4), 32–46. doi:10.1353/csd.2007.0037

Griffiths, A. J., Lilles, E., Furlong, M. J., & Sidhwa, J. (2012). The relations of adolescent student engagement with troubling and high-risk behaviors. In S. Christenson, A. L. Reschly, & C. Wylie (Eds.), *Handbook of research on student engagement* (Vol. 840). Springer. doi:10.1007/978-1-4614-2018-7_27

Grills-Taquechel, A. E., Norton, P., & Ollendick, T. H. (2010). A longitudinal examination of factors predicting anxiety during the transition to middle school. *Anxiety, Stress, and Coping*, *23*(5), 493–513. doi:10.1080/10615800903494127 PMID:20711893

Gross, J. P., Mommaerts, C. D., Earl, D., & De Vries, R. G. (2008). Perspective: After a century of criticizing premedical education, are we missing the point? *Academic Medicine*, *83*(5), 516–520. doi:10.1097/ACM.0b013e31816bdb58 PMID:18448911

Grotan, K., Sund, E. R., & Bjerkeset, O. (2019). Mental health, academic self-efficacy and study progress among college students - The SHoT study, Norway. *Frontiers in Psychology*, *10*(JAN), 1–11. doi:10.3389/fpsyg.2019.00045 PMID:30733694

Grzybowski, J., & Brinthaupt, T. M. (2022). Trait Mindfulness, Self-Compassion, and Self-Talk: A Correlational Analysis of Young Adults. *Behavioral Sciences (Basel, Switzerland)*, *12*(9), 300. doi:10.3390/bs12090300 PMID:36135104

Guan, S.-S. A., & Fuligni, A. J. (2015). Changes in parent, sibling, and peer support during the transition to young adulthood. *Journal of Research on Adolescence*, *26*(2), 286–299. doi:10.1111/jora.12191

Guilliver, A., Griffiths, K. M., & Christensen, H. (2010). Perceived barriers and facilitators to mental health-help seeking in young people. *Systematic Reviews*, *1*, 32–45.

Guinta, M. R., & John, R. M. (2018). Social media and adolescent health. *Pediatric Nursing*, *44*(4), 196–201.

Gulliver, A., Farrer, L., Bennet, K., & Griffiths, K. M. (2019). University staff mental health literacy, stigma and their experience of students with mental health problems. *Journal of Further and Higher Education*, *43*(3), 434–442. doi:10.1080/0309877X.2017.1367370

Gulliver, A., Wysoke, T., Calear, A. L., & Farrer, L. M. (2023). Factors Associated with Engagement in University Life, and Help Seeking Attitudes and Behaviour in First Year Undergraduate Students. *International Journal of Environmental Research and Public Health*, *20*(1), 120. doi:10.3390/ijerph20010120 PMID:36612442

Gunn, H. E., & Eberhardt, K. R. (2019). Family dynamics in sleep health and hypertension. *Current Hypertension Reports*, *21*(5), 39. doi:10.100711906-019-0944-9 PMID:30982174

Guo, F., Liu, J., & Li, L. (2022). Student support and services in Chinese higher education institutions: Practices and impacts. *Student Support Services*, 113–143. doi:10.1007/978-981-16-5852-5_45

Gupta, K., Parimal, B. S., & Narang, N. (2023). Academic stress among first-year undergraduate college students: role of emotional intelligence in coping with academic stress. In P. Aloka & K. Mukuna (Eds.), *Handbook of Research on Coping Mechanisms for First-Year Students Transitioning to Higher Education* (pp. 191–210). IGI Global. doi:10.4018/978-1-6684-6961-3.ch004

Gustems-Carnicer, J., Calderón, C., & Calderón-Garrido, D. (2019). Stress, coping strategies and academic achievement in teacher education students. *European Journal of Teacher Education*, *42*(3), 375–390. doi:10.1080/02619768.2019.1576629

Guszkowska, M., & Dąbrowska-Zimakowska, A. (2022). Coping with stress during the second wave of the COVID-19 pandemic by Polish university students: Strategies, structure, and relation to psychological well-being. *Psychology Research and Behavior Management*, *15*, 339–352. doi:10.2147/PRBM.S345648 PMID:35210882

Guthrie, S., Lichten, C., van Belle, J., Ball, S., Knack, A., & Hofman, J. (2017). *Understanding mental health in the research environment*. Rand Corporation. Retrieved fromhttps., www.rand.org/pubs/research_reports/RR2022.html

Gutman, L. M., & Schoon, I. (2013). *The Impact of Non-Cognitive Skills on Outcomes for Young People*. Education Endowment Foundation. Leading Education and Social Research.

Gyawali, K. (2021). Sexual harassment and its effects on mental health of the teenage school girls in lalitpur and Rupandehi District. *Journal of Balkumari College*, *10*(1), 39–47. doi:10.3126/jbkc.v10i1.42092

Haile, Y. G., Senkute, A. L., Alemu, B. T., Bedane, D. M., & Kebede, K. B. (2019). Prevalence and associated factors of burnout among Debre Berhan University medical students: A cross-sectional study. *BMC Medical Education*, *19*(1), 1–11. doi:10.118612909-019-1864-8 PMID:31703674

Haile, Y., Alemu, S., & Habtewold, T. (2017). Common mental disorder and its association with academic performance among Debre Berhan University students, Ethiopia. *International Journal of Mental Health Systems*, *11*(1), 34–45. doi:10.118613033-017-0142-6 PMID:28473869

Hako, A. N., & Mbongo, E. N. (2018). Beneficiaries' satisfaction with the School Counselling Services in Namibia: A case study of a selected region. *Namibia CPD Journal for Educators*, *4*(1), 20–35.

Haleh-Heizomi, H., Allahverdipour, H., Hejazi, S. B., Jafarabadi, M. A., & Shirazi', A. (2018). Factors Associating Perceived Stress and Psychological Well-being among Iranian Female Adolescents. *Int J Depress Anxiety*, *1*(1), 1–6.

Hall, R. (2017). *The rise of academic ill-health*. Wonkhe. https://wonkhe.com/blogs/therise-of-academic-ill-health/

Halland, E., De Vibe, M., Solhaug, I., Friborg, O., Rosenvinge, J., Tyssen, R., Sørlie, T., & Bjørndal, A. (2015). Mindfulness training improves problem-focused coping in psychology and medical students: Results from a randomized controlled trial. *College Student Journal*, (49), 387–398.

Hall, G. S. (1904). Adolescence in literature, biography, and history. In G. S. Hall (Ed.), *Adolescence: Its psychology and its relations to physiology, anthropology, sociology, sex, crime, religion and education* (Vol. 1, pp. 513–589). D Appleton & Company. doi:10.1037/10616-008

Hamad, E. O. (2022). Psychological well-being among Saudi adults during the context of COVID-19 lockdown: A psychometric analysis of the 12-item General Health Questionnaire. *BMC Psychology*, *10*(1), 319. doi:10.118640359-022-01030-0 PMID:36572926

Hamdan-Mansour, A. M., Puskar, K., & Bandak, A. G. (2009). Effectiveness of Cognitive-Behavioral Therapy on Depressive Symptomatology, Stress and Coping Strategies among Jordanian University Students. *Issues in Mental Health Nursing*, *30*(3), 188–196. doi:10.1080/01612840802694577 PMID:19291496

Hamilton, J. E. (2019). Cash or Kudos: Addressing the Effort-Reward Imbalance for Academic Employees. *International Journal of Stress Management*, *26*(2), 193–203. doi:10.1037tr0000107

Hamza, C. A., Ewing, L., Heath, N. L., & Goldstein, A. L. (2021). When social isolation is nothing new: A longitudinal study on psychological distress during COVID-19 among university students with and without pre-existing mental health concerns. *Canadian Psychology*, *62*(1), 20–30. doi:10.1037/cap0000255

Han, H. (2018). The VIA inventory of strengths, positive youth development, and moral education. *The Journal of Positive Psychology*, *14*(1), 32–40. doi:10.1080/17439760.2018.1528378

Hanley, A. W., de Vibe, M., Solhaug, I., Gonzalez-Pons, K., & Garland, E. L. (2019). Mindfulness training reduces neuroticism over a 6-year longitudinal randomized control trial in Norwegian medical and psychology students. [CrossRef]. *Journal of Research in Personality*, *82*, 103859. doi:10.1016/j.jrp.2019.103859

Hans-Werner, R. (2015). Students' mental health and psychological counselling in Europe. *Mental Health & Prevention*, *3*(1–2), 34–40. doi:10.1016/j.mhp.2015.04.006

Harari, Y. N. (2018). Yuval Noah Harari on what 2050 has in store for humankind. *WIRED UK*. https://www.wired.co.uk/article/yuval-noah-harari-extract-21-lessons-for-the-21st-century

Harari, Y. N. (2016). *Sapiens: A Brief History of Humankind*. Signal.

Harding, T., Lopez, V., & Klainin-Yobas, P. (2019). Predictors of Psychological Well-Being among Higher Education Students. *Psychology (Irvine, Calif.)*, *10*(10), 578–594. doi:10.4236/psych.2019.104037

Hardy, J. (2006). Speaking clearly: A critical review of the self-talk literature. *Psychology of Sport and Exercise*, *7*(1), 81–97. doi:10.1016/j.psychsport.2005.04.002

Hardy, J., Gammage, K., & Hall, C. (2001). A descriptive study of athlete self-talk. *The Sport Psychologist*, *15*(3), 306–318. doi:10.1123/tsp.15.3.306

Hardy, J., Hall, C. R., & Hardy, L. (2004). A Note on Athletes' Use of Self-Talk. *Journal of Applied Sport Psychology*, *16*(3), 251–257. doi:10.1080/10413200490498357

Harrington, A., & Dunne, J. D. (2015). When mindfulness is therapy: Ethical qualms, historical perspectives. *The American Psychologist*, *70*(7), 621–631. doi:10.1037/a0039460 PMID:26436312

Harrison, E. D., Hulme, J. A., & Fox, C. L. (2022). A Thematic Analysis of Students' Perceptions and Experiences of Bullying in UK Higher Education. *Europe's Journal of Psychology*, *18*(1), 1841–0413. ejop.psychopen.eu. doi:10.5964/ejop.3669 PMID:35330856

Hartrey, L., Denieffe, S., & Wells, J. S. (2017). A systematic review of barriers and supports to the participation of students with mental health difficulties in higher education. *Mental Health & Prevention*, *6*, 26–43. doi:10.1016/j.mhp.2017.03.002

Harvard Health. (2021). *Protect your brain from stress*. https://www.health.harvard.edu/mind-and-mood/protect-your-brain-from-stress

Hascher, T., & Waber, J. (2021). Teacher well being: A systematic review of the research literature from the Year 2000-2019. *Educational Research Review*, *34*(8), 10041. doi:10.1016/j.edurev.2021.100411

Hassan, S. U. N., Algahtani, F. D., Atteya, M. R., Almishaal, A. A., Ahmed, A. A., Obeidat, S. T., Kamel, R. M., & Mohamed, R. F. (2022). The impact of extended E-Learning on the emotional well-being of students during the COVID-19 pandemic in Saudi Arabia. *Children (Basel, Switzerland)*, *9*(1), 13. doi:10.3390/children9010013 PMID:35053638

Hassanzadeh, A., Heidari, Z., Feizi, A., Hassanzadeh Keshteli, A., Roohafza, H., Afshar, H., & Adibi, P. (2017). Association of stressful life events with psychological problems: A large-scale community-based study using grouped outcomes latent factor regression with latent predictors. *Computational and Mathematical Methods in Medicine*, *3457103*, 1–12. doi:10.1155/2017/3457103 PMID:29312459

Hassel, S., & Ridout, N. (2018). An Investigation of First-Year Students' and Lecturers' Expectations of University Education. *Frontiers in Psychology*. doi:10.3389/fpsyg.2017.02218

Hatzigeorgiadis, A. (2006). Instructional and motivational self-talk: An investigation on perceived self-talk functions. *Hellenic Journal of Psychology*, *3*(2), 164–175. https://www.researchgate.net/publication/284903463_instructional_and_motivational_self-talk_An_investigation_on_perceived_self-talk_funvtion

Havik, T., & Westergård, E. (2020). Do teachers matter? Students' perceptions of classroom interactions and student engagement. *Scandinavian Journal of Educational Research*, *64*(4), 488–507. doi:10.1080/00313831.2019.1577754

Hawkins, Y. (2019). Mental wellbeing: let's find new ways to support students. *Office for Students*. https://www.officeforstudents.org.uk/news-blog-and-events/blog/mental-wellbeing-let-s-find-new-ways-to-support-students/

Hayden, M., Hemmens, A., Mcintosh, S., Sandoval-Hernandez, A., & Thompson, J. (2017). *The impact of creativity, activity, and service (CAS) on students and communities: Non-technical report for the International Baccalaureate Organization.* University of Bath. https://www.ibo.org/globalassets/publications/ib-research/dp/cas-finalreport-2017-en.pdf

Heavey, C. L., & Hurlburt, R. T. (2007). The phenomena of inner experience. *Consciousness and Cognition*. doi:10.1016/j.concog.2007.12.006 PMID:18258456

Heck, K. E., & Subramaniam, A. (2009). Youth development frameworks [Monograph]. *4-H Center for Youth Development Monograph: University of California.* https://youthrex.com/wp-content/uploads/2019/02/1224.pdf

He, F. X., Turnbull, B., Kirshbaum, M. N., Phillips, B., & Klainin-Yobas, P. (2018). Assessing Stress, Protective Factors and Psychological Well-Being among Undergraduate Nursing Students. [CrossRef]. *Nurse Education Today*, *68*, 4–12. doi:10.1016/j.nedt.2018.05.013 PMID:29870871

Hefner, J. L., & Eisenberg, D. (2009). Social support and mental health among college students. *The American Journal of Orthopsychiatry*, *79*(4), 491–499. doi:10.1037/a0016918 PMID:20099940

Henry, A. (2016, August 11). Why we should all spend more time staring out of the window. *Lifehacker*. https://lifehacker.com/why-we-should-all-spend-more-time-staring-out-of-the-wi-1784903049

Henry, T. L., Jetty, A., Petterson, S., Jaffree, H., Ramsay, A., Heiman, E., & Bazemore, A. (2020). Taking a closer look at mental health treatment differences: Effectiveness of mental health treatment by provider type in racial and ethnic minorities. *Journal of Primary Care & Community Health*, *11*, 2150132720966403. doi:10.1177/2150132720966403 PMID:33089752

Herbert, C., Meixner, F., Wiebking, C., & Gilg, V. (2020). Regular physical activity, short-term exercise, mental health, and well-being among university students: The results of an online and a laboratory study. *Frontiers in Psychology*, *11*, 509. doi:10.3389/fpsyg.2020.00509 PMID:32528333

Hernández, C., Jiménez, M., & Guadarrama, E. (2015). La percepción del hostigamiento y acoso sexual en mujeres estudiantes en dos instituciones de educación superior. *Revista de la Educación Superior*, *44*(176), 63–82. doi:10.1016/j.resu.2015.12.004

Hernández-Torrano, D., Ibrayeva, L., Sparks, J., Lim, N., Clementi, A., Almukhambetova, A., Nurtayev, Y., & Muratkyzy, A. (2020). Mental Health and Well-Being of University Students: A Bibliometric Mapping of the Literature. *Frontiers in Psychology*, *11*, 1226. doi:10.3389/fpsyg.2020.01226 PMID:32581976

Herzog-Punzenberger, B., Altrichter, H., Brown, M., Burns, D., Nortvedt, G. A., Skedsmo, G., Wiese, E. F., Nayır, F., Fellner, M., McNamara, G., & O'Hara, J. (2020). Teachers responding to cultural diversity: Case studies on assessment practices, challenges and experiences in secondary schools in Austria, Ireland, Norway and Turkey. *Educational Assessment, Evaluation and Accountability*, *32*(3), 395–424. doi:10.100711092-020-09330-y

Hinami, K., & Wetterneck, T. B. (2017). For individuals and practices: Career sustainability and avoiding burnout. In McKean S.C., & Ross J.J., & Dressler D.D., & Scheurer D.B.(Eds.), Principles and Practice of Hospital Medicine (2nd ed.). McGraw Hill.

Hinderaker, D. J. (2013). *Counseling center college student mental health and use of counseling center services.* St. Catherine University Repository. https://sophia.stkate.edu/cgi/viewcontent.cgi?article=1191&context=msw_papers

Hirsch, J., & Khan, S. (2020). *Sexual citizens: A landmark study of sex, power and assault on Campus*. W.W. Norton and Company Independent Publishers.

Hobson, J. (2009, November 4). *Danish pupils use web in exams.* BBC. http://news.bbc.co.uk/2/hi/uk_news/education/8341886.stm

Hoen, P. W., Denollet, J., de Jonge, P., & Whooley, M. A. (2013). Positive affect and survival in patients with stable coronary heart disease: Findings from the Heart and Soul Study. [PubMed: 23945449]. *The Journal of Clinical Psychiatry, 74*(7), 716–722. doi:10.4088/JCP.12m08022 PMID:23945449

Hofmann, S. G., Grossman, P., & Hinton, D. E. (2011). Loving-kindness and compassion meditation: Potential for psychological interventions. *Clinical Psychology Review, 31*(7), 1126–1132. doi:10.1016/j.cpr.2011.07.003 PMID:21840289

Hogan, V., Hogan, M., & Hodgins, M. (2016). A study of workaholism in Irish academics. *Occupational Medicine, 66*(6), 460–465. doi:10.1093/occmed/kqw032 PMID:27170737

Holloway, S. D., & Jonas, M. (2016). Families, culture, and schooling: A critical review of theory and research. In K. R. Wentzel & G. B. Ramani (Eds.), *Handbook of social influences in school contexts: Socio-emotional, motivation, cognitive outcomes* (pp. 258–272). Taylor & Francis.

Holt, E. W., Lombard, Q. K., Best, N., Smiley-Smith, S., & Quinn, J. E. (2019). Active and passive use of green space, health, and well-being amongst university students. *International Journal of Environmental Research and Public Health, 16*(3), 424. doi:10.3390/ijerph16030424 PMID:30717193

Holt, M. K., Vivolo-Kantor, A. M., Polanin, J. R., Holland, K. M., Degue, S., Matjasko, J. L., & Reid, G. (2015). Bullying and Suicidal Ideation and Behaviors: A Meta-Analysis. *Pediatrics, 135*(2), E496–E509. doi:10.1542/peds.2014-1864 PMID:25560447

Holt, R. J., Graham, J. M., Whitaker, K. J., Hagan, C. C., Ooi, C., Wilkinson, P. O., & Suckling, J. (2016). Functional MRI of emotional memory in adolescent depression. *Developmental Cognitive Neuroscience, 19*, 31–41. doi:10.1016/j.dcn.2015.12.013 PMID:26802367

Hoogwegt, M. T., Versteeg, H., Hansen, T. B., Thygesen, L. C., Pedersen, S. S., & Zwisler, A.-D. (2013). Exercise mediates the association between positive affect and 5-year mortality in patients with ischemic heart disease. [PubMed: 24021694]. *Circulation: Cardiovascular Quality and Outcomes, 6*(5), 559–566. doi:10.1161/CIRCOUTCOMES.113.000158 PMID:24021694

Hope, J. (2017). Comprehensive student support efforts lead to impressive outcomes. *Student Affairs Today, 20*(10), 6–6. doi:10.1002ay.30422

Hornby, G., & Blackwell, I. (2018). Barriers to parental involvement in Education: An Update. *Educational Review, 70*(1), 109–119. doi:10.1080/00131911.2018.1388612

Horwitz, A. G., McGuire, T., Busby, D. R., Eisenberg, D., Zheng, K., Pistorello, J., & King, C. A. (2020). Sociodemographic differences in barriers to mental health care among college students at elevated suicide risk. *Journal of Affective Disorders, 271*, 123–130. doi:10.1016/j.jad.2020.03.115 PMID:32479307

Houston, J. B., First, J., Spialek, M. L., Sorenson, M. E., Mills-Sandoval, T., Lockett, M. K., First, N. L., Nitiéma, P., Allen, S. F., & Pfefferbaum, B. (2017). Randomized controlled trial of the Resilience and Coping Intervention (RCI) with undergraduate university students. *Journal of American College Health, 65*(1), 1–9. doi:10.1080/07448481.2016.1227826 PMID:27559857

Huang, L., Xu, F., & Liu, H. (2020). Emotional responses and coping strategies of nurses and nursing college students during the COVID-19 outbreak. MedRxiv, 2020-03. doi:10.1101/2020.03.05.20031898

Huffman, J. C., DuBois, C. M., Mastomauro, C. A., Moore, S. V., Suarez, L., & Park, E. R. (2014). Positive psychological states and health behaviours in acute coronary syndrome patients: A qualitative study. *Journal of Health Psychology*. PMID:25114026

Hughes, G. (2021). The challenge of student mental wellbeing: Reconnecting students services with the academic universe. *Student Support Services*, 1–23. doi:10.1007/978-981-13-3364-4_6-1

Hughes, G., & Spanner, L. (2019). The University Mental Health Charter. *Student Minds*. https://www.studentminds.org.uk/uploads/3/7/8/4/37845 84/191208_umhc_artwo rk.pdf

Hughes, G., & Spanner, L. (2019). *The University Mental Health Charter*. Student Minds. https://www.studentminds.org.uk/uploads/3/7/8/4/3784584/191208_umhc_artwork.pdf

Hughes, G., Panjwani, M., Tulcidas, P., & Byrom, N. (2018). *Student mental health: The role and experience of academics*. Student Minds.

Hughes, G., & Spanner, L. (2019). *The university mental health charter*. Student Minds.

Hughes, G., & Spanner, L. (2019). *The University Mental Health Charter*. Student Minds.

Huijser, H., Kek, M. Y., & Padró, F. F. (2022). Introduction: Student support services in an overall ecology for learning. *Student Support Services*, 3–10. doi:10.1007/978-981-16-5852-5_49

Hunt, J., & Eisenberg, D. (2010). Mental Health Problems and Help-Seeking Behavior Among College Students. *The Journal of Adolescent Health*, *46*(1), 3–10. doi:10.1016/j.jadohealth.2009.08.008 PMID:20123251

Huppert, F. A. (2017). *Challenges in defining and measuring well-being and their implications for policy. In future directions in well-being*. Springer.

Hutcherson, C. A., Seppala, E. M., & Gross, J. J. (2008). Lovingkindness meditation increases social connectedness. *Emotion (Washington, D.C.)*, *8*(5), 720–724. doi:10.1037/a0013237 PMID:18837623

Hyde, J. S., & Mezulis, A. H. (2020). Gender differences in depression: Biological, affective, cognitive, and sociocultural factors. *Harvard Review of Psychiatry*, *28*(1), 4–13. doi:10.1097/HRP.0000000000000230 PMID:31913978

Hyseni Duraku, Z., Davis, H., & Hamiti, E. (2023). Mental health, study skills, social support, and barriers to seeking psychological help among university students: A call for mental health support in higher education. *Frontiers in Public Health*, *11*, 1220614. doi:10.3389/fpubh.2023.1220614 PMID:37920583

Iddon, J. L., & Grant, L. (2013). Behavioural and cognitive treatment interventions in depression:An analysis of the evidence base. *Open Journal of Depression*, *2*(2), 1–10. doi:10.4236/ojd.2013.22003

Idowu, A., Olawuyi, D. A., & Nwadioke, C. O. (2020). Impacts of the COVID-19 pandemic on the psychological well-being of students in a Nigerian university. *Journal of Medical and Surgical Research*, *7*, 798–806. doi:10.46327/msrjg.1.000000000000173

Ikeda, M. (2022). What can we do to ensure a level playing field for all students? In *PISA in Focus, No. 117*. OECD Publishing. oi:10.1787/e297c355-

Immordino-Yang, M. H., Christodoulou, J. A., & Singh, V. (2012). Rest is not idleness. *Perspectives on Psychological Science*, *7*(4), 352–364. doi:10.1177/1745691612447308 PMID:26168472

Ingrum, A. (2006). High School Dropout Determinants: The Effect of Socioeconomic Status And Learning Disabilities. *Honors Projects, 24*.

International, Q. S. (2021). Brain food: What to eat when revising. *Top Universities.* https://www.topuniversities.com/blog/brain-food-what-eat-when-revising

Ishii, T., Tachikawa, H., Shiratori, Y., Hori, T., Aiba, M., Kuga, K., & Arai, T. (2018). What kinds of factors affect the academic outcomes of university students with mental disorders? A retrospective study based on medical records. *Asian Journal of Psychiatry, 32*, 67–72. doi:10.1016/j.ajp.2017.11.017 PMID:29216609

Itani, T., Jacobsen, K.H., & Kraemer, A. (2017). Suicidal ideation and planning among Palestinian middle school students living in Gaza Strip, West Bank, and United Nations Relief and Works Agency (UNRWA) camps. *Int J Pediatr Adolesc Med. 4*(2), 54–60. https://doi.org/. 003. doi:10.1016/j.ijpam.2017.03

Izutsu, T., Tsutsumi, A., Minas, H., Thornicroft, G., Patel, V., & Ito, A. (2015). Mental health and wellbeing in the Sustainable Development Goals. *The Lancet. Psychiatry, 2*(12), 1052–1054. doi:10.1016/S2215-0366(15)00457-5 PMID:26613844

Jabbari, B., & Rouster, A. S. (2023). *Family dynamics.* StatPearls Publishing.

Jackson, C., & Sundaram, V. (2020). *Lad culture in Higher Education: Sexism, sexual harassment and violence.* Routledge. doi:10.4324/9780203702901

Jafari, F. (2020). The mediating role of self-compassion in relation between character strengths and flourishing in college students. *International Journal of Happiness and Development, 6*(1), 76–93. doi:10.1504/IJHD.2020.108755

Jaffery, A., & Kishwar, M. (2019). Student's perception of educational environment and their academic performance; Are they related? *Pakistan Armed Forces Medical Journal, 69*(6), 1267–1271.

Jameson, J., Rumyantseva, N., Cai, M., Markowski, M., Essex, R., & McNay, I. (2022). A systematic review, textual narrative synthesis and framework for digital leadership research maturity in Higher Education. *Computers and Education Open, 100115.* Advance online publication. doi:10.1080/03075079.2022.2145278

JCTP. (n.d.). *Code of FairTesting Practices in Education.* APA. https://www.apa.org/science/programs/testing/fair-testing.pdf

Jehi, T., Khan, R., Dos Santos, H., & Majzoub, N. (2022). Effect of COVID-19 outbreak on anxiety among students of higher education; A review of literature. *Current Psychology (New Brunswick, N.J.)*, 1–15. doi:10.100712144-021-02587-6 PMID:35018081

Jemmer, P. (2010). Self-talk: The spells of Psycho-chaotic Sorcery. *European Journal of Clinical Hypnosis, 9*(1), 51–58.

Jeoung, B., Hong, M., & Lee, Y. C. (2013). The relationship between mental health and health-related physical fitness of university students. *Journal of Exercise Rehabilitation, 9*(6), 544–548. doi:10.12965/jer.130082 PMID:24409433

Jessop, D. C., Herberts, C., & Solomon, L. (2005). The impact of financial circumstances on student health. *British Journal of Health Psychology, 10*(3), 421–439. doi:10.1348/135910705X25480 PMID:16238857

Jirek, S. L., & Saunders, D. G. (2018). Cumulative adversity as a correlate of posttraumatic growth: The effects of multiple traumas, discrimination, and sexual harassment. *Journal of Aggression, Maltreatment & Trauma, 27*(6), 612–630. doi:10.1080/10926771.2017.1420720

Jitaru, O., Axinte, R., & Vatavu, C. (2022). The role of personal development in students adapting to the academic life. *Scientific Research and Education in the Airforce.* doi:10.19062/2247-3173.2021.22.10

Joan, C., Finson, B., & Wilson, K. (2021). Challenges that Students Face at The University that May Require Counselling. *International Journal of Academic Research in Business & Social Sciences*, *11*(9), 18–34. doi:10.6007/IJARBSS/v11-i9/10968

Joanna Briggs Institute. (2017). JBI critical appraisal checklist for analytical cross sectional studies. 2017. *Diakses Pada*, *22*, 2019–05.

Jochman, J. C., Cheadle, J. E., Goosby, B. J., Tomaso, C., Kozikowski, C., & Nelson, T. (2019). Mental health outcomes of discrimination among college students on a predominately White campus: A prospective study. *Socius: Sociological Research for a Dynamic World*, *5*, 1–16. doi:10.1177/2378023119842728 PMID:31819906

John N.M., Page O., Martin S.C. &Whittaker P. (2018). Impact of peer support on student mental wellbeing: a systematic review. *MedEdPublish*, *7*, 170 (https://doi.org/ doi:10.15694/mep.2018.0000170.1

Johnson, A. P., & Lester, R. J. (2022). Mental health in academia: Hacks for cultivating and sustaining wellbeing. *American Journal of Human Biology*, *34*(S1), e23664. doi:10.1002/ajhb.23664 PMID:34357661

Johnson, S. J., Willis, S. M., & Evans, J. (2019). An Examination of Stressors, Strain, and Resilience in Academic and Non-Academic U.K. University Job Roles. *International Journal of Stress Management*, *26*(2), 162–172. doi:10.1037tr0000096

Joing, I., Vors, O., & Potdevin, F. (2020). The subjective well-being of students in diferent parts of the school premises in French middle schools. *Child Indicators Research*, *13*(4), 1469–1487. doi:10.100712187-019-09714-7

Jones, M. G., & Ennes, M. (2018). *High-stakes testing* [Dataset]. doi:10.1093/obo/9780199756810-0200

Jones, G. A. (2012). Why Chunking Should be Considered as an Explanation for Developmental Change before Short-Term Memory Capacity and Processing Speed. *Frontiers in Psychology*, *3*. doi:10.3389/fpsyg.2012.00167 PMID:22715331

Jordan, L. (2021). *Disillusioned, Disenchanted, Disembodied? Towards a Collective Imagination of the University. In the Promise of the University*. Springer. doi:10.1007/978-981-16-5277-6_14

Joyce-Beaulieu, D., & Zaboski, B. (2020). Raising the emotional wellbeing of students with anxiety and depression. *Fostering the Emotional Wellbeing of our Youth*, (pp. 435–458). Oxford press. doi:10.1093/med-psych/9780190918873.003.0022

Juergens, J. (2020). *Prescription study aid abuse*. Addiction Center. https://www.addictioncenter.com/college/prescription-study-aid-abuse/

Jumani, N. B., Bhatti, A. J., & Malik, S. (2013). Student Support in Higher Education: Lessons Learnt and Challenges Ahead. *International Journal of Technology and Educational Marketing*, *3*(1), 77–88. doi:10.4018/ijtem.2013010106

Kabagenyi, A., Baiden, F., Schmied, V., & Javanparast, S. (2020). The impact of the COVID-19 pandemic on academic performance and wellbeing of university students: Implications for policy and practice. *International Journal of Educational Development*, *85*, 102388. oi:10.1016/j.ijedudev.2020.102388

Kahneman, D. (2011). *Thinking, fast and slow*. NII. http://ci.nii.ac.jp/ncid/BB2184891X

Kajjimu, J., Kaggwa, M. M., & Bongomin, F. (2021, January). Burnout and associated factors among medical students in a Public University in Uganda: A cross-sectional study. *Advances in Medical Education and Practice*, *12*, 63–75. doi:10.2147/AMEP.S287928 PMID:33531852

Kalagher, S. S., & Curran, R. D. (2023). Crafting and revising your student conduct code. *Student Conduct Practice*, (pp. 36–57). Taylor & Francis. doi:10.4324/9781003447177-4

Kalkan, F., & Dağlı, E. (2021). The relationships between school climate school belonging and school burnout in secondary school students. *International Journal of Contemporary Educational Research*, *8*(4), 59–79. doi:10.33200/ijcer.878682

Kalkbrenner, M. T., Jolley, A. L., & Hays, D. G. (2019). Faculty Views on College Student Mental Health: Implications for Retention and Student Success. *Journal of College Student Retention*, *23*(3), 636–658. doi:10.1177/1521025119867639

Kalra, G., Christodoulou, G. N., Jenkins, R., Tsipas, V., Christodoulou, N., Lečić-Toševski, D., Mezzich, J. E., & Bhugra, D. (2012). Mental health promotion: Guidance and strategies. *European Psychiatry*, *27*(2), 81–86. doi:10.1016/j.eurpsy.2011.10.001 PMID:22197146

Kamaludin, K., Chinna, K., Sundarasen, S., Khoshaim, H. B., Nurunnabi, M., Baloch, G. M., Sukayt, A., & Hossain, S. F. A. (2020). Coping with COVID-19 and movement control order (MCO): Experiences of university students in Malaysia. *Heliyon*, *6*(11), e05339. doi:10.1016/j.heliyon.2020.e05339 PMID:33134570

Kandasamy, N., Indraah, K., Tukiman, N. A., Khalil Kusairi, F. W. K., Amir Sjarif, S. I., & Shahrul Nizar, M. S. S. (2020). Factors that influence mental illness among students in public universities. *Journal of Business and Economic Analysis*, *3*(1), 77–90. doi:10.1142/j_10.36924sbe.2020.3106

Karaman, M. A., Lerma, E., Vela, J. C., & Watson, J. C. (2019). Predictors of academic stress among college students. *Journal of College Counseling*, *22*(1), 41–55. doi:10.1002/jocc.12113

Karimzadeh, M., Rostami, M., Teymouri, R., Moazzen, Z., & Tahmasebi, S. (2017). The association between parental mental health and behavioral disorders in pre-school children. *Electronic Physician*, *9*(6), 4497–4502. doi:10.19082/4497 PMID:28848622

Karugahe, W., & Lambert, J. (2021). Gender, role in domestic violence as victim or perpetrator and coping strategies in Uganda: Implications for gender-inclusive counsellors. *Asia Pacific Journal of Counselling and Psychotherapy*, *12*(1), 58–72. doi:10.1080/21507686.2021.1876113

Katz, D. S., & Davison, K. (2014). Community College Student Mental Health: A Comparative Analysis. *Community College Review*, *42*(4), 307–326. doi:10.1177/0091552114535466

Kaur, S., Christian, H., Cooper, M. N., Francis, J., Allen, K. L., & Trapp, G. (2020). Consumption of energy drinks is associated with depression, anxiety, and stress in young adult males: Evidence from a longitudinal cohort study. *Depression and Anxiety*, *37*(11), 1089–1098. doi:10.1002/da.23090 PMID:32845046

Kayla, N., Kayla, S., Amy, M., & Samuel, A. (2018). College students' pereption of family influence impacting their health and lifestyle. *TEACH Journal of Christian Educ*, *12*(2), 10.

Kearns, M., Muldoon, O. T., Msetfi, R. M., & Surgenor, P. W. G. (2015). Understanding help-seeking amongst university students: The role of group identity, stigma, and exposure to suicide and help-seeking. *Frontiers in Psychology*, *6*, 6. doi:10.3389/fpsyg.2015.01462 PMID:26483722

Kebede, M. A., Anbessie, B., & Ayano, G. (2019). Prevalence and predictors of depression and anxiety among medical students in Addis Ababa, Ethiopia. *International Journal of Mental Health Systems*, *13*(1), 30. doi:10.118613033-019-0287-6 PMID:31080499

Keeling, R. P. (2014). An Ethic of Care in Higher Education: Well-Being and Learning. *Journal of College and Character*, *15*(3), 141–148. doi:10.1515/jcc-2014-0018

Kennedy, D. R., Clapp, P., DeLuca, J. L., Filtz, T. M., Kroon, L., Lamberts, J. T., Oliphant, C. M., Prescott, W. A., & Ray, S. D. (2022). Enhancing Pharmacy Faculty Well-Being and Productivity While Reducing Burnout. *American Journal of Pharmaceutical Education*, *86*(5), 8764. doi:10.5688/ajpe8764 PMID:34507961

Kenney, M., & Müller, R. (2017). Of rats and women: Narratives of motherhood in environmental epigenetics. *Biosocieties*, *12*(1), 23–46. doi:10.105741292-016-0002-7

Kerr, H. (2013). *Mental distress survey overview.* MRS Evidence Matters: United Kingdom. https://www.nus.org.uk/Global/Campaigns/20130517%20Mental%20Distress%20Survey%20%20Overview.pdf.

Kessler, R. C., Aguilar-Gaxiola, S., Alonso, J., Chatterji, S., Ormel, J., Üstün, T. B., & Wang, P. S. (2011). *The global burden of mental disorders: An update from the WHO World Mental Health (WMH).* Surveys.

Keyes, C. L. M., Eisenberg, D., Perry, G. S., Dube, S. R., Kroenke, K., & Dhingra, S. S. (2012). The Relationship of level of positive mental health with current mental disorders in predicting suicidal behavior and academic impairment in college students. *Journal of American College Health*, *2*(2), 34–46. doi:10.1080/07448481.2011.608393 PMID:22316409

Khatoon, A., & Sharma, M. (2021). Relationship between family environment and academic achievement. *Elementary Education Online*, *20*(1), 3202–3207.

Khodabakhsh, M., Kiani, F. K., & Ahmedbookani, S. (2014). Psychological Well-being and Parenting Styles as Predictors of Mental Health among Students: Implication for Health Promotion. *International Journal of Pediatrics*, *2*, 39–46.

Kibbe, M. R., Pellegrini, C. A., Townsend, C. M. Jr, Helenowski, I. B., & Patti, M. G. (2016). Characterization of Mentorship Programs in Departments of Surgery in the United States. *JAMA Surgery*, *151*(10), 900–906. doi:10.1001/jamasurg.2016.1670 PMID:27383863

Kiburi, R. K. (2022). *Challenges, Coping Mechanisms and the Support Accorded to Student Mothers in Academic Pursuit: A Case Study of Egerton University, Nakuru County, Kenya.* [Thesis, Egerton University].

Kidd, I. J. (2021). *Character, Corruption, and 'Cultures of Speed' in Higher Education. In the Promise of the University.* Springer. doi:10.1007/978-981-16-5277-6_2

Kierstead, J. (1980). *Montessori and Dewey: A comparison of their theory and practice* (ED198506). ERIC. https://eric.ed.gov/?id=ED198506

Kılıç, C., & Karahan, F. Ş. (2023). Mental health problems among graduate students in Turkey: A cross-sectional study. *International Journal for the Advancement of Counseling*, *45*(4), 634–650. doi:10.100710447-023-09514-3 PMID:37359032

Kimbrough, E., Magyari, T., Langenberg, P., Chesney, M., & Berman, B. (2010). Mindfulness intervention for child abuse survivors. *Journal of Clinical Psychology*, *66*(1), 17–33. doi:10.1002/jclp.20624 PMID:19998425

Kim, J., Kim, D., & Kamphaus, R. W. (2022). *Early Detection of Mental Health Through Universal Screening at Schools.* Georgia Educational Researcher. doi:10.20429/ger.2022.190104

Kindred, R., & Bates, G. W. (2023). The Influence of the COVID-19 Pandemic on Social Anxiety: A Systematic Review. *International Journal of Environmental Research and Public Health*, *20*(3), 2362. doi:10.3390/ijerph20032362 PMID:36767728

King, L., & Nicolson, M. (2019). *DP ATL Skills Student Workbook: DP ATL Skills. 3i Deal effectively with pressure, stress and anxiety.*

King, V., Boyd, L. M., & Pragg, B. (2018). Parent–adolescent closeness, family belonging, and adolescent well-being across family structures. *Journal of Family Issues*, *39*(7), 2007–2036. doi:10.1177/0192513X17739048 PMID:29805189

Kinman, G. (2014). Doing more with less? Work and wellbeing in academics. *Somatechnics*, *4*(2), 219–235. doi:10.3366oma.2014.0129

Kinman, G. (2019). Effort-reward imbalance in academic employees: Examining different reward systems. *International Journal of Stress Management*, *26*(2), 184–192. doi:10.1037tr0000128

Kinman, G., & Johnson, S. (2019). Special section on well-being in academic employees. *International Journal of Stress Management, 26*(2), 159–161. doi:10.1037tr0000131

Kirby, N., Wright, B., & Allgar, V. (2020). Child mental health and resilience in the context of socioeconomic disadvantage: Results from the Born in Bradford cohort study. *European Child & Adolescent Psychiatry, 29*(4), 467–477. doi:10.100700787-019-01348-y PMID:31243580

Kitzrow, M. A. (2009). The Mental Health Needs of Today's College Students: Challenges and Recommendations. *NASPA Journal, 46*(4), 646–660. doi:10.2202/1949-6605.5037

Kiziela, A., Viliūnienė, R., Friborg, O., & Navickas, A. (2018). Distress and resilience associated with workload of medical students. *Journal of Mental Health (Abingdon, England), 28*(3), 319–323. doi:10.1080/09638237.2018.1521922 PMID:30449227

Klainin-Yobas, P., Ramirez, D., Fernandez, Z., Sarmiento, J., Thanoi, W., Ignacio, J., & Lau, Y. (2016). Examining the Predicting Effect of Mindfulness on Psychological Well-Being among Undergraduate Students: A Structural Equation Modelling Approach. Personal. *Individ.* [CrossRef]. *Personality and Individual Differences, 91*, 63–68. doi:10.1016/j.paid.2015.11.034

Klein, G. (2014). Performing a project premortem. *Harvard Business Review*. https://hbr.org/2007/09/performing-a-project-premortem

Klein, J. T. (2010). A taxonomy of Interdisciplinary. The oxford handbook of Interdisciplinary. In R. Frodeman, J. T. Klein, & C. Mitcham (Eds.), *The Oxford Handbook of Interdisciplinarity* (pp. 15–30). Oxford University Press.

Klein, L. B., Stoner, M. C. D., Bhushan, N. L., Mulholland, G. E., Fisher, B. S., Kupper, L. L., Alam, I. Z., & Martin, S. L. (2022). Sexual harassment of students at institutions of Higher Education: Variations in students' experiences, knowledge, and perceptions across institutions. *Feminist Criminology, 17*(3), 322–342. doi:10.1177/15570851211062572

Klemenčič, M., & Park, B. (2018). *Student politics: Between representation and activism. (Handbook on Politics and Higher Education)*. Edward Edgar.

Kloss, J. D., Nash, C. O., Walsh, C. M., Culnan, E., Horsey, S., & Sexton-Radek, K. (2016). A "Sleep 101" program for college students improves sleep hygiene knowledge and reduces maladaptive beliefs about sleep. *Behavioral Medicine (Washington, D.C.), 42*(1), 48–56. doi:10.1080/08964289.2014.969186 PMID:25268924

Knifsend, C. A. (2020). Intensity of activity involvement and psychosocial well-being among students. *Active Learning in Higher Education, 21*(2), 116–127. doi:10.1177/1469787418760324

Koehler, C., & Schneider, J. (2019). Young refugees in education: The particular challenges of school systems in Europe. *Comparative Migration Studies, 7*(1), 28. doi:10.118640878-019-0129-3

Kong, F., Wang, X., Song, Y., & Liu, J. (2016). Brain regions involved in dispositional mindfulness during resting state and their relation with well-being. *Social Neuroscience, 11*(4), 331–343. doi:10.1080/17470919.2015.1092469 PMID:26360907

Kons, K., Biney, A. A., & Sznajder, K. (2022). Factors associated with adolescent pregnancy in sub-Saharan Africa during the COVID-19 pandemic: A review of socioeconomic influences and essential interventions. *International Journal of Sexual Health, 34*(3), 386–396. doi:10.1080/19317611.2022.2084199

Koopmans, T. A., Geleijnse, J. M., Zitman, F. G., & Giltay, E. J. (2010). Effects of happiness on all-cause mortality during 15 years of follow-up: The Arnhem Elderly Study. *Journal of Happiness Studies, 11*(1), 113–124. doi:10.100710902-008-9127-0

Kotera, Y., Green, P., & Sheffield, D. (2019). Mental health of therapeutic students: Relationships with attitudes, self-criticism, self-compassion, and caregiver identity. *British Journal of Guidance & Counselling, 49*(5), 701–712. doi:10.1080/03069885.2019.1704683

Kowal, M., Coll-Martín, T., Ikizer, G., Rasmussen, J., Eichel, K., Studzińska, A., Koszałkowska, K., Karwowski, M., Najmussaqib, A., Pankowski, D., Lieberoth, A., & Ahmed, O. (2020). Who is the most stressed during the COVID-19 pandemic? Data from 26 countries and areas. *Applied Psychology. Health and Well-Being, 12*(4), 946–966. doi:10.1111/aphw.12234 PMID:32996217

Kukoyi, O., Orok, E., Oluwafemi, F., Oluwadare, T., Oni, O., Bamitale, T., Jaiyesimi, B., Ojo, T., & Eze, H. (2022). *Factors affecting the utilization of mental health services among undergraduate students in a Nigerian University. Heliyon.* Cell Press. doi:10.1016/j.heliyon.2022.e11476

Kumar, N. (2022). Mental health and well-being. Mental. *Applied Psychology. Health and Well-Being*, 1–23. doi:10.4324/9781003350651-1

Kumar, P. A., & Mohideen, F. (2021). Strengths-Based Positive Schooling Interventions: A Scoping Review. *Contemporary School Psychology, 25*(1), 86–98. doi:10.100740688-019-00260-1

Kunjiapu, S., & Kunasegaran, M. (2021). Psychological Wellbeing Among Undergraduates of Higher Learning Institutions in Malaysia. *Psychology and Education, 58*(2), 9179–9187.

Kurki, M., Gilbert, S., Mishina, K., Lempinen, L., Luntamo, T., Hinkka-Yli-Salomäki, S., & Sourander, A. (2021). Digital mental health literacy-program for the first-year medical students' wellbeing: A one group quasi-experimental study. *BMC Medical Education, 21*, 1–11.

Kurniawati, K. D., & Hafina, A. (2020). *The analysis of classroom climate in the perspective of peace psychology.* Atlantis Press. doi:10.2991/assehr.k.200130.093

Kustiani, A., & Fauziyah, P. Y. (2019). Analysis of factors affecting parental participation towards early childhood education program. *Journal of Nonformal Education, 5*(1), 47–56. doi:10.15294/jne.v5i1.18333

Kutcher, S., Wei, Y., & Coniglio, C. (2016). Mental health literacy: Past, present and future. *Canadian Journal of Psychiatry, 61*(3), 154–158. doi:10.1177/0706743715616609 PMID:27254090

Kwaah, C. Y., & Essilfie, G. (2017). Stress and coping strategies among distance education students at the University of Cape Coast, Ghana. *Turkish Online Journal of Distance Education, 18*(3), 120–134. doi:10.17718/tojde.328942

Kyvik, S. (2013). The academic researcher role: Enhancing expectations and improved performance. *Higher Education, 65*(4), 525–538. doi:10.100710734-012-9561-0

Lai, K., Guo, S., Ijadi-Maghsoodi, R., Puffer, M., & Kataoka, S. (2016). Bringing Wellness to Schools: Opportunities for and Challenges to Mental Health Integration in School-Based Health Centers. *Psychiatric Services (Washington, D.C.), 67*(12), 1328–1333. doi:10.1176/appi.ps.201500401 PMID:27417895

Lang, A. (2019). Analysis of burnout and career calling in undergraduate pre-medical students. *Journal of Interdisciplinary Undergraduate Research, 11*(1), 1.

Langley, E. (2018). *Study on triggers that lead to student protests and violent behaviours at the University of Kwazulu-Natal.* [Unpublished Master of Commerce Dissertation, University of Kwa Zulu Natal, South Africa].

Larcombe, W., Finch, S., Sore, R., Murray, C. M., Kentish, S., Mulder, R. A., & Williams, D. (2016). Prevalence and socio-demographic correlates of psychological distress among students at an Australian university. *Studies in Higher Education, 41*(6), 1074–1091. doi:10.1080/03075079.2014.966072

Larson, J. S. (1996). The World Health Organization's Definition of Health: Social Versus Spiritual Health. *Social Indicators Research, 38*(2), 181–192. doi:10.1007/BF00300458

Larson, L. R., Mullenbach, L. E., Browning, M. H., Rigolon, A., Thomsen, J., Metcalf, E. C., Reigner, N. P., Sharaievska, I., McAnirlin, O., D'Antonio, A., Cloutier, S., Helbich, M., & Labib, S. M. (2022). Greenspace and park use associated with less emotional distress among college students in the United States during the COVID-19 pandemic. *Environmental Research, 204*, 112367. doi:10.1016/j.envres.2021.112367 PMID:34774510

Larson, R. W. (2000). Toward a psychology of positive youth development. *The American Psychologist, 55*(1), 170–183. doi:10.1037/0003-066X.55.1.170 PMID:11392861

Laschinger, H. K. S., & Leiter, M. P. (2006). The impact of nursing work environments on patient safety outcomes: The mediating role of burnout engagement. *The Journal of Nursing Administration, 36*(5), 259–267. doi:10.1097/00005110-200605000-00019 PMID:16705307

Lashuel, H. A. (2020). What about faculty? *eLife, 9*, e54551. doi:10.7554/eLife.54551 PMID:31912781

Latcheva, R. (2017). Sexual harassment in the European Union: A Pervasive But Still Hidden Form of Gender-Based Violence. *Journal of Interpersonal Violence, 32*(12), 1821–1852. doi:10.1177/0886260517698948 PMID:30156991

Lattie, E. G., Adkins, E. C., Winquist, N., Stiles-Shields, C., Wafford, Q. E., & Graham, A. K. (2019). Digital mental health interventions for depression, anxiety, and enhancement of psychological well-being among college students: Systematic review. *Journal of Medical Internet Research, 21*(7), e12869. doi:10.2196/12869 PMID:31333198

Lattie, E. G., Cohen, K. A., Hersch, E., Williams, K. D., Kruzan, K. P., MacIver, C., Hermes, J., Maddi, K., Kwasny, M., & Mohr, D. C. (2022). Uptake and effectiveness of a self-guided mobile app platform for college student mental health. *Internet Interventions : the Application of Information Technology in Mental and Behavioural Health, 27*, 100493. doi:10.1016/j.invent.2021.100493 PMID:35036331

Lattie, E. G., Lipson, S. K., & Eisenberg, D. (2019). Technology and college student mental health: Challenges and opportunities. *Frontiers in Psychiatry, 10*(15), 246. doi:10.3389/fpsyt.2019.00246 PMID:31037061

Lauria, M. J., Gallo, I. A., Rush, S., Brooks, J., Spiegel, R., & Weingart, S. D. (2017). Psychological Skills to Improve Emergency Care Providers' Performance Under Stress. *Annals of Emergency Medicine, 70*(6), 884–890. doi:10.1016/j.annemergmed.2017.03.018 PMID:28460863

Lazarus, R. S., & Folkman, S. (2013). Stress: appraisal and coping. In Springer eBooks (pp. 1913–1915). doi:10.1007/978-1-4419-1005-9_215

Lazarus, R. S. (1985). The Psychology of stress and coping. *Issues in Mental Health Nursing, 7*(1–4), 399–418. doi:10.3109/01612848509009463 PMID:3854019

Lazurenko, N., Korolyova, K., Voloshina, I Svischeva (2021). The role of family in the students' educational achievement. *Revista on line de Política e Gestão Educacional,* 2(7), 3986-3997.

Lea, V., & Sims, E. J. (2008). Imaging Whiteness Hegemony in the Classroom: Undoing Oppressive Practice and Inspiring Social Justice Activism. *Counterpoints, 321,* 185–202. https://www.jstor.org/stable/42979967

Lee, M. F. & Syaid, S. (2017). Factors contributing towards Malaysian Technical University (MTU) students' mental health. *Pertanika J. Soc. Sci. & Hum. 25*(S), 93 – 100.

Leong, D., & Bodrova, E. (2006). Developing self-regulation: The vygotskian view. *Academic Exchange Quarterly, 10*(4), 1–10.

Leshner, A. (2021). Target student mental well-being. *Science*, *371*(6527), 325–325. doi:10.1126cience.abg5770 PMID:33479127

Lessard, A., Fortin, L., Butler-Kisber, L., & Marcotte, D. (2014). Analysing the discourse of dropouts and resilient students. *The Journal of Educational Research*, *107*(2), 103–110. doi:10.1080/00220671.2012.753857

LeSueur, I. (2019). An investigation of existential and positive psychological resources in college students. City: Seton Hall University.

Levi-Belz, Y., Gvion, Y., & Apter, A. (2019). The psychology of suicide: From research understandings to intervention and treatment. *Frontiers in Psychiatry*, *10*, 214. doi:10.3389/fpsyt.2019.00214 PMID:31019475

Levi-Belz, Y., Gvion, Y., Grisaru, S., & Apter, A. (2018). When the pain becomes unbearable: A case-control study of mental pain characteristics among medically serious suicide attempters. *Archives of Suicide Research*, *22*(3), 380–393. doi:10.1080/13811118.2017.1355288 PMID:28786756

Levin, D. J. (2021). *Academic stressors, perceived stress, and coping strategies among undergraduate students* [Senior Honours Projects, James Madison University]. https://commons.lib.jmu.edu/honors202029/128

Levitt, J. M., Saka, N., Romanelli, L. H., & Hoagwood, K. E. (2007). Early identification of mental health problems in schools: The status of instrumentation. *Journal of School Psychology*, *45*(2), 163–191. doi:10.1016/j.jsp.2006.11.005

Levula, A., Wilson, A., & Harré, M. (2016). The association between social network factors and mental health at different life stages. *Quality of Life Research: An International Journal of Quality of Life Aspects of Treatment, Care and Rehabilitation*, *25*(7), 1725–1733. doi:10.100711136-015-1200-7 PMID:26669317

Li,C.T., Cao,J., & Li,T.M.H.(2016). *Eustress or distress: an empirical study of perceived stress in everyday college life*, 1209-1217. ACM. doi:10.1145/2968219.2968309

Liao, C., Nong, L., Wu, Y.-F., Wu, Y.-T., & Ye, J.-H. (2023). The relationships between university students' physical activity needs, involvement, flow experience and sustainable well-being in the post-pandemic era. *Sustainability (Basel)*, *15*(11), 8719. doi:10.3390u15118719

Lilienfeld, S. O. (2007). Psychological treatments that cause harm. *Perspectives on Psychological Science*, *2*(1), 53–70. doi:10.1111/j.1745-6916.2007.00029.x PMID:26151919

Lim, A. Y., Lee, S. H., Jeon, Y., Yoo, R., & Jung, H. Y. (2018). Job-seeking stress, mental health problems, and the role of perceived social support in university graduates in Korea. *Journal of Korean Medical Science*, *33*(19), e149. doi:10.3346/jkms.2018.33.e149 PMID:29736162

Limone, P., & Toto, G. A. (2021). Psychological and emotional effects of digital technology on children in Covid-19 pandemic. *Brain Sciences*, *11*(9), 1126. doi:10.3390/brainsci11091126 PMID:34573148

Limone, P., & Toto, G. A. (2022). Factors that predispose undergraduates to mental issues: A cumulative literature review for future research perspectives. *Frontiers in Public Health*, *10*, 10. doi:10.3389/fpubh.2022.831349 PMID:35252101

Limone, P., Zefffferino, R., Toto, G. A., & Tomei, G. (2021). Work stress, mental health and validation of professional stress scale (PSS) in an Italian-speaking teachers' sample. *Healthcare (Basel)*, *9*(11), 1434. doi:10.3390/healthcare9111434 PMID:34828481

Lindell, A. K., & Nicole, C. (2018). Continuity and change in the family system across the transition from adolescence to emerging adulthood. *Marriage & Family Review*, *53*(4), 388–416. doi:10.1080/01494929.2016.1184212

Lipson, S. K., & Eisenberg, D. (2018). Mental health and academic attitudes and expectations in university populations: Results from the healthy minds study. *Journal of Mental Health (Abingdon, England), 27*(3), 205–213. doi:10.1080/09638237.2017.1417567 PMID:29265935

Lipson, S. K., Lattie, E. G., & Eisenberg, D. (2019). Increased Rates of Mental Health Service Utilization by U.S. College Students: 10-Year Population-Level Trends (2007–2017). *Psychiatric Services (Washington, D.C.), 70*(1), 60–63. doi:10.1176/appi.ps.201800332 PMID:30394183

Lipson, S. K., Zhou, S., Abelson, S., Heinze, J., Jirsa, M., Morigney, J., Patterson, A., Singhd, M., & Eisenberg, D. (2022, June 01). Trends in College Student Mental Health and Help-Seeking by Race/Ethnicity: Findings from the national Healthy Minds Study, 2013–2021. *Journal of Affective Disorders, 306*, 138–147. doi:10.1016/j.jad.2022.03.038 PMID:35307411

Lisiecka, A., Chimicz, D., & Lewicka-Zelent, A. (2023). Mental Health Support in Higher Education during the COVID-19 Pandemic: A Case Study and Recommendations for Practice. *International Journal of Environmental Research and Public Health, 20*(6), 4969. doi:10.3390/ijerph20064969 PMID:36981877

Lister, K., Seale, J., & Douce, C. (2021). Mental health in distance learning: A taxonomy of barriers and enablers to student mental wellbeing. *Open Learning*. doi:10.1080/02680513.2021.1899907

Liu, C. H., Stevens, C., Wong, S., Yasui, M., & Chen, J. A. (2019). The prevalence and predictors of mental health diagnoses and suicide among U.S. college students: Implications for addressing disparities in service use. *Depression and Anxiety, 36*(1), 8–17. doi:10.1002/da.22830 PMID:30188598

Liu, J. (2012). Does cram schooling matter? Who goes to cram schools? Evidence from Taiwan. *International Journal of Educational Development, 32*(1), 46–52. doi:10.1016/j.ijedudev.2011.01.014

Livana, P. H., Mubin, M. F., & Basthomi, Y. (2020). "Learning Task" Attributable to Students' Stress During the Pandemic Covid-19. *Jurnal Ilmu Keperawatan Jiwa, 3*(2), 203–208. oi:10.32584/jikj.v3i2.590

Liviatan, I., Trope, Y., & Liberman, N. (2008). Interpersonal similarity as a social distance dimension: Implications for perception of others' actions. *Journal of Experimental Social Psychology, 44*(5), 1256–1269. doi:10.1016/j.jesp.2008.04.007 PMID:19352440

Li, X., Zhang, C., & Li, W. (2015). Does the visibility of greenery increase perceived safety in urban areas? Evidence from the place pulse 1.0 Dataset. *ISPRS International Journal of Geo-Information, 4*(3), 1166–1183. doi:10.3390/ijgi4031166

Li, Z.-S., & Hasson, F. (2020). Resilience, stress, and psychological well-being in nursing students: A systematic review. *Nurse Education Today, 90*(104440), 104440. doi:10.1016/j.nedt.2020.104440 PMID:32353643

Loades, M. E., Chatburn, E., Higson-Sweeney, N., Reynolds, S., Shafran, R., Brigden, A., Linney, C., McManus, M. N., Borwick, C., & Crawley, E. (2020). Rapid systematic review: The impact of social isolation and loneliness on the mental health of children and adolescents in the context of COVID-19. *Journal of the American Academy of Child and Adolescent Psychiatry, 59*(11), 1218–1239. doi:10.1016/j.jaac.2020.05.009 PMID:32504808

Longworth, C., Deakins, J., Rose, D., & Gracey, F. (2016). The nature of self-esteem and its relationship to anxiety and depression in adult acquired brain injury. *Neuropsychological Rehabilitation*, 1–17. PMID:27580356

Loosen, P. T., & Shelton, R. C. (2019). Mood disorders. In M. H. Ebert, J. F. Leckman, & I. L. Petrakis (Eds.), *Current Diagnosis & Treatment: Psychiatry* (3rd ed.). McGraw Hill.

Lopez, V., Yobas, P., Chow, Y. L., & Shorey, S. (2018). Does building resilience in undergraduate nursing students happen through clinical placements? A qualitative study. *Nurse Education Today, 67*, 1–5. doi:10.1016/j.nedt.2018.04.020 PMID:29704800

Ludeman, R. B., Osfield, K. J., Hidalgo, E. I., Oste, D., & Wang, H. S. (Eds.). (2009). *Student Affairs and Services in Higher Education: Global Foundations, Issues and Best Practices*. UNESCO.

Ludmerer, K. M. (1999). *Time to heal: American medical education from the turn of the century to the era of managed care*. Oxford University Press.

Luescher-Mamashela, T., Moja, T., & Schreiber, B. (2013). Towards a professionalisation of student affairs in Africa. *Journal of Student Affairs in Africa*, *1*(1&2). oi:10.14426/jsaa.v1i1-2.181q1

Luescher, T., Loader, L., & Mugume, T. (2017). Feesmustfall: An internet-age student movement in South Africa and the case of The University of The Free State. *Politikon: South African Journal of Political Studies*, *44*(2), 231–245. do i:10.1080/02589346.2016.1238644

Luo, L. (2022). The practice of psychological well-being education model for poor university students from the perspective of positive psychology. *Frontiers in Psychology*, *13*, 951668. doi:10.3389/fpsyg.2022.951668 PMID:35978785

Macaskill, A. (2013). The mental health of university students in the United Kingdom. *British Journal of Guidance & Counselling*, *41*(4), 426–441. doi:10.1080/03069885.2012.743110

Maddux, J. E. (2016). Self-efficacy. In *Interpersonal and intrapersonal expectancies* (pp. 41–46). Routledge. doi:10.4324/9781315652535-5

Madsen, T. (2020). Between frustration and education: Transitioning students' stress and coping through the lens of semiotic cultural psychology. *Theory & Psychology*, *31*(1), 61–83. doi:10.1177/0959354320944496

Magnusson, J. E., & van Roon, C. A. (2013). Determining the Effectiveness of Personalized Versus Prescribed Self-Talk on Athletic Performance for Elite and Novice Athletes. *American Journal of Applied Psychology*, *1*(1), 1–6. oi:10.12691/ajap-1-1-1

Mahon, Á. (2021). *The Promise of the University: Reclaiming Humanity, Humility, and Hope* (Vol. 10). Springer Nature. doi:10.1007/978-981-16-5277-6_1

Maier, S. L., & DePrince, B. T. (2020). College students' fear of crime and perception of safety: The influence of personal and University prevention measures. *Journal of Criminal Justice Education*, *31*(1), 63–81. doi:10.1080/10511253.2019.1656757

Maina, G., Mauri, M., & Rossi, A. (2016). Anxiety and depression. *Journal of Psychopathology*, (22), 236–250.

Makarowski, R., Piotrowski, A., Predoiu, R., Görner, K., Predoiu, A., Mitrache, G., & Nikkhah-Farkhani, Z. (2020). Stress and coping during the COVID-19 pandemic among martial arts athletes: A cross-cultural study. *Archives of Budo*, *16*, 161–171.

Malkoc, A., & Yalcin, I. (2015). Relationships among Resilience, Social Support, Coping, and Psychological Well-Being among University Students. *Turk. Psychol. Couns. Guid. J.*, *5*, 35–43.

Mamun, M. A., Hossain, M. S., & Griffiths, M. D. (2019). Mental health problems and associated predictors among Bangladeshi students. *International Journal of Mental Health and Addiction*, 1–15. doi:10.100711469-019-00144-8

Manalo, E. (2018). Teaching and learning support services. *Wellbeing in Higher Education*, (pp. 161-173). Taylor & Francis. doi:10.4324/9781315641539-16

Manap, R., Hamid, A. S., & Ghani, A. M. (2019). Depression, Anxiety and Stress Among Undergraduate Students. *Journal of Social Sciences and Humanities*, *16*(2), 1–7.

Manap, R., Hamid, S. A., & Ghani, M. A. (2018). Depression, anxiety and stress among undergraduate students. *Journal of Social Sciences and Humanities*, *16*(2), 1–7.

Mangus, L., Somers, C., Yoon, J., Partridge, T., & Pernice, F. (2021). Examination of college student achievement within an ecological framework. *Journal of Adult and Continuing Education*, *27*(2), 231–247. doi:10.1177/1477971420963434

Manwell, L. A., Barbic, S. P., Roberts, K., Durisko, Z., Lee, C., Ware, E., & McKenzie, K. (2015). What is mental health? Evidence towards a new definition from a mixed methods multidisciplinary international survey. *BMJ Open*, *007079*(6), e007079. doi:10.1136/bmjopen-2014-007079 PMID:26038353

Marandet, E., & Wainwright, E. (2010). Invisible Experiences: Understanding the Choices And Needs of University Students with Dependent Children. *British Educational Research Journal*, *36*(5), 787–805. doi:10.1080/01411920903165595

Mardhiyah, S. A. (2021). Mental health literacy and psychological distress as predictors of psychological well-being in Sriwijaya University students. *Mental Health: Global Challenges*, *4*(1), 49–60. doi:10.32437/mhgcj.v4i1.114

Maringe, F., & Chiramba, O. (2022). Disruptions in higher education: Mitigating issues of access and success in the COVID-19 pandemic. *South African Journal of Higher Education*, *36*(4), 6–20. doi:10.20853/36-4-5382

Markovits, D. (2019). The Meritocracy Trap: How America's foundational myth feeds inequality, dismantles the middle class, and devours the elite. https://openlibrary.org/books/OL28209037M/The_Meritocracy_Trap

Marquez, C. G. (2019). A review on first-generation college students: Challenges they face in college when dealing with mental health issues. *UC Merced Undergraduate Research Journal*, *11*(2). doi:10.5070/M4112043709

Mart'ınez-Fern'andez, M. J., Díaz-Aguado, M. J., Chacón, J. C., & Martín-Babarro, J. (2021). Student misbehaviour and school climate: A multilevel study. *Psicologia Educativa*, *27*(1), 1–11. doi:10.5093/psed2020a10

Marthoenis,. (2018). Cultural background, social support and mental health of college students. *Proceedings of the Aceh International Nursing Conference*. ScitePress. doi:10.5220/0008396702210227

Martineau, M., Beauchamp, G., & Marcotte, D. (2017). Efficacy of mental health prevention and promotion strategies in higher education. *Sante Mentale au Quebec*, *42*, 165–182. doi:10.7202/1040249ar PMID:28792567

Martínez-Líbano, J., & Yeomans Cabrera, M. M. (2021). Suicidal ideation and suicidal thoughts in university students during the COVID-19 pandemic. *Systematic Reviews*, *XXX*(2), 390–405. oi:10.24205/03276716.2020.4038

Martínez-Martí, M. L., & Ruch, W. (2016). Character strengths predict resilience over and above positive affect, self-efficacy, optimism, social support, self-esteem, and life satisfaction. *The Journal of Positive Psychology*, *12*(2), 110–119. doi:10.1080/17439760.2016.1163403

Martin, J., Martin, W., & Slemon, A. G. (1989). Cognitive-mediational models of action-act sequences in counseling. *Journal of Counseling Psychology*, *36*(1), 8–16. doi:10.1037/0022-0167.36.1.8

Massey, K. D. (2019). Student affairs and services in Canadian higher education. *Preparing Students for Life and Work*, (pp. 78–97). Brill. doi:10.1163/9789004393073_005

Maunah, B. (2019). The contribution of family and community education in realizing the goals of school education. *American Journal of Education and Learning*, *4*(2), 292–301. doi:10.20448/804.4.2.292.301

Maunder, R. E., & LaMothe, J. (2020). Using mobile phones to capture emotions and experiences in situation: A study of feasibility and user experience. *Journal of Mixed Methods Research*, *14*(4), 416–435.

Ma, X., Shen, J., Krenn, H. Y., Hu, S., & Yuan, J. (2016). A meta-analysis of the relationship between learning outcomes and parental involvement during early childhood education and early elementary education. *Educational Psychology Review*, *28*(4), 771–801. doi:10.100710648-015-9351-1

Mayaba, N. N., Ralarala, M. K., & Angu, P. (2018). Student voice: Perspectives on language and critical pedagogy in South African higher education. *Educational Research for Social Change*, *7*(1), 1–12. doi:10.17159/2221-4070/2018/v7i1a1

Mayo Clinic. (2019). *Anxiety disorders-Symptoms and causes.* Mayo Clinic. www.mayoclinic.org/diseases-conditions/anxiety/symptoms-causes/sync-20350961

Mbongo, E.N., Möwes, A.D. & Chata, C.C. (2016). Factors impacting the implementation of guidance and counselling in secondary schools in the Ohangwena Region of Namibia. *International Journal for innovation, education and research, 4*(5).

McCreary, D. R. (2021). Psychology of Men and Masculinities: Implications for Men's Experiences of Posttraumatic Stress Disorder. In authors Handbook of Posttraumatic Stress (pp. 177-197). Routledge.

McGill. (2023). *Current applicant statistics*. Undergraduate Medical Admissions. https://www.mcgill.ca/medadmissions/after-youve-applied/currentapplicantstats

McGorry, P. D., Mei, C., Chanen, A., Hodges, C., Alvarez-Jimenez, M., & Killackey, E. (2022). Designing and scaling up integrated youth mental health care. *World Psychiatry; Official Journal of the World Psychiatric Association (WPA)*, *21*(1), 61–76. doi:10.1002/wps.20938 PMID:35015367

McIntyre, N. A., Mulder, K. T., & Mainhard, M. T. (2020). Looking to relate: Teacher gaze and culture in student-rated teacher interpersonal behaviour. *Social Psychology of Education*, *23*(2), 411–431. doi:10.100711218-019-09541-2

McKinney, C., Morse, M., & Pastuszak, J. (2016). Effective and Ineffective Parenting: Associations with Psychological Adjustment in Emerging Adults. *Journal of Family Issues*, *37*(9), 1203–1225. doi:10.1177/0192513X14537480

McKinnon-Crowley, S. (2021). College belonging: How first-year and first-generation college students navigate campus life by Lisa M. Nunn. *Review of Higher Education*, *45*(2), 270–273. doi:10.1353/rhe.2021.0024

McMahon, G., Creaven, A., & Gallgher, S. (2020). Stressful life events and adolescent well being: The role of parents and peer relationships. *Stress and Health*, *36*(3), 299–310. doi:10.1002mi.2923 PMID:31920010

McNally, A., & Susan, M. (2018). *Early Alert Programme Presentation Orientation.* NUST.

McPhillips, D. (2023). *Mental health struggles are driving more college students to consider dropping out, survey.* Finds Edition. finds.edition.cnn.com/2023/03/23/health/mental-health-college-dropout-survey-wellness/index.html

Meeus, W. (2016). Adolescent psychosocial development: A review of longitudinal models and research. *Developmental Psychology*, *52*(12), 1969–1993. doi:10.1037/dev0000243 PMID:27893243

Mehnert, A., Berg, P., Henrich, G., & Herschbach, P. (2009). Fear of cancer progression and cancer-related intrusive cognitions in breast cancer survivors. *Journal Of The Psychological. Psycho-Oncology*, *18*(12), 1273–1280. doi:10.1002/pon.1481 PMID:19267364

Mellins, C. A., Walsh, K., Sarvet, A. L., Wall, M., Gilbert, L., Santelli, J. S., Thompson, M., Wilson, P. A., Khan, S., Benson, S., Bah, K., Kaufman, K. A., Reardon, L., & Hirsch, J. S. (2017). Sexual assault incidents among college undergraduates: Prevalence and factors associated with risk. *PLoS One*, *12*(11), 1–23. doi:10.1371/journal.pone.0186471 PMID:29117226

Mercier, J., Powell, C., Langdon-Pole, G., Finau, D., Hicks, K., Bourchier, L., & Hampton, J. (2019). The five Cs of positive youth development in an Aotearoa/New Zealand program context. *Journal of Youth Development, 14*(4), 36–58. doi:10.5195/jyd.2019.774

Mergler, A., & Boman, P. (2020). Promoting good mental health and supporting social and emotional wellbeing. *Developing Positive Classroom Environments*, (pp. 228-244). Taylor & Francis. doi:10.4324/9781003115335-18

Merriam-Webster. (2020). All-nighter. *Merriam-Webster.* https://www.merriamwebster.com/dictionary/all-nighter

Mhata, N.T., Ntlantsana, V., Tomita, A.M., Mwambene, K., & Saloojee, S. (2023). Prevalence of depression, anxiety and burnout in medical students at the University of Namibia. *S Afr J Psychiatr, 31*(29), 2044. doi: . v29i0.2044. PMID: 37292521; PMCID: PMC10244924. doi:10.4102/sajpsychiatry

Mhata, N. T., Ntlantsana, V., Tomita, A. M., Mwambene, K., & Saloojee, S. (2023). Prevalence of depression, anxiety and burnout in medical students at the University of Namibia. *The South African Journal of Psychiatry : SAJP : the Journal of the Society of Psychiatrists of South Africa, 31*(29). doi:10.4102ajpsychiatry.v29i0.2044 PMID:37292521

Mihai, A. (2021). *Mental health stigma on campus: The promotion of mental wellbeing to Ryerson students.* Toronto Metropolitan University. doi:10.32920/ryerson.14668134.v1

MijsJ. J. B. (2018). The Unfulfillable Promise of Meritocracy: Three Lessons and their Implications for Justice in Education. SocArXiv *Papers.* https://doi.org/ doi:10.31235/osf.io/6w9rg

Miller, D. N., Gilman, R., & Martens, M. P. (2008). Wellness promotion in the schools: Enhancing students' mental and physical health. *Psychology in the Schools, 45*(1), 5–15. doi:10.1002/pits.20274

Minasi, P., Jr. (2022, January 24). *Reflecting on the Kaplan med school admissions officers survey.* Med Educators Blog. https://www.kaptest.com/blogs/med-educators/author/petros-minasi

Mindell, J. A., Bartle, A., Abd Wahab, N., Ahn, Y., Ramamurthy, M. B., Huong, H. T. D., Kohyama, J., Ruangdaraganon, N., Sekartini, R., Teng, A., & Goh, D. Y. (2011). Sleep education in medical school curriculum: A glimpse across countries. *Sleep Medicine, 12*(9), 928–931. doi:10.1016/j.sleep.2011.07.001 PMID:21924951

Mirza, A. A., Baig, M., Beyari, G. M., Halawani, M. A., & Mirza, A. A. (2021). Depression and anxiety among medical students: A brief overview. *Advances in Medical Education and Practice, 12*, 393–398. doi:10.2147/AMEP.S302897 PMID:33911913

Mischel, W., Cantor, N., & Feldman, S. (1996). Principles of self-regulation: The nature of willpower and self-control. In E. T. Higgins & A. W. Kruglanski (Eds.), *Social Psychology: Handbook of basic principles* (pp. 329–360). Guilford.

Mishra, J., Samanta, P., Panigrahi, A., Dash, K., Behera, M. R., & Das, R. (2023). Mental health status, coping strategies during Covid-19 pandemic among undergraduate students of healthcare profession. *International Journal of Mental Health and Addiction, 21*(1), 562–574. doi:10.100711469-021-00611-1 PMID:34393684

Misra, R., & Castillo, L. G. (2004). Academic Stress among College Students: Comparison of American &b International Students. *International Journal of Stress Management, 3*(2), 1–10. doi:10.1037/1072-5245.11.2.132

Misra, R., & McKean, M. (2000). College students' academic stress and its relation to their anxiety, time management, and leisure satisfaction. *American Journal of Health Studies, 16*(1), 41–51.

Misra, R., McKean, M., West, S., & Russo, T. (2000). Academic Stress of College Students: Comparison of student and faculty perceptions. *College Student Journal, 34*(2), 236–245.

*Mission Laïque Française , (*2020, May 17). *Réinventer l'éducation, une nécessité - Mission laïque française.* Mission Laïque Française. https://www.mlfmonde.org/tribunes/reinventer-leducation-une-necessite/

Mitra, S. (2013). Should students be allowed to use the internet in exams? The Guardian. https://www.theguardian.com/teacher-network/teacher-blog/2013/jun/17/ipads-exams-teaching-test-schools

Mofatteh, M. (2021). Risk factors associated with stress, anxiety, and depression among university undergraduate students. *AIMS Public Health, 8*(1), 36–65. doi:10.3934/publichealth.2021004 PMID:33575406

Mohammad, M.S., Kobra, K., Ebrahim, M., & Farhad, F.A. (2015). *The Role of Mental Health on Academic Performance of University Students with the Meditation of Academic Achievement Motivation.*

Mohd, N. M. N., Nahar, H. S., Alrazi, B., & Taha, R. (2019). Stress among accounting students: A preliminary study of Malaysian Universities. *Journal of Business and Social Development, 7*(1), 9–19.

Molla- Jafar, H., Salabifard, S., Mousavi, S. M., and Sobhani, Z. (2015). The effectiveness of group training of CBT-based stress management on anxiety, psychological hardiness and general self-efficacy among university students. *Glob. J. Health Sci.* 8, 47–54. doi: . v8n6p47. doi:10.5539/gjhs

Mollah Jérusalem. (2019, September 20). *Comment notre alimentation influence notre santé mentale | ARTE* [Video]. YouTube. https://www.youtube.com/watch?v=IM-YhqnybJM

Mónaco, E., Schoeps, K., & Montoya-Castilla, I. (2019). Attachment styles and well-being in adolescents: How does emotional development affect this relationship? *International Journal of Environmental Research and Public Health, 16*(14), 2554. doi:10.3390/ijerph16142554 PMID:31319570

Montagni, I., Tzourio, C., Cousin, T., Sagara, J. A., Bada-Alonzi, J., & Horgan, A. (2020). Mental health-related digital use by university students: A systematic review. *Telemedicine Journal and e-Health, 26*(2), 131–146. doi:10.1089/tmj.2018.0316 PMID:30888256

Morales-Rodríguez, F. M., Espigares-López, I., Brown, T., & Pérez-Mármol, J. M. (2020). The Relationship between Psychological Well-Being and Psychosocial Factors in University Students. *International Journal of Environmental Research and Public Health, 17*(13), 4778. doi:10.3390/ijerph17134778 PMID:32630816

Moreau, M. P., & Kerner, C. (2015). Care In Academia: An Exploration of Student Parents' Experiences. *British Journal of Sociology of Education, 36*(2), 215–233. doi:10.1080/01425692.2013.814533

Morgan, J. (2021). International student perceptions of the UK higher education experience during the pandemic. *International Student Barometer.* https://services.isb.world/reports/2021/ISB_UK_HEI_COVID_19_Whitepaper_2021.pdf

Morgan, B., & Simmons, L. (2021). A 'PERMA' response to the pandemic: an online positive education programme to promote wellbeing in university students. In *Frontiers in Education, 6.* Frontiers Media South Africa. doi:10.3389/feduc.2021.642632

Morgan, D., & Hoffman, K. (2018). Focus groups. In *U. Flick The sage handbook of qualitative data collection* (pp. 250–263). SAGE Publications Ltd. doi:10.4135/9781526416070.n16

Morin, A. (1993). Self-talk and self-awareness:On the nature of the relation. *Journal of Mind and Behavior, 14*(3), 223–234. https://philpapers.org/rec/MORSAS

Morin, A. (1995). Preliminary data on a relation between self-talk and complexity of the self-concept. *Psychological Reports, 76*(1), 1–10. doi:10.2466/pr0.1995.76.1.267 PMID:7770579

Morrish, L. (2019). *Pressure Vessels: The Epidemic of poor mental health among higher education staff.* Higher Education Policy Institute. https://www.hepi.ac.uk/wp-content/uploads/2019/05/HEPI-Pressure-Vessels-Occasional-Paper-20.pdf

Mshenga, R. (2022). Effect of sexual harassment affect students. *International Journal of Novel Research in Healthcare and Nursing*, *9*(3), 160–165.

Mubita, K. (2021). Understanding school safety and security: Conceptualization and definition. *Journal of Lexicography and Terminology*, *5*(1), 76–86.

Muhammad Asyraf Haziq Rossli, K. M. (2021). Determinants of academic fraud in higher education institutions: A fraud triangle perspective. *Psychology (Savannah, Ga.)*, *58*(2), 3879–3892. doi:10.17762/pae.v58i2.2653

Muhammad, B. M.(2020). The effect of learning environment towardspsychological wellbeing and academic achievement of University Students. *Palarch's Journal of Archaeology of Egypt/Egyptology 17*(2), 1-11.

Murphy, B. (2021). *How the pandemic has spiked stress for many med school applicants.* American Medical Association. https://www.ama-assn.org/medical-students/preparing-medical-school/how-pandemic-has-spiked-stress-many-med-school-applicants

Murray, J., & DeBerard, S. (2022). *Biopsychosocial model and health.* Biopsychosocial Model and Health., doi:10.4324/9780367198459-REPRW63-1

Musika, F., & Bukaliya, R. (2015). The Effectiveness of Counseling on Students' Learning Motivation in Open and Distance Education. *International Journal of Research in Humanities and Social Studies*, *2*(7), 85.

Muthonde, C. K. (2022). Sexual harassment and related policy in Higher Institutions of Learning in Kenya. In L. A. Wakiaga (Ed.), *Women's contribution to Higher Education and social transformation. Implications for policy and praxis from Kenya* (pp. 51–67). Springer International Publishing. doi:10.1007/978-3-030-95622-6_4

Mutinta, G. (2022). undefined. *BMC Psychology*, *10*(1). doi:10.118640359-022-00903-8 PMID:35982493

Muynck, G., Vansteenkiste, M., Delrue, J., & Aelterman, N. (2017). The effects of feedback valence and style on need satisfaction, self-talk, and perseverance among tennis players: An experimental study. *Journal of Sport & Exercise Psychology*, *39*(1), 1–38. doi:10.1123/jsep.2015-0326 PMID:28253062

Naeemi, S., & Tamam, E. (2017). The relationship between emotional dependence on Facebook and psychological well-being in adolescents aged 13–16. *Child Indicators Research*, *10*(4), 1095–1106. doi:10.100712187-016-9438-3

Naidoo, P., Theron, L., & Esterhuizen, T. M. (2021). Mental health outcomes during the COVID-19 pandemic among South African university students. *South African Journal of Psychology. Suid-Afrikaanse Tydskrif vir Sielkunde*, *51*(2), 204–216. oi:10.1177/00812463211017913

Nair, B., & Otaki, F. (2021). Promoting university students' mental health: A systematic literature review introducing the 4M-model of individual-level interventions. *Frontiers in Public Health, 9.* httpss:// doi:10.3389/fpubh.2021.699030

Namibia Council of Higher Education (NCHE). (2020). *2019 Namibia higher education statistical yearbook.* Ministry of Higher Education, Technology and Innovation.

Namibia Council of Higher Education (NCHE). (2021). *2020 Namibia higher education statistical yearbook.* Ministry of Higher Education, Technology and Innovation.

Namibia University of Science and Technology. (2023). *NUST social welfare services.* NUST. https://www.nust.na/dss/social-welfare

Nami, Y., Nami, M. S., & Eishani, K. A. (2014). The Students' Mental Health Status. *Procedia: Social and Behavioral Sciences, 114*, 840–844. doi:10.1016/j.sbspro.2013.12.794

Naom, O. (2020). *Influence of sexual harassment on High School Students' self-esteem in selected Secondary Schools in Nyamira and Kiambu Counties, Kenya*. [Unpublished PhD Thesis, Kenyatta University, Kenya].

National Academies of Science, Engineering, and Medicine. (2016). *Preventing Bullying through Science, Policy, and Practice*. Washington, DC: The National Academies Press.

National Academies of Sciences. (2021). Engineering; and Medicine, Health and Medicine Division, Policy and Global Affairs, Board on Health Sciences Policy, Board on Higher Education and Workforce, & Committee on Mental Health; Substance Use; and Wellbeing in STEM Undergraduate and Graduate Education. Mental health, substance use, and wellbeing in higher education: Supporting the whole student. National Academies Press.

National College Health Assessment. (2015). *Annual Report sponsored by the American College Health Assessment*. ACHA-NCHA.

National Institute of Mental Health (NIMH). (n.d.). *Suicide. Bethesda, MD*. NIMH. https://www.nimh.nih.gov/ health/ statistics/suicide.shtml

National Institute on Alcohol Abuse and Alcoholism (NIH). (2020). College Drinking. *National Institute on Alcohol Abuse and Alcoholism*. https://www.niaaa.nih.gov/publications/brochures-and-fact-sheets/college-drinking

Neck, C. P., & Manz, C. C. (1992). Thought self-leadership: The influence of self-talk and mental imagery on performance. *Journal of Organizational Behavior, 13*(7), 681–699. doi:10.1002/job.4030130705

Neff, K. D., & Dahm, K. A. (2015). Self-compassion: What it is, what it does, and how it relates to mindfulness. Handbook of mindfulness and self-regulation, 121-137.

Neff, K. D., & Costigan, A. P. (2014). Self-compassion, well-being, and happiness. *Psychologie in Österreich, 2*(3), 114–119.

Neupert, S. (2022). *Mental health, stress and student wellbeing*. Wicked Problems, Wolfpack Solutions. doi:10.52750/300976

Newhart, S. (2019). *The influence of family functioning on social competence, social support, and mental health among college students*. [Unpublished Doctor of Education Dissertation, The College of William and Mary, Virginia].

Ng, K. Y., & Earley, P. C. (2006). Cultural intelligence as predictor of individuals adaptive performance. *International Area Studies Review, 17*(4), 394–413. doi:10.1177/2233865914550727

Nguyen-Feng, V.N., Greer, C.S., & Frazier, P. (2017). Using online interventions to deliver college student mental health resources: Evidence from randomized clinical trials. *Psychol. Serv, 14*, 481.

Nguyen, H. T. L., Nakamura, K., Seino, K., & Vo, V. T. (2020). Relationships among cyberbullying, parental attitudes, self-harm and suicidal behaviour among adolescents: Results from a school-based survey in Vietnam. *BMC Public Health, 20*(1), 476. doi:10.118612889-020-08500-3 PMID:32276608

NHS England. (2021). *Children and Young People with an Eating Disorder Waiting Times*. NHS England. https://www.england.nhs.uk/statistics/statistical-work-areas/cyped-waiting-times/

NHS. (2023). *Tips on preparing for exams*. nhs.uk. https://www.nhs.uk/mental-health/children-and-young-adults/help-for-teenagers-young-adults-and-students/tips-on-preparing-for-exams/

Nicholls, H., Nicholls, M., Tekin, S., Lamb, D., & Billings, J. (2022). The impact of working in academia on researchers' mental health and well-being: A systematic review and qualitative meta-synthesis. *PLoS One*, *17*(5), e0268890. doi:10.1371/journal.pone.0268890 PMID:35613147

Nielsen, I., Newman, A., Smyth, R., Hirst, G., & Heilemann, B. (2017). The influence of instructor support, family support and psychological capital on the well-being of postgraduate students: A moderated mediation model. *Studies in Higher Education*, *42*(11), 2099–2115. doi:10.1080/03075079.2015.1135116

Nilson, L. B. (2010). *Teaching at its best: A research-based resource for college instructors* (2nd ed.). Jossey-Bass.

Ning, X., Wong, J. P. H., Huang, S., Fu, Y., Gong, X., Zhang, L., Hilario, C., Fung, K. P. L., Yu, M., Poon, M. K. L., Cheng, S., Gao, J., & Jia, C.-X. (2022). Chinese University Students' Perspectives on Help-Seeking and Mental Health Counseling. *International Journal of Environmental Research and Public Health*, *19*(14), 8259. doi:10.3390/ijerph19148259 PMID:35886103

Niu, X., & Snyder, H. R. (2022). The role of maladaptive emotion regulation in the bidirectional relation between sleep and depression in college students during the COVID-19 pandemic. *Anxiety, Stress, and Coping*, *36*(1), 83–96. doi:10.1080/10615806.2022.2073441 PMID:35536737

Ni, Y., Yao, X., Leung, K., Yau, C., Leung, C., Lun, P., & Leung, G. (2020). Depression and post-traumatic stress during major social unrest in Hong Kong: A 10-year prospective cohort study. *Lancet*, *395*(10220), 273–284. doi:10.1016/S0140-6736(19)33160-5 PMID:31928765

Noor, K. M. (2011). Work-life balance and intention to leave among academics in Malaysian public higher education institutions. *International Journal of Business and Social Science*, *2*(11), 1–12.

Norman, L. B., & Ford, J. A. (2019). Undergraduate prescription stimulant misuse and academic strain: The role of college major and graduate school plans. *Journal of Drug Issues*, *49*(4), 756–771. doi:10.1177/0022042619870504

Norman, L., & Ford, J. (2018). Undergraduate prescription stimulant misuse: The impact of academic strain. *Substance Use & Misuse*, *53*(9), 1482–1491. doi:10.1080/10826084.2017.1413393 PMID:29313737

Norrish, J. M., Williams, P., O'Connor, M., & Robinson, J. (2013). An applied framework for positive education. *International Journal of Wellbeing*, *3*(2), 147–161.

Ntshoe, I., Higgs, P., Higgs, L. G., & Wolhuter, C. C. (2008). The changing academic profession in higher education and new managerialism and corporatism in South Africa. *South African Journal of Higher Education*, *22*(2), 391–403. doi:10.4314ajhe.v22i2.25793

Nurrokhmanti, H., Claramita, M., & Utomo, P. S. (2016). Among students' internal factors, should motivation be used as one of recruitments for admission of medical students in Indonesia? *Indosesian Journal of Medical Education*, *5*(2), 59–66.

Nwoke, C. N., Okpalauwaekwe, U., & Bwala, H. (2020). Mental health professional consultations and the prevalence of mood and anxiety disorders among immigrants: Multilevel analysis of the Canadian community health survey. *JMIR Mental Health*, *7*(9), e19168. doi:10.2196/19168 PMID:32801115

Nyamberega (2018). Factors influencing student unrest in Kenya's Secondary Schools:A survey of selected Counties. *The International Journal of Humanities & Social Studies*, *6*(4), 346-356.

O'Keeffe, P. (2013). Mental Illness within Higher Education: Risk Factors, Barriers to Help Seeking and Pressures on Counselling Centres. *JANZSSA. Journal of the Australian and New Zealand Student Services Association*, 1–12.

O'Keeffe, P., Haralambous, B., Egan, R., Heales, E., Baskarathas, S., Thompson, S., & Jerono, C. (2023). Reimagining social work placements in the COVID-19 pandemic. *British Journal of Social Work, 53*(1), 448–470. doi:10.1093/bjsw/bcac124

O'Mahony, H. (2017). The revision diet: what's the best food and drink to help students focus? *The Guardian.* https://www.theguardian.com/education/2017/may/29/the-revision-diet-whats-the-best-food-and-drink-to-help-students-focus

O'Neill, S., McLafferty, M., Ennis, E., Lapsley, C., Bjourson, T., Armour, C., Murphy, S., Bunting, B., & Murray, E. (2018). Socio-demographic, mental health and childhood adversity risk factors for self-harm and suicidal behaviour in College students in Northern Ireland. *Journal of Affective Disorders, 239*, 58–65. doi:10.1016/j.jad.2018.06.006 PMID:29990663

O'Sullivan, K., Clark, S., McGrane, A., Rock, N., Burke, L., Boyle, N., Joksimovic, N., & Marshall, K. (2021). A qualitative study of child and adolescent mental health during the COVID-19 pandemic in Ireland. *International Journal of Environmental Research and Public Health, 18*(3), 1062. doi:10.3390/ijerph18031062 PMID:33504101

Oaes, J. (2023). Namibia. Mental Health Conversation-Stress and Depression among Children and Adolescents is Real. *New Era, 21*(May), 1–3.

Oberle, E., & Schonert-Reichl, K. A. (2016). Stress contagion in the classroom? The link between classroom teacher burnout and morning cortisol in elementary school students. *Social Science & Medicine, 159*, 30–37. doi:10.1016/j.socscimed.2016.04.031 PMID:27156042

Oberst, U., Wegmann, E., Stodt, B., Brand, M., & Chamarro, A. (2017). Negative consequences from heavy social networking in adolescents: The mediating role of fear of missing out. *Journal of Adolescence, 55*(1), 51–60. doi:10.1016/j.adolescence.2016.12.008 PMID:28033503

Odebode, A. (2019). Factors responsible for students' unrest in Nigerian tertiary institutions: Implications for counselling practices. *Mimbar Pendidikan: Jurnal Indonesia untuk Kajian Pendidikan, 4*(2), 93–102.

OECD. (2015). *Helping immigrant students to succeed at school – and beyond.* OECD. https://www.oecd.org/education/Helping-immigrant-students-to-succeed-at-school-and-beyond.pdf

OECD. (2016). Education and training for doctors and nurses: What's happening with numerus clausus policies? In *Health Workforce Policies in OECD Countries: Right Jobs, Right Skills, Right Places.* OECD Publishing. oi:10.1787/9789264239517-6-

Oettingen, G. (2014). *Rethinking Positive Thinking: Inside the New Science of Motivation.* Penguin.

Ogunji, C. V., Nwajiuba, C. A., & Uwakwe, R. C. (2019). Student-Mothers in Higher Education: An Exploratory Study of Challenges and Support System for Inclusion. *Journal of the Nigerian Academy of Education, 15*(2), 278–294.

Oh, H., Marinovich, C., Jay, S., Marsh, J., Zhou, S., & DeVylder, J. E. (2022). COVID-19 factors and self-injurious behaviors among us college students: Findings from the healthy minds study 2020. *Journal of American College Health*, 1–5. doi:10.1080/07448481.2022.2081059 PMID:35728007

Ojediran, T. D., & Emeka, E. A. (2021). Prevalence and predictors of poor mental health outcomes among Nigerian university students during the COVID-19 pandemic. *Frontiers in Psychiatry, 12*, 652028. oi:10.3389/fpsyt.2021.652028

Oladipo, S. A., Awoyinfa, J. O., & Adefarakan, O. S. (2018). Institutional critical factors in University Personnel Security. [IJIBS]. *International Journal of Innovative Business Strategies, 4*(2), 219–227. doi:10.20533/ijibs.2046.3626.2018.0031

Oliffe, J. L., Kelly, M. T., Montaner, G. G., Seidler, Z. E., Ogrodniczuk, J. S., & Rice, S. M. (2022). Masculinity and mental illness in and after men's intimate partner relationships. *SSM. Qualitative Research in Health, 2*, 100039. doi:10.1016/j.ssmqr.2022.100039

Olingo, A. (2020 April 29th). The economy hit hard as services slow down. *Daily Nation P.2*. Nation Media Group: Nairobi, Kenya.

Omodan, B. I. (2016). *Influence of trade unionism on management of Tertiary Institutions in Ekiti State.* [M.Ed. Thesis, Ekiti State University, Ado Ekiti, Nigeria].

Omodan, B. (2023). Addressing the underside of student unrest in South African universities using collegial leadership as approach. *Transformation in Higher Education*, *8*(0), 27. doi:10.4102/the.v8i0.273

Omodan, B. I., & Dube, B. (2019). Bridging the dichotomous gaps between trade unions and management of Tertiary Institutions in Nigeria. *Journal of Social Studies Education Research*, *10*(1), 285–300.

Ondicho, N. K., Njuguna, F. W., & Kombo, K. (2019). Prevalence of students' sexual harassment in Secondary Schools in Nyamira and Kiambu Counties, Kenya. *Journal of Education*, *7*(3), 1–21.

Ong, B., & Cheong, K. C. (2009). Sources of Stress among College Students—The Case of a Credit Transfer Program. *College Student Journal*, *43*, 1279–1286.

Oni, H., Tshitangano, T., & Akinsola, H. (2019). Sexual harassment and victimization of students: A case study of a higher Education Institution In South Africa. *African Health Sciences*, *19*(1), 1478–1485. doi:10.4314/ahs.v19i1.21 PMID:31148975

Onivehu, A. (2021). Causes, consequences and control of student protests. *Sociální Pedagogika. Social Education*, *9*(1), 8–21.

Orfan, S., Ibrahim, F., & Noori, A. (2022). Sexual harassment of higher education female students in Afghanistan: A case study. *Issues in Educational Research*, *32*(2), 659–680.

Organization for Economic Co-operation and Development. (2017). PISA 2015 Results (Volume III). Paris, France.

Ormel, J., Kessler, R. C., & Schoevers, R. (2019). Depression: more treatment but no drop in prevalence: How effective is the treatment? And can we do better? *Current Opinion in Psychiatry*, *32*(4), 348–354. doi:10.1097/YCO.0000000000000505 PMID:30855297

Orth, U., & Robins, R. (2018). Development of self-esteem across the lifespan. *Handbook of personality development,* 328-344. Research Gate. https://www.researchgate.net/publication/329512803_Development_of_SelfEsteem_Across_the_Lifespan

Orth, U., Robins, R. W., & Roberts, B. W. (2008). Low self-esteem prospectively predicts depression in adolescence and young adulthood. *Journal of Personality and Social Psychology*, *95*(3), 695–708. doi:10.1037/0022-3514.95.3.695 PMID:18729703

Orth, U., Robins, R. W., Widaman, K. F., & Conger, R. D. (2014). Is low self-esteem a risk factor for depression? Findings from a longitudinal study of Mexican-origin youth. *Developmental Psychology*, *50*(2), 622–633. doi:10.1037/a0033817 PMID:23895172

Orygen. ((2017)). *Under the radar.* The mental health of Australian university students. Melbourne: Orygen, The National Centre of Excellence in Youth Mental Health.

Oswalt, S. B., Lederer, A., Chestnut-Steich, K., Day, C., Halbritter, A., & Ortiz, D. (2020). Trends in college students' mental health diagnoses and utilization of services, 2009–2015. *Journal of American College Health*, *68*(1), 41–51. doi:10.1080/07448481.2018.1515748 PMID:30355071

Otálora, A. R., & Barros, A. S. S. (2014). Psychological well-being (PWB) and personal problems (PP) in university students: A descriptive study in a distance learning context, preliminary results. *Procedia: Social and Behavioral Sciences, 132*, 427–433. doi:10.1016/j.sbspro.2014.04.332

Ouzzani, M., Hammady, H., Fedorowicz, Z., & Elmagarmid, A. (2016). Rayyan—A web and mobile app for systematic reviews. *Systematic Reviews, 5*(1), 1–10. doi:10.118613643-016-0384-4 PMID:27919275

Owusu, G. A., Akoto, J. S., & Abnory, M. M. (2016). Is our safety and security guaranteed on University of Cape Coast Campus? Undergraduates Students' Perceptions. *International Journal of Higher Education, 5*(4), 75–85.

Oyoo, E. (2017). *Indicators of Mental Status of University Students at the onset of Unrest: A Case of Kisii University, Kenya*. [Unpublished Phd Thesis, Rongo University, Kenya].

Pacheco, J. P., Giacomin, H. T., Tam, W. W., Ribeiro, T. B., Arab, C., & Bezerra, I. M. (2017). Mental health problems among medical students in Brazil: a systematic review and meta-analysis. *Brazillian Journal of Psychiatry*. https://www.scielo.br/j/rbp/a/FsKx7VwgRVSvwS638BqhbmK/#

Pachucki, M. C., Ozer, E. J., Barrat, A., & Cattuto, C. (2015). Mental health and social networks in early adolescence: A dynamic study of objectively-measured social interaction behaviors. *Social Science & Medicine, 125*, 40–50. doi:10.1016/j.socscimed.2014.04.015 PMID:24797692

Pacifici, L. B., & Thomson, N. (2011). Undergraduate science research: A comparison of influences and experiences between premed and non-premed students. *CBE Life Sciences Education, 10*(2), 199–208. doi:10.1187/cbe.11-01-0005 PMID:21633068

Panahi, R. (2018). The factors associated to high risk behaviors in Sanandaj city students based on health belief model. *Journal of Health Education and Health Promotion*, 393-402. doi:10.30699/acadpub.ijhehp.6.4.393

Panahi, S., Yunus, A. S. M., Roslan, S., Jaafar, R. A. K., Jaafar, W. M. W., & Panahi, M. S. (2016). Predictors of Psychological Well-being among Malaysian Graduates. *The European Journal of Social and Behavioural Sciences, 16*(2), 2067–2083. doi:10.15405/ejsbs.186

Pandya, A., & Lodha, P. (2022). Mental health consequences of COVID-19 pandemic among college students and coping approaches adapted by higher education institutions: A scoping review. *SSM. Mental Health, 2*, 100122. doi:10.1016/j.ssmmh.2022.100122 PMID:35665095

Pankowski, D., & Wytrychiewicz-Pankowska, K. (2023). Turning to religion during COVID-19 (Part I): A systematic review, meta-analysis and meta-regression of studies on the relationship between religious coping and mental health throughout COVID-19. *Journal of Religion and Health, 62*(1), 510–543. doi:10.100710943-022-01703-5 PMID:36592322

Paque, K., Vander Stichele, R., Elseviers, M., Pardon, K., Dilles, T., Deliens, L., & Christiaens, T. (2019). Barriers and enablers to deprescribing in people with a life-limiting disease: A systematic review. *Palliative Medicine, 33*(1), 37–48. doi:10.1177/0269216318801124 PMID:30229704

Park, N. (2004). Character strengths and positive youth development. *The Annals of the American Academy of Political and Social Science, 591*(1), 40–54. doi:10.1177/0002716203260079

Park, N., Park, M., & Peterson, C. (2010). When is the search for meaning related to life satisfaction? *Applied Psychology. Health and Well-Being, 2*(1), 1–13. doi:10.1111/j.1758-0854.2009.01024.x PMID:23457083

Pascob, M. C., Hetrick, S. E., & Parker, A. G. (2020). The Impact of stress on students in Secondary School and higher education. *International Journal of Adolescence Psychology, 3*, 46–56.

Pascoe, M. C., Hetrick, S. E., & Parker, A. G. (2020). The impact of stress on students in secondary school and higher education. *International Journal of Adolescence and Youth, 25*(1), 104–112. doi:10.1080/02673843.2019.1596823

Patel, V., Saxena, S., Lund, C., Thornicroft, G., Baingana, F., & Bolton, P. (2018). The Lancet Commission on Global Mental Health and Sustainable Development. *Lancet, 392*(10157), 1598. Doi: 31612-x. doi:10.1016/S0140-6736(18)

Patel, V., Belkin, G. S., & Chockalingham, A. (2013). Grand challenges; integrating mental health services into priority care platforms. *PLoS Medicine, 10*(5), e1001448. doi:10.1371/journal.pmed.1001448 PMID:23737736

PatientPop. (2019, April 16). *Why doctors are stressed and how to lower stress at your practice.* PatientPop. https://www.patientpop.com/blog/lessen-stress-and-physician-burnout/

Paton, G. (2014). Allow pupils to use Google in GCSE exams, says academic. *The Telegraph.* https://www.telegraph.co.uk/education/educationnews/11275200/Allow-pupils-to-use-Google-in-GCSE-exams-says-academic.html

Paton, G. (2021). Students' mental health and motivation hit by pandemic; UK survey finds. *Times Higher Education.* https://bit.ly/41ZZZQk

Patterson, Z.R., Gabrys, R.L., Prowse, R.K., Abizaid, A.B., Hellemans, K.G. & McQuaid, R. J. (2021). The influence of COVID-19 on stress, substance use, and mental health among postsecondary students. Emerging Adulthood, 9(5), pp.516-530. https://doi.org/10.1177/21676968211014080 doi:10.1177/21676968211014080

Patton, L. D., Renn, K. A., Guido, F. M., & Quaye, S. J. (2016). *Student development in college: Theory, research, and practice*. John Wiley & Sons.

Paul, R., & Kumar, A. (2021). Creating a positive school culture through new educational practices. In C. B. Gaines & K. M. Hutson (Eds.), *Promoting Positive Learning Experiences in Middle School Education* (pp. 149–166). IGI Global. doi:10.4018/978-1-7998-7057-9.ch008

Payne, H. (2022). Teaching Staff and Student Perceptions of Staff Support for Student Mental Health: A University Case Study. *Education Sciences*, *12*(4), 237–249. doi:10.3390/educsci12040237

Pedersen, A. L., Lindekilde, C. R., Andersen, K., Hjorth, P., & Gildberg, F. A. (2020). Health behaviours of forensic mental health service users, in relation to smoking, alcohol consumption, dietary behaviours and physical activity—A mixed methods systematic review. *Journal of Psychiatric and Mental Health Nursing*, *28*(3), 444–461. doi:10.1111/jpm.12688 PMID:32916759

Pedrelli, P., Nyer, M., Yeung, A., Zulauf, C., & Wilens, T. (2015). College Students: Mental Health Problems and Treatment Considerations. *Academic Psychiatry*, *39*(5), 503–511. doi:10.100740596-014-0205-9 PMID:25142250

Pengpid, S., & Peltzer, K. (2018). Parental involvement and health risk behaviours among school-going adolescents in six African countries. *Journal of Psychology in Africa*, *28*(3), 212–217. doi:10.1080/14330237.2017.1409481

Pereira, S., Reay, K., Bottell, J., Walker, L., Dzikiti, C., Platt, C., & Goodrham, C. (2019). *University Student Mental Health Survey 2018: A large scale study into the prevalence of student mental illness within UK universities*. Insight Network.

Perez-Trujillo, M., Jaramillo-Sierra, A., & Quintane, E. (2019). Connectedness as a protective factor of sexual victimisation among University Students. *Victims & Offenders*, *14*(7), 895–919. doi:10.1080/15564886.2019.1655121

Perron, N. C. (2017). Bronfenbrenner's ecological systems theory. *College student Development. Applying Theory to Practice on the Diverse Campus*, *197*(23), 1–10.

Petersen, A. M., Riccaboni, M., Stanley, H. E., & Pammolli, F. (2012). Persistence and uncertainty in the academic career. *Proceedings of the National Academy of Sciences of the United States of America, 109*(14), 5213–5218. doi:10.1073/pnas.1121429109 PMID:22431620

Peterson, C., & Seligman, M. E. (2004). *Character strengths and virtues: A handbook and classification.* Oxford University Press.

Phang, C. K., Mukhtar, F., Ibrahim, N., & Keng, S. L., & Mohd- Sidik, S. (2015). Effects of a brief mindfulness-based intervention program for stress management among medical students: The Mindful-Gym randomized controlled study. *Advances in Health Sciences Education : Theory and Practice, 20,* 1115–1134. doi:10.100710459-015-9591-3 PMID:25697124

Phatudi-Mphahlele, B., & Mashele, M. (2021). South African students' experience of online learning during the Covid-19 pandemic: A case of a higher education institution. *International Journal of Educational Technology in Higher Education, 18*(1), 1–19. oi:10.118641239-021-00278-2

Pillay, J. (2022). University students' mental health: A concern for all. In S. Deb & B. A. Gerrard (Eds.), *Handbook of health and wellbeing* (pp. 277–293). doi:10.1007/978-981-16-8263-6_12

Pluut, H., Curşeu, P. L., & Ilies, R. (2015). Social and study related stressors and resources among university entrants: Effects on well-being and academic performance. *Learning and Individual Differences, 37,* 262–268. doi:10.1016/j.lindif.2014.11.018

Polanczyk, G.V., Salum, G.A., Sugaya, L.S., Caye, A., Rohde, L.A. (2015). Annual research review: a meta-analysis of the worldwide prevalence of mental disorders in children and adolescents. *J Child Psychol Psychiatry, 56*(3), 345–65.

Porru, F., Schuring, M., Bultmann, U., Portoghese, I., Busdorf, A., & Robroek, S. J. N. (2022). Associations of university student life challenges with mental health and self-rated health: A longitudinal study with 6 months follow-up. [CrossRef]. *Journal of Affective Disorders, 296,* 250–257. doi:10.1016/j.jad.2021.09.057 PMID:34624809

Porter, L. (2020). Safeguarding students: Physical and emotional security. *Student Behaviour,* (pp. 209-224). Taylor & Francis. doi:10.4324/9781003117520-11

Porter, S. (2018). *A descriptive study of post-secondary student mental health crises.*

Potgieter, M., Pilcher, L. A., Tekane, R. R., Louw, I., & Fletcher, L. (2019). Lessons learnt from teaching and learning during disruptions. In: Schultz, M., Schmid, S., Lawrie, G. (eds) Research and practice in Chemistry Education. Springer, Singapore. doi:10.1007/978-981-13-6998-8_6

Priesack, A., & Alcock, J. (2015). Well-Being and Self-Efficacy in a Sample of Undergraduate Nurse Students: A Small Survey Study. [CrossRef]. *Nurse Education Today, 35*(5), e16–e20. doi:10.1016/j.nedt.2015.01.022 PMID:25702848

Priestley, M., Broglia, E., Hughes, G., & Spanner, L. (2022). Student Perspectives on improving mental health support services at University. *Counselling & Psychotherapy Research, 22*(1), 197–206. doi:10.1002/capr.12391

Priestley, M., Hall, A., Wilbraham, S. J., Mistry, V., Hughes, G., & Spanner, L. (2022). Student perceptions and proposals for promoting wellbeing through social relationships at university. *Journal of Further and Higher Education, 46*(9), 1243–1256. doi:10.1080/0309877X.2022.2061844

Prince, J. P. (2015). University student counseling and mental health in the United States: Trends and challenges. *Mental Health & Prevention, 3*(1-2), 5–10. doi:10.1016/j.mhp.2015.03.001

Prowse, R., Sherratt, F., Abizaid, A., Gabrys, R. L., Hellemans, K. G., Patterson, Z. R., & McQuaid, R. J. (2021). Coping with the COVID-19 pandemic: Examining gender differences in stress and mental health among university students. *Frontiers in Psychiatry*, *12*, 650759. doi:10.3389/fpsyt.2021.650759 PMID:33897499

Puckett, K. (2022). Safety and Security On Campus: *Student perceptions and influence on enrollment.* [Unpublished MA Thesis, Electronic Theses and Dissertations. East Tennessee State University, USA].

Putrah, A. (2023). Students' reception towards sexual harassment case of Gen-Z At a Private Universityin Depok. *IJAMESC*, *1*(2), 35–44.

Quick, J. C., & McFadyen, M. A. (2017). Sexual harassment: Have we made any progress? *Journal of Occupational Health Psychology*, *22*(3), 286–298. doi:10.1037/ocp0000054 PMID:27732009

Rafferty, K. A., Beck, G., & McGuire, M. (2020). When facing hopeful and hopeless experiences: Using snyder's hope theory to understand parents' caregiving experiences for their medically complex child. *Journal of Pediatric Health Care*, *34*(6), 542–549. doi:10.1016/j.pedhc.2020.06.003 PMID:32771340

Rafsanjani, M. A., Pamungkas, H. P., & Rahmawati, E. D. (2019). Does teacher-student relationship mediate the relation between student misbehavior and teacher psychological well-being? *Journal of Accounting And Business Education*, *4*(1), 34–44. doi:10.26675/jabe.v4i1.8411

Ramluggun, P., Kozlowska, O., Mansbridge, S., Rioga, M., & Anjoyeb, M. (2022). Mental health in higher education: Faculty staff survey on supporting students with mental health needs. *Health Education*, *122*(6), 601–616. doi:10.1108/HE-02-2022-0011

Ramshe, M. H., Ghazanfari, M., & Ghonsooly, B. (2019). The Role of Personal Best Goals in EFL Learners' Behavioural, Cognitive, and Emotional Engagement. *International Journal of Instruction*, *12*(1), 1627–1638. doi:10.29333/iji.2019.121103a

Ranganathan, M., Wamoyi, J., Pearson, I., & Stockl, H. (2020). Measurement and Prevalence of Sexual Harassment In Low- And Middle-Income Countries: A Systematic Review and Meta-Analysis. *BMJ Open*, *11*(6), 1–15. PMID:34168030

Rao, C. R., Darshan, B. B., Das, N., Rajan, V., Bhogun, M., & Gupta, A. (2012). Practice of physical activity among future doctors: A cross-sectional analysis. *International Journal of Preventive Medicine*, *3*(5), 365–369. PMID:22708033

Ray, D. C., & Radimer, S. (2019). Preparing student affairs professionals to serve in urban institutions. *Student Affairs in Urban-Serving Institutions*, (pp. 128–150). Taylor & Francis. doi:10.4324/9781351043366-7

Reaves, S., McMahon, S. D., Duffy, S. N., & Ruiz, L. (2018). The Test of Time: A Meta-Analytic Review of The Relation Between School Climate And Problem Behavior. *Aggression and Violent Behavior*, *39*, 100–108. doi:10.1016/j.avb.2018.01.006

Reddy, K. J., Menon, K. R., & Thattil, A. (2018). Academic stress and its sources among university students. *Biomedical & Pharmacology Journal*, *11*(1), 1. doi:10.13005/bpj/1404

Regehr, C., Glancy, D., & Pitts, A. (2013). Interventions to reduce stress in university students: A review and meta-analysis. *Journal of Affective Disorders*, *148*(1), 1–11. doi:10.1016/j.jad.2012.11.026 PMID:23246209

Rehman, A. U., Bhuttah, T. M., & You, X. (2020). Linking burnout to psychological well-being: The mediating role of social support and learning motivation. *Psychology Research and Behavior Management*, *13*, 545–554. doi:10.2147/PRBM.S250961 PMID:32753983

Reimers, F., Schleicher, A., Saavedra, J., & Tuominen, S. (2020). Supporting the continuation of teaching and learning during the COVID-19 Pandemic. *Oecd*, *1*(1), 1–38.

Report, N. I. H. (2018). Emotional Well-Being: Emerging Insights and Questions for Future Research. Bethesda, MD.

Rettew, D. C., McGinnis, E. W., Copeland, W., Nardone, H. Y., Bai, Y., Rettew, J., Devadenam, V., & Hudziak, J. J. (2021). Personality trait predictors of adjustment during the COVID pandemic among college students. *PLoS One*, *16*(3), e0248895. doi:10.1371/journal.pone.0248895 PMID:33730075

Rheeder, C. (2022). Student affairs and services leadership in trying times: Student social behaviour project and psycho-social support interventions at a comprehensive university in South Africa. *Journal of Student Affairs in Africa*, *10*(2). doi:10.24085/jsaa.v10i2.4369

Ribeiro, I. J. S., Freire, I. V., & de Araújo, T. M. (2020). Are stress management interventions effective in reducing stress, anxiety, and depression in college students? *Clinical Psychology : a Publication of the Division of Clinical Psychology of the American Psychological Association*. doi:10.1111/cpsp.12385

Richardson, A. (2019). Can food improve your exam performance? *BBC Food*. https://www.bbc.co.uk/food/articles/food_exam_performance

Rickwood, D., Deane, F. P., Wilson, C. J., & Ciarrochi, J. (2005). Young people's help-seeking for mental health problems. *Australian e-Journal for the Advancement of Mental Health*, *4*(3), 218–251. doi:10.5172/jamh.4.3.218

Riehm, K. E., Feder, K. A., Tormohlen, K. N., Crum, R. M., Young, A. S., Green, K. M., Pacek, L. R., La Flair, L. N., & Mojtabai, R. (2019). Associations between time spent using social media and internalizing and externalizing problems among US youth. *JAMA Psychiatry*, *76*(12), 1266. doi:10.1001/jamapsychiatry.2019.2325 PMID:31509167

Riekie, H., Aldridge, J. M., & Afari, E. (2017). The Role of the School Climate in High School Students' Mental Health and Identity Formation: A South Australian study. *British Educational Research Journal*, *43*(1), 95–123. doi:10.1002/berj.3254

Riley, (2004), Understanding the stresses and strains of being a doctor, *MJA*, *181*(7). doi:10.5694/j.1326-5377.2004.tb06322.x

Riley, R., Spiers, J., Buszewicz, M., Taylor, A., Thorton, G., & Chew-Graham, C. (2018). What are the sources of stress and distress for general practitioners working in England? A qualitative study. *BMJ Open*, *8*(1), e017361. doi:10.1136/bmjopen-2017-017361 PMID:29326181

Rink, J., & Lipinska, G. (2020). Evidence of Distinct Profiles Of ICD-11 Post-Traumatic Stress Disorder (PTSD) And Complex PTSD In A South African Sample. *European Journal of Psychotraumatology*, *11*(1), 1818965. doi:10.1080/20008198.2020.1818965 PMID:33282146

Ríos-Risquez, M. I., García-Izquierdo, M., Sabuco-Tebar, E., Carrillo-Garcia, C., & Solano-Ruiz, C. (2018). Connections between academic burnout, resilience, and psychological well-being in nursing students: A longitudinal study. *Journal of Advanced Nursing*, *74*(12), 2777–2784. doi:10.1111/jan.13794 PMID:29992596

Riva, E., Freeman, R., Schrock, L., Jelicic, V., Ozer, C.-T., & Caleb, R. (2020). Student Wellbeing in the Teaching and Learning Environment: A Study Exploring Student and Staff Perspectives. *Higher Education Studies*, *10*(4), 103–115. doi:10.5539/hes.v10n4p103

Robbins, A., Kaye, E., & Catling, J. C. (2018). Predictors of student resilience in higher education. *Psychology Teaching Review*, *24*(1), 44–52. doi:10.53841/bpsptr.2018.24.1.44

Robertson, I., & Cooper, C. L. (2013). Resilience. *Stress and Health*, *29*(3), 175–176. doi:10.1002mi.2512 PMID:23913839

Roberts, R., Golding, J. F., Towell, T., Reid, S., Woodford, S., Vetere, A. L., & Weinreb, I. (2000). Mental and physical health in students: The role of economic circumstances. *British Journal of Health Psychology*, *5*(3), 289–297. doi:10.1348/135910700168928

Robinson, K., & Aronica, L. (2015). How schools kill creativity: Forget standardized tests, here's how we really engage our kids. *Salon.* https://www.salon.com/2015/04/26 how_schools_kill_creativity_forget_standardized_tests_heres_how_we_really_engage_our_kids/)

Robinson, K. (2017). *Out of our minds: The Power of Being Creative.* John Wiley & Sons.

Robson, D. (2022). How interior design choices can boost your mental and physical health. *New Scientist.* https://www.newscientist.com/article/mg25433823-000-how-interior-design-choices-can-boost-your-mental-and-physical-health/

Rochin Demong, N. A., Shahrom, M., Abdul Rahim, R., Omar, E. N., & Yahya, M. (2023). Personalized recommendation classification model of students' social well-being based on personality trait determinants using machine learning algorithms. *Journal of Information and Communication Technology*, *22*(4), 545–585. doi:10.32890/jict2023.22.4.2

Rodríguez, S., Piñeiro, I., Gómez-Taibo, M. L., Regueiro, B., Estévez, I., & Valle, A. (2017). An explanatory model of maths achievement: Perceived parental involvement and academic motivation. *Psicothema*, *29*(2), 184–190. 10.7334 PMID:28438240

Rogowska, A. M., Kuśnierz, C., & Bokszczanin, A. (2020). Examining anxiety, life satisfaction, general health, stress and coping styles during COVID-19 pandemic in Polish sample of university students. *Psychology Research and Behavior Management*, *13*, 797–811. doi:10.2147/PRBM.S266511 PMID:33061695

Roksa, J., & Kinsley, P. (2019). The Role of Family Support in Facilitating Academic Success of Low-Income. *Research in Higher Education*, *60*(4), 415–437. doi:10.100711162-018-9517-z

Rosario, M. G. L. D. (2023). Stress and coping strategies and academic performance of teacher education students. *Journal for Educators, Teachers and Trainers, 14*(3). https://jett.labosfor.com/

Rosenthal, M., Smidt, A., & Freyd, J. (2016). Still Second Class: Sexual Harassment of Graduate Students. *Psychology of Women Quarterly*, *40*(3), 364–377. doi:10.1177/0361684316644838 PMID:27821904

Rosenthal, S. R., Clark, M. A., Marshall, B. D., Buka, S. L., Carey, K. B., Shepardson, R. L., & Carey, M. P. (2018). Alcohol consequences, not quantity, predict major depression onset among first-year female college students. *Addictive Behaviors*, *85*, 70–76. doi:10.1016/j.addbeh.2018.05.021 PMID:29860191

Rosli, I. N., & Harun, M. M. (2023). The relationship between mental health, coping strategies and attitudes towards seeking counselling services among University students. *International Journal of Academic Research in Business & Social Sciences*, *13*(7). doi:10.6007/IJARBSS/v13-i7/17443

Ross, S. E., Niebling, B. C., & Heckert, T. M. (1999). Sources of stress among college students. *College Student Journal*, *33*, 312–317.

Rotenstein, L. S., Ramos, M. A., Torre, M., Segal, J. B., Peluso, M. J., Guille, C., Sen, S., & Mata, D. A. (2016). Prevalence of depression, depressive symptoms, and suicidal ideation among medical students: A systematic review and meta-analysis. *Journal of the American Medical Association*, *316*(21), 2214–2236. doi:10.1001/jama.2016.17324 PMID:27923088

Roth, J. L., & Brooks-Gunn, J. (2003). What exactly is a youth development program? Answers from research and practice. *Applied Developmental Science*, *7*(2), 94–111. doi:10.1207/S1532480XADS0702_6

Rowe, N. (2015). *Creating a Healing Campus: A Partnership between a University and a Provider of Mental Health Services.*

Rudasill, K. M., Snyder, K. E., Levinson, H., & Adelson, J. L. (2018). Systems View of School Climate: A Theoretical Framework for Research. *Educational Psychology Review, 30*(1), 35–60. doi:10.100710648-017-9401-y

Rupert, P. A., & Dorociak, K. E. (2019). Self-care, stress, and well-being among practicing psychologists. *Professional Psychology, Research and Practice, 50*(5), 343–350. doi:10.1037/pro0000251

Rush, A. J. (2022, November 28). Unipolar major depression in adults: Choosing initial treatment. *Up to Date.* https://www.uptodate.com/contents/unipolar-major-depression-in-adults-choosing-initial-treatment

Rutkowska, A., Liska, D., Cieślik, B., Wrzeciono, A., Broďáni, J., Barcalová, M., Gurín, D., & Rutkowski, S. (2021). Stress levels and mental well-being among Slovak students during e-learning in the COVID-19 pandemic. *Health Care, 9*(10), 1356. doi:10.3390/healthcare9101356 PMID:34683036

Ruzhenkova, V. V. (2020). Prevalence and dynamics of depression and anxiety in local and foreign medical students for a 6- year training period. *International Journal of Early Childhood Special Education, 12*(1), 606–611. doi:10.9756/INT-JECSE/V12I1.201044

Ryan, T., & Ryan, T. (2022). A Study Guide To Getting Sleep During Final Exams. *Sleep Foundation.* https://www.sleepfoundation.org/school-and-sleep/final-exams-and-sleep

Ryan, T., Marangell, S., & Baik, C. (2023). Examining Mental Health and Wellbeing Policies in Australian Universities. In K. Coleman, D. Uzhegova, B. Blaher, & S. Arkoudis (Eds.), *The Educational Turn. Rethinking Higher Education.* Springer. doi:10.1007/978-981-19-8951-3_12

Ryff, C. D. (2023). A new direction in mental health: Purposeful life engagement. Encyclopedia of Mental Health (3rd ed.). Science Direct. doi:10.1016/B978-0-323-91497-0.00096-5

Ryff, C. (1989). Happiness is Everything, or Is It? Exploration of the Meaning of Psychological Well-Being. *Journal of Personality and Social Psychology, 57*(2), 1069–1081. doi:10.1037/0022-3514.57.6.1069

Saade, S., Lamarche, A. P., Khalaf, T., Makke, S., & Legg, A. (2023). What barriers could impede access to mental health services for children and adolescents in Africa? A scoping review. *BMC Health Services Research, 23*(1), 348. doi:10.118612913-023-09294-x PMID:37024835

Sadri Damirchi, E., Mojarrad, A., Pireinaladin, S., & Grjibovski, A. M. (2020). The Role of Self-Talk in Predicting Death Anxiety, Obsessive-Compulsive Disorder, and CopingStrategies in the Face of Coronavirus Disease (COVID-19). *Iranian Journal of Psychiatry, 15*(3), 182–188. doi:10.18502/ijps.v15i3.3810 PMID:33193766

Sæther, M. H., Sivertsen, B., & Bjerkeset, O. (2021). Mental Distress, Help Seeking, and Use of Health Services Among University Students. The SHoT-Study 2018, Norway. *Frontiers in Psychiatry, 12*, 727237. doi:10.3389/fpsyt.2021.727237 PMID:34744820

Safran, W. (1990). Review: The French and Their National Identity: The Quest for an Elusive Substance? on JSTOR. Vol. 8, No. 1 (Winter 1990), pp. 56-67 (12 pages). https://doi.org/ doi:10.2307/42844146

Sakhelashvili, I., & Spruyt, K. (2023). The interaction between stress and sleep disorders among foreign medical students in Georgia. *Sleep Medicine, 110*, 225–230. doi:10.1016/j.sleep.2023.08.021 PMID:37647713

Saleh, D., Camart, N., & Romo, L. (2017). Predictors of stress in college students. *Frontiers in Psychology, 8*, 19. doi:10.3389/fpsyg.2017.00019 PMID:28179889

Saleh, D., Camart, N., & Romo, L. (2017). Predictors of Stress in College Students. *Frontiers in Psychology*, 8. PMID:28179889

Salgar, S. (2014). Stress in first year medical students. *International Journal of Biomedical and Advance Research, 5*(1), 1. doi:10.7439/ijbar.v5i1.580

Salik, I., & Marwaha, R. (2022). *Electroconvulsive Therapy*. StatPearls Publishing. https://www.ncbi.nlm.nih.gov/books/NBK538266/

Salois, D. J. M. (2021). Promoting well-being among college students: the effects of a positive psychology course. *Graduate student theses, dissertations, & professional papers*. Https://scholarworks.umt.edu/etd/1179

Sampath, H., Biswas, A. G., Soohinda, G., & Dutta, S. (2019). Mindfulness and Its Role in Psychological Well-Being among Medical College Students. *Open Journal of Psychiatry & Allied Sciences, 10*(1), 52. doi:10.5958/2394-2061.2019.00013.2

Sanci, L., Williams, I., Russell, M., Chondros, P., Duncan, A., Tarzia, L., Peter, D., Lim, M. S. Y., Tomyn, A., & Minas, H. (2022). Towards a health promoting university: Descriptive findings on health, wellbeing and academic performance amongst university students in Australia. *BMC Public Health, 22*(1), 2430. doi:10.118612889-022-14690-9 PMID:36575509

Sandel, M. J. (2021). *The tyranny of merit: Can We Find the Common Good?* Picador.

Sandoval, S., Dorner, A., & Véliz, A. (2017). Psychological well-being of students taking health degree courses]. *Investigación en Educación Médica, 6*, 260–266.

Sanjay, K. (2019). Causes and Consequences of Unrest Among Phd Scholars: A Study On Regular Phd Students in Himachal Pradesh. *The Journal of Progressive Education, 12*(2), 119–127.

SantiagoP. H.SoaresG. H.SmithersL. G.RobertsR.JamiesonL. (2022). Psychological network of stress, coping and social support in an Aboriginal population. https://doi.org/ doi:10.31234/osf.io/cz59w

Sapiro, B., & Ward, A. (2020). Marginalized youth, mental health, and connection with others: A review of the literature. *Child & Adolescent Social Work Journal, 37*(4), 343–357. doi:10.100710560-019-00628-5

Savitsky, B., Findling, Y., Ereli, A., & Hendel, T. (2020). Anxiety and coping strategies among nursing students during the covid-19 pandemic. *Nurse Education in Practice, 46*, 102809. doi:10.1016/j.nepr.2020.102809 PMID:32679465

Savolainen, T. (2023). A Safe Learning Environment from The Perspective of Laurea University of Applied Sciences Safety, Security and Risk Management Students and Staff. *Heliyon, 9*(3), 1–14. doi:10.1016/j.heliyon.2023.e12836 PMID:36895344

Sawatzky, R. G., Ratner, P. A., Richardson, C. G., Washburn, C., Sudmant, W., & Mirwaldt, P. (2012). Stress and depression in students: The mediating role of stress management self-efficacy. *Nursing Research, 61*(1), 13–21. doi:10.1097/NNR.0b013e31823b1440 PMID:22166906

Schelvis, R. M. C., Wiezer, N. M., Blatter, B. M., van Genabeek, J. A., Oude Hengel, K. M., Bohlmeijer, E. T., & van der Beek, A. J. (2016). Evaluating the implementation process of a participatory organizational level occupational health intervention in schools. *BMC Public Health, 16*(1), 1212. doi:10.118612889-016-3869-0 PMID:27905904

Schmits, E., Dekeyser, S., Klein, O., Luminet, O., Yzerbyt, V., & Glowacz, F. (2021). Psychological Distress among Students in Higher Education: One Year after the Beginning of the COVID-19 Pandemic. *International Journal of Environmental Research and Public Health, 18*(14), 7445. doi:10.3390/ijerph18147445 PMID:34299896

Schonert-Reichl, K. A. (2017). Social and Emotional Learning and Teachers. *The Future of Children, 27*(1), 137–155. doi:10.1353/foc.2017.0007

Schreiber, K. R., & Cunningham, F. O. (2016). Nutrition education in the medical school curriculum: A review of the course content at the Royal College of Surgeons in Ireland-Bahrain. *Irish Journal of Medical Science, 185*(4), 853–856. doi:10.100711845-015-1380-8 PMID:26563109

Schuck, A. M. (2016). Evaluating the Impact of Crime and Discipline on Student Success in Postsecondary Education. *Research in Higher Education, 58*(1), 77–97. doi:10.100711162-016-9419-x

Schütte, S., Chastang, J. F., Parent-Thirion, A., Vermeylen, G., & Niedhammer, I. (2014). Social inequalities in psychological well-being: A European comparison. *Community Mental Health Journal, 50*(8), 987–990. doi:10.100710597-014-9725-8 PMID:24664367

Schwieger, D., & Ladwig, C. (2018). Reaching and retaining the next generation: Adapting to the expectations of Gen Z in the classroom. *Information Systems Education Journal, 16*(3), 45–54.

Scott, B., Modna, Y., Khashchuk, D., & Duke, J. (2019). The Interrelationship between perceived stress level, sleep quality, and academic performance among students of a Caribbean Medical School. *Anatomy Physiology & Biochemistry International Journal, 6*(1), 555676.

Scullin, M. K., MacGregor, J., & King, E. (2019). 0096 Sleep in college students during final exams week: The Eight Hour challenge. *Sleep, 42*(Supplement_1), A39–A40. Advance online publication. doi:10.1093leep/zsz067.095

Seehuus, M., Moeller, R. W., & Peisch, V. (2021). Gender effects on mental health symptoms and treatment in college students. *Journal of American College Health, 69*(1), 95–102. doi:10.1080/07448481.2019.1656217 PMID:31513464

Seemiller, C., & Clayton, J. (2019). Developing the strengths of generation Z college students. *Journal of College and Character, 20*(3), 268–275. doi:10.1080/2194587X.2019.1631187

Segametsi, B. (2017). Students' Unrest in Tertiary Institutions of Botswana: Implications on Teaching and Learning. [Unpublished Masters in Higher Education, Botho University, Botswana].

Sekibo, I., Tinibu, J., & Balogun, M. (2022). School Counselling Programme and Students' Academic Development. *Journal Educational Verkenning, 3*(1), 1–9. https://hdpublication.com/index.php/jev/article/view/140

Seligman, M. (2018). PERMA and the building blocks of well-being. *The Journal of Positive Psychology, 13*(4), 333–335. doi:10.1080/17439760.2018.1437466

Seligman, M. E. P., & Csikszentmihalyi, M. (2000). Positive psychology: An introduction. *The American Psychologist, 55*(1), 5–14. doi:10.1037/0003-066X.55.1.5 PMID:11392865

Seligman, M. E., Ernst, R. M., Gillham, J., Reivicha, K., & Linkinsd, M. (2009). Positive education: Positive psychology and classroom interventions. *Oxford Review of Education, 35*(3), 293–311. doi:10.1080/03054980902934563

Seppälä, E. (2021). Research: Why Breathing Is So Effective at Reducing Stress. *Harvard Business Review*. https://hbr.org/2020/09/research-why-breathing-is-so-effective-at-reducing-stress

Sevlever, M., & Rice, K. G. (2010). Perfectionism, depression, anxiety, and academic performance in premedical students. *Canadian Medical Education Journal, 1*(2), e96–e104. doi:10.36834/cmej.36537

Shafer, L. (2017). *Making student feedback work*. Harvard Graduate School of Education. https://www.gse.harvard.edu/ideas/usable-knowledge/17/11/making-student-feedback-work

Shah, K. M. D., Padli, J., Talib, J. A., & Mukhta, F. (2020). The Psychological Well-Being from The University Students' Perspective and Culture– Palarch's. *Journal of Archaeology of Egypt/Egyptology 17*(2), 1- 11.

Shahar, G., & Davidson, L. (2003). Depressive symptoms erode self-esteem in severe mental illnesss:A three-wave, cross-lagged study. *Journal Of Consulting and Clinical, 71*(5), 21-31. oi:10.1037/0022-006X.71.5.890

Shahira, M. N., Hanisshya, H., Lukman, Z. M., Normala, R., Azlini, C., & Kamal, M. Y. (2018). Psychological Well-Being among University Students in Malaysia. *International Journal of Research and Innovation in Social Science*, (2), 133–137.

Shankar, N. L., & Park, C. (2016). Effects of stress on students' physical and mental health and academic success. *International Journal of School & Educational Psychology*, *4*(1), 5–9. doi:10.1080/21683603.2016.1130532

Shariati, A., & Guerette, R. T. (2019). Resident students' perception of safety in on- campus residential facilities: Does crime prevention through environmental design (CPTED) make a difference? *Journal of School Violence*, *18*(4), 570–584. doi:10.1080/15388220.2019.1617721

Sharma, A., & Sharma, R. (2018). Internet addiction and psychological well-being among college students: A cross-sectional study from Central India. *Journal of Family Medicine and Primary Care*, *7*(1), 147–151. doi:10.4103/jfmpc.jfmpc_189_17 PMID:29915749

Sharma, A., Singh, T. P., Sharma, R., Dhakar, J. S., & Bharti, A. (2022). Psychological well-being among college students: A study from Central India. *Asian Journal of Medical Sciences*, *13*(1), 46–51. doi:10.3126/ajms.v13i1.39350

Sharp, J., & Theiler, S. (2018). A Review of Psychological Distress Among University Students: Pervasiveness, Implications and Potential Points of Intervention. *International Journal for the Advancement of Counseling*, *40*(3), 193–212. doi:10.100710447-018-9321-7

Shatimwene, G. P., Ashipala, D. O., & Kamenye, E. (2020). Experiences of student nurses on the use of the two-week block system at the satellite campus of a higher education institution in Namibia. *International Journal of Higher Education*, *9*(3), 222–231. doi:10.5430/ijhe.v9n3p222

Shek, D. T., Dou, D., Zhu, X., & Chai, W. (2019). Positive youth development: Current perspectives. *Adolescent Health, Medicine and Therapeutics*, *10*, 131–141. doi:10.2147/AHMT.S179946 PMID:31572041

Sheldon, E., Simmonds-Buckley, M., Bone, C., Mascarenhas, T., Chan, N., Wincott, M., Gleeson, K., Sow, D., Hind, M., & Barkham, M. (2021). Prevalence and risk factors for mental health problems in university undergraduate students: A systematic review with meta-analysis. *Journal of Affective Disorders*, *287*, 282–292. doi:10.1016/j.jad.2021.03.054 PMID:33812241

Sheroun, D., Wankhar, D. D., Devrani, A., Lissamma, P. V., & Chatterjee, K. (2020). A study to assess the perceived stress and coping strategies among B. Sc. nursing students of selected colleges in Pune during COVID-19 pandemic lockdown. *International Journal of Science and Healthcare Research*, *5*(2), 280–288.

Sheyapo, M., Haihambo, C. K., & Mbongo, E. N. (2023). The roles of institutions in addressing the needs of students from marginalised backgrounds in higher education in Namibia. Edulearn23 Proceedings.

Shikulo, L., & Lekhetho, M. (2020). undefined. *Cogent Social Sciences*, *6*(1). doi:10.1080/23311886.2020.1737401

Shim, G., & Jeong, B. (2018). Predicting suicidal ideation in college students with mental health screening questionnaires. *Psychiatry Investigation*, *15*(11), 1037–1045. doi:10.30773/pi.2018.08.21.3 PMID:30380820

Shoshani, A., & Slone, M. (2013). Middle school transition from the strengths perspective: Young adolescents' character strengths, subjective well-being, and school adjustment. *Journal of Happiness Studies*, *14*(4), 1163–1181. doi:10.100710902-012-9374-y

Shrivastava, A., & Rajan, D. (2019). Assessmen Competitive Exams. *International Journal of Healthcare Sciences*, 2348-5728. doi:10.13140/RG.2.2.10711.42406

Shukla, K. D., Waasdorp, T. E., Lindstrom Johnson, S., Orozco Solis, M. G., Nguyen, A. J., Rodríguez, C. C., & Bradshaw, C. P. (2019). Does School Climate Mean the Same Thing in The United States as in Mexico? A Focus On Measurement Invariance. *Journal of Psychoeducational Assessment*, *37*(1), 55–68. doi:10.1177/0734282917731459

Siddiqui, Z. U., & Khan, M. I. (2016). Psychological Well-Being among University Students. *International Journal of Indian Psychology*, *3*(4), 114–118.

Simkins, C. (2016). Funding. South African higher education reviewed: two decades of democracy. In: Kagisano, (10), 39-115.

Simons, G., & Baldwin, D. S. (2021). A Critical Review Of The Definition Of 'Wellbeing' for Doctors and Their Patients In A Post Covid-19 Era. *The International Journal of Social Psychiatry*, *67*(8), 984–991. doi:10.1177/00207640211032259 PMID:34240644

Simons, J., Beaumont, K., & Holland, L. (2018). What factors promote student resilience on a level 1 distance learning module? *Open Learning*, *33*(1), 4–17. doi:10.1080/02680513.2017.1415140

Simonsmeier, B. A., Peiffer, H., Flaig, M., & Schneider, M. (2020). Peer Feedback Improves Students' Academic Self-Concept in Higher Education. *Research in Higher Education*, *61*(6), 706–724. doi:10.100711162-020-09591-y

Simpson, O. (2018). Student support face to face. I O. Simpson, O. (Ed.), Supporting students in online, open and distance learning (pp. 78–87). Taylor & Francis. doi:10.4324/9780203417003-7

Singh, S. (2018). Positive schooling and resilience. *Indian Journal of Positive Psychology*, *9*(2), 311–316.

Sin, N. L., Moskowitz, J. T., & Whooley, M. A. (2015). Positive Affect and Health Behaviors across Five Years in Patients with Coronary Heart Disease: The Heart and Soul Study. *Psychosomatic Medicine*, *77*(9), 1058–1066. doi:10.1097/PSY.0000000000000238 PMID:26428445

Siqi, J., & Siqi, J. (2023b). What is 'lying flat', and why are Chinese officials standing up to it? *South China Morning Post*. https://www.scmp.com/economy/china-economy/article/3153362/what-lying-flat-and-why-are-chinese-officials-standing-it

Sivertsen, B., Hysing, M., Knapstad, M., Harvey, A. G., Reneflot, A., Lønning, K. J., & O'Connor, R. C. (2019). Suicide attempts and non-suicidal self-harm among university students: Prevalence study. *BJPsych Open*, *5*(2), e26. doi:10.1192/bjo.2019.4 PMID:31068238

Skilbred-Fjeld, S., Reme, S. E., & Mossige, S. (2020). Cyberbullying involvement and mental health problems among late adolescents. *Cyberpsychology (Brno)*, *14*(1), 1–16. doi:10.5817/CP2020-1-5

Slavin, S. J., Schindler, D. L., & Chibnall, J. T. (2014). Medical student mental health 3.0: Improving student wellness through curricular changes. *Academic Medicine*, *89*(4), 573–577. doi:10.1097/ACM.0000000000000166 PMID:24556765

Snyder, C. R., & Lopez, S. J. (2007). *Positive psychology: The scientific and practical explorations of human strengths*. Sage Publications, Inc.

Soldevila-Domenech, N., Forero, C. G., Alayo, I., Capella, J., Colom, J., Malmusi, D., Mompart, A., Mortier, P., Puértolas, B., Sánchez, N., Schiaffino, A., Vilagut, G., & Alonso, J. (2021). Mental well-being of the general population: Direct and indirect effects of socioeconomic, relational and health factors. *Quality of Life Research: An International Journal of Quality of Life Aspects of Treatment, Care and Rehabilitation*, *30*(8), 2171–2185. doi:10.100711136-021-02813-5 PMID:33847868

Sommet, N., Pulfrey, C., & Butera, F. (2013). Did my M.D. really go to university to learn? Detrimental Effects of Numerus Clausus on Self-Efficacy, Mastery Goals and learning. *PLoS One*, *8*(12), e84178. doi:10.1371/journal.pone.0084178 PMID:24376794

SOS Samaritans of Singapore. (n.d.). *Suicide facts and figures*. SOS. https://www.sos.org.sg/learn-about-suicide/quick-facts

Sowani, D., & Lavalekar, A. (2020). Exploring Psychological Well-Being of College Students In Maharashtra in Relation to Their Family Environment. *Indian Journal of Positive Psychology*, *11*(3), 197–202.

Sowislo, J. F., & Orth, U. (2013). Does low self-esteem predict depression and anxiety? A meta-analysis of longitudinal studies. *Psychological Bulletin*, *139*(1), 213–240. doi:10.1037/a0028931 PMID:22730921

Spielberger, C. D. (2013). *Anxiety: Current trends in theory and research*. Elsevier.

Spies, J. (2022). *Exploring Teacher Experiences of Subjective Well-Being During a Pandemic*. [Master's thesis, University of Pretoria]. https://hdl.handle.net/2263/82445

Srabstein, J. C., & Leventhal, B. L. (2010). Prevention of Bullying-Related Morbidity and Mortality: A Call for Public Health Policies. *Bulletin of the World Health Organization*, *88*(6), 403–403. doi:10.2471/BLT.10.077123 PMID:20539848

Srikanth, A. (2018). Incidents of Sexual Harassment at Educational Institutions in India: Preventive Measures and Grievance Handling. *Asian Review of Social Sciences*, *7*(3), 108–113. doi:10.51983/arss-2018.7.3.1458

Stancin, T., Wade, S. L., Walz, N. C., Yeates, K. O., & Taylor, H. G. (2010). Family Adaptation. 18 Months after Traumatic Brain Injury in Early Childhood. *Journal of Developmental and Behavioral Pediatrics*, *31*(4), 317–325. doi:10.1097/DBP.0b013e3181dbaf32 PMID:20431399

Stanton, A., Zandvliet, D., Dhaliwal, R., & Black, T. (2016). Understanding students" experiences of wellbeing in learning environments. *Higher Education Studies*, *6*(3), 90–99. doi:10.5539/hes.v6n3p90

Stawarz, K., Preist, C., & Coyle, D. (2019). Use of smartphone apps, social media, and Web-based resources to support mental health and well-being: Online survey. *JMIR Mental Health*, *6*(7), e12546. doi:10.2196/12546 PMID:31301126

Steinberg, L., & Silk, J. S. (2002). *Parenting adolescents* (Vol. 1). Handbook of parenting.

Stein, K. F. (2013). DSS and Accommodations in Higher Education: Perceptions of Students with Psychological Disabilities. *Journal of Postsecondary Education and Disability*, *26*(2), 145–161.

Stephenson, B. C. (2013). Guidance and Counselling. In *Schools and Colleges*. University of London Press.

Stiles, W. B., Honos-Webb, L., & Surko, M. (1998). Responsiveness in psychotherapy. *Clinical Psychology : a Publication of the Division of Clinical Psychology of the American Psychological Association*, *5*(4), 439–458. doi:10.1111/j.1468-2850.1998.tb00166.x

Stolzenberg, E. B., Aragon, M. C., Romo, E., Couch, V., McLennan, D., Eagan, M. K., & Kang, N. (2019). The American freshman: National norms fall 2018. *Higher Education Research Institute, UCLA*. https://www.pushkin.fm/wp-content/uploads/imported-files/TheAmericanFreshman2018.pdf

Storrie, K., Ahern, K., & Tuckett, A. (2010). A systematic review: Students with mental health problems—A growing problem. *International Journal of Nursing Practice*, *16*(1), 1–6. doi:10.1111/j.1440-172X.2009.01813.x PMID:20158541

Stringer, P., Saqr, S., & Tennant, L. (2014). Challenges and Support Factors of Married Emirati Students in Teacher Education. *Journal of Research in Humanities and Social Science*, *2*(8), 46–56.

Stuart-Edwards, A. (2023). Good begets good? Reciprocal relationships between mindfulness, approach coping, and subjective vitality. *Personality and Individual Differences, 202*, 111970. doi:10.1016/j.paid.2022.111970

Stults-Kolehmainen, M., Gilson, T., SantaBarbara, N., McKee, P., Sinha, R., Bartholomew, J., Boullosa, D., Budnick, C., Bueno, F. A., Haughton, A., Barker, J., & Ash, G. (2022). Qualitative and quantitative evidence of motivation states for physical activity, exercise and being sedentary from university student focus groups. *SportRxiv.* doi:10.51224/SRXIV.189

Substance Abuse and Mental Health Services Administration (SAMHSA). (2021). *Prevention and Treatment of Anxiety, Depression, and Suicidal Thoughts and Behaviors Among College Students*. SAMHSA Publication No. PEP21-06-05-002. Rockville, MD: National Mental Health and Substance Use Policy Laboratory.

Suh, H., Liou, P., Jeong, J., & Kim, S. Y. (2022). Perfectionism, Prolonged stress reactivity, and Depression: A Two-Wave Cross-Lagged Analysis. *Journal of Rational-Emotive & Cognitive-Behavior Therapy*. doi:10.100710942-022-00483-x PMID:36406657

Suldo, S. M., Shaunessy, E., & Hardesty, R. B. (2008). Relationships among Stress, Coping, and Mental Health in High-Achieving High School Students. *Psychology in the Schools, 45*(4), 273–290. doi:10.1002/pits.20300

Suprihatin & Azis, A. (2020). Pelecehan Seksual pada Jurnalis Perempuan di Indonesia. *Jurnal Studi Gender, 13*(2), 413–434.

Sutcliffe, K. M., & Vogus, T. (2003). Organizing for resilience. In K. S. Cameron, J. E. Dutton, & R. E. Quinn (Eds.), *Positive organizational scholarship: Foundations of a new discipline*. Berrett-Koehler Press.

Sutton, A. (2020). Living the good life: A meta-analysis of authenticity, well-being and engagement. *Personality and Individual Differences, 153*, 109645. doi:10.1016/j.paid.2019.109645

Svane, D., Evans, N. S., & Carter, M.-A. (2019). Wicked Wellbeing: Examining The Disconnect Between The Rhetoric and Reality of Wellbeing Interventions In Schools. *Australian Journal of Education, 63*(2), 209–231. doi:10.1177/0004944119843144

Svoboda, E. (2021, August 9). What is mental skills coaching? *The New York Times*. https: www.nytimes.com/2021/08/05/well/move/mental-skills-coaching-olympics.html

Tagoe, M., Quarshie, E. N. B., Ahiaku, A. E., & Ansong, E. (2020). Utilization of mental health services among university students in Ghana. *Journal of College Student Psychotherapy, 34*(2), 109–124. oi:10.1080/87568225.2019.1674669

Tam, W., Lo, K., & Pacheco, J. (2019). Prevalence of depressive symptoms among medical students: Overview of systematic reviews. Med Educ. *Medical Education, 53*(4), 345–354. doi:10.1111/medu.13770 PMID:30474128

Tang, Y. Y. (2017). *The Neuroscience of Mindfulness Meditation: How the Body and Mind Work Together to Change Our Behavior*. Springer Nature. doi:10.1007/978-3-319-46322-3

Tang, Y. Y., Hölzel, B. K., & Posner, M. I. (2016). Traits and states in mindfulness meditation. *Nature Reviews. Neuroscience, 17*(1), 59. doi:10.1038/nrn.2015.7 PMID:26631928

Tang, Y. Y., Tang, R., & Gross, J. J. (2019). Promoting Psychological Well-Being through an Evidence-Based Mindfulness Training Program. *Frontiers in Human Neuroscience, 13*(1), 1–5. doi:10.3389/fnhum.2019.00237 PMID:31354454

Taseer, N. A., Khan, S. A., Yasir, W., Kishwer, R., & Iqbal, K. (2023). Impact of Family Involvement on Academic Achievement at Higher Secondary Level. *Journal of Social Sciences Review, 3*(2), 1–10. doi:10.54183/jssr.v3i2.231

Tasnim, R., Islam, M. S., Sujan, M. S. H., Sikder, M. T., & Potenza, M. N. (2020). Suicidal ideation among Bangladeshi university students early during the COVID-19 pandemic: Prevalence estimates and correlates. *Children and Youth Services Review*, *119*, 105703. doi:10.1016/j.childyouth.2020.105703 PMID:33204046

Tauken, S. (2014). The Main Challenges Student Mothers Experience to Manage Their Dual Roles. [IJAP]. *International Journal of Advances in Psychology*, *3*(3), 94–98. doi:10.14355/ijap.2014.0303.04

Tavolacci, M. P., Wouters, E., Van de Velde, S., Buffel, V., Déchelotte, P., Van Hal, G., & Ladner, J. (2021). The impact of COVID-19 lockdown on health behaviors among students of a French university. *International Journal of Environmental Research and Public Health*, *18*(8), 4346. doi:10.3390/ijerph18084346 PMID:33923943

Taylor, H. G., Yeates, K. O., Wade, S. L., Drotar, D., Stancin, T., & Minich, M. (2006). A Prospective Study of Short- and Long-Term Outcomes after Traumatic Brain Injury in Children: Behavior and Achievement. *Neuropsychology*, *16*(1), 15–27. doi:10.1037/0894-4105.16.1.15 PMID:11853353

Teague, R. G. (2023). Infusing KM in global higher education: How effective KM program supports critical tacit knowledge retention within a US higher education institution. In L. J. Jones-Esan, V. Nadda, & K. S. Albright (Eds.), *Knowledge management and research innovation in global higher education institutions* (pp. 236–250). IGI Global.

TED-Ed. (2018a, May 21). *How to stay calm under pressure - Noa Kageyama and Pen-Pen Chen* [Video]. YouTube. https://www.youtube.com/watch?v=CqgmozFr_GM

TEd-Ed. (2022). *Why you procrastinate even when it feels bad* [Video]. TED Talks. https://www.ted.com/talks/ted_ed_why_you_procrastinate_even_when_it_feels_bad/comments/transcript

Teh, C. K., Ngo, C. W., Binti Zulkifli, R. A., Vellasamy, R., & Suresh, K. (2015). Depression, anxiety and stress among undergraduate students: A cross-sectional study. [Crossref]. *Open Journal of Epidemiology*, *5*(04), 260–268. doi:10.4236/ojepi.2015.54030

Teixeira, R. J., Brandão, T., & Dores, A. R. (2021). Academic stress, coping, emotion regulation, affect and psychosomatic symptoms in higher education. *Current Psychology (New Brunswick, N.J.)*, 1–10. doi:10.100712144-020-01304-z

Tennant, L., & Dickson, M. (2019). Challenges Facing Emirati College Student Mothers Post Childbirth. *Journal of Research on Women and Gender*, *9*, 76–90.

Tennant, L., Stringer, P., & Saqr, S. (2013). Motivation and Challenges of Married Emirati Students in Teacher Education. *International Review of Contemporary Learning Research*, *2*(2), 99–109. doi:10.12785/irclr/020205

Terhart, H., & Von Dewitz, N. (2017). Newly arrived migrant students in German schools: Exclusive and inclusive structures and practices. *European Educational Research Journal*, *17*(2), 290–304. doi:10.1177/1474904117722623

Tett, L., Cree, V. E., & Christie, H. (2017). From Further to Higher Education: Transition as an on-Going Process. *Higher Education*, *73*(3), 389–406. doi:10.100710734-016-0101-1

Tezza, S. F., & Gulanhem, O. P. (2010). Parents' Involvement in Managing Adolescent Mothers' Psychological Stress. *The Journal of Psychology*, *4*(2), 215–221.

Thamtanajit, K. (2022). Prolonged Protests And Student Achievement: Evidence From Political Unrest In Thailand. *Eastern Economic Journal*, *48*(2), 226–250. doi:10.105741302-022-00216-z

Thanoi, W., Vongsirimas, N., Sitthimongkol, Y., & Klainin-Yobas, P. (2023). Examining Predictors of Psychological Well-Being among University Students: A Descriptive Comparative Study across Thailand and Singapore. *International Journal of Environmental Research and Public Health*, *20*(3), 1875. doi:10.3390/ijerph20031875 PMID:36767238

The Museum of British Colonialism. (2023, April 10). *Education*. MBC. https://museumofbritishcolonialism.org/education/

Thomas, J., Raynor, M., & Al-Marzooqi, A. (2012). Marital Status and Gender as Predictors Of Undergraduate Academic Performance: United Arab Emirates Context. *Learning And Teaching in Higher Education: Gulf Perspectives, 9*(2).

Thomas, J., & Harden, A. (2008). Methods for the thematic synthesis of qualitative research in systematic reviews. *BMC Medical Research Methodology, 8*(1), 1–10. doi:10.1186/1471-2288-8-45 PMID:18616818

Thomas, L. (2012). Building Student Engagement and Belonging in Higher Education at a Time of Change. *Paul Hamlyn Foundation, 100*, 1–99.

Thomas, P. A., Liu, H., & Umberson, D. (2017). Family Relationships and Well-Being. *Innovation in Aging, 1*(3), 1–11. doi:10.1093/geroni/igx025 PMID:29795792

Thomas, S., Jose, K. A., & Kumar, A. (2018). *Child Friendly Schools: Challenges and Issues in Creating a Positive and Protective School Environment. Positive Schooling and Child Development, 233*. Springer.

Thomas, V., Muls, J., De Backer, F., & Lombaerts, K. (2020). Middle school student and parent perceptions of parental involvement: Unravelling the associations with school achievement and wellbeing. *Educational Studies, 46*(4), 404–421. doi:10.1080/03055698.2019.1590182

Thompson, S. (2010). Complexities of Supporting Teenagers in Pregnancy. *The Journal of School Nursing: the Official Publication of the National Association of School Nurses, 5*(8), 388–392. doi:10.12968/bjsn.2010.5.8.78911

Thorley, C. (2017). *Not By Degrees: Not by degrees: Improving student mental health in the UK's universities*. IPPR.

Thuraiselvam, S., & Thang, R. B. (2015). Factors That Affect Students' Mental Health: A Study at Taylor's University School of Hospitality. *Tourism and Culinary Arts Final Year Students*. Springer, Singapore. 10.1007/978-981-287-399-6_10

Tian-Ci Quek, T., & Wai-San Tam, W. (2019). The global prevalence of anxiety among medical students: A meta-analysis. *Int J Environ Res Public Health, 16*(15), 2735. 10.3390/ijerph16152735

Tolsgaard, M. G. (2013). Clinical skills training in undergraduate medical education using a student-centered approach. *Danish Medical Journal, 60*(8), B4690. PMID:23905573

Tomai, M., & Lauriola, M. (2019). Biopsychosocial correlates of adjustment to cancer during chemotherapy: The key role of health-related quality of life. *TheScientificWorldJournal, 2019*(5), 1–12. doi:10.1155/2019/9750940 PMID:30983914

Tommasi, M., Grassi, P., Balsamo, M., Picconi, L., Furnham, A., & Saggino, A. (2018). Correlations between personality, affective and filial self-efficacy beliefs, and psychological well-being in a sample of Italian adolescents. *Psychological Reports, 121*(1), 59–78. doi:10.1177/0033294117720698 PMID:28750584

Tone, S. (2020, November 5). *How one obscure word captures urban China's unhappiness*. #SixthTone. https://www.sixthtone.com/news/1006391/how-one-obscure-word-captures-urban-chinas-unhappiness

Toni Bernhard, J. D. (2011, September 11). 4 Tips for Slowing Down to Reduce Stress. *psychologytoday.com*. https://www.psychologytoday.com/us/blog/turning-straw-gold/201109/4-tips-slowing-down-reduce-stress

Torres, V. M. R., Sangala, L. J. T., Jose, A. E. S., & Mortos, A. R. (2020). Untold Stories of Student-Mothers' Academic Journey: A Phenomenology. *Journal of Studies in Social Sciences and Humanities, 6*(4), 58–169.

Tran, A., Tran, L., Geghre, N., Darmon, D., Rampal, M., Brandone, D., Gozzo, J.-M., Haas, H., Rebouillat-Savy, K., Caci, H., & Avillach, P. (2017). Health assessment of French university students and risk factors associated with mental health disorders. *PLoS One, 12*(11), e0188187. doi:10.1371/journal.pone.0188187 PMID:29176864

*Tremendously, adv*. (2023). Oxford English Dictionary. doi:10.1093/OED/4986167386

Trullàs, J. C., Blay, C., Sarri, E., & Pujol, R. (2022). Effectiveness of problem-based learning methodology in undergraduate medical education: A scoping review. *BMC Medical Education*, *22*(1), 104. doi:10.118612909-022-03154-8 PMID:35177063

Truschel, J. (2020). *Depression Definition and DSM-5 Diagnostic Criteria: What is Depression?* PsyCom. https://www.psycom.net/depression-definition-dsm-5-diagnostic-criteria/

Tsai, A., & William, R. (2016). Prospective Study of The Mental Health Consequences of Sexual Violence Among Women Living With HIV In Rural Uganda. *Journal of Interpersonal Violence*, *31*(8), 1531–1553. doi:10.1177/0886260514567966 PMID:25586914

Tudge, J. R. H., Mokrova, I., Hatfield, B. E., & Karnik, R. B. (2009). Uses and Misuses of Bronfenbrenner's Bioecological Theory of Human Development. *Journal of Family Theory & Review*, *1*(4), 198–210. doi:10.1111/j.1756-2589.2009.00026.x

Turner, C.S., Ro, H.K., Loya, K.I., Rhoads, R.A., Camacho, M.S., Toven-Lindsey, B., Lozano, J.B., Cowan, J., Goldhaber, D., Lopez, H.D., Ream, T.C., Hurst, A.L., Crisp, G., Curette, A., Hansen, T.I., & Nehls, K. (2015). Lessons from the Field: Cultivating Nurturing Environments in Higher Education. *The Review of Higher Education.*

Twenge, J. M., Cooper, C., & Thomas, E. (2021). Anxiety And Depressive Symptoms In US Census Bureau Assessments of Adults: Trends From 2019 To Fall 2020 across Demographic Groups. *Journal of Anxiety Disorders*, *83*, 102455. doi:10.1016/j.janxdis.2021.102455 PMID:34332230

Tyson, P. J., Wilson, K. L., Crone, D. M., Brailsford, R., & Laws, K. R. (2010). Physical activity and mental health in a student population. *Journal of Mental Health (Abingdon, England)*, *19*(6), 492–499. doi:10.3109/09638230902968308 PMID:20812852

Tytherleigh, M. Y., Webb, C., Cooper, C. L., & Ricketts, C. (2007). Occupational stress in UK higher education institutions: A comparative study of all staff categories. *Higher Education Research & Development*, *24*(1), 41–61. doi:10.1080/0729436052000318569

UCLA. (2012). Cramming for a test? Don't do it, say UCLA researchers. *UCLA Health*. https://www.uclahealth.org/news/cramming-for-a-test-dont-do-it-say-ucla-researchers

Udah, H., & Francis, A. (2022). COVID-19 and mental health and wellbeing of higher education international students. In H. Udah & A. Francis (Eds.), *Mental health and higher education in Australia* (pp. 303–320). Routledge. doi:10.1007/978-981-16-8040-3_18

Udhayakumar, P., & Illango, P. (2018). Psychological Wellbeing among College Students. *Journal of Social Work Education and Practice*, *3*(2), 79–89.

Ulla, D., & Lena, R. (2023). Sustainable development work aimed at promoting mental health among municipal adult students with mental health problems. *Insights on the Depression and Anxiety, 7*(1), 016–017. doi:10.29328/journal.ida.1001037

UNC-Chapel Hill Learning Center. (2022, July 12). *Study Groups – Learning Center*. Learning Center. https://learningcenter.unc.edu/tips-and-tools/study-partners/

UNICEF. (2020, March 10). *A third of youth surveyed globally by UNICEF say their education is not preparing them with the skills to get jobs*. aunicef.org. https://aunicef.org/press-releases/third-youth-surveyed-globally-unicef-say-their-education-not-preparing-them-skills

University of International Management (IUM). (2023). *Administrative departments*. IUM. https://ium.edu.na/

University of Namibia (UNAM). (2023). *Directorate of student affairs*. UNAM. https://www.unam.edu.na/student-affairs

Upali, P. (2017). Impact of Family on Children's Wellbeing. *Journal of Sociology and Social Work*, *5*(1), 149–158.

US Department of Health and Human Services. (2018). *President's council on sports, fitness & nutrition.* US DoHHS.

Utami, N. A., Maharani, W., & Atastina, I. (2021). Personality classification of Facebook users according to Big Five personality using SVM (Support Vector Machine) Method. *Procedia Computer Science*, *179*, 177–184. doi:10.1016/j.procs.2020.12.023

Utkina,V & Efimova, A. (2022). *Career Barriers In Ghana: Evidence From Female Civil Servants.*

Vallejo- Slocker, L., Fresneda- Sánchez, F. J., & Vallejo -Pareja, M. Á. (2020). Psychological well-being of vulnerable children during the COVID-19 pandemic. *Psicothema.*

Van Der Feltz-Cornelis, C. M., Varley, D., Allgar, V. L., & De Beurs, E. (2020). Workplace stress, presenteeism, absenteeism, and resilience amongst university staff and students in the COVID-19 lockdown. *Frontiers in Psychiatry*, *11*, 588803. doi:10.3389/fpsyt.2020.588803 PMID:33329135

van Herpen, S. G. A., Meeuwisse, M., Hofman, W. H. A., & Severiens, S. E. (2020). A head start in higher education: The effect of a transition intervention on interaction, sense of belonging, and academic performance. *Studies in Higher Education*, *45*(4), 862–877. doi:10.1080/03075079.2019.1572088

van Hooijdonk, K. J., Rubio, M., Simons, S. S., van Noorden, T. H., Luijten, M., Geurts, S. A., & Vink, J. M. (2022). Student-, Study-and COVID-19-Related Predictors of Students' Smoking, Binge Drinking and Cannabis Use before and during the Initial COVID-19 Lockdown in The Netherlands. *International Journal of Environmental Research and Public Health*, *19*(2), 812. doi:10.3390/ijerph19020812 PMID:35055634

Van Rijswijk, L., & Haans, A. (2018). Illuminating For Safety: Investigating The Role Of Lighting Appraisals on The Perception Of Safety In The Urban Environment. *Environment and Behavior*, *50*(8), 889–912. doi:10.1177/0013916517718888 PMID:30245528

Vargas-Tonsing, T. M., Myers, N. D., & Feltz, D. L. (2004). Coaches' and Athletes' Perceptions of Efficacy-Enhancing Techniques. *The Sport Psychologist*, *18*(4), 397–414. doi:10.1123/tsp.18.4.397

Velasco, A. A., Cruz, I. S. S., Billings, J., Jimenez, M., & Rowe, S. (2020). What are the barriers, facilitators and interventions targeting help-seeking behaviours for common mental health problems in adolescents? A systematic review. *BMC Psychiatry*, *20*(1), 293. doi:10.118612888-020-02659-0 PMID:32527236

Venugopal-Wairagade, G. (2016). Creating a supportive learning environment for better student engagement. *2016 International Conference on Learning and Teaching in Computing and Engineering (LaTICE).* IEEE. 10.1109/LaTiCE.2016.26

Verrocchio, M. C., Carrozzino, D., Marchetti, D., Andreasson, K., Fulcheri, M., & Bech, P. (2016). Mental pain and suicide: A systematic review of the literature. *Frontiers in Psychiatry*, *7*, 108. doi:10.3389/fpsyt.2016.00108 PMID:27378956

VIA Institute on Character. (n.d.). *The 24 Character Strengths.* VIA. https://www.viacharacter.org/character-strengths

Vidas, D., Larwood, J. L., Nelson, N. L., & Dingle, G. A. (2021). Music listening as a strategy for managing COVID-19 stress in first-year university students. *Frontiers in Psychology*, *12*, 647065. doi:10.3389/fpsyg.2021.647065 PMID:33868120

Visser, M. M., Aben, L., Heijenbrok-Kal, M. H., Busschbach, J. J., & Ribbers, G. M. (2014). The relative effect of coping strategy and depression on health-related quality of life in patients in the chronic phase after stroke. *Journal of Rehabilitation Medicine*, *4*(6), 514–519. doi:10.2340/16501977-1803 PMID:24687167

Vloo, A., Alessie, R. J. M., Mierau, J. O., Boezen, M. H., Mierau, J. O., Franke, L., Dekens, J., Deelen, P., Lanting, P., Vonk, J. M., Nolte, I., Ori, A. P. S., Claringbould, A., Boulogne, F., Dijkema, M. X. L., Wiersma, H. H., Warmerdam, R., & Jankipersadsing, S. A. (2021). Gender differences in the mental health impact of the COVID-19 lockdown: Longitudinal evidence from the Netherlands. *SSM - Population Health, 15*, 100878. doi:10.1016/j.ssmph.2021.100878 PMID:34471666

Vongsirimas, N., Thanoi, W., & Klainin-Yobas, P. (2017). Evaluating Psychometric Properties of the Connor-Davidson Resilience Scale (10-Item CD-RISC) among University Students in Thailand. *Journal of Nursing Science, 35*, 25–35.

Voth Schrag, R. J. (2017). Campus based sexual assault and dating violence: A review of study contexts and participants. *Affilia, 32*(1), 67–80. doi:10.1177/0886109916644644

Votruba, N., & Thornicroft, G. (2016). Sustainable development goals and mental health: Learnings from the contribution of the FundaMentalSDG global initiative. *Global Mental Health (Cambridge, England), 3*, e26. doi:10.1017/gmh.2016.20 PMID:28596894

Vryonides, M., & Vitsilakis, C. (2008). Widening Participation in Postgraduate Studies in Greece: Mature Working Women Attending An E-Learning Programme. *Journal of Education Policy, 23*(3), 199–208. doi:10.1080/02680930801923781

Vuckovic, M., Altvater, A., Helgesson, S., & Kloss, K. (2017). Sexual harassment and gender-based violence in Tanzania's public service. *International Journal of Workplace Health Management, 10*(2), 116–133. doi:10.1108/IJWHM-02-2015-0011

Vujcic, M. T., Brajsa-Zganec, A., & Franc, R. (2019). Children And Young Peoples' Views On Well-Being: A Qualitative Study. *Child Indicators Research, 12*(3), 791–819. doi:10.100712187-018-9559-y

Walker, J. G. (2022). *Towards improving the mental health of students at South African universities.* Universities South Africa. https://www.usaf.ac.za/towards-improvingthe-mental-health-of-students-at-south-african-universities/

Walker, R., Usher, K., Jackson, D., Reid, C., Hopkins, K., Shepherd, C., Smallwood, R., & Marriott, R. (2021). Connection to... Addressing digital inequities in supporting the well-being of young Indigenous Australians in the wake of COVID-19. *International Journal of Environmental Research and Public Health, 18*(4), 2141. doi:10.3390/ijerph18042141 PMID:33671737

Wallick, W. T. (2023). *Pre-med mentorship program proposal.* Boise State University. https://scholarworks.boisestate.edu/cgi/viewcontent.cgi?article=1220&context=mds495_proj

Wang, X. (2018). Research on college students' mental health and crisis intervention. *International Workshop on Advances in Social Sciences (IWASS 2018).* SAMHSA.

Wang, X. Q., Ren, T. R., & Wang, J. C. (2017). The Construction of University Aid-receiving Students Gratitude Education Model from the Perspective of Positive Psychology. *Educ. Teach. Forum, 3*, 94–103.

Wang, C., Boyanton, D., Ross, A. S. M., Liu, J. L., Sullivan, K., & Anh Do, K. (2018). School Climate, Victimization, and Mental Health Outcomes Among Elementary School Students In China. *School Psychology International, 39*(6), 587–605. doi:10.1177/0143034318805517

Wang, M. T., & Degol, J. L. (2016). School climate: A review of the construct, measurement, and impact on student outcomes. *Educational Psychology Review, 28*(2), 315–352. doi:10.100710648-015-9319-1

Wang, M. T., & Eccles, J. S. (2012). Adolescent behavioral, emotional, and cognitive engagement trajectories in school and their differential relations to educational success. *Journal of Research on Adolescence, 22*(1), 31–39. doi:10.1111/j.1532-7795.2011.00753.x PMID:22822296

Wango, G. (2023). Psychological Health. Counselling Diary. University of Nairobi: Kenya.

Wang, X., Hegde, S., Son, C., Keller, B., Smith, A., & Sasangohar, F. (2020). Investigating mental health of US college students during the COVID-19 pandemic: Cross-sectional survey study. *Journal of Medical Internet Research, 22*(9), e22817. doi:10.2196/22817 PMID:32897868

Wang, Y. (2020). College students' trait gratitude and subjective well-being mediated by basic psychological needs. *Social Behavior and Personality, 48*(4), 1–10. doi:10.2224bp.8904

Wang, Y., & Guan, H. (2020). Exploring Demotivation Factors Of Chinese Learners Of English As a Foreign Language Based on Positive Psychology. *Revista Argentina de Clínica Psicológica, 29*(1), 851.

Warren, J. M. (2017). *School consultation for student success*. Springer. doi:10.1891/9780826177780

Waters, S. K., Cross, D. S., & Runions, K. (2009). Social and ecological structures supporting adolescent connectedness to school: A theoretical model. *The Journal of School Health, 79*(11), 516–524. doi:10.1111/j.1746-1561.2009.00443.x PMID:19840228

Weinberg, J., & Nielsen, L. (2017). What is sexual harassment? An empirical study of perceptions of ordinary people and judges. *Saint Louis University Public Law Review, 36*(1), 39–58.

Weinberg, R. S., Smith, J., Jackson, A., & Gould, D. (1984). Effect of association, dissociation and positive self-talk strategies on endurance performance. *Canadian Journal of Applied Sport Sciences, 9*(1), 25–32. https://psycnet.apa.org/record/1985-00646-001 PMID:6705126

Weissberg, R. P., Durlak, J. A., Domitrovich, C. E., & Gullotta, T. P. (2015). Social and emotional learning: Past, present, and future. In J. A. Durlak, C. E. Domitrovich, R. P. Weissberg, & T. P. Gullotta (Eds.), *Handbook of social and emotional learning: Research and practice* (pp. 3–19).

Wen, C. I. (2019). Factors affecting students' subjective well-being: The relationship between religion, cultural intelligence, personality traits and subjective well-being (SWB) (December 30, 2019). *J. Mgt. Mkt. Review, 4*(4), 234–241. doi:10.35609/jmmr.2019.4.4(2)

Wessels, E., & Wood, L. (2019). Fostering teachers' experiences of well-being: A participatory action learning and action research approach. *South African Journal of Education, 39*(1), 1–10. doi:10.15700aje.v39n1a1619

West, M. (2022, April 21). *What to know about guided imagery*. https://www.medicalnewstoday.com/articles/guided-imagery#techniques

Westerhof, G. J., & Keyes, C. L. M. (2010). Mental illness and mental health: The two continua model across the lifespan. *Journal of Adult Development, 17*(2), 110–119. doi:10.100710804-009-9082-y PMID:20502508

White, K., Morrison, S. P., & Jane, V. V. (2011). Basics in Education Research. London: Lawrence Erlbaum Associates.

White, L. B. (2004). *The Psychological well-being and academic achievement of children raised by single parents* [Master dissertation, University of Wisconsin Stout]. http://www.uwstout.edu/lib /thesis/2004

Whitlock, J. (2007). The role of adults, public space, and power in adolescent community connectedness. *Journal of Community Psychology, 35*(4), 499–518. doi:10.1002/jcop.20161

WHO. (2019 May 28). *Burn-out an "occupational phenomenon": International classification of diseases*. World Health Organization. https://www.who.int/news/item/28-05-2019-burn-out-an-occupational-phenomenon-international-classification-of-diseases

WHO. (2022). *World mental health report: transforming mental health for all*. Geneva: World Health Organization.

Wickrama, T., Wickrama, K., Banford, A., & Lambert, J. (2016). PTSD symptoms among tsunami exposed mothers in Sri Lanka: The role of disaster exposure, culturally specific coping strategies, and recovery efforts. *Anxiety, Stress, and Coping, 30*(4), 415–427. doi:10.1080/10615806.2016.1271121 PMID:27960534

Widdicks, K. (2020). When the good turns ugly: Speculating next steps for digital well-being tools. *Proceedings of the 11th Nordic Conference on Human-Computer Interaction: Shaping Experiences*, Shaping Society, Tallinn, Estonia. 10.1145/3419249.3420117

Wiedemann, K. (2015). Anxiety and anxiety disorders. International Encyclopedia of the Social & Behavioral Sciences, (2nd ed) 804-810.

Wiederkehr, V., Bonnot, V., Krauth-Gruber, S., & Darnon, C. (2015). Belief in school meritocracy as a system-justifying tool for low-status students. *Frontiers in Psychology, 6.* doi:10.3389/fpsyg.2015.01053 PMID:26283991

Wiens, K., Williams, J. V., Lavorato, D. H., Duffy, A., Pringsheim, T. M., Sajobi, T. T., & Patten, S. B. (2017). Is the prevalence of major depression increasing in the Canadian adolescent population? Assessing trends from 2000 to 2014. *Journal of Affective Disorders, 210,* 22–26. doi:10.1016/j.jad.2016.11.018 PMID:28012349

Wilczenski, F. L., & Cook, A. L. (2009). How service learning addresses the mental health needs of students in urban school. *Journal of School Counseling, 7,* 1–20.

Williams, S. A. (2011). Graduate Students/Mothers Negotiating Academia and Family Life: Discourses, Experiences, and Alternatives Education, Implication, Counselling and Education. *Edo Journal of Counselling, 4*(1, 2).

Williams, J., & Kumar, A. (2018). *From Deficit to a Strength Model. Character Strength Development: Perspectives from Positive Psychology, 353.* Sage Publication.

Wilson, M. J., Seidler, Z. E., Oliffe, J. L., Toogood, N., Kealy, D., Ogrodniczuk, J. S., Walther, A., & Rice, S. M. (2022). "Appreciate the little things": A qualitative survey of men's coping strategies and mental health impacts during the COVID-19 pandemic. *American Journal of Men's Health, 16*(3), 15579883221099794. doi:10.1177/15579883221099794 PMID:35608377

Winkle-Wagner, R., McCallum, C. M., Luedke, C., & Ota-Malloy, B. (2019). Instrumental or meaningful friendships: Black alumnae perspectives on peer relationships during college. *Journal of Women and Gender in Higher Education, 12*(3), 283–298. doi:10.1080/19407882.2019.1593201

Wong, D., & Kulwant, K. (2021). The longitudinal relationship of school climate with adolescent social and emotional health. *BMC Public Health, 21*(1), 207–215. doi:10.118612889-021-10245-6 PMID:33485308

Wood, L., Hoefer, S., Kammer-Kerwick, M., Parra-Cardona, J. R., & Busch-Armendariz, N. (2021). Sexual harassment at institutions of higher education: Prevalence, risk, and extent. *Journal of Interpersonal Violence, 36*(9-10), 4520–4544. doi:10.1177/0886260518791228 PMID:30071790

Worland, J. (2014, December 4). How your cell phone distracts you even when you're not using it. *Time.* https://time.com/3616383/cell-phone-distraction/

World Bank Group. (2022, July 14). Financing for Education Stagnant or Declining Despite Chronic Learning Needs Post-COVID-19. *World Bank.* https://www.worldbank.org/en/news/press-release/2022/06/28/financing-for-education-stagnant-or-declining-despite-chronic-learning-needs-post-covid-19

World Conference on Higher Education (WCHE). (1998). Higher Education in the Twenty-first Century: Vision and Action. *World Declaration on Higher Education for the Twenty-first Century; Framework for Priority Action for Change and Development in Higher Education.* UNESCO.

World Health Organization (2014). *Fact Sheet.* WHO. Http:Wen.Tvv.Stats. 1421ysr.Adyi/Od/

World Health Organization. (2009). Promoting Gender Equality to Prevent Violence against. *Women.*

World Health Organization. (2016). Working for health and growth: investing in the health workforce. Report of the High- Level Commission on Health Employment and Economic Growth, Geneva, Switzerland. WHO.

World Health Organization. (2018). *Mental health atlas 2017.* WHO Regional Office for the Eastern Mediterranean.

World Health Organization. (2020). *Mental Health and Substance Use.* Geneva: WHO https://www.who.int/teams/mental-health-and-substance-use/overview

World Health Organization. (2021). *Mental health and COVID-19.* WHO. https://www.who.int/teams/mental-health-and-substance-use/covid-19

World Health Organization. (2021). *Mental Health.* WHO. https://www.who.int/healthtopics/mental-health/#tab=tab

Wornast, T. (2018). *Exploring student well-being in Higher Education.* [Unpublished PhD Thesis, Canteburry Christ University, UK].

Worobetz, A., Retief, P. J., Loughran, S., Walsh, J., Casey, M., Hayes, P., Bengoechea, E. G., O'Regan, A., Woods, C., Kelly, D., Connor, R. O., Grath, D. M., & Glynn, L. G. (2020). A feasibility study of an exercise intervention to educate and promote health and well-being among medical students: The 'MED-WELL' programme. *BMC Medical Education, 20*(1), 183. doi:10.118612909-020-02097-2 PMID:32493427

Wray, S., & Kinman, G. (2021). *Supporting Staff Wellbeing in Higher Education.* Education Support. https://www.educationsupport.org.uk/media/x4jdvxpl/es-supporting-staff-wellbeing-in-he-report.pdf

Wren-Lewis, S., & Alexandrova, A. (2021, December). Mental health without well-being. *Journal of Medicine and Philosophy: A Forum for Bioethics and Philosophy of Medicine, 46*(6), 684–703.

Wright, C. N. (2013, August 29). *Examining the silence of academic disappointment: A typology of students' reasons for not discussing disappointing grades with instructors.* ScholarWorks. https://scholarworks.iu.edu/journals/index.php/josotl/article/view/3513

Wright, R. R. (2020). Directed coping: A key to coping effectively? *Stress and Health, 37*(3), 466–475. doi:10.1002mi.3009 PMID:33220167

WulandariP. H. (2021). Nothing good happens after midnight: The relationship between circadian disruption due to insomnia and lack of sleep to increased risk of cardiovascular diseases. doi:10.22541/au.161360164.47679831/v1

Wyatt, T. J., Oswalt, S. B., & Ochoa, Y. (2017). Mental Health and Academic Performance of First-Year College Students. *International Journal of Higher Education, 6*(3), 178–187. doi:10.5430/ijhe.v6n3p178

Xiong, P., Ming, W. K., Zhang, C., Bai, J., Luo, C., Cao, W., Zhang, F., & Tao, Q. (2021). Factors influencing mental health among Chinese medical and non-medical students in the early stage of the COVID-19 pandemic. *Frontiers in Public Health, 9,* 603331. doi:10.3389/fpubh.2021.603331 PMID:34095044

Xu, J., & Lee, S. G. (2023). Problems with complex college admissions policies and overloaded after-school private education on middle- and high-school students' mental health in South Korea. *Journal of Global Health Reports, 7.* doi:10.29392/001c.84099

Yang, Y., Liu, K., Li, M., & Li, S. (2022). Students' affective engagement, parental involvement, and teacher support in emergency remote teaching during the COVID-19 pandemic: Evidence from a cross-sectional survey in China. *Journal of Research on Technology in Education, 54*(sup1), S148-S164.

Yang, J., Zhang, Y., Li, P., Zhang, H., & Liu, T. (2022). College students' academic stressors on mental health during the COVID-19 pandemic: A comparison between graduating students and non-graduating students. *International Journal of Mental Health Promotion*, *24*(4), 603–618. doi:10.32604/ijmhp.2022.019406

Yanos, P. T., & Rosario, A. (2014). Preventive coping among people with severe mental illness in daily life: Strategies used and associations with mood. *The International Journal of Social Psychiatry*, *60*(5), 489–491. doi:10.1177/0020764013501291 PMID:24004616

Yao, F., & Zhang, A. (2021). Integration of education management and mental health in psychological crisis intervention in colleges and universities. *ASP Transactions on Psychology and Education*, *1*(1), 31–38.

Yao, J. (2023). Starting with the mental health of students. In J. Yao (Ed.), *Psychological communication between teachers and students* (pp. 3–22). Routledge. doi:10.4324/9781003360094-2

Yap, M.B.H., Pilkington, P.D., Ryan, S.M., Jorm, A.F. (2014). Parental factors associated with depression and anxiety in young people: a systematic review and meta-analysis. *J Affect Disord. 156*(8), 23. https://doi.org/. jad.2013.11.007. doi:10.1016/j

Yaratan, H., & Yucesoylu, R. (2010). Self-esteem,self-concept,self-talk and significant others statements in fifth grade students: Differences according to gender and school type. *Procedia: Social and Behavioral Sciences*, *2*(2), 3506–3518. doi:10.1016/j.sbspro.2010.03.543

Yasmin, H., Khalil, S., & Mazhar, R. (2020). COVID 19: Stress management among students and its impact on their effective learning. *International Technology and Education Journal*, *4*(2), 65–74.

Yates, S. (2019). Physician stress and burnout. *The American Journal of Medicine*, *133*(2), 160–164. doi:10.1016/j.amjmed.2019.08.034 PMID:31520624

Yeung, J., & Karasawa, M. (2023, April 7). *Japan was already grappling with isolation and loneliness. The pandemic made it worse.* CNN. https://edition.cnn.com/2023/04/06/asia/japan-hikikomori-study-covid-intl-hnk/index.html

Yomtov, D., Plunkett, S. W., Efrat, R., & Marin, A. G. (2015). Can peer mentors improve first-year experiences of university students? *Journal of College Student Retention*, *19*(1), 25–44. doi:10.1177/1521025115611398

Yu, R. (2015). Choking under pressure: The neuropsychological mechanisms of incentive-induced performance decrements. *Frontiers in Behavioral Neuroscience*, *9*. doi:10.3389/fnbeh.2015.00019 PMID:25713517

Yurayat, P., & Seechaliao, T. (2021). Effectiveness of Online Positive Psychology Intervention on Psychological Well-Being among Undergraduate Students. *J. Educ. Learn. 10*, 143–155. doi: . v10n4p143. doi:10.5539/jel

Yusoff, M. S. B., Mat Pa, M. N., Esa, A. R., & Abdul Rahim, A. F. (2013). Mental health of medical students before and during medical education: A prospective study. *Journal of Taibah University Medical Sciences*, *8*(2), 86–92. doi:10.1016/j.jtumed.2013.03.004

Yusof, H. M., Rahman, R. H., Noordin, N. F., Patah, S. A., Yunus, W. M., & Fei, G. C. (2019). Does University Students' Stress Have an Impact on their Psychological Well-Being? *Indian Journal of Public Health Research & Development*, *10*(6), 1290. doi:10.5958/0976-5506.2019.01473.6

Yusufov, M., Nicoloro-SantaBarbara, J., Grey, N. E., Moyer, A., & Lobel, M. (2019). A meta-analytic evaluation of stress reduction interventions for undergraduate and graduate students. *International Journal of Stress Management*, *26*(2), 132–145. doi:10.1037tr0000099

Zadow, C., Houghton, S., Hunter, S. C., Rosenberg, M., & Wood, L. (2017). Associations between Positive Mental Well-Being and Depressive Symptoms in Australian Adolescents. [CrossRef]. *Educ. Dev. Psychol*, *34*, 95–105.

Zariatu, I. (2018). Back to School—Resilience among Student Mothers in Ghana: The case of Nkawkaw. *Scientific Research Journal (SCIRJ), 6*(11), 68.

Zastrow, C. (1988). What really causes psychotherapy change? *Journal of Independent Social Work, 2*(3), 5–16. doi:10.1300/J283v02n03_02

Zepke, N. (2014). Student engagement research in higher education: Questioning an academic orthodoxy. *Teaching in Higher Education, 19*(6), 697–708. doi:10.1080/13562517.2014.901956

Zepke, N., & Leach, L. (2010). Improving student engagement: Ten proposals for action. *Active Learning in Higher Education, 11*(3), 167–177. doi:10.1177/1469787410379680

Zhai, Y., & Du, X. (2023). Trends and prevalence of suicide 2017–2021 and its association with COVID-19: Interrupted time series analysis of a national sample of college students in the United States. *Psychiatry Research*, 1–7. www.elsevier.com/locate/psychres PMID:35987067

Zhang, C., Kuncel, N. R., & Sackett, P. R. (2020). The process of attrition in pre-medical studies: A large-scale analysis across 102 schools. *PLoS One, 15*(12), e0243546. doi:10.1371/journal.pone.0243546 PMID:33370336

Zhao, K. L., Yang, M. Y., Miao, L. T., Liu, S., & Zhang, L. (2017). The effect of attachment on college students' internet altruistic behavior: Mediating model of trust and empathy. *Chinese J. Ergon, 23*, 23–28.

Zheng, G., Zhang, Q., & Ran, G. (2023). The association between academic stress and test anxiety in college students: The mediating role of regulatory emotional self-efficacy and the moderating role of parental expectations. *Frontiers in Psychology, 14*, 1008679. Advance online publication. doi:10.3389/fpsyg.2023.1008679 PMID:36824305

Zhigunova, M. (2017). Matrimonial installations of modern students (On the Example of the City of Barnaul). *Herald of Omsk University. Series. Historical Studies (Melbourne, Vic.), 3*(15), 183–188.

Zhou, S. J., Wang, L. L., Qi, M., Yang, X. J., Gao, L., Zhang, S. Y., Zhang, L.-G., Yang, R., & Chen, J. X. (2021). Depression, anxiety, and suicidal ideation in Chinese university students during the COVID-19 pandemic. *Frontiers in Psychology, 12*, 669833. doi:10.3389/fpsyg.2021.669833 PMID:34421725

Zungu, S. (2022). *Student support services: Opening TVET education in South Africa through the provision of student support.* ScienceOpen.com. doi:10.47622/9781928502425_P07

Zysberg, L. (2012). *Emotional antecedents of psychological loneliness. In book: Loneliness: Psychosocial Risk Factors, Prevalence and Impacts on Physical and Emotional Health. Publisher*. Nova Science Publishers.

# About the Contributors

**Peter J.O. Aloka** is a senior lecturer at Wits school of Education, University of the Witwatersrand South Africa. He holds a PhD in Educational Psychology from the University of the Western Cape. He has published over 50 articles and supervised several masters and PhD students in the area of Educational Psychology.

***

**Vivek Ahuja** is a PhD in Business from Aligarh Muslim University. He also holds an MBA, and a Bachelor of Engineering in Information Technology. He is an experienced education administrator with teaching and leadership experience at leading universities in India and is currently the Associate Director of Accreditation, Ranking & Compliance, and Doctoral Programs at FLAME University Pune, India. Additionally, he is also the in-charge of Alumni Relations. Prior to joining FLAME, Vivek worked with Ashoka University, spearheading the academics and peer learning verticals at the Young India Fellowship. He also worked with Shiv Nadar University, leading academic program operations at the business school and taught Global Entrepreneurship Simulation Capstone in the MBA and Executive MBA Programs. Vivek has research interests in the field of Education and Entrepreneurship. He has published papers in indexed and peer reviewed international journals.

**Daniel Opotamutale Ashipala** (MN Sc) is a senior lecturer and Head of Department for the School of nursing and Public Health (SoNPH), General Nursing Science department in the Faculty of Health Sciences and Veterinary Medicine (FHSVM) at the University of Namibia, Namibia. His research interests include Primary health Care, Health care services and Nursing education, and Mental health. He has published a quite number of peer reviewed articles on the delivery of teaching and learning in higher education studies. He is a doctoral candidate at Stellenbosch University in Cape Town, South Africa. His doctoral work focuses on developing a framework to facilitate the implementation of a task shifting approach for nurses in the Namibia PHC services.

**Enos Barasa Mukadi** is the Dean of School of Education cum Teacher Educator in Laikipia University, Kenya. He is an associate professor of Educational Counselling Psychology, a very dedicated, well organized, action oriented and a problem solver who delights in offering unique solutions to issues plus being a team player with outstanding interpersonal and communication skills. Prof. Mukadi is a professional psychotherapist, counselling educator and has served as an external examiner at several universities for a number of years. He is experienced in teaching Inclusive Education, Counseling Psychology and has also an extensive understanding of child protection rights and Gender Based Issues. He has been contracted by World Vision, Kenya on numerous advocacy projects on school education in rural districts of Kenya. In addition to working with youths in the Kenya National Youth Service, he has also conducted study with members of underprivileged and marginalized populations, such as women and children. Prof. Enos Barasa Mukadi began his academic/professional career as a secondary school teacher in Kenya, his native country. He attended National Youth Service (NYS) in Kenya and subsequently Maseno University and Egerton University where he obtained his Bachelor of Education and Master of Education degrees respectively. Upon successfully completion of M.Ed. degree in Guidance and Counseling he joined Laikipia University where he taught Psychology and Guidance and Counseling courses as Assistant Lecturer. In 2013, he earned his PhD degree in Educational Counseling Psychology from Kabarak University. Thereafter, (2014) he was promoted to Lecturer grade while teaching in Laikipia University. He was promoted to the rank of senior lecturer in 2017 and associate professor in 2022 which is his current professional cum academic. Prof Mukadi has successfully served as a departmental Exam officer and Chair of Department for 4 years and is currently the Dean School of Education. He teaches counseling psychology at postgraduate level and has supervised 20 masters and 8 PhD students to completion. He has published 35 papers on internationally refereed journals on Guidance and Counseling psychology profession.

**Anna Niitembu Hako**, PhD., is a Senior Lecturer for Guidance and Counselling at the University of Namibia, Hifikepunye Pohamba Campus-Namibia. She holds a PhD in Educational Psychology from the University of the Western Cape and a Master's degree in Counsellor Education from Emporia State University, USA. She also holds a Bachelor of Education degree from the University of Namibia. Her research areas are general education, guidance and counselling, psycho-social support and inclusive education.

**Aneesh Kumar P.** is currently working as Assistant Professor of Psychology and Coordinator of MPhil and Undergraduate Programmes at the Department of Psychology, CHRIST (Deemed to be University), Bengaluru, India. He is also involved in research projects like incorporating character strengths into the early school curriculum, student mental health through positive schooling program, trauma-informed teaching program and developing culturally competent and evidence-based mental health care training model for diverse societies. His research interests include child development, positive psychology and student mental health. He teaches child and adolescent counselling, counselling interventions for special population, developmental psychology, and qualitative research methods. Dr Kumar has published and presented papers in various national and international forums.

**Robert Lubin**, PsyD, is the Managing Director of the American Medical Program at the Technion School of Medicine in Haifa, Israel. He provides personal counseling and guidance as well as academic support to the American and Canadian medical students who choose to study medicine in Israel. Dr. Lubin is an adjunct Professor of Psychology at Touro University Worldwide and Fairleigh Dickinson University.

**Emilia Mbongo** is a lecturer in the Department of Educational Psychology and Inclusive Education at the University of Namibia. Her research interests are in the areas of School Guidance and Counselling, Inclusive Education and HIV and AIDS. Dr Mbongo served as a Regional School Counsellor for 10 years and has immense experience in the guidance and counselling system in Namibian schools.

**Fransisco Chindongo Ntjamba** is a graduate of Bachelor of Nursing Science (Clinical) (Honours) degree in Nursing Science at the University of Namibia, School of Nursing and Public Health, General Nursing department in the Faculty of Health Sciences and Veterinary Medicine (FHSVM) at the University of Namibia, Namibia. He actually has a greater interest of partaking in all the heath care research fields. His research interests would specifically focus, in Primary Health Care, Health care services, Nursing education, and Mental health.

**Damaris Ochanda** is the current Chairperson, Department of Nursing Research, Education and Management in the School of Nursing, Midwifery and Paramedical Sciences of Masinde Muliro University of Science and Technology, Kenya. She holds Bsc (Nursing) from University of Nairobi, Hons. BA (Health Studies) from University of South Africa (UNISA), MA (Health Studies) from UNISA and a doctorate in Public Health from Jaramogi Oginga Odinga University of Science and Technology. She is a registered nurse with over 8 years clinical nursing experience and 15 years in teaching of nursing programmes in higher education for both undergraduate and postgraduate. Her research interests include, public health nursing and research. She has published several articles in peer reviewed journals and has participated in collaborative research focusing in solutions that address public health problems including mental health.

**Calvins Okongo** holds a PhD degree in Educational Psychology from Rongo University.

**Pamela Awuor Onyango** is a lecturer of psychology at the University of Nairobi, Kenya. Pamela holds a doctorate degree in Educational Psychology from Jaramogi Oginga Odinga University of Science and Technology, masters in Educational Psychology from Maseno University and bachelor's degree in education from Egerton university. She is a member of Kenyan Guidance, Counseling and Psychological Association and Association of Behavioural Scientist, Kenya, Africa, who has authored several journals in addition to attending conferences. Pamela's research interest is in the field of Psychology.

**Joshua Owino** holds PhD in Educational Psychology. He is temporary lecturer in Educational Psychology at the Jaramogi Oginga Odinga University of Science and Technology - (Kenya)

**Sindu Padmanabhan** is a highly skilled researcher in Education & Health Psychology with experience in educational institutions and organizations and possessing a strong interest in health and cognitive psychology. I have a proven track of various research work, education delivery, as well as outstanding analytical and observational skills. Reviewer for International Journals. Highly proficient in using industry research software packages. Now seeking to advance my research career and take on further responsibilities.

**Rithu Paul** is a Mental Health Professional and a researcher with a Masters' degree in Clinical Psychology from CHRIST (Deemed to be University), Bangalore, India. Her areas of interest are in child and adolescent mental health, positive psychology, well-being, strength- based education and positive school relationships. She has experience with conducting trainings, webinars, creating modules, and moderating group discussions in these areas. She is currently involved in various research projects.

**S.C. Vetrivel** is a faculty member in the Department of Management Studies, Kongu Engineering College (Autonomous), Perundurai, Erode Dt. Having experience in Industry 20 years and Teaching 16 years. Awarded with Doctoral Degree in Management Sciences in Anna University, Chennai. He has organized various workshops and Faculty Development Programmes. He is actively involved in research and consultancy works. He acted as a resource person to FDPs & MDPs to various industries like, SPB ltd, Tamilnadu Police, DIET, Rotary school and many. His areas of interest include Entrepreneurship, Business Law, Marketing and Case writing. Articles published more than 100 International and National Journals. Presented papers in more than 30 National and International conferences including IIM Bangalore, IIM Kozhikode, IIM Kashipur and IIM Indore. He was a Chief Co-ordinator of Entrepreneurship and Management Development Centre (EMDC) of Kongu Engineering College, he was instrumental in organizing various Awareness Camps, FDP, and TEDPs to aspiring entrepreneurs which was funded by NSTEDB – DST/GoI

**Jamie Sharabani** is a third-year undergraduate student at the University of Miami. She is currently studying Public Health and is on a pre-Physician Assistant track. Her previous work includes research at The American University on neurotransmitters and their effects through FSCV and clinical work through Technion University and the Rambam Hospital.

**Mirjam Sheyapo** is a Lecturer and doctoral candidate in the Department of Intermediate and Vocational Education at the University of Namibia. Her research interests include mental health care for marginalised students at higher education institutions.

**Sruthi Suresh** is a doctoral research scholar in Psychology at CHRIST (Deemed to be University). In 2018, she completed her M.Sc. in Counseling Psychology and worked as an IB DP Psychology Faculty for the next two years. After joining the Ph.D. program in 2020, she has been an active scholar and engaged with the department as a Research Assistant, Teaching Assistant, Impact Assessment Research Team Lead, and Department Magazine Editor. She writes and presents widely on issues related to child and adolescent mental health, teacher education, and social emotional learning.

**Mohanasundaram Thangamuthu** completed his Doctoral degree in Management from Anna University. He has done his Master of Business Administration (MBA) from Bharathiar University. He has 20 years of total experience in Industry and Academics. He has published 40 research articles in reputed Journals and presented many research papers at International Conferences organized by IIMs, IITs, IISC and other reputed institutions. He is actively involved in research and consultancy works for Government, public and private institutions. He has received grants and financial assistance from various agencies like AICTE, ICSSR, AIMS, ICWA and NHRC for research projects and for organizing research programmes. He is a recognized Research Supervisor in Visvesvaraya Technological University, Belagavi. He has organized many FDPs/Workshops and MDPs. He has acted as a resource person for more than 60 programmes related to Management research that are organised across the country (including BITS Pilani, IMS Gaziabad, VESIM Mumbai, Osmania University, Hyderabad). His favourite subjects of teaching are; Predictive Analytics, International Finance, Financial Management, Bank Management, Financial and Management Accounting,SecurityAnalysis&PortfolioManagementandBusinessRe searchMethodology.Heisacertifiedfinancialeducation Resource Person of the Securities and Exchange Board of India (SEBI). He has received thenational level ‘Best Young Teacher Award-2018’ from the Association of Indian Management Schools(AIMS) and Best Young Faculty award from Nehru Group of Institutions,Coimbatore.

**Theolinda N. Tomas** is an occupational nurse with extensive hands-on experience in General nursing, Primary Health, and Occupational nursing. She currently works at Ohlthaver & List, Hangana clinic. She have interest in nursing education and management and currently pursuing her Master's degree in nursing education

**Theodore Tran** is a medical student at the California University of Science and Medicine. He graduated Magna Cum Laude with a Bachelor of Science in Human Biology from the University of California, San Diego. His research interests include healthcare administration optimization and promoting equitable care

**Elana Weiss** is a dedicated and motivated pre-medical undergraduate student with a strong interest in medicine. She is now pursuing a major in Biochemistry and is committed to academic success as well as learning the essential skills in order to make a significant difference in the healthcare profession. Elana continues to pursue education, growth, and the opportunity to make a meaningful contribution to the field of medicine while advocating for the importance of mental health awareness.

# Index

## G



## H



## I



## M



## N



## P



## Q



## R



## S

# T



# U



# V



# W

www.ingramcontent.com/pod-product-compliance
Lightning Source LLC
LaVergne TN
LVHW080119011026
849160LV00013B/1136